A PHILOSOPHICAL PATH FOR PARACELSIAN MEDICINE

To my sons,

Gorm Eirik and Leif Harald

The past is always most important for one's hopes for the future.

EMBLEMA XLII. *De secretis Naturæ.*

In Chymicis versanti Natura, Ratio, Experientia & lectio, sint Dux, scipio, perspicilia & lampas,

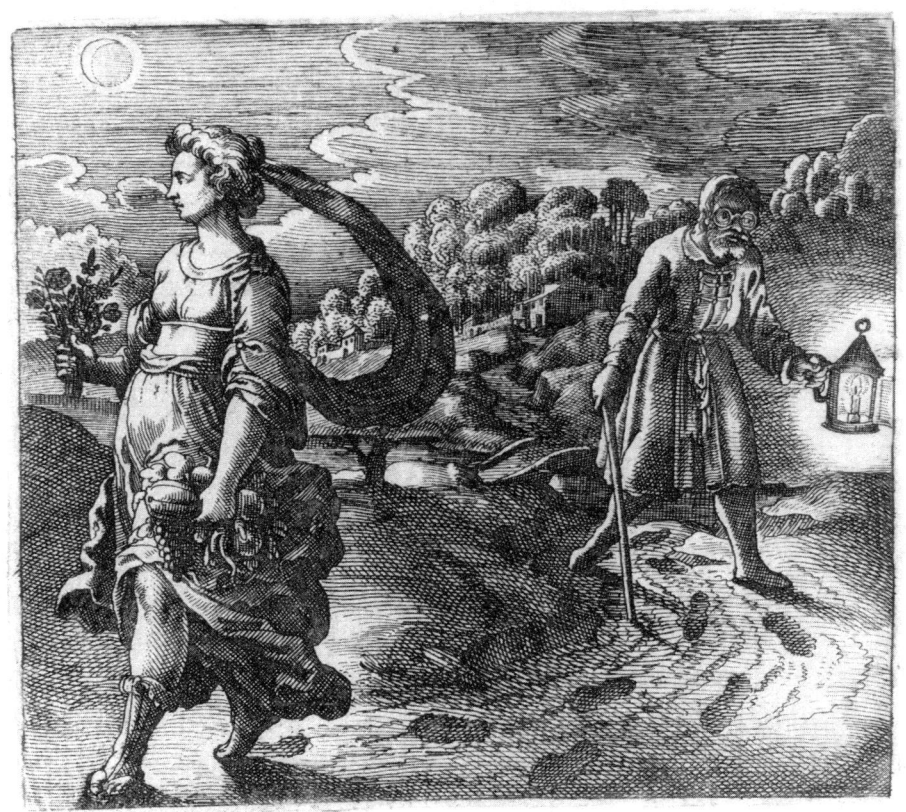

EPIGRAMMA XLII.

This emblem from Michael Maier's Atalanta Fugiens *(1618; reprint Frankfurt: Oehrling, 1687) illustrates a motif common among early modern natural philosophers, namely that their quest for the truth, indicated here by the Diogenes-like figure, required following in Nature's footsteps, using both reasoning and experiment. The emblem reads: "In the examination of chemical matters, let Nature, Reason, Experience, and reading be your Leader, walking stick, spectacles, and lantern." Courtesy of the University of Chicago Library.*

A PHILOSOPHICAL PATH FOR PARACELSIAN MEDICINE

THE IDEAS, INTELLECTUAL CONTEXT, AND INFLUENCE OF

PETRUS SEVERINUS (1540/2-1602)

by Jole Shackelford

MUSEUM TUSCULANUM PRESS
UNIVERSITY OF COPENHAGEN
2004

A Philosophical Path for Paracelsian Medicine.
The Ideas, Intellectual Context, and Influence of Petrus Severinus (1540/2-1602)
© Museum Tusculanum Press and Jole Shackelford
Consultant on Latin texts: Fritz S. Pedersen
Cover design: Henrik Maribo
Composition: Narayana Press, Denmark
Printed in Denmark by Narayana Press, www.narayanapress.dk
ISBN 87 7289 817 8

Published as vol. 46 in the series *Acta Scientiarum Naturalium et Medicinalium*
ISSN 0065 1311
Series editors: Mette Stockmarr and Torsten Schlichtkrull

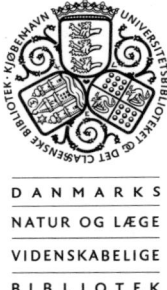

DANMARKS
NATUR OG LÆGE
VIDENSKABELIGE
BIBLIOTEK

Cover illustrations details. See pages: 36, 371, 405 and 416

Published with financial support from:

The Danish Research Council for the Humanities
Lillian og Dan Finks Fond
Nordea Danmark Fonden

Museum Tusculanum Press
Njalsgade 94
DK-2300 Copenhagen S

www.mtp.dk

CONTENTS

Acknowledgments

This book has been in the making for well over a decade, during which time I have benefitted from the assistance of numerous people in various capacities. My study of Petrus Severinus and Paracelsian medicine began with my doctoral research in the history of science and medicine at the University of Wisconsin, and I will always fondly remember the faculty of that institution and the collegiality of the graduate students in those fields during those years, when it was still acceptable to follow one's intellectual curiosity rather than a marketing stratagem. All of those people and institutions who aided me in my doctoral work also contributed to this study, which grew organically from it, and again deserve my thanks, especially David C. Lindberg, who whetted my appetite for history of science as an undergraduate, and Harold J. Cook, who helped me give form to my research aspirations. The University of Wisconsin remains a source of academic fellowship for me and an excellent place to undertake research, and I am particularly grateful to the staffs of the Middleton Health Sciences Library and the Memorial Library, especially the departments of special collections and microforms. In particular, I wish to acknowledge the assistance of John Neu, Robin Rider, Ed Duesterhoeft, and Micaela Sullivan-Fowler.

Deep scrutiny of the ideas of Petrus Severinus entailed a careful reading of his main work, the language and concepts of which I believe have deterred past scholars. The award of a Rockefeller postdoctoral scholarship at the University of Oklahoma enabled me to devote an academic year to studying Severinus' writings in detail, and I am grateful to Ken Taylor and the staff of the Degolyer collection for making me welcome there. Pursuit of Severinus' influence on the history of ideas has taken me to many other libraries, whose staff have helped me locate books and manuscripts, and I wish to acknowledge these, too. Foremost among research venues for my work are the Royal Library in Copenhagen, the Danish State Archive, The Danish National Library of Science and Medicine, the Norwegian State Archive, The Oslo City Archive, The

University of Oslo Library, The British Library, the History of Medicine Division at the National Library of Medicine, and the Libraries of the University of Minnesota. I also want to thank Susan Alons, then at Washington University School of Medicine Library, for providing me information on a particular edition of Paracelsus. Several people at the University of Minnesota warrant my special thanks: Charles Spetland of the Wilson Library has been a long-time friend and a constant source of information about the mysteries of collection practices and obtaining information; Elaine Challacombe, curator of the Wangensteen Library at the University of Minnesota, Carol Urness, director of the James Ford Bell Library, and Tim Johnson, curator of rare books have made available to me rare books and reference materials that have helped me to finish this project. Finally, I must thank Torsten Schlichtkrull of the Danish National Library of Science and Medicine for helping me find illustrations and facilitating the publication of this book, and Fritz Saaby Pedersen of the University of Southern Denmark, whose mastery of classical languages and careful scrutiny alerted me to several mistakes before this book went to press. Those errors that remain are, of course, my responsibility.

Academic research would be much less satisfying without the friendship and fellowship of one's academic colleagues, and I should especially like to thank Allen Debus, whose seminar at the Newberry Library many years ago provided a subtle but enduring foundation for my continued interest in Paracelsian studies. Allen has long argued for the importance of the Paracelsians to the development of early science and medicine, and most of us who engage in Paracelsian studies today habitually return to his books and articles for guidance. I have enjoyed the comradery of many historians associated with such studies, for whom Paracelsian medical, philosophical, and religious ideas are not a ridiculously arcane subject for scrutiny, including Bruce Moran, Bill Newman, Larry Principe, Bill Eamon, Chad Gunnoe, John Christianson, Anita Guerrini, Mike Walton, Pam Long, Mike Shank, and many others, too numerous to mention. But most of all I owe my thanks to Hal Cook and Faye Getz, who have been persistent friends and supporters.

Besides the Rockefeller postdoctoral fellowship that I enjoyed at the University of Oklahoma in 1989-90, I have received no research grants or other financial assistance to pursue the work behind this study and, consequently, my greatest debt of gratitude for financial resources as well as moral support is to my friends and family: to the Kolstrup and Kjeldsen families in Denmark, who always seem to welcome me into their homes as an itinerant scholar abroad; to my parents, who never goaded me to abandon my scholarship and seek a more remunerative career; to Frankie Shackelford, who has steadfastly taught Norwegian to help support our family, while her husband has been reading old books and struggling with recurrent underemployment; and to Terry Shackelford, whose untimely, violent death in 1983 provided his brother with economic resources that continue to sustain my scholarship. I wish that he were here to see the results. Lastly, I hope that my sons, whose childhoods are an indelible backdrop to my work on Severinus, and who have grown up watching me fret over the academic marketplace, are not dissuaded from strenuously pursuing whatever kind of study drives their imaginations and finds outlets for their talents.

Introduction

PETRUS SEVERINUS AND THE ASSIMILATION OF PARACELSIAN MEDICINE

FOR MANY readers of this book, Petrus Severinus will be an un-known name, but this was not the case in the seventeenth century, when his reputation as an important Paracelsian author was widespread. His obscurity today is owing to several factors, not the least of which is the difficulty that his written work presents to the modern reader. Furthermore, Severinus' fame rested on his success in interpreting and presenting certain concepts that were introduced by Paracelsus, which, despite the strenuous efforts of Walter Pagel, Allen Debus, and several other twentieth-century historians of science and medicine, often remain peripheral to the grand narratives of early modern intellectual development. This book, an intellectual biography of Petrus Severinus, offers the reader an introduction to Severinus' ideas and their social and intellectual context and an assessment of who read his work and what they made of it. An underlying assumption is that once we better understand the work of Paracelsus' followers – those who brought his ideas to a wide intellectual audience – we will better understand the significance of Paracelsian ideas, both in relation to early modern science and medicine and also as forming an ideology. The latter is especially important for assessing seventeenth-century reactions to Paracelsian ideas, which were frequently viewed in a religious frame and accepted or rejected on religious grounds.[1]

---

[1] For a recent summary of the historiography of Paracelsus and Paracelsianism and current problems in Paracelsian research, see Stephen Pumfrey, "The Spagyric Art; Or, the Impossible Work of Separating Pure from Impure Paracelsianism: A Historiographical Analysis," in Ole Peter Grell, ed., *Paracelsus: The Man and His Reputation, His Ideas and Their Transformation* (Leiden: Brill, 1998), pp. 21-51.

The ideas associated with Philippus Aureolus Bombastus von Hohenheim (1493-1541), the German medical and religious reformer generally known as Paracelsus, were a significant contribution to the intellectual ferment of early modern Europe. Paracelsian theories found an audience among physicians and pharmacists, who used them to explain the operation of diseases and drugs and as a rationale for prescribing new kinds of remedies. They were debated by astronomers and chemists and natural philosophers, who were groping for a new theoretical basis to explain the changes that are evident as the things of this world appear and disappear, grow and move, age and decay. They were taken up by theologians and lay religious writers, who sought to explain the natural world and its creation in ways that were compatible with their views of Christ, the Bible, and the church. In short, the ideas of Paracelsus were of interest to healers, whether they were ministers to the sick, ministers of a faith, or menders of natural philosophy, which many in the early modern period saw as in need of repair. Thus we find Paracelsian concepts embedded in a variety of social and intellectual contexts, providing an ideological justification and a metaphysical foundation for a medical *praxis*, a chemical philosophy, and a spiritual doctrine that united man to God and both to the universe. It is in part owing to their breadth of application that Paracelsian doctrines – and indeed the world view that they supported – became the subject of bitter debate and a salient component of the early modern dialogue of reform.

It is unlikely that many university-educated physicians and natural philosophers of seventeenth-century Europe were in ignorance of at least the basic precepts of Paracelsian theory. These ran counter to the traditional medical doctrines of Galen and the medieval Arabic writers, upon which academic medicine was largely based, and were therefore controversial throughout the period. They challenged the Aristotelian metaphysics on which all the sciences depended. Moreover, Paracelsian methodology rejected much of the book-learning and scholastic methods of the universities and urged the physician to rely on his senses and intuition when investigating nature: the physician – and by implication everyone – should learn the wisdom of God directly from the book of nature, rather than rely on the mediation of questionable written authority, namely the dead letters of the ancient pagans and their scholastic commentators.

The Paracelsian rhetoric of empirical observation and laboratory experience complemented the Reformation ideal that the pious Christian should seek to know the word of God directly from Holy Scripture, without the dubious mediation of the church. For Paracelsus, piety was one of the four pillars upon which true medicine rested, and just as the Paracelsian physician should be illuminated by the light of nature, through his study of the "anatomy of the world," so too should he be spiritually enlightened. Paracelsian medicine, like Paracelsian religion, was rooted firmly in the religious reform of the sixteenth century, and both found acceptance among the Rosicrucians, Puritans, and Pietists of the seventeenth century. In the minds of some observers, these ideas threatened the status quo, even as they promised reformation and renewal to others. For all of these reasons, the doctrines and historical development of Paracelsianism have been objects of interest, curiosity, and study for historians of science and medicine, who continue to evaluate the place of Paracelsian and Hermetic thought in the emergence of a new approach to natural philosophy in the early modern period.[2] Paracelsus is also coming to be appreciated by Reformation scholars as well, who are finding his writings to have been an inspiration to radical Protestants of the sixteenth century and the pietistic movements of the seventeenth and eighteenth centuries.

A key problem facing those who seek to understand Paracelsian ideas and the influence that they have had on the course of social and intellectual history is to learn how they were developed and disseminated. Investigating this subject entails an enquiry into the editing, translating, and printing of Paracelsus' texts themselves, but it also demands study of the works of the Paracelsians, that is, those who followed Paracelsus, adopted his ideas, and adapted them to different contexts. In a sense, Paracelsianism was invented by these followers, who forged Paracelsus' inchoate teachings into a workable mass of chemical medicine. The present book is an intellectual biography of one of these Paracelsians,

---

2 William R. Newman, *Gehennical Fire: The Lives of George Starkey, an American Alchemist in the Scientific Revolution* (Cambridge, Massachusetts: Harvard University Press, 1994), p. 94, gives the Paracelsians a critically important role in the transition from scholastic natural philosophy to the new science of the early modern period: "One could argue not only that the scientific revolution in chemistry was not 'postponed' until Lavoisier, but that Paracelsus himself inaugurated the scientific revolution per se."

Petrus Severinus, and an investigation of the influence of his work, which will illuminate an important stage in the assimilation and diffusion of Paracelsian theory in early modern Europe.

How important was Severinus? Daniel Sennert, a respected medical author and professor at Wittenberg, wrote in 1619 that most chemical physicians followed the lead of Petrus Severinus, who had succeeded in bringing together the ideas of Paracelsus into a coherent philosophy; that indeed one could speak of a new "Severinian" school of medical theory. A century later, Johann Conrad Barchusen identified Petrus Severinus as the first to hand down Paracelsian theory to posterity. Kurt Polycarp Sprengel, the great German medical historian of the late Enlightenment, referred to Severinus as the most famous of the sixteenth-century Paracelsians. Modern historians have echoed this assessment of Severinus, calling him "the most important Paracelsian theorist in the sixteenth century," and "the clearest expositor and follower of Paracelsian natural philosophy."[3] Yet few of them treated Severinus in any detail, and none ventured to explore his influence on seventeenth-century medicine.[4]

Petrus Severinus was a Danish physician, roughly contemporary with the well-known Danish astronomer Tycho Brahe, and was one of the early members of the first generation of Paracelsian writers. His *Idea medicinæ philosophicæ* (Ideal of Philosophical Medicine) brought together many of the key metaphysical concepts of Paracelsian medicine, which were scattered about in diverse texts left by Paracelsus, and introduced them to learned philosophers and physicians of the late sixteenth and early seventeenth centuries. The Elizabethan physician and entomologist Thomas Moffet, for instance, solicited Severinus' help in defending

---

3 Allen Debus, "Mathematics and Nature in the Chemical Texts of the Renaissance," *Ambix* 15(1968), p. 22; Walter Pagel, *The Smiling Spleen: Paracelsianism in Storm and Stress* (Basel: Karger, 1984), p. 18.

4 Kurt Polycarp Sprengel briefly surveyed the main points of Severinus' doctrine in 5 pages in his *Versuch einer pragmatischen Geschichte der Arnzneikunde*; Walter Pagel, *Smiling Spleen*, devoted ten pages to placing Severinus between Paracelsus and William Harvey and identifying him as an important interpreter of Paracelsian and Neoplatonic doctrine. Severinus' recent biographer, Eyvind Bastholm, provided a thirty two page introduction to Hans Skov's Danish translation of Severinus' works, but did not investigate Severinus' influence on his contemporaries and followers. See Eyvind Bastholm and Hans Skov, *Petrus Severinus og hans Idea medicinæ philosophicæ* (Odense: Odense Universitetsforlag, 1979). Furthermore, no proper effort was made to investigate the subsequent history of Paracelsianism – in part the legacy of Severinus – within the kingdom of Denmark.

Paracelsian theory against the onslaught of anti-Paracelsianism that was unleashed by Thomas Erastus, whose scathing attack on Paracelsian medicine encompassed doctrines espoused by Severinus, too. Four decades later, Severinus' theory was singled out for specific criticism by Andreas Libavius, who crusaded against occult sciences of all kinds, but especially against the Paracelsians. His attack on Johann Hartmann, considered to be the first European professor of chemistry, recognized that Hartmann's philosophy was largely based on the *Idea medicinæ.* Francis Bacon, who held Paracelsus in low esteem, but has been shown to have adopted some of his metaphysical suppositions, praised Severinus' genius, but thought that he had wasted it on the doctrines of Paracelsus. Even John Donne, the erudite poet and incisive observer of the intellectual life of early seventeenth-century England, knew of Severinus and made a place for him in *Ignatius his Conclave.* An examination of references to Severinus and the *Idea medicinæ* in the literature of the period reveals that Severinus' book was extensively read and very successful, particularly as a source of theory about the generation and elimination of diseases, but also as an introduction to the new Paracelsian theories. For this reason, Severinus and his work merit consideration by all those who wish to understand how Paracelsian ideas were interpreted, enlarged, and propagated in early modern Europe.

In his Danish homeland specifically, Petrus Severinus was an important figure in the last quarter of the sixteenth century and warrants study as a member of the intellectual elite that was renewing the university and bringing Denmark up to a continental standard of cultural and intellectual development during the reigns of King Frederik II and Christian IV. Throughout his career Severinus maintained close ties with the medical faculty at the University of Copenhagen, to which he was appointed immediately prior to his death. His education had been supported by the crown, and his work as a Paracelsian must be viewed within the context of royal patronage of learning and the encouragement of chemical philosophy and medicine in particular. As royal physician, he was an insider and advisor at the Danish court as well as a leader in the Danish medical community. Moreover, his position conferred authority to his work, which continued to be read and recommended by the next generation of Danish physicians.

Petrus Severinus had personal and intellectual ties with Tycho Brahe,

whose efforts to reform astronomy have interested historians of science
since the time of Pierre Gassendi. Their worlds intersected at many
points, including the Danish royal court, and for this reason, Tycho's
involvement in natural philosophy and religion are an important part
of Severinus' historical context. Like Severinus, Tycho had also enjoyed
royal patronage, which enabled him to build Uraniborg and Stjærneborg,
his "castle of the stars," not far from Copenhagen. But Tycho was not
merely an astronomer – he was also a chemist engaged in the preparation of chemical medicines. He, too, was affected by the philosophy of
Paracelsus, and Uraniborg not only served as a platform for observing
the heavens, but also housed a chemical laboratory that rivaled those of
the late sixteenth-century kings and princes. The two, astronomy and
chemistry – or celestial astronomy and terrestrial astronomy, as Tycho
termed them – were complementary parts of the worldview that Tycho
and Severinus shared. This world view also had a religious dimension,
as is clear from the published treatises of Kort Aslakssøn, whose work
reflects a commitment to fitting together chemical philosophy and
Scriptural accounts of the creation of the world. Aslakssøn, who joined
the theological faculty at the University of Copenhagen after Severinus
and Brahe were dead, had plainly been influenced by his years as an
assistant at Uraniborg and by his reading of Severinus' *Idea medicinæ*.
An enquiry into Severinus' ideas is therefore of interest to historians
of science who wish to know more about the ideological background
to Tycho Brahe's planned renovation of astronomy and, of course, to
students of late-Reformation Denmark as well.

The *Idea medicinæ* was a widely read and influential book in the
early modern period, but is unread today, partly because of the linguistic barriers that the Latin text and its Danish translation present to
most would-be readers, and partly because the ideas expressed within
it are themselves arcane and embedded in a mental framework that is
alien to a modern audience. To understand Severinus' importance to
early modern theorists and thereby secure his place in the history of
science and medicine, it is necessary to turn to the *Idea medicinæ* to
characterize the author's approach and explain his chief doctrines, a task
undertaken in part two of this book. Many of these doctrines are Paracelsian, but Severinus related them in terms of Neoplatonist philosophy
and grounded them in the authority of Hippocrates and other ancient

authors, a feat that gave the *Idea medicinæ* and the Paracelsian ideas it purveyed credibility. It is important to realize that the philosophy that Severinus constructed and expounded in the *Idea medicinæ* is not just a medical theory, but a metaphysical system, which applies generally to change in the natural world. This accounts for why Severinus was so widely admired as a Paracelsian author and why his formulations found application among diverse writers.

At the core of Severinus' theory is his doctrine of efficient causation, which I have called his *semina* theory, after the seed-like principles (*semina*) that lay at the foundation of his system and connected Paracelsus' medicine to a venerable intellectual heritage stretching back through the Middle Ages to the work of St. Augustine. Severinus considered these *semina* to be the loci of the generation and corruption of all physical reality, complementary processes that produced all material existence through emanation from these centers under the direction of immaterial agents. *Semina* theory is interesting in its own right as a formulation of Paracelsus' perception that certain diseases have an existence that is ontologically distinct from the host. Severinus' "seeds of disease" (*semina morborum*), perhaps more than any other concept in the *Idea medicinæ*, grabbed the attention of medical posterity and, consequently, have interested historians of medicine who wish to trace the origins of modern pathology. But *semina* are even more compelling for their theological dimension and the role they play within Severinus' natural philosophy, which made the theory attractive to certain Christian philosophers.

To the extent that Severinus elaborated an entire theory of generation and corruption based on the seminal principle, his work can be viewed as an advanced form of immaterial metaphysics, a kind of matterless atomism, which was eclipsed by the materialist philosophies of the seventeenth century, or perhaps was coopted by them. There is a striking resemblance between Severinus' seminal centers and the inertial, material corpuscles endowed with active principles that characterized the natural hypotheses of Walter Charleton, Robert Boyle, and other representatives of the new scientific spirit of the seventeenth century. However, there is an essential difference: Severinus permitted his *semina*, the loci for all change in the subvisible world, to take on a material nature, but they were intrinsically formal and immaterial, and were both logically and ontologically prior to matter. By contrast, the corpuscularians believed in a material basis for reality, even if some of them permitted corpuscles to be endowed with active principles and plastic forces. Severinus was a Neoplatonist, not a Democritus or an Epicurus, and his "seeds" were neither atoms nor corpuscles, but an elaboration and extrapolation of Paracelsian idealism. Indeed, the *Idea medicinæ* represents an extreme development of Paracelsian metaphysics, which remained viable into the second half of the seventeenth century, when William Davidson used it as a basis for his philosophical system, which, although more elaborate in some ways, lacks the simple elegance and coherence of Severinus' theory.

A FEW WORDS ON SCOPE AND METHOD

This book is mainly concerned with Severinus as an expositor and for-mulator of Paracelsian ideas and the influence that these ideas had on the philosophical, medical, and religious world of the late sixteenth and seventeenth centuries. Yet it is not *merely* intellectual history, inasmuch as all ideas must be contextualized, in order to have meaning to the historian. Nevertheless, this is unabashedly and self-consciously a study of ideas and their influence upon the framers of theory, the sources that they used, and the practical expressions that they gave their theories. As such, I have relied on the principal tools of the intellectual historian – texts and their interpretation – which are subject to the vagaries of time, the marketplace, and a host of other factors that introduce biases into the historical record and how we come to view it centuries after the event. Not the least of these is the well-known fact that early modern authors exhibited little regularity in their citation of other authors, who may have influenced their thinking. Nevertheless, it is the web of causes and effects – including ideas and their reception – that make history interesting and meaningful, and ferreting out these intellectual con-nections is a useful preliminary step to understanding Severinus' role as midwife to Paracelsian medicine, both as philosophy and practice.

I have made an attempt to collate as many references to Severinus as I could find in order to fairly demonstrate not only the use of his ideas by medical authors, but also the diversity of contexts in which

Severinus' conceptions are found — in poetry and geology as well as in medical theory. The reader will find Severinus mentioned by a host of writers whose names are familiar to scholars of early modern science and medicine — men such as Tycho Brahe, Andreas Libavius, Jean Baptiste van Helmont, Walter Charleton, Robert Boyle, and Pierre Gassendi. But Severinus' influence extended well beyond these leading figures to affect early modern natural philosophy more generally, and the full impact of his work can only be appreciated by viewing the many contexts in which the influence of the *Idea medicinæ* is manifest. The method I have employed is to trace references and examine commentaries in detail, which the reader may find tedious on occasion, but I am committed to presenting the full extent of the diffusion of Severinus' ideas in the intellectual world of early modern Europe in a way that is factually sound and will permit readers to see how these unfamiliar Paracelsian terms and concepts were received and interpreted.

Since both of the authors who published book-length monographs specifically explaining and defending the *Idea medicinæ* are today obscure, I have devoted considerable space in part four to presenting samples of how they used and explained Severinus' ideas in their texts. The first of these, Ambrosius Rhodius, is unknown to historians of medicine, and therefore deserves some introduction. Copies of his commentary on the *Idea medicinæ* are relatively rare and, to my knowledge, he and his work have not been treated in any English-language publication prior to my own studies.[5] The second writer, a Scot named William Davidson, is somewhat better known, but his voluminous commentaries on Severinus' *Idea medicinæ* have received scant attention. For this reason, and because he filled more pages clarifying Severinus' meanings than any other author, I have devoted an entire chapter to an assessment of his work. Moreover, Davidson did something with *semina* theory that Severinus did not — he considered its specific application to disease, in this case fevers. Study of this portion of Davidson's work will therefore

---

5 Selected details of his life and work are presented in Jole Shackelford, "Paracelsianism in Denmark and Norway in the 16th and 17th centuries, (Ph.D. Dissertation, University of Wisconsin, 1989); "Hans Jochum Scharff: A Paracelsian Apothecary in Seventeenth-Century Norway," *Norges Apotekerforenings Tidsskrift* 95 (1987): 212-217; "A Reappraisal of Anna Rhodius: Religious Enthusiasm and Social Unrest in Seventeenth-Century Christiania, Norway," *Scandinavian Studies* 65(1993): 349-89.

help illuminate an aspect of Paracelsian medicine that has hitherto re-ceived insufficient scholarly attention, namely how Paracelsian theory was brought to bear on particular therapeutic problems. Investigation of how Rhodius and Davidson read and used the *Idea medicinæ* enhances our perception of the meanings found in it by his seventeenth-century successors, which provides a historical insight that is not obtainable from study of the original text alone. The novelty and importance of these two authors warrants the lengthy treatment they receive in this book, and I hope that the reader's patience will be rewarded with a rich understanding of Severinus and the historical significance of his philosophical medicine and a deepened appreciation for the place of Paracelsian theory in early modern science and medicine.

PART ONE

Paracelsianism in Tycho Brahe's Denmark

Chapter One

THE EDUCATION
OF A DANISH PHYSICIAN

PEDER SØRENSEN, later known by his Latinized name, Petrus Severinus, was born in the Danish provincial town of Ribe in either 1542 or 1540.[1] Ribe, which is today a small, remarkably well-preserved town on the west coast of Jutland, is perhaps Denmark's oldest town. It was built on several small islands, high ground in the marshland where various streams run into the Ribe River before it resumes its winding course to the sea. Astride a main trade route, Ribe was well located to benefit from the flourishing commerce between the farmers of Jutland and the markets for their cattle and horses to the south. It was a prosperous town, sustaining at its peak ten churches and four cloisters, including a leprosarium. At the time of Severinus' birth it was still an important

---

1 Severinus is a Latinization of Sørensen or Severinsen, and the name is treated variously by historians. Rørdam, ed., *Kjøbenhavns Universitets Historie fra 1537 til 1621* (hereafter *KUH*), vol. 2, p. 573, states that 1542 is commonly given as his birthyear ("almindelig angives 1542 som hans Fødeaar"), and finds the probable source of this tradition in Thomas Bartholin, *Cista medica Hafniensis* (Copenhagen: Haubold, 1662), p. 114. He notes, however, that Peder Hansen Resen, *Inscriptiones Hafnienses Latinæ* (Copenhagen: Godicchenius, 1668), p. 105, reported that Severinus' grave inscription indicated he was 62 years old when he died in 1602, hence he must have been born in 1540. Eyvind Bastholm, *Petrus Severinus*, p. 2, n. 13, echos Rørdam ("almindeligvis angives 1542 som hans fødselsår"). Both dates are in fact given in *Cista medica*. Given this, I find no reason to prefer 1542 over 1540, as did Vilhelm Ingerslev, *Danmarks Læger og Lægevæsen fra de ældste Tider indtil Aar 1800*, vol. 1 (Copehagen: E. Jespersen, 1873), p. 176, and Johan D. Herholdt and Frederik V. Mansa, *Samlinger til den danske Medicinal-Historie*, vol. 1 (Copenhagen: Gyldendal, 1835), p. 14. The fact that Bartholin states that Severinus died 29 July 1602 at age 62 on the same page where he gives the death dates for Severinus' wife and children (*Cista medica*, p. 120), suggests that 1540, if any, has the better claim for authority. Dated 1615, the grave-inscription may have been erected by Severinus' surviving children.

seaport, supporting regular trade with Holland, England, and the port town of the Frisian coast. It was also an administrative center: the cathedral at Ribe governed one of the most powerful sees in sixteenth-century Denmark, and the fortification built to defend the town, called Riberhus, was the official residence of the local military authority. In the early seventeenth century, the silting up of the Ribe River conspired with the growing commercial vitality of Copenhagen and the Baltic Sea routes to eclipse Ribe economically, but the decline was not obvious in Severinus' lifetime. Riberhus was rebuilt in the years after the Reformation swept through Denmark (1537) and remained a military stonghold until the seventeenth-century wars with Sweden proved its vulnerability to a large army that was well equipped with field artillery.[2]

Petrus Severinus' parents, Bodil (Botilda) Sørensdatter and Søren (Severin) Jessen, were probably prosperous and socially well-positioned, and Severinus was able to join the ranks of the other sons of Ribe who attended the local Latin school before moving on to Copenhagen and positions of influence in the Danish church, university, and state.[3] Not a few of the people who shaped Danish history hailed from Ribe, often suffixing *Ripensis* to the Latin form of their names in order to distinguish them from the Sørensens, Petersens, and Jensens from other parts of the north.[4] The Latin school in Ribe was, like others in Denmark, the old

---

2   On Ribe see Hugo Matthiessen, *Gamle Huse i Ribe* (Copenhagen: Reitzel, 1937); Christian Axel Jensen, *Riberhus Slotsbanke* (Copenhagen: Gyldendal, 1942); Ole Degn, *Rig og fattig i Ribe: Økonomiske og sociale forhold i Ribe-samfundet 1560-1660* (Aarhus: Universitetsforlaget, 1981); and Ingrid Nielsen, ed., *Ribe Bys Jordebog: Grundlagt i 1450erne og videreført til omkring 1600* (Esbjerg: Sydjysk Universitetsforlag, 1979). For a complete socio-historical study of Ribe's geography see Ole Degn, *Scandinavian Atlas of Historic Towns*, vol. 3, *Ribe 1500-1950* (Odense: Odense University Press, 1983).

3   Rørdam and other historians, going back to Bartholin's *Cista medica* (p. 114), claim that Søren Jessen was a councilman of Ribe (*senator* or *rådmann*), but his name does not appear in the list of councilmen, nor in any of the court proceedings surviving from 1527-76. See Erik Kroman, ed., *Ribe Rådstuedombøger 1527-1576 og 1580-1599* (Copenhagen: Selskabet for udgivelse af kilder til dansk historie, 1974). The surviving records of land ownership indicate that Severin Jessen owned a lot along the river, upon which some sort of structure was built ("som hans brwhwss paa staar") in the 1540s and 1550s, but there is no other mention of him. See Ingrid Nielsen, *Ribe Bys Jordebog*, p. 48.

4   A number of the professors at the University of Copenhagen in the sixteenth century came from Ribe. Hans Frandsen (Johannes Franciscus Ripensis) and Anders Christensen (Andreas Christianus Ripensis), for example, were professors of medicine at Copenhagen during Severinus' career as Royal Physician.

cathedral school. Until the founding of the University of Copenhagen in 1479, the cathedral schools had provided the highest level of education in the kingdom and were intended primarily to train young boys in Latin, to enable them to serve the church or to continue their education abroad. After the Reformation dismantled the Catholic administrative hierarchy, the schools continued in this role, but now under Lutheran masters.

No records exist of what was actually taught at Ribe Latin School in the 1540s and 1550s, but by 1548 there were five courses or grades and by 1552-3 six grades, each with its own teacher. This corresponded to the ideal set out in the Church Ordinance of 1537 and described by Bishop Petrus Palladius, himself from Ribe, in his "Tabula de exercitiis scholasticis" of 1546, and the curriculum at Ribe presumably followed Palladius' prescriptions in other respects. Through five grades of primary schooling, students such as Severinus would be taught to read, speak, sing, and write in Latin, using both traditional and newer, humanist primers and grammars written by Donatus, Cato, Torrentinus, Mosella-nus, and Philipp Melanchthon. Exemplary texts were drawn from the classical stylists Terence, Plautus, Cicero, Ovid, and Virgil, and from the pedagogical reformers Erasmus and Melanchthon. The upper grades introduced the young Danish Lutherans to texts that were essential to Protestant doctrine, including the Pauline Epistles. All instruction in grades three through five was conducted in Latin, and in the final grade the schoolmaster introduced the students to the fundamentals of Greek.[5] According to the Church Ordinance, the school day began at 6 a.m. (7 in the winter) and lasted until 4 p.m. Advanced students were expected to attend both morning and afternoon church services. Instruction was given on Mondays, Tuesdays, Thursdays, and Fridays, with Wednesdays being reserved for examinations and special assignments. Schooling on Saturdays was limited to religious instruction.[6]

The Cathedral at Ribe was administered by some of the most learned and competent humanist reformers in sixteenth and seventeenth century Denmark – Hans Tausen, Peder Hegelund, and Jens Dinesen Jersin rank among the most important of Denmark's early Lutheran bishops. Under

5 Bjørn Kornerup, *Ribe Katedralskoles Historie: Studier over 800 Aars dansk Skolehistorie*, vol. 1 (Copenhagen: Gyldendal, 1947), pp. 265-7.
6 Ibid., p. 268.

their regime the old cathedral school was maintained at the highest level of excellence. Therefore, in Ribe Severinus had access to the best primary education available in Denmark at mid-century. From there he travelled to Copenhagen to attend the University.

The University of Copenhagen in these years was financially weak. Chartered in 1479, it was refounded in 1537 under the guidance of the Lutheran reformer Johan Bugenhagen to provide the advanced education required by the reformed church. But despite some improvements made in the 1550s, its finances were not secure until Frederik II undertook to set the institution on a solid footing in the late 1560s, well after Severinus had left the university to study abroad.[7] According to the articles of the new foundation (1539), the university was patterned after the university at Wittenberg. There were four faculties, in keeping with the medieval academic system: an arts faculty (philosophy) and the three higher faculties of Theology, Law, and Medicine. The form of teaching was the familiar lecturing, disputation, and declamation that characterized academic life in the late Middle Ages.[8] But if the refounded university was strongly medieval in form, its purpose was suited to the needs of the Reformation. It was not so much a collection of faculties, as it was a unified system in the service of the church and state.[9] The Reformation fostered an atmosphere of Biblical humanism which was strongly influenced by the ideas of the Lutheran reformer Philipp Melanchthon, for whom philosophy and medicine were seen as important aspects of a well rounded education rather than merely as preparation for professional careers in these subjects. It is not surprising, then, that theological concerns dominated university activities and that philosophical concerns entered into religious debate and are reflected in the theological literature. This interpenetration of natural philosophy

7 Christian III took the initial steps by attaching the incomes from certain churches and a farm in 1555 and 1557, which Frederik confirmed in 1560. See Rørdam, *KUH*, vol. 2, p. 6.

8 Oluf Friis, *Den Danske Litteraturs Historie* (hereafter *DDLH*), vol. 1 (Copenhagen: Hirschsprung, 1945), p. 329; P. L. Panum, "Vort medicinske Fakultets Oprinelse og Barnedom: et Bidrag til Kundskab om Lægevidenskabens og Naturvidenskabernes Udvikling i Danmark," in *Festskrifter udgivne af Det Lægevidenskabelige Fakultet ved Kjøbenhavns Universitet i Anledning af Universitets Firehunderedaarsfest Juni 1879* (Copenhagen: Gyldendal, 1879), p. 42.

9 O. Friis, *DDLH*, vol. 1, p. 331.

(cosmology) and theology is of great importance to understanding the intellectual issues confronting Severinus and his late-sixteenth century colleagues.

We do not know what year Severinus was matriculated into the University of Copenhagen, but it was likely sometime in the late 1550s. Once there, he would have followed a fairly standardized undergraduate curriculum, based in large part on the Aristotelian texts and commentaries that had ruled European arts faculties since the late thirteenth century. Philippist humanism, so named after Philipp Melanchthon, left room for natural philosophy in the curriculum of the reformed universities, and we see this at Copenhagen. Petrus Palladius, Bishop of Sjælland, defined philosophy at the University of Copenhagen in 1555 as comprising three branches: logic (grammar, dialectic, and rhetoric), physics, and ethics (special, political, and economic). Physics was the study of natural phenomena and included mathematics, physiology (the study of nature), and metaphysics. Severinus' first exposure to the basic study underlying academic medicine must have been in physiology and metaphysics at Copenhagen, and according to Palladius' description these were fundamentally Aristotelian. Physiology was to be taught mainly from Aristotle's *Physics, On the Heavens and Earth*, and *On Generation and Corruption*. However, theoretical medicine, meteorology, the study of metals (alchemy), and astrology were also included in physiology.[10]

According to the Church Ordinance and articles of the university's foundation (1539), lectures were to be held Monday through Friday beginning at 6 a.m. and ending at 5 p.m., except for Wednesdays, which were set aside for disputations (8-10 a.m.). Such a schedule would have been quite familiar to the Latin school graduate. Each professor was to hold four lectures a week, presumably one each day. Two hours every day (10-12) were designated as free time, and no lectures were to be held in the month of August, one week in October, and on holidays.[11]

The early historians reported that Severinus was himself holding lectures on Latin poetry at the University of Copenhagen before he reached the age of 20, and this has led to speculation that he was granted

---

10 Petrus Palladius, *Formula visitationis provincialis*, 1555, after Panum, "Vort medicinske Fakultets," pp. 24-5.
11 Ibid., pp. 26 and 42.

a bachelor's degree already in 1561.[12] Certainly there was a need for teachers competent in Latin poetry, which was fundamental to humanistic
education. Even in the 1570s Dr. Hans Frandsen, professor of medicine,
lectured on poetry, indicating that the arts faculty drew on members of
the higher faculties.[13] It was not unusual for a clever advanced student
such as Severinus to hold undergraduate lectures as a means of support
until he attained the master's degree, which would certify him to teach
anywhere in Europe. However, possibilities for advanced study were
no doubt hampered by the shaky economy and consequent low salaries
of the faculty, which resulted in vacancies and encouraged students to
look to foreign universities for instruction. Thus, Severinus travelled to
France to begin his study of medicine in 1562, but returned the very next
year, most likely because he did not have enough money to sustain him
abroad. In 1563 King Frederik II offered Severinus a canonry intended
to support a doctor in Viborg, but with the specific instruction that
he be allowed to study for three years before taking up that provincial
post.[14] The salary had been used for a stipend before: in 1559 two medical
students were supported on it.[15] What became of Severinus' preferment
is uncertain. Although another man was appointed physician in Viborg
in 1564, references to Severinus as a Canon of Viborg exist for 1569 and
1574.[16] Conceivably, the king funded a physician for this town in Jutland
by other means, permitting Severinus to retain the attached benefice.
Or perhaps more than one canonry was involved.

    Severinus was promoted to master in 1564 under the direction of

---

12 Wilhelm Reymann wrote that Severinus became a student about 1560 and received his
bachelor's degree in Copenhagen in 1561. See V. Gaunø-Jensen, "Wilhelm Reymann:
Undersøgelser over Peder Sørensens Liv og Lære," *Bibliotek for Læger* 166, no. 3 (1974),
p. 115. Reymann's chronology assumes Severinus was born in 1542. If in fact he was
born in 1540, then he may have been promoted to bachelor already by 1559. Rørdam,
KUH, vol. 2, p. 573, stated that Severinus lectured on Latin poetry, which was part of
the foundation curriculum in the arts faculty.

13 Rørdam, *KUH*, vol. 2, p. 326.

14 Ibid., p. 573; L. Laursen, ed., *Kancelliets Brevbøger*, vol. 3 (Copenhagen: Reitzel, 1393-
95), p. 352. Ingerslev, *Danmarks Læger*, vol. 1, p. 177, states that Severinus received the
canonry while abroad.

15 Rørdam, *KUH*, vol. 2, p. 9.

16 Daniel Henrik Otto Cold, *Lægevæsenet og Lægerne under Christian IV's Regiering (1588-
1648)* (Copenhagen: C.G. Iversen, 1858), p. 84, and Rørdam, *KUH*, vol. 2, p. 574, n. 1,
and p. 576.

Nicolaus Laurentius Scavenius. Scavenius had been educated in Copenhagen, Wittenberg, and Paris, and after he returned to Copenhagen he held first the chair in Mathematics (1555) and then the one in Physics (1564).[17] These disciplines covered the basic philosophical groundwork for medicine, including the problems of generation and corruption to which Severinus was to return throughout his lifetime. It was in fact Severinus' theory of generation and corruption as the flowing forth of being from an invisible seed, and its subsequent return to that seed, that attracted international attention to him.

Sometime before 1564 Severinus met Johannes Pratensis, and during the next ten years the two became close friends and travelling companions.[18] Johannes Pratensis (Hans Filipsen du Pré) was born 27 November 1543 in Århus, another episcopal seat in Jutland. His father, Master Philippe du Pré (Philippus Pratensis) had come to Denmark from Rouen in Normandy with Christian II's queen, Elisabeth, and for support he was given a canonry at Århus Cathedral. Through the efforts of his father, young Johannes Pratensis was also made a canon to finance his education, with the provision that he hire a chaplain to fulfill the religious obligations associated with the prebend. Presumably he received his primary education at the Latin school in Århus. Pratensis was promoted to master under Scavenius in 1564, along with Severinus, and afterwards he was appointed Rector of his old Latin school in Århus, a post generally intended to support scholars until there was further opportunity for advancement.[19]

Meanwhile, Severinus was hired as a "professor pædagogicus" at the university, one of two such positions in the arts faculty. The already poor economy of the university was further stressed by the Seven Years' War with Sweden, which commenced in 1563. The currency was debased, forcing the lower rank professors to seek financial assistance from the university. The 100 rigsdalers and free housing a professor pædagogicus received was unattractive, and the turnover was frequent until the two positions were merged into one in 1567.[20] To make a bad situation worse,

17 On Scavenius see Rørdam, *KUH*, vol. 2, pp. 486-490.
18 On Pratensis see Ibid., pp. 598-604; Anker Aggebo, "Hans Philipsen Pratensis 1543-76," *Arosia* 17, no. 1 (Aarhus, 1938).
19 Rørdam, *KUH*, vol. 2, p. 600.
20 Ibid., pp. 54-61.

epidemic disease appeared in Copenhagen during the winter of 1563-64, and by mid summer mortality had climbed to alarming numbers. In September the king issued an order suspending lectures, permitting professors and students to leave town. Despite the epidemic, which is estimated to have killed 1800 citizens, about one person in seven, Severinus stayed in Copenhagen and lectured on meteorology.[21]

It must have been clear to Severinus and Pratensis at this point in their education that they must finish their studies abroad, because the University of Copenhagen was too small, too parochial, and under-staffed. The refounded university provided for two chairs in medicine, two in theology, and one in law, indicating both the modest size of the higher faculties and the relative importance assigned to medicine. But in practice it was difficult to retain medical professors in one of the chairs for more than a year or two, a fact partly owing to the lack of native Danish medical doctors. The first chair in medicine was rather stable, being occupied successively by three Danes from the refounding of the university in 1537 until after Severinus' death in 1602. Thus, with the exception of the semester after Christiern Torkelsen Morsing died (Fall 1560), there was always one qualified professor of medicine on the faculty. In contrast, the second medical chair was in almost constant flux before 1571, and in the comparable period (1537-1602) there were eleven names associated with the position, which stood empty for all or part of at least thirteen academic years. In particular, in the eleven years after the death of Jacob Bording in September 1560, the position was intermittently filled in the first several years, and wholly vacant from 1565 to 1570! Elias Rempolt, a German who nominally held the post 1561-63, was so often away from Copenhagen in the service of the queen mother that the university complained. His death in August 1563 solved their problem, and in late Spring the following year a Dutchman named Adrian de Jonge (Hadrianus Junius) was appointed to the chair. However, it seems he wandered back to Holland before the year was out,

---

21 Bastholm, *Petrus Severinus*, p. 3, says that about 1800 of an estimated 13,000 citizens died that year, about 14% mortality. Meteorology was one of the topics listed in the 1555 curriculum for the University of Copenhagen under physics, one of the three branches of philosophy (logic, physics, and ethics). See Panum, "Vort medicinske Fakultets," pp. 24-25. These lecturers were therefore outside the duties of a professor pædagogicus.

disappointed with the low salary and poor standard of living in Denmark.[22] Thus, for all practical purposes there was only one professor of medicine at the University of Copenhagen while Severinus and Pratensis were studying there. They could have learned the basics of mathematics and natural philosophy from the arts' masters, Anders Pedersen Kjøge (Andreas Petreius Coagius) and Nicolaus Scavenius, but what actual medicine was taught must have been done by Hans Frandsen of Ribe (Johannes Franciscus Ripensis).

In the preface to his 1579 edition of Galen's *De ossibus*, Hans Frandsen summarized his activities over his first eighteen years on the job.[23] First, he says that to the extent that his official duties and medical practice have permitted, he has attended to that other part of his position, namely teaching the fundamentals of medicine to the medical students at the university. For this he began with Hippocrates' *Aphorisms* and then explained and interpreted Galen's *Liber ad Glauconem* concerning the symptoms and curing of fevers. Since mathematics (astronomy) was also part of medicine, he lectured on Regiomontanus' *Tabulæ directionum*. After that he lectured on plants, to enable his students to read Macer's poem, which was a traditional medieval text on herbal drugs.[24] Regarding the theory of critical days, he explicated several treatises by Philipp Melanchthon (1497-1560) and Guillaume Rondelet (1507-1566). Since plague has been raging in the country, he also wrote a tract on that subject, though more out of regard for what his audience demanded than for his own opinion. But now, in 1579, he has decided to approach medicine systematically, beginning with the skeleton (after the manner of humanist medicine). Considering the state of the medical faculty and what Frandsen said

22 On Elias Rempolt and Adrian de Jonge see Rørdam, *KUH*, vol. 2, pp. 540-43 and 567-69.

23 This preface is printed in Rørdam, *KUH*, vol. 4, #214, pp. 301-3, and summarized in Panum, "Vort medicinske Fakultets" pp. 44-5.

24 *Macer Floridus de virtutibus herbarum* was a 2269-line herbal poem composed probably by Odo of Meung sometime in the late eleventh century under the pen name Macer Floridus. It was widely used and translated in Europe from the High Middle Ages into the sixteenth century, when it began to decline in popularity with the printing of more comprehensive herbals. See Bruce P. Flood, "The Medieval Herbal Tradition of Macer Floridus," *Pharmacy in History* 18(1976): 62-66.

about his own teaching, it is clear that Severinus and Pratensis could have gotten in Copenhagen only the most rudimentary acquaintance with what constituted learned medicine in mid-16th-century Europe – a smattering of what was taught about Hippocrates, Galen, and herbalism in the late Middle Ages. It is no wonder they readily seized the opportunity to study abroad when finances permitted.

In 1565 the university offered Severinus and Pratensis a stipend to study abroad, and Severinus departed from Copenhagen that fall.[25] He left Denmark by way of his home town in South Jutland, where his friend Peder Hegelund noted the occasion in his almanac for 7 November: "Master Petrus Severinus met me on his way to Italy."[26] Pratensis joined his friend *en route* and they matriculated at the University of Padua 13 January 1566.[27]

Padua was perhaps the leading place to study medicine in Europe in the sixteenth century. It enjoyed the protection and economic well-being of the Republic of Venice and attained a preeminence in anatomy with a series of brilliant professors of surgery, including Andreas Vesalius, Gabriele Fallopio, and Realdo Columbo. These men were dead by the time Severinus matriculated, but Hieronymus Fabricius of Aquapendente, who was himself a product of Paduan anatomical training, had recently been appointed Professor of Surgery. We do not know what course of study Severinus and Pratensis followed, but they in any case had access to Europe's best-trained physicians at Padua, and they would likely have been exposed to the forefront of the debate over discrepancies in the teachings of Galen and Aristotle regarding the fine points of human anatomy and physiology – debate that led to the discovery of the circulation of blood in the human body by an English student of Fabricius, William Harvey. Neither Severinus nor Pratensis showed much inclination toward anatomy in their later careers as physicians, and in his writing Severinus treats the study of human anatomy as an

---

25 Rørdam, *KUH*, vol. 2, p. 574.

26 "Obuius mihi fuit M: Petrus Seuerinus abiturus in Italiam." Bue Kaae, ed., *Peder Hegelunds Almanakoptegnelser 1565-1613* (Ribe: Historisk Samfund for Ribe Amt, 1976), vol. 1, p. 14, entry for 7 November 1565.

27 Ingerslev, *Danmarks Læger*, vol. 1, p. 157, cites a list of Danish names on the matriculation list for the German nation (arts faculty) at Padua that was compiled by Henrik Fuiren in 1641-42.

idle science that has little to do with the true end of medicine, namely curing the sick. More likely they were inspired by another tradition in medicine at Padua, the revival of Hippocratism.

The medicine portrayed in the Hippocratic Corpus, a collection of treatises by Hippocrates that later physicians associated with the ancient medical school at Cos, had been incorporated into the authoritative texts of Galen in late antiquity, but there the emphasis was on theory. In the fifteenth and sixteenth centuries attention was again directed to the Hippocratic writings themselves, which encouraged the development of clinical medicine at Padua under the leadership of Girolamo Fracastoro and Giambattista da Monte.[28] Da Monte took his students into the houses of his patients, linking theory with bedside observation. This attention to symptoms, a kind of empirical tradition, is clearly evident in Severinus' book, *Idea medicinæ philosophicæ*, which was perhaps written in Northern Italy at the end of the decade. The date on the letter of dedication indicates that the book was essentially complete in 1570, when he was in Florence. However, the Hippocratic revival had also taken root in the Paris medical faculty, and Severinus may have been influence by it while he was studying there, too.[29]

The stipend that Severinus and Pratensis had been awarded was drawn from the salary (200 rigsdalers) attached to one of the two chairs in medicine at the University of Copenhagen. The professorship was vacant, and the university temporarily allotted the money to the students. Frederik II confirmed the stipend in a royal letter issued 19 June 1566, in which he also expressed the expectation that one or both of the young Danes would return to hold chairs in medicine at the university. This letter officially relieved the university of its obligation to fill the vacant second chair in medicine, and divided the associated salary between Severinus and Pratensis, allowing them to remain abroad until their studies were complete.[30] This was not a unique practice, in that

---

28 Charles Donald O'Malley, *Andreas Vesalius of Brussels 1514-1564* (Berkeley: University of California Press, 1964), p. 76.

29 On the Hippocratic revival, specifically in Paris, see I. M. Lonie, "The 'Paris Hippocratics': teaching and research in Paris in the sixteenth century," in A. Wear, R.K. French, and I. M. Lonie (eds.), *The Medical Renaissance of the Sixteenth Century* (Cambridge: Cambridge University Press, 1985), pp. 155-174.

30 This letter is printed in Herholdt and Mansa, *Samlinger*, pp. 16-17.

the salary intended for a professor of law was later used to finance two medical students in Italy in 1578 and 1579.[31]

In 1568 the king apparently changed his mind about the stipend, or had forgotten about the young students, for he appointed Dr. Martinus Ædituus, his personal physician, to the vacant position by royal letter of 21 October. The faculty quickly reminded the king of his earlier commitment, and he soon retracted the appointment by a royal letter of 28 November.[32] In this second letter the king stated that the young Danes should be supported through the end of their study and return to serve the fatherland, rather than have cause to seek service under foreign lords.[33] This points out the problem the king was having retaining well educated scholars, because of the then relatively low salaries, academic isolation, and, for physicians, the limited opportunities to earn money from medical practice. The attractiveness of living abroad, where a physician could supplement his salary with a lucrative private medical practice, was clearly expressed by Christiern Morsing already in 1556, when he wrote that many learned doctors in Venice and Florence earned 1000 ducats or more a year. Thus, it was unremunerative for well-trained *medici* to work in Denmark in the 1550s.[34] It is doubtful that conditions changed much in the decade following.

It had been the desire of Frederik II's father, Christian III, to expand learned medicine in Denmark by having the church support a physician at each of the episcopal seats. But Frederik made no progress in this direction until after the end of the Seven Years' War (1570), and this must have contributed to the continued dearth of employment opportunities for learned physicians in Denmark. Without a sufficiently wealthy and cultured aristocracy and upper middle class to support private practice, and without publicly financed positions, there can have been little incentive for foreign physicians to stay, or Danes educated abroad to return.

---

31 Anders Christensen and Eskil Christensen were given the salary as a stipend by a royal letter of 10 December 1579. See Rørdam, *KUH*, vol. 4, p. 303, and vol. 2, p. 654. The previous year the stipend had been assigned to Eskil Christensen and Jacob Hasebart. See Ingerslev, *Danmarks Læger*, vol. 1, p. 151.

32 Rørdam, *KUH*, vol. 4, #148 and #149, pp. 214-16.

33 Ibid., #149, p. 216.

34 Bastholm, *Petrus Severinus*, p. 5. On medical salaries at the University of Copenhagen, see Panum, "Vort medicinske Fakultets," pp. 40-41.

The details of the travels of Severinus and Pratensis are sparse, making it difficult to discern where they might have studied, what, and with whom. We can assume they were students for some time in Padua after matriculating, perhaps through 1566 and into the spring of 1567, when Severinus, at least, headed for France. On the basis of a manuscript preserved in the British Library we can infer that Severinus was studying in Paris in 1567, but perhaps not at the university.[35] For even then the Catholic and conservative medical faculty of Paris was beginning to take on a hostile attitude to the ideas, drugs, and rhetoric of Paracelsus, whose theories already attracted the young Dane. It is further evident from Severinus' treatise, the title of which promises to explain "philosophical, astronomical, medical, and cabalistical questions," that Severinus had already become deeply interested in the medical ramifications of a Renaissance complex of philosophy associated with the *prisci theologi* and the Hermetic revival, particularly as espoused by Paracelsus.[36] This treatise is our best evidence that Severinus was drawn to the doctrines of Paracelsus very early in his career, and that these ideas formed the core of his more expansive and philosophically sophisticated *Idea medicinæ* several years later. But to understand the importance of Paracelsianism to Severinus and how his work would be shaped and received, some background is necessary.

"First among the students of Paracelsus"

Paracelsianism takes its name from the German medical reformer and iconoclast, Theophrastus Paracelsus (1493-1541).[37] The mass of manuscript treatises and several printed volumes that Paracelsus produced

35 Petrus Severinus, "Exercitationum liber in qua quæstiones philosophicæ, astronomicæ, medicæ, cabalisticæ explicantur," dated Paris, July 1567. British Library, Sloane MS 3005, ff. 1r-37v. This manuscript appears to be a copy.

36 Frances Yates has most forcefully drawn attention to the importance of Hermetism to Renaissance Platonism in her study of Severinus' contemporary, Giordano Bruno. See Frances Yates, *Giordano Bruno and the Hermetic Tradition* (Chicago: University of Chicago Press, 1964).

37 Philippus Aureolus Theophrastus Bombastus von Hohenheim was born in Einsiedeln, Switzerland, and died in Salzburg, Austria. The literature on Paracelsus is immense. The standard biography and treatment of his medical philosophy remains Walter
→

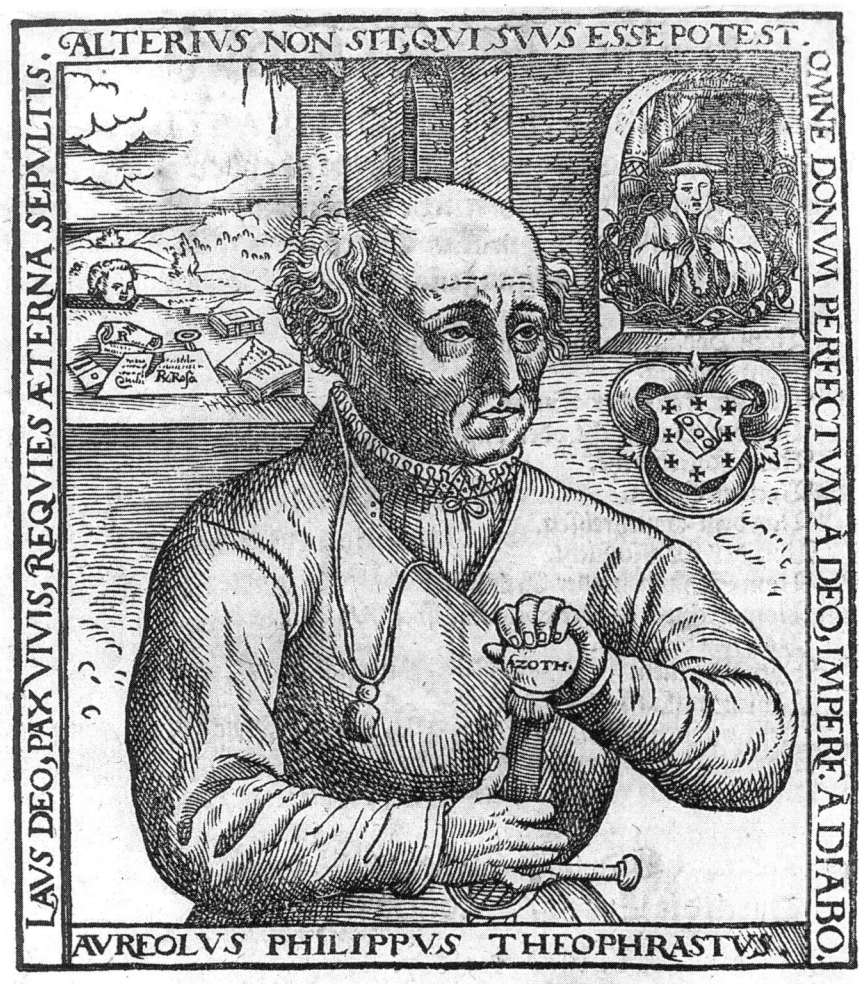

ALTERIVS NON SIT,QVI SVVS ESSE POTEST.

LAVS DEO, PAX VIVIS, REQVIES ÆTERNA SEPVLTIS.

OMNE DONVM PERFECTVM Â DEO,IMPERF. Â DIABO.

AVREOLVS PHILIPPVS THEOPHRASTVS

AV.PH.TH.PARACELSI,NATI ANNO 1493. MORTVI ANNO 1541. ÆTA
TIS SVÆ 47.EFFIGIES.

This image of Paracelsus, published in his Etliche Tractaten *(1567), is notable for
the inclusion of "Rosicrucian" emblems, shown through the window at the upper left.
It illustrates the widely understood connection between Paracelsian medicine and
Rosicrucian ideals. Courtesy of the Wangensteen Historical Library of Biology and
Medicine, University of Minnesota.*

in his troubled, itinerant life contain a rich stew of ancient and novel ideas drawn from such widely differing sources as the Hippocratic and Hermetic writings, German mysticism, the Renaissance Platonism of Marsilio Ficino, the medieval European alchemical tradition, and the common superstitions of central European miners.[38] Although it was difficult to find a coherent doctrine in these texts, Paracelsus' severe criticism of established university medicine was clear: school medicine was grounded in a dead literary tradition developed by Aristotle and Galen and elaborated by their Islamic commentators, pagans all.[39] True medicine ought to be founded on Christian piety and a personal knowledge of nature's fundamentals, which were celestial and chemical. Such knowledge was not gained by reading books, but by learning the properties of things through direct observation in the laboratory and field. Experience and piety, neither of which is attained from the dead words of the scholastic physicians, were the keys to true medicine.

These generalizations, though useful for grasping the tone of Paracelsian rhetoric, hide the fact that the ideas themselves were buried in texts that were mostly unpublished and written in a language and style that defied easy understanding. Riddled with linguistic novelties, mysterious doctrines, and self-contradictions, Paracelsus' tracts appeared to some to be the work of a poorly educated madman. Yet scholars were drawn to Paracelsus' ideas because they offered an alternative to the traditional body of medical theory that not only was firmly rooted in medieval Aristotelianism, but also seemed to be unable to cope well with diseases that were perceived to be new, many of which were epidemic fevers.[40] That is, Paracelsian medicine was attractive for its therapeutic use as well as for ideological reasons.

→ Pagel, *Paracelsus: An Introduction to Philosophical Medicine in the Era of the Renaissance*, 2nd ed. (Basel: Karger, 1982). A more recent study of his formative years, stressing his religious ideas, is Andrew Weeks, *Paracelsus: Speculative Theory and the Crisis of the Early Reformation* (Albany, NY: SUNY Press, 1997).

38 Pagel, *Paracelsus*, treats Paracelsus' doctrines in some detail. Concerning Paracelsus' belief in kobolds, etc., see Charles Webster, "Paracelsus and Demons: Science as a Synthesis of Popular Belief," in *Scienze Credenze Occulte Livelli di Cultura* (Florence: Leo Olschki, 1982), pp. 3-20.

39 This attitude is symbolized by Paracelsus' reputed casting of Avicenna's *Canon* onto the St. John's day bonfire at Basel in 1527. By wantonly destroying such an expensive volume, Paracelsus indicated the worthlessness of such Pagan literature.

40 Lloyd G. Stevenson, "'New diseases' in the Seventeenth Century," *Bulletin of the History of Medicine* 39 (1965): 1-21.

Paracelsian medicine emphasized the use of carefully prepared chemical drugs. Some of these were mineral-based substances, which were quite toxic and very effective against infected wounds and skin diseases. Others, taken internally, produced dramatic effects that indicated their power, although great controversy arose over whether they were helpful or harmful. These drugs gained popularity in the sixteenth century, elevating the status of the chemists, surgeons, and pharmacists who made them and used them. Stories of the successful curing of patients who were given up as lost by university-educated physicians soon made "Paracelsians" attractive to nobles and well-to-do citizens.

When Severinus and Pratensis set off to learn medicine in the 1560s, controversy was brewing over the validity of Paracelsus' philosophical ideas and the effectiveness of chemical medicines, when taken internally. The intellectual excitement surrounding the new doctrines and the possiblility of employment (and protection) by rich and powerful patrons would have made Paracelsian medicine mighty attractive to the young Danish students. But how did one go about studying Paracelsus' works?

A couple of Paracelsus' texts were published in his lifetime, but it was the task of the generation following him to publish, translate, interpret, adapt, and extend his work. The most important of Paracelsus' medical manuscripts lay unpublished until the 1560s, when Adam von Bodenstein (in Basel), Michael Toxites (in Strassburg), Gerhard Dorn (in Frankfurt), and Theodor Birckmann (in Cologne) undertook to codify the master's work.[41] These texts were being readied for the presses in some of the towns through which Severinus and Pratensis travelled to and from Italy and France, and the young Danes may have perused some of them in passing. The earliest books to interpret and extend Paracelsus' ideas were also beginning to appear at that time. A Frenchman named Jacques Gohory was one of the first to publish a treatise explaining Paracelsus' doctrine, *Theophrasti Paracelsi philosophiæ et medicinæ ... compendium* (Basel 1568), which was a commentary on Paracelsus' *De vita longa*. The next important publications were Albert Wimpinæus' *De concordia Hippocraticorum et Paracelsistarum* (Basel 1569), Guinter von Andernach's *De medicina veteri et nova* (Basel 1571), and then Severinus'

---

41 Hugh Trevor-Roper, "The Paracelsian movement," pp. 149-199 in his *Renaissance Essays* (London: Secker and Warburg, 1985), pp. 152-3 and 159-60. This essay provides a very readable introduction to the development of Paracelsianism.

Idea medicinæ philosophicæ, which also came out at Basel in 1571. After Severinus, Paracelsian authors began to publish in increasing numbers: Thomas Moffet, Joseph Duchesne (Quercetanus), Johannes Hartmann, and Oswald Croll, to name but a few. It was these people who created Paracelsian doctrine as it was presented and argued in the centuries following the master's death.

From this chronology it is evident that Petrus Severinus was among the first to attempt a synthesis of Paracelsus' doctrines, to make sense of them in light of accepted philosophies, and to support them with the authority of the ancients. It is for this reason that Severinus was regarded by subsequent medical writers as "the first among the students of Paracelsus," and even a "second Paracelsus," by admirers and critics alike.[42] Even in our own age, when the history of Paracelsianism has been examined more closely, his book is regarded as "the most important and influential in all the Paracelsian literature ... a milestone."[43] The timing of Severinus' visit to Paris strongly suggests that he may have been influenced by Jacques Gohory (1520-1576) and his associates. The years antecedent to the foundation of Gohory's philosophical circle, the *Lyceum*, were the very years during which Severinus was forming his Paracelsian philosophy.[44] Gohory was one of several philosophers interested in Florentine Platonism in mid sixteenth-century Paris, and his studies encompassed Paracelsianism as well, no doubt because Paracelsus' writings reflected the influence of Ficino's Platonism. Indeed, Ficino's

42 O.H. Moller, *Cimbria literata sive scriptorum ducatus utriusque Slesvicensis et Holsatici historia literata tripartita*, vol. 1 (Copenhagen, 1744), pp. 623 ff. lists various assessments of Severinus under the rubrics "elogia" and "censuræ." The above two, "Qui sane inter discipulos Paracelsi præcipuus est, Pet. Severinus, Danus" and "Paracelsus secundus," come respectively from Hermann Conring, who disliked Paracelsianism, and Johan Kozackius (*Anatomia vitalis Macrocosmi*), who had a more favorable opinion.

43 Sten Lindroth, *Paracelsismen i Sverige till 1600-tallets mitt.* Lychnos Bibliotek, no. 7 (Uppsala: Almqvist & Wiksell, 1943), pp. 21-22: "Detta arbete måste otvivelaktigt betecknas som det viktigaste och inflytelserikaste i hela den paracelsistiska litteraturen ... Severinus' verk är en milstolpe i paracelsismens historia." More recently Allen Debus, *The French Paracelsians: The Chemical Challenge to Medical and Scientific Tradition in Early Modern France* (Cambridge: Cambridge University Press, 1991), p. 18, has written that "perhaps the most distinguished early defender of the Paracelsian system was Petrus Severinus" and "Severinus presented a theoretical defense of Paracelsian medicine that spread the concept of a chemical medicine far beyond the confines of central Europe."

44 D.P. Walker, *Spiritual and Demonic Magic from Ficino to Campanella* (London: Warburg Institute, 1958), p. 99.

De triplici vita (1489) was an important source for Paracelsus' *De vita longa* (1562).[45] We know that Gohory was engaged in study of Paracelsian ideas already in the 1550s, because he refers to his long discussions on Paracelsianism with the famous physician Jean Fernel, who died in 1558. By the early 1560s he had become an enthusiast.[46] Gohory's *Theophrasti Paracelsi philosophiæ et medicinæ ... compendium*, which included a commentary on Paracelsus' *De vita longa*, was published in 1568, and although there is no evidence linking Gohory and Severinus, we do know from Severinus' manuscript (Sloane MS 3005) that he was writing in Paris when Gohory was at work on the *Compendium*, so perhaps the two were acquainted. Since Gohory drew attention to the similarity between Paracelsian doctrine in *De vita longa* and Ficino's Platonism on many points, it is tempting to speculate that he may have influenced the Platonic orientation of Severinus' exposition of Paracelsian doctrine in the *Idea medicinæ* (1571).[47]

Severinus may have returned to Copenhagen in the autumn of 1568 to seek a continuation of his stipend, which was then threatened by the above-mentioned royal letter. In late March 1569 he was staying at Langesø, a manor on the Danish island of Fyn, where Sidsel Bryske gave him an old manuscript book of the Jutish Law. Why she should give this particular book to Severinus is unclear, although such artifacts seem to have been dear to natural philosophers.[48] We might well conjecture that

45 Pagel, *Paracelsus*, pp. 218-227, discusses Ficino's *De triplici vita* as a source for Neoplatonic elements of Paracelsus' thought.

46 D.P. Walker, *Spiritual and Demonic Magic*, p. 101, and Trevor-Roper, "The Paracelsian Movement," pp. 166-7.

47 Jacques Gohory, *Theophrasti Paracelsi philosophiæ et medicinæ ... compendium* (Basel: Perna, 1568), summarized Paracelsus' main doctrines. On Gohory see Owen Hannaway, "Gohory," *Dictionary of Scientific Biography* (hereafter *DSB*), vol. 5, pp. 447-8, and Debus, *The French Paracelsians*, pp. 26-28. Wilhelm Reymann, who studied Severinus in the nineteenth century, considered Severinus and Gohory to have been old friends by the time Severinus was promoted to M.D. Reymann seldom cited the sources of his information and admitted that he did not have access to the materials he needed, so we must view his scholarship with skepticism. See Gaunø-Jensen, "Wilhelm Reymann: Undersøgelser over Peder Sørensens Liv og Lære."

48 Rørdam, *KUH*, vol. 2, p. 575. The book, written in a runic alphabet, was inscribed by Sidsel Bryske to "Mester Peder Seurinsen Canich vdi Wiburge ... thend 29 dag Martij ... 1569." It subsequently came into the possession of Ole Worm, Villum Worm, Ole Borch, and finally Arne Magnusson. See Lauritz Nielsen, *Danmarks Middelalderlige Haandskrifter* (Copenhagen: Gyldendal, 1937), pp. 116-19.

Severinus was already practicing medicine among the nobility at this time, and that the manuscript was the sort of gift that constituted polite patronage.[49] Where Pratensis was during this period we do not know, but in April 1569 both students were in Wittenberg with the intention of travelling to Cologne, according to an almanac entry by his townsman from Ribe, Peder Hegelund. Hegelund noted that Severinus performed a venesection on him on 2 May, the first surviving reference to Severinus' medical practice. A month later Hegelund accompanied Severinus, Pratensis, and several other Danes to Leipzig.[50] From Leipzig, Severinus went to Basel, where he became friends with Theodor Zwinger, who was very interested in Paracelsianism, but not uncritically so.[51] Thereafter Severinus and Pratensis went to Italy, perhaps by way of France, where Severinus may have taken his doctorate.

When and where Severinus received his M.D. remains a mystery. Thomas Bartholin, drawing on the University of Copenhagen's program at Severinus' death, claimed that he was promoted in France while on his way home from Italy in 1571.[52] This has been generally accepted by historians, but is not supported by the evidence. We know from both Sidsel Bryske's inscription on her gift to Severinus and Hegelund's almanac entries that Severinus was still a Master as late as June 1569. In the dedication of the *Idea medicinæ*, dated 1 November 1570, Florence, Severinus refers to himself as *"philosophiæ et medicinæ doctor,"* suggesting

49 Herholdt and Mansa, *Samlinger*, p. 17, claimed that Severinus not only practiced in Denmark but also in Italy, especially in Venice, and in several of Germany's larger towns, so that he was "een af de meest berømte Læger paa de Tider" (one of the most famous physicians in those times). What the sources of these claims were is not evident, except that the reputation goes back to the seventeenth-century historians. On gift giving as a way of cementing patron-client relationships, see Paula Findlen "The Economy of Scientific Exchange in Early Modern Italy," in *Patronage and Institutions: Science, Technology, and Medicine at the European Court 1500-1750*, ed. Bruce Moran. (Woodbridge, Suffolk: Boydell, 1991), pp. 5-24.

50 Kaae, *Almanakoptegnelser*, vol. 1., p. 51, entry for 29 April 1569: "Aduenerunt Witebergam profecturi Coloniam M: Petrus Seuerinus, M: Ioh: Philippus Pratensis." Ibid., 2 May 1569: "Misi sanguinem, incidente mihi venam M: Petro Seuerino Ripensi." Ibid., p. 52, 4 June 1569: "Expatiabar Lipsiam cum M: Petro Seuerino, M: Iohanne Philippo, M: Iacobo Mathiæ, M: Desiderio Fossio, M: Iohanne Hemmingio."

51 Bastholm, *Petrus Severinus*, p. 5.

52 "In itinere domum versus, dum Galliam transiret gradu Doctoratus Anno 1571 ornatus est." Bartholin, *Cista medica*, p. 115.

that he took his doctorate in Italy or on his way there, therefore in fall 1569 or 1570. He could not have received the degree on his way home from Italy, unless this preface was dated in anticipation of the actual promotion. In any case, when Hegelund refered to him in his 22 June 1571 entry he called him "D.D. Petrus Seuerinus," indicating that Severinus was presenting himself as having attained the rank of doctor.[53]

If Severinus received his M.D. in France, it was probably not at the University of Montpellier. The medical faculty there was amenable to Paracelsian medicine, but his name does not appear in the matriculation list, which seems quite complete for that period.[54] Since we know from a manuscript in the British Library that Severinus was working on "cabalistic" and medical matters in Paris in 1567, and therefore probably had both personal and academic contacts there, it might be supposed that he was awarded an M.D. at the University of Paris on his way from Ribe to Florence. However, the medical faculty at Paris was already opposed to any Paracelsian challenge to Galen's hegemony and was beginning to take action. In 1566 the faculty placed a ban on the use of antimony as a medicine, claiming it to be a poison that could not be corrected – this was the first shot of the "antimony wars" that would for the rest of the century increasingly divide the Galenic (and Catholic) academic physicians from the community of Paracelsians, mostly Huguenots, who were supported by the crown and aristocracy.[55] It is not, however, impossible that Severinus received his degree at Paris, since his theoretical work, as evident in Sloane MS 3005, was heavily influenced by what we might

---

53 Kaae, *Almanakoptegnelser*, vol. II, p. 71. It is my speculation that Severinus had a manuscript draft of the *Idea medicinæ* completed by early spring 1570, to which he added the dated preface dedicating the book to Frederik II. As noted below, the Chancellory promised Severinus a canonry at Roskilde, a benefice typical for professors (and which he would eventually receive), already in May of 1570. This may have been awarded after receipt of the manuscript of the *Idea medicinæ* and therefore after Severinus had attained the doctorate. There is, however, no surviving manuscript to support this speculation. D.D. is the abbreviation for Dominus Doctor, the title then used for a person granted the doctorate degree.

54 Marcel Gouron, *Matricule de L'Université de Médicine de Montpellier (1503-1599)* (Geneva: Droz, 1957).

55 Debus, *The French Paracelsians*, pp. 25-26; Trever-Roper, "The Paracelsian Movement," p. 168.

call the "Hermetic" aspects of Paracelsus' medicine, which was not yet the principle object of the Parisian medical faculty's ire. It seems that opposition to Paracelsianism first erupted as a controversy over prescriptions – specifically toxic ones like those involving antimony – and the threat they posed to purveyors of Galenic drugs. Attacks on the doctrinal orthodoxy of Paracelsianism had already begun by this time, but did not become really prominent until after Thomas Erastus' biting charges that Paracelsian doctrine contained heresy were published in 1574, well after the publication of Severinus' work.[56] Thus, it is possible that Severinus received his M.D. at Paris *en route* to Italy in 1569 or 1570, since his development of Paracelsian theory might not at that point have appeared threatening. However, in the absence of more compelling evidence, the possibility must be admitted that he received his doctorate at a smaller French university, or in Italy, or even at a German university, such as Basel or Heidelberg.[57]

Pratensis, at least, is reported to have received his M.D. in Padua, but when is not known.[58] Although Severinus likely first became familiar with the ideas of Paracelsus in France or Germany, even more likely at Basel, the possibility that the intellectual milieu of northern Italy helped shape his medicine cannot be excluded. In the *Idea medicinæ* Severinus turns again and again to the precepts of Hippocrates as an authoritative source – not the corrupt version of Hippocrates' ideas seen through Galen's eyes, but the "authentic" Hippocratic medicine that

---

56 Johan Wier's *De præstigiis dæmonum et incantationibus, ac veneficiis* (Basel: Oporinus, 1563), which attacked Paracelsus and his followers, was translated into French as *Cinq livres de l'imposture et tromperie des diables: des enchantemenets & sorcelleries* in 1567 – exactly when Severinus was finishing his manuscript. Paracelsian cosmology was hotly debated in the years immediately following, but the use and rationale of chemical medicines, rather than the theological orthodoxy of Paracelsus' doctrines, dominated the controversy. See Debus, *The French Paracelsians*, p. 26-30.

57 Given the importance of Basel as a center of Paracelsian publishing, one might think that Severinus had studied there. However, Severinus' name does not appear on the published matriculation list for the University of Basel. See H.G. Wackernagel, ed., *Die Matrikel Der Universität Basel*, vol. 2 (1532/3-1600/1) (Basel: Universitätsbibliothek, 1956). Thomas Moffet wrote to Severinus that Peter Turner sends his greetings and would probably write to him (see chapter six, below). If this means that Severinus and Turner were acquainted, it may be that they met at Heidelberg, where Turner received his M.D. in 1571.

58 Ingerslev, *Danmarks Læger*, vol. 1, p. 157.

springs directly from the treatises.[59] This attitude is wholly in agreement with late Renaissance humanistic attention to texts as well as with the Hippocratic revival at Padua and Paris, which has been mentioned.

Sixteenth-century Italians were experimenting with a variety of physical and metaphysical explanations for how nature operated and how nature was related to its creator. Perhaps the most famous of these were propounded by Bernardo Telesio (1509-1588), Giordano Bruno (1548-1600), and Francesco Patrizi (1529-1597).[60] Although the work of the last two came too late to have directly affected Severinus, it nevertheless reflects the type of thinking going on in Italy at that time. Both, for example, put forth theories that are characterized by an attempt to find some common ground between scholastic Aristotelianism and Platonic ideas, and both were particularly interested in how the dimensional world of body and the unextended world of soul interact.

Telesio studied in Padua, but had returned to southern Italy before Severinus and Pratensis entered Italy. His magnum opus, *De rerum natura iuxta propria principia* (Rome 1565), may have been available to Severinus while he was forming the metaphysical foundations of his theory of medicine. Telesio rejected the traditional Aristotelian concept of form, preferring to conceive of soul or spirit as a corporeal substance arising from some sort of seed. The similarity of this idea with Severinus' *semina* theory, at least superficially, shows that Severinus' captivation with this kind of metaphysics was well grounded in the newest trends in sixteenth-century philosophy.[61]

Patrizi's theory, published well after the *Idea medicinæ*, also reveals a commitment to the general Neoplatonist metaphysics underlying Severinus' work. However, whereas Severinus was preoccupied with generation and corruption primarily in a biological context, with application

---

59 However, Severinus took as authentic certain texts that today are considered not to have been written by Hippocrates. On Severinus' use of Hippocrates, see Jole Shackelford, "The Chemical Hippocrates: Paracelsian and Hippocratic Theory in Petrus Severinus' Medical Philosophy," in *Reinventing Hippocrates*, in David Cantor, ed. *Reinventing Hippocrates*. (Aldershot, Hampshire: Ashgate, 2002), pp. 59-88.

60 Paul Oskar Kristeller, *Eight Philosophers of the Italian Renaissance* (Stanford, CA: Stanford University Press, 1964), pp. 94-96 groups these three as "Renaissance philosophers of nature," sixteenth-century philosophers primarily concerned with nature and natural explanation. He also includes Cardano, Fracastoro, and Paracelsus under this rubric.

61 Niel Gilbert, "Telesio," *DSB* vol. 13 (1976), pp. 277-280.

to human pathology, Patrizi built a more abstract philosophy that was based on a tradition of light metaphysics that was well established in medieval philosophy.[62] But even so, there is some compatibility between the two: for Patrizi, light is a creative agency mediating between divine ideas and corporeal creation, bringing with it the seeds of all things. We therefore cannot rule out that Severinus' main doctrine of *semina* as the *fontes* (sources) of beings and recepticles for their passing away into oblivion may have developed in a northern Italian context.[63]

Giordano Bruno's theory also exhibits certain general affinities to that of Severinus. Bruno was, as far as we know, in southern Italy until he left his monastery and fled north in 1576. But when he finally ex-pounded his metaphysics in writing, most clearly in *De la causa, principio e uno* (1584), it reminds one of the *Idea medicinæ*. For Bruno there was a common matter that underlies both corporeal and incorporeal reality. He compared this matter to a pregnant woman, an abyss that sends forth dimensions to form bodies, as if from a womb. Although Bruno knew something of Paracelsus' matter theory, the formulation he gave to generation, namely a springing forth of form from the oneness of the seed, suggests Neoplatonic roots further back in history.[64]

The metaphysical line of thinking evident in the works of Telesio, Bruno, Patrizi, and the other sixteenth-century Italian "Renaissance phi-losophers of nature," as Kristeller termed them, could well have nurtured Severinus' basic doctrine of generation and corruption, which particularly addresses this very problem of the relation of the visible and extended to the invisible and dimensionless. These writers were inspired by the Neoplatonist metaphysics of Plotinus' *Enneads*, which probably was an important source for Severinus as well.[65] Severinus' achievement was to

---

62 On the importance of Neoplatonic light metaphysics to 16th-century philosophy, see David C. Lindberg, "The Genesis of Kepler's Theory of Light: Light Metaphysics from Plotinus to Kepler," *Osiris* ser. 2, 2(1986): 5-42.

63 On Patrizi see Benjamin Brickman, "An Introduction to Francesco Patrizi's *Nova de universis philosophia*" (Ph.D. Diss., Columbia University, 1941).

64 Giordano Bruno, *Cause, Principle and Unity*, trans. Jack Lindsay (New York: Interna-tional, 1964), pp. 128 and 140. P.H. Michel, *The Cosmology of Giordano Bruno*, trans. R.E.W. Maddison (Paris: Hermann, 1973), p. 46, notes that Bruno rejected Paracelsus' *tria prima* (salt, sulphur, and mercury) because this implied a triple, not a unitary, material substratum for bodies.

65 Severinus' theories will be examined in detail in chapter 4, below.

take these ideas and apply them specifically to medical theory. His writing does not merely use medical examples to illuminate his metaphysics, but consistently uses his theory to explain medicine, whether it is the normal functioning of the human body or the nature and treatment of disease. This is immediately evident in Severinus' earliest surviving text, his "Exercitationum liber in qua quæstiones philosophicæ, astronomicæ, medicæ, cabalisticæ explicantur" from 1567. In this manuscript one finds the metaphysical, causal mechanisms that are central to the *Idea medicinæ* already well developed and applied to different classes of diseases.

Besides Hippocratism and Renaissance Platonism, one must also consider the possibility that the young Danes were exposed to Paracelsian ideas in Italy. The nature and extent of Paracelsianism in northern Italy in the late 1560s is far from clear, and many factors discouraged the spread of Paracelsian ideas into Italy. Most of Paracelsus' treatises were written in German, including the early printed collections by Huser, and language may have inhibited ready transmission. Furthermore, much of the printing of Paracelsus' texts occurred after 1560 and coincided with post-Tridentine restrictions on the circulation of books. For example, the Venetian Holy Office confiscated, as heretical texts, the Paracelsian books belonging to the Paduan surgeon Nicolo Bucella when he was leaving Italy for Poland in 1574.[66] Nevertheless, transalpine connections within the printing and bookselling industry were strong, and Paracelsian books found their way into Italian hands.

Indeed, one of the main early printers of Paracelsian texts, Pietro Perna in Basel, was an Italian expatriate, and it is likely that Paracelsian texts came into Italy through his contacts there. Girolamo Donzellini, a "heretical physician" in the 1550s, has been mentioned in this regard. Through him Paracelsian books reached Ulisse Aldrovandi and Tommaso Bovio.[67] Leonardo Fioravanti, perhaps the best known Italian

66 Richard Palmer, "Pharmacy in the Republic of Venice in the Sixteenth Century," in *The Medical Renaissance of the Sixteenth Century*, ed. Andrew Wear, R.K. French, and I.M. Lonie, pp. 100-117 and 303-312 (Cambridge: Cambridge University Press, 1985), pp. 110-111. Eventually, in 1599, Paracelsus' works were placed on the Roman Index of Prohibited Books. See Trevor-Roper, "The Paracelsian Movement," p. 173.

67 Marco Ferrari, "Alcune vie di diffusione in Italia di idee e di testi di Paracelso," *Scienze credenze occulte livelli di cultura* (Florence: Olschki, 1982), p. 23ff. Another article on Paracelsianism in Italy appears in that book: Paolo Galluzzi, "Motivi Paracelsiani nella Toscana di Cosimo II e di Don Antonio Dei Medici: alchimia, medicina 'chimica' e riforma del sapere," pp. 31-62.

chemical physician of this period, praised Paracelsus for his alchemical skill, especially in the preparation of antimony. Although he was not himself a Paracelsian, he greatly influenced the popularity of Paracelsianism in Italy.[68] Fioravanti mentioned several persons interested in Paracelsianism already in the 1560s: At the University of Padua there was Alberto Cimerlino, rector of the university 1567-69 (when Pratensis and perhaps Severinus were students there), who was regarded as an "expert in the doctrine of Paracelsus"; Albertino Bottoni, a professor at Padua, was likewise noted for his Paracelsian expertise, as were others for their interest in Paracelsianism.[69] Although his period of active publication was a decade or more after Severinus and Pratensis had left Italy, Tommaso Bovio stands out for his attention to Paracelsus' works, thirty seven of which he claimed to have read.[70] These references tell us that Paracelsian treatises were available and read, at least by some, in northern Italy during the time Severinus was finishing the *Idea medicinæ*.

We can speculate on the basis of Severinus' 1567 manuscript and his 1571 *Idea medicinæ* that Severinus became acquainted with many of the medical and chemical ideas expressed in Paracelsus' writings rather early in his studies abroad and began to give them the philosophical basis that one finds in the *Idea* by drawing on Platonist metaphysics. The 1567 treatise reveals Severinus' familiarity with Paracelsian medical theory and his rationale for the use of chemical drugs. In this manuscript Severinus used and developed ideas characteristic of Paracelsus' writings, for example the concept that there are "stomachs" in various parts of the body, which are responsible for the diverse "separations" or purifications that comprise human chemistry. Severinus' early presentation of these ideas is couched in the familiar Paracelsian terms: the *archeus*, *vulcan*, *astrum*, *iliaster*, and even *semina*. Severinus was content to describe and

---

68 Palmer, "Pharmacy in the Republic of Venice," p. 113. Even though Fioravanti was an avid iatrochemist and praises Paracelsus, William Eamon, who has studied Fioravanti's work in detail, does not think that Paracelsus was a primary influence on Fioravanti. See William Eamon, *Science and the Secrets of Nature: Books of Secrets in Medieval and Early Modern Culture* (Princeton: Princeton University Press, 1994), p. 191.

69 Palmer, "Pharmacy in the Republic of Venice," p. 114.

70 Ibid., p. 114, and Marco Ferrari, "Alcune vie di diffusione," p. 23.

develop specific Paracelsian doctrines in 1567. By 1571 he had given these doctrines a general explanation in terms of seminal (and astral) causation and placed Paracelsian pathology into his own general theory of generation and corruption, which explained human reproduction and growth, normal physiology, the nature and action of diseases, and the operation of drugs in rooting out diseases. Furthermore, between 1567 and 1571 Severinus saw the need to emphasize the historical roots of his theories – to validate them by tracing them back to Hippocratic writings. While one finds references to Hippocrates in the 1567 treatise, it as a whole lacks the rhetoric of the *Idea medicinæ*, specifically the criticism of Galenic medicine. The *Idea medicinæ* clearly offers both a self-consciously defensive treatment and a more generalized presentation of Paracelsus' medical theory than does the earlier document. But whether he encountered these ideas first in France or in Italy is unknown. By that time the general culture of Florentine Platonism, the love of Plotinus that Pratensis would express to a close friend while awaiting death, was alive in learned circles in Paris and Lyons as well as in Italy.[71]

We might suppose that the bulk of the *Idea medicinæ* was in draft by the time Severinus wrote the letter of dedication, dated Florence, 1 November 1570. Severinus was no doubt very grateful for the support he and Pratensis had enjoyed, without which they would have been sitting out the war with Sweden as underpaid lecturers in the arts faculty at Copenhagen, or as canons of cathedrals in Denmark's provincial towns. Nevertheless, the dedication of a major treatise – which costs a good deal to print – to a king implies the expectation of patronage. It therefore seems warranted to conclude that Severinus' book was essentially finished by the time he wrote the dedication, and that either patronage had been offered, or he was getting ready to send a fair copy off to the the king to win it.

After a decade of study and research, Severinus and Pratensis headed for home, probably with the expectation that they would be called into

---

71 See Pratensis' poem to the French ambassador to Denmark, Charles Danzay, printed in Holger Rørdam, "Charles de Danzay, fransk Resident ved det danske Hof," pp. 252-333 in *Historiske Samlinger og Studier vedrørende danske Forhold og Personligheder, især i det 17. Aarhundrede*, ed. Rørdam, vol. 3 (Copenhagen: Gad, 1898), appendix 5, pp. 324-326.

service at the university or at court. Severinus was not formally appointed Physician to the King until fall 1571, but he may well have been promised a position of some sort already in the spring of the previous year, over a year before they returned to Denmark. Such is suggested by the "letter of expectation" drafted by the Chancellory 28 May 1570, which put Severinus in line for a canonry at Roskilde Cathedral, an offer that was affirmed later in his contract.[72] Furthermore, Severinus refers to himself on the title page of the *Idea medicinæ* as "Philosopher and Physician to Frederik II, King of Denmark and the North," indicating that he was confident of his appointment before the book was ready for the market. Severinus presumably oversaw the printing at Basel on the way home from Italy, that is, in the fall of 1570 or spring of 1571, again implying that he was offered a job before coming home. Pratensis may well have hoped to occupy the vacant professorship at Copenhagen, since their stipend was intended to train one of them for this position. After eleven years of neglect, it was high time that the second chair in medicine – which had supported them for these five years of study abroad – be filled.

It hardly seems likely that the two young Danes, Severinus in particular, could have travelled more than what has been indicated and still have had time left for study and writing. Two poems written to commemorate Johannes Pratensis' life imply that he, and therefore by implication Severinus, also visited Spain, Greece, and Hungary before returning to Denmark, but corroborative evidence is lacking.[73] The seventeenth-century Danish physician and medical historian of sorts,

---

72 Laursen, *Kancelliets Brevbøger*, vol. 4 (1896), p. 589.
73 In an elegaic epitaph, Tycho Brahe refers to Pratensis' determination to travel:

Non rapere hunc bellax poterat Germania, non hunc
    Gallia, dum mutua cæde timenda furit:
Nil nocuere Alpes, nec celsior Appenninus,
    Dum Latii, procul hinc, celsa Theatra videt:
Obfuit haud sæuis vicina Vngaria Turcis,
    Nilque alia a nostris dissita Regna focis;

J.L.E. Dreyer, ed., *Tychonis Brahe Dani opera omnia* (hereafter *TBDOO*), vol. 9, p. 177, lines 7-12. A similar poem by Isak Mouritsen mentions "Pratensis Danus, Germanus, Gallus, Iberus; / Idem Romanus, Græcus et Οὐράνιος" the last, "Uranius," referring to his now being a citizen of heaven. See Rørdam, *KUH*, vol. 4, #79, p. 114.

Thomas Bartholin, mentions only travel to Italy, France, and Germany in his biographical entry for Pratensis, and this seems more reasonable.[74] To this list must be added the low countries, since a note left by Severinus in the personal album of Johannes Vivianus in early June 1571 indicates that he returned to Jutland by way of Antwerp.[75] Before the end of the month they were home.

74 Thomas Bartholin, *Cista medica*, p. 57: "post tam longinqvas, in Italia, Gallia, Germania, peregrinationes."
75 "Album amicorum Joannis Viviani," The Hague, Kon. Bibl. MS 74 F 19 f. 21. I have not seen this manuscript.

Chapter Two

PARACELSIANISM IN SIXTEENTH-CENTURY DENMARK

T HE DENMARK to which Johannes Pratensis and Petrus Severinus returned was in some ways different from the one they had left. The 1560s were a decade of transition, during which the generation of political and intellectual leaders that had wrought the Reformation in Denmark was giving way to a new generation, which sought to bring Danish culture into the European mainstream. The new cultural elite acquired a Renaissance taste for the artistic expression of fundamental truths that could only be fully grasped through intuition. It was the beginning of a period characterized by poetry and ornamental architecture, by symbols and by ritual; a period characterized by the poetry of Erasmus Lætus, the architecture of "Hamlet's Castle," Kronborg, and both the art and artifices of Denmark's most famous scientific mind of the period, Tycho Brahe.

Paracelsianism was also a part of this cultural matrix. Its speculative nature and fanciful ideas fit well with the poetry of the young Danish intellectuals. Certainly Severinus and Pratensis were known for their sensitivity to poetic form. Severinus had a reputation for Latin skills, which earned him recognition as a teacher of poetry at a young age, and the long poem that Pratensis wrote to decorate his friend's book bears witness to the importance these men and their peers assigned to poetic expression as a key element of their ideology. This same aesthetic impulse pervades the letters of Tycho Brahe and his sister, Sophie, and attained concrete form in the design of Tycho's "philosophical" house, Uraniborg. Paracelsianism first appeared in Denmark with this new generation of Danes – Tycho Brahe's generation – and it appeared as part of their attempt to reform their intellectual world.[1] There is a real excitement evident in these years, when new ideas were brought to old institutions, and new institutions were forged to extend education beyond the walls of the university. Tycho Brahe's Uraniborg was the first of these. Indeed, Tycho's presence so dominated natural philosophy that his laboratory and observatory served as a post-graduate research institution of sorts, where Danish students could seek instruction beyond what was offered at the University of Copenhagen. The intellectual circle around Tycho, which included Pratensis and Severinus, was therefore of primary importance to the reception of Severinus' ideas in Denmark and warrants detailed investigation here.

Government support for learning

With the war against Sweden drawing to a close, Frederik II was free to concentrate the energy and resources of the kingdoms of Denmark and Norway on internal development. Not only was he personally interested in learned culture, but he was surrounded by noble advisors who favored the growth of the university and the apparatus of state. These were the cream of an aristocratic crop that had sought scholarly education for their sons in numbers unprecedented in Denmark.[2] The nobles did not themselves flock to the University of Copenhagen (Tycho being a no-

1 Peter Zeeberg, "Science versus Secular Life: A Central Theme in the Latin Poems of Tycho Brahe," in *Acta Conventus Neo-Latini Torontonensis: Proceedings of the Seventh International Congress on Neo-Latin Studies, Toronto 8 August to 13 August 1988* (Binghamton, NY: Medieval and Renaissance Texts and Studies, 1991), pp. 831-838, discusses the tension between the old medieval culture, strongly maintained by the conservative nobility, and the new Renaissance culture, which offered Platonic philosophy and aesthetics to Tycho and his generation. On Tycho Brahe's education and ability as a Latin poet, see Peter Zeeberg, *Den praktiske muse: Tycho Brahes brug af latindigtningen.* Studier fra Sprog- og Oldtidsforskning #321 (Copenhagen: Museum Tusculanums Forlag, 1993).
2 Degn, *Rig og fattig i Ribe*, vol. 1, p. 338, table 91, has reduced the information presented in Birte Andersen, *Adelig Opfostring: Adelsborns opdragelse i Danmark 1536-1660* (Copenhagen: Gad, 1971) appendix 4, pp. 114-19. This table shows that aristocratic enrollment in provincial Latin Schools increased from 7 in the 1530s to 14 in the 1550s and 21 in the 1570s before beginning to decline again to fewer than 10 per decade in the half century after 1600. Birte Andersen (p. 101) notes that few Danish nobles proceeded to the University of Copenhagen.

table exception), but prefered to seek out foreign universities, a practice that was consistent with the traditional education of the aristocracy for service in matters of statecraft, where the experience of foreign courts and cultures would be useful. Nevertheless, as the nobles who supported the Danish crown became more learned, they sought to emulate their peers to the south and promoted higher education at home.

With the backing of noblemen such as Johann Friis and Peder Oxe, Frederik II (1559-1588) was finally able to put the University of Copenhagen on a secure financial footing. The first decisive steps were the establishment in 1569 of the *kommunitet*, to provide beer and two meals per day for 100 students, and the *stipendium regium*, to furnish travel expenses and maintenance abroad for four doctoral students; three in theology and one in medicine.[3] Encouraged by the relative political stability in the north after the Peace of Stetin (1570) had ended the the Seven Years War with Sweden, economic growth continued through the reign of Frederik's successor, Christian IV (1588-1648). During these years Copenhagen was greatly enlarged and modernized, as were the chief provincial towns of the realm. With expansion came better opportunities for learned physicians. In 1571 the king issued new articles of foundation for the university, which included increases in professorial salaries.[4] The government created positions for regional physicians in the provincial cities, augmenting employment opportunities in the public sector.[5] Likewise, other sorts of medical services increased in this period. The officially sanctioned

---

3 Rørdam, *KUH*, vol. 2, pp. 74 ff. Frederik's support followed similar moves taken by his relative, the Elector of Saxony, for the University of Wittenberg. The significance of royal support for the university was recognized by contemporaries. In his 1594 description of the University of Copenhagen, Jonas Kolding, *Daniæ descriptio nova* (Frankfurt am Main: Feyrabendt, 1594), p. 115, says about Frederik II: "Maximum vero, & immortale decus, Friderico II. ante omnes tribuendum: qui eam omnibus modis studiosus exornavit, & ampliavit: tum numero professorum, tum eorundem stipendio adaucto. Anno Christi 1569." [But the greatest and most enduring credit should be given to Frederik II before all others, for he assiduously furnished and expanded the university in many ways: both the numbers of professors and their salaries were increased.] See also Cold, *Lægevæsenet og Lægerne*, p. 110, note 2.

4 For details of Frederik II's improvements in the university, see Ingerslev, *Danmarks Læger*, vol. 1, pp. 136-139.

5 The numbers, however, remained small. Only seven such regional *medici* are noted during Frederik II's reign, according to Panum, "Vort medicinske Fakultets," p. 31. Yet this is a different situation from that of mid-sixteenth-century Denmark.

pharmacists and barber-surgeons, at first found only in Copenhagen, gradually spread to the provincial cities.[6]

Although the modernization and growth that defined Denmark's renaissance is most closely associated with Frederik's son and successor, Christian IV, it was Frederik II himself who sponsored the betterment of the university and patronized learning. It was during his reign and with his support that a significant amount of royal income was siphoned off and given to Tycho Brahe to build his remarkable home, laboratory, and observatory on the island of Hven. Clearly the king was concerned to prevent the best educated minds from leaving the country to seek patronage elsewhere, and this included his unprecedented subsidy of a member of the high nobility for what amounted to purely academic pursuits. His support of Tycho's plans for astronomical and alchemical research show a willingness to develop these subjects as well as the natural philosophy traditionally found within the university's walls, presumably because they were viewed as assets to the crown. In any case, the kind of research and the funding astronomy and alchemy would require were clearly beyond the financial means and curricular limits of the university.

The fact that Tycho Brahe, a Danish nobleman born and bred into the political and military leadership of the feudal realm, could and would hold a series of lectures at the University of Copenhagen in the fall of 1574 indicates both the interest in higher education among the younger aristocrats and the academics' desire for a liberalized curriculum. Pratensis and his friend the French ambassador, and quite possibly Severinus (since he was near the king), were influential in arranging for Tycho to hold these lectures, and we can suspect that this new generation of academics was eager to reform learning and free it from the shackles of scholastic forms and social norms that governed education.[7] These

6 We can see the pattern of growth from the licensing of apothecaries. The first privilege was granted in 1514 for a pharmacy in Copenhagen. The next licenses were for Odense (1549), Viborg (1573), Helsingør (1577), Kolding (1585), Aarhus (1596), Sorø (1606), a second in Copenhagen (1609), and so on. In Norway the first were in Bergen (1588) and Christiania (1628). See Nicolai Aagaard Sverre, *Et studium av farmasiens historie*, 2nd edition (Oslo: Norges Apotekerforening, 1982), pp. 81, 84, and 86; also Ingerslev, *Danmarks Læger*, vol. 1, pp. 209ff.

7 Victor Thoren, *The Lord of Uraniborg: A Biography of Tycho Brahe* (Cambridge: Cambridge University Press, 1990), has convincingly shown that Tycho's noble birth discouraged his teaching at the University of Copenhagen, the series of lectures he held there in the fall of 1574 being an important exception.

were the times recalled by Caspar Bartholin, professor at the University of Copenhagen in the early seventeenth century, as the institution's golden years.[8]

It was during these golden years that Severinus and Pratensis came home to Denmark to take positions in the new order, Severinus as Royal Physician and Pratensis as Professor of Medicine. The fact that they had become proponents of Paracelsian medicine quite likely aided them in acquiring the patronage that helped them win continued support for their studies and, finally, remunerative positions in Denmark.[9] An interest in Paracelsian chemistry accompanied Paracelsian cosmology to Denmark, as elsewhere, and certainly the promise of powerful new medicines to heal the sick and prolong life made Paracelsian ideas attractive to noble patrons. Yet Severinus' book, the *Idea medicinæ*, is no cookbook, but a lengthy philosophical discussion of the fundamental causes of change in natural bodies, including those accounting for normal and pathological physiology. Severinus was clearly attractive to the crown not just as a chemical physician, but as a theoretician.

Certainly Severinus' and Pratensis' Paracelsian leanings were public knowledge at the time they were hired, for on his way back to Denmark, Severinus published not only the *Idea medicinæ*, but also a short "letter to Paracelsus" (*Epistola scripta Theophrasto Paracelso*),[10] which identifies

---

8   Caspar Bartholin, *Oratio de ortu, progressu, et incrementis Regiæ Academiæ Hafniensis*, sig. c1v, (Wittenberg: Michael Wendt, 1645): "Tempora Frederici II, quæ Academiæ vere fuerunt aurea." [The times of Frederik II, which for the royal university were golden.]

9   I have specifically discussed the role of Patronage in furthering Paracelsianism in Denmark in Jole Shackelford, "Paracelsianism and Patronage in Early Modern Denmark," in *Patronage and Institutions: Science, Technology and Medicine at the European Court, 1500-1750*, ed. Bruce T. Moran (Woodbridge, Suffolk: Boydell, 1991), pp. 85-109. Some of that material is reproduced here.

10 Petrus Severinus, *Epistola scripta Theophrasto Paracelso, in qua ratio ordinis et nominum, adeoque totius Philosophiæ Adeptæ Methodus compendiose et erudite ostenditur a Petro Severino Dano Philosophiæ et Medicinæ Doctore*, hereafter *Epistola* (Basel, no date), unpaginated. *Epistola* was included in *Paracelsi opera omnia medico-chemico-chirurgica*, ed. Bitiskius (Geneva: de Tournes, 1658), vol. 1. No publication date is given for *Epistola*, but Bastholm (*Petrus Severinus*, p. 34) is surely correct in rejecting earlier claims that it was printed in 1572. A printer's note on the verso of the title page indicates it was printed and distributed before *Idea medicinæ*. My conjecture is that Severinus delivered both manuscripts to Henric Petri in late 1570 or early 1571, and that *Epistola* was put on the market while *Idea medicinæ* was still being printed for distribution in the fall of 1571. The lack of a date on the title page suggests to me that *Epistola* may have been set into type in late 1570, when the date of printing would

→

its author as a well-read Paracelsian: besides lauding Paracelsus for bringing together "the piety of Orpheus, the majesty of Pythagoras and his secret knowledge of Creation, the humanity of Socrates, and the eloquence and subtle inquiry of Plato," the author praised him for drawing his philosophy from fresh, living sources, rather than from dead literature.[11] References to no fewer than thirteen of Paracelsus' treatises give support to Severinus' claim that he had expended great mental effort and many sleepless nights (*immensis meditationibus & diuturnis vigiliis*) trying to sort out the obscure and often variable terminology in Paracelsus' various works. This entailed finding a common ground between Paracelsus' theories and similar doctrines manifest in texts by "Geber, Alphicinus, Rhasis, Plotinus, Senior, Rosinus, Morienus, Villanova, Raymund, Isaac," and "Orpheus, Pythagoras, Plato, Synesius, Iamblichus, ... Proclus, Porphyry, and the other Platonists."[12]

Given the epistolic form and rhetorical content of the *Epistola*, we cannot but conclude that it was meant to identify Severinus as a Paracelsian philosopher. Considering the timing of its publication, namely shortly before the *Idea medicinæ* and bearing the publisher's promise to have the *Idea medicinæ* out at the next Frankfurt book fair, we might view this piece as an advertisement. The *Idea medicinæ* was, as we shall see, Severinus' attempt to explain Paracelsian teaching and resolve those discrepancies and contradictions already identified in the *Epistola*, which

---

→   have been as yet undetermined, but this is just a guess. This view is supported by Sudhoff's dating of "wahrscheinlich Herbstmesse 1570." Karl Sudhoff, *Bibliographia Paracelsica, Besprechung der unter Hohenheims Namen 1527-1893 erschienen Druckschriften* (1894; reprint, Graz: Akademische Druck- und Verlagsanstalt, 1958), p. 588.

11   Severinus, *Epistola*: "Orphei admiramur pietatem, Pythagoræ maiestatem, & absconditam totius Creaturæ scientiam, Socratis humanitatem, Platonis eloquentiam, & inquisitionum subtilitatem: tibi uero hæc omnia, uel plurima certe, uni contigisse, etiam nostro hoc seculo gratulamur. Nec dubito quin ex uiuentibus uigentibusque riuulis, non ex mortuis & silentibus literis ut nos solemus, horum arcanorum thesaurum receperis."

12   Ibid. "Balsami naturalis naturam & proprietates, ... apud Hermetem, ... apud Gebrum, Alphidium, Rhasin, Seniorem, Rosinum, Morienum, Villanouanum, Raymundum, Isaacum, descriptas vidimus. Tria uero Principia tua, toties sunt apud Raymundum, Isaacum, Gebrum & cæteros, tam clare posita, depicta ac declarata .... Similiter Balsami supranaturalis ..., de quo agis in omnibus tuis contemplationibus Magicis & Cabalisticis, ab eodem Hermete, trinæ Philosophiæ Monarcha, ab Orpheo, Pythagora, Platone, Synesio, Iamblicho, Plotino, Proclo, Porphyrio, & reliquis Platonicis descripta uidimus."

serves as a harbinger. From it, it is clear that Severinus was strongly attracted to aspects of Paracelsus' philosophy. He saw Paracelsus as the latest in the line of *prisci theologi*, one of the few who was given the mental keenness to "ascend to the inner chambers of the Mosaic mysteries."[13] It follows from this panegyric that Severinus viewed himself as a disciple of the Hermetic lineage and was not afraid to advertize this to the academic world.

RESISTANCE TO PARACELSIANISM?

I have argued above that when Severinus and Pratensis returned from their peregrinations in 1571 to accept appointments to the most influential posts in the medical establishment, namely Royal Physician and Professor of Medicine, they were not at all secretive about their Paracelsian sympathies. This raises questions of importance to understanding the sixteenth-century reception of Paracelsian ideas: What was the prevailing attitude toward Paracelsianism at court and among Danish academicians at this time? To what extent did Severinus' and Pratensis' commitment to Paracelsian doctrine affect their professional life, as practitioners and as philosophers of medicine? Although evidence is not as plentiful as one would like, it can be argued that both of them advocated and used Paracelsian drugs, and that their knowledge of Paracelsianism enhanced their reputation and careers.

Peder Hegelund wrote in his almanac for 22 June 1571 that "about this time Doctor Petrus Severinus of Ribe and Doctor Johannes Philippus Pratensis returned to this country."[14] Less than two weeks later, on 3 July, there was an administrative meeting at the University of Copenhagen. One of the topics raised concerned filling the still-vacant second chair in medicine. Here is an extract from the consistorial record.

---

13 Ibid. "Et quamuis aliorum Philosophorum ingenia ijsdem implicata fuisse difficultatibus sciam: paucis tamen datum fuit æquali mentis acie, ad Mosaicorum mysteriorum penetralia ascendere."

14 Kaae, *Almanakoptegnelser*, vol. 1, p. 71: "22. June, 1571: Circa hoc tempus reuersi sunt in patriam D. D. Petrus Seuerinus Ripensis et D. D. Iohannes Philippus Pratensis."

The Lord Rector [Niels Hemmingsen] proposed calling M. Johannes Pratensis to the chair in medicine, saying: "I was recently in Roskilde, and Master Nicolas of Kolding [Court Priest and Royal Librarian] pointed out to me that Doctor Petrus Severinus had been called to serve the king, but Doctor Johannes Pratensis still had no employment, and that [therefore] we were free to call him (or not) to the university. With regard to this I ask you to give me your votes on these two points:

1. Whether you wish Doctor Johannes Pratensis to be called to a chair at this school.

2. And whether it would seem reasonable, if you called him, that he not teach other than Hippocratic and Galenic doctrine in our school, just as the medical professors do at the schools in Wittenberg and Leipzig."

The votes were given thus: Doctor Erasmus Lætus [said], "In truth I judge both that Doctor Johannes Philippus should be called to a chair and that the doctrine of Galen and Hippocrates be taught by him at the university, just as is, in general, customarily done at other universities." The rest of the professors unanimously subscribed to this judgement.[15]

15 These passages from *Acta consistorii* are printed in Herholdt and Mansa, *Samlinger*, pp. 148-49, as well as in Holger Rørdam, ed., "Uddrag af Konsistoriets Forhandlinger 1543-1599," *[Ny] Kirkehistoriske Samlinger*, 2d ser., 1 (1857-59), pp. 44-45. There is some discrepancy between these two transcriptions, but the meaning is not affected. I have taken Rørdam's as the more correct transcription, with the exception of the first reference to "ad lectionem" (Rørdam = "ad Actionem"), where I have followed Herholdt and Mansa: "Dnus Rector de Doctore Johanne Pratensi Medico vocando ad Lectionem Medicam proposuit, inquiens: Ego nuper fui Roschildiæ et mihi a M. Nicolao Coldingio significatum est, Doctorem Petrum Severini vocatum esse ad serviendum Regi, sed Doctorem Johannem Pratensem adhuc non habere vocationem, nobisque liberum esse ipsum ad Academiam vocare vel non vocare. Quare ad hæc duo velim mihi dari vestra suffragia.
I. Utrum velitis vocari ad lectionem in hac schola Doctorem Johannem Pratensem.
II. Anne videatur vobis utile, ut si eum vocaveritis, alium non tradat in schola nostra doctrinam, quam Hypocratis et Galeni, sicut quoque faciunt Medici scholæ Vitebergensis et Lipsiensis. →

This record has been taken by scholars as a measure of academic opposition to Paracelsianism at this time, an interpretation compatible with reactions elsewhere. Yet this conclusion must not be taken too far. For example, it is not justified to suppose on this basis that Pratensis was chosen over Severinus for the chair *because* he had a lower profile as a Paracelsian than did the author of openly Paracelsian tracts.[16] In fact we can conclude from the consistorial record that Pratensis *was* recognized as a Paracelsian proponent, that teaching Paracelsian doctrine would be inappropriate, but that they hired him, anyway, knowing his inclinations.

I offer a different interpretation of the university's restriction on Pratensis' teaching. The organizational structure and curriculum of medieval and Renaissance universities was codified to a degree uncommon in our own time. Which authors were to be lectured on, and when, was defined for each subject in official documents. For example, the *Ordinatio lectionum* set forth by the first rector of the reformed University of Copenhagen, Christiern Terkelsen Morsing, M.D., specifies that there be two medical professors. One should teach *theory*, from Galen and Hippocrates, and the other should teach *practice*, from "Ægineta and other well chosen moderns."[17] My interpretation of the professors' stipulation that Pratensis teach only Galenic and Hippocratic medicine, as done at the other universities, is that it was a conservative statement

→ Data hoc pacto suffragia.
  D. Erasmus Lætus. Ego re vera iudico et vocandum ad lectionem Doct. Johannem Philippi, et ab eo in schola proponendam esse doctrinam Galeni et Hypocratis, sicut in aliis Academiis communiter solet fieri.
  Huic suffragio professores reliqui unanimiter subscripserunt."

16 This was the position taken by Eyvind Bastholm, *Petrus Severinus*, p. 6: "At Pratensis og ikke Sørensen fik professoratet, kan måske skyldes at han ikke i samme grad som denne havde markeret sig som aktiv paracelsist, selv om man naturligvis var klar over hans sympati for de nye tanker." Bastholm notes that Pratensis did, in fact, indicate his Paracelsian leaning in a laudatory poem affixed to the *Idea medicinæ*, which may have been printed by that time.

17 This part of the consistorial record is reproduced by Panum, "Vort medicinske Fakultets," p. 26: "Duo erunt imprimis Medicinæ Professores et Doctores, quorum unus theoriam ex Galeno et Hypocrate græce, alter practicam ex Ægineta et Neotericis aliis selectioribus latine prælegit." Although Paulus Ægineta was not actually a "modern," his work was popular with sixteenth-century *moderni*. See Nancy Siraisi, *Avicenna in Renaissance Italy: The* Canon *and Medical Teaching in Italian Universities after 1500* (Princeton: Princeton University Press, 1987), pp. 77-78.

of a bureaucratic reality: a professor was bound to teach within the prescribed academic limits of his position. There was no doubt a difference between what was mandated and what was actually taught at the universities, and possibly also a discrepancy between what needed to be stipulated in a contract or official record and what was actually expected from a professor. Therefore, Pratensis may have been expected to formally satisfy the curricular requirements, with the realization that he would be an available resource for the new medicine, which had not yet gained a foothold in European education.

This interpretation is in accordance with the fact that the professors did *unanimously* approve the hiring of a known Paracelsian physician to fill the vacant chair that had supported his education abroad. It is also in accord with the "negative" phrasing of the restriction, that is, that Pratensis was not proscribed from teaching Paracelsian doctrine, but rather required to teach Galenic and Hippocratic.[18] It is doubtful whether this was enforced, anyway. The university program on the occasion of Pratensis' death, just five years after he was hired, says that "his dexterity, skill, success, and diligence in performing both Galenic and Paracelsian medicine was remarkable and admirable."[19] This eulogy supports Pratensis' own admission, in a declaration enclosed with a letter to Severinus, that he had violated the university's restriction. He said he had followed Galen's teaching in good conscience, but that "from the very beginning I secretly rejoiced, while by means of the obscure and skillful

18 The question of what was taught at the universities and how this differed from the prescribed curricula is of central importance to our understanding of the universities' reception and reaction to new ideas in the sixteenth and seventeenth centuries. John Gascoigne, "A Reappraisal of the Role of the Universities in the Scientific Revolution," in *Reappraisals of the Scientific Revolution*, ed. David C. Lindberg and Robert S. Westman (Cambridge: Cambridge University Press, 1990), pp. 207-260, has begun to address this problem with regard to the reception of the kinds of science that led to modern science (mathematics, physics, anatomy, Copernicanism, etc.), but does not address the universities' response to chemical philosophy, except to suggest that the establishment of chairs in chemistry was due to the medical faculties' wresting the subject away from alchemy and metallurgy. Paracelsianism is not mentioned, but, as we see in the case of Pratensis, some accommodation may have been attempted by the back door, as it were.

19 Bartholin, *Cista medica*, p. 57: "Fuit præclara ac divina ejus in facienda medicina utraque, Galenica et Paracelsica, dexteritas, solertia, felicitas, et industria."

art of Proteus I patched sweet and sumptuous flowers from foreign gardens onto Galen's darnel and oats."[20] Now that others are visiting those foreign gardens, Pratensis continued, he feels he must "without modesty embrace the path of truth and conscientiousness."[21] The implication is that Pratensis was at the cutting edge of a reform of academic medicine that failed to succeed at the University of Copenhagen, perhaps because his early death deprived it of a resident champion.

The hiring of Pratensis, a recognized Paracelsian, cannot be taken to indicate a decided sympathy for neoteric medicine or a distinct atmosphere of medical reform among the members of the faculty. Rather it should be seen as a symptom of the eclecticism that dominated academic medicine in late sixteenth and seventeenth-century Denmark and the result of the king's desire to encourage Paracelsian ideas within academic medicine, much as his German peers were doing.[22] Galenism and Aristotelianism continued to dominate natural philosophy (including medicine), and there are even some hints of low-level friction between the Galenists and the Paracelsians. When Niels Kaas died in 1594, Professor Hans Slangerup gave a funeral oration in which he commented on the deplorable state of medicine: "Who does not know of those barbaric upstarts who are preferred by the physicians over the ancient Greeks and some of the Arabic physicians?"[23] Presumably he was referring to the Paracelsians.

20 Letter from Pratensis to Severinus, 14 March (1574?): "Ab initio quidem gaudebam in sinu meo, dum obscura & callida Prothei arte ex alienis hortis tam suaues et opulentos flores Galenicis loliis et auenis assuerem." The letter is not dated as to year, but the enclosed declaration is dated 1 October 1573, likely the previous year. Printed in "Tychonis Brahe, Ioh. Pratensis, ... Epistolæ ad Petrum Severinum," chapter 11 of *Altes und Neues von Gelehrten Sachen aus Dännemark*, vol. 2 (Copenhagen and Leipzig, 1768), p. 480.

21 Ibid., p. 480: "Sine pudore ueritatis et fidei uiam candide amplecti."

22 Bruce T. Moran, "Court Authority and Chemical Medicine: Moritz of Hessen, Johannes Hartmann, and the Origin of Academic Chemiatria," *Bulletin of the History of Medicine* 63 (1989), p. 246, refers to a similar "court-prescribed role within the university" in his discussion of the Landgraf of Hessen's appointment of professors to the university at Marburg. Moran deepens his analysis of how Hermetic philosophy and Paracelsian chemistry were integrated into court culture in Hessen-Kassel in *The Alchemical World of the German Court: Occult Philosophy and Chemical Medicine in the Circle of Moritz of Hessen (1572-1632)* (Stuttgart: Franz Steiner, 1991).

23 *Oratio funebris de vita et obitu Nic. Kaasii*: "Quis ignorat, a medicis, barbaros quosdam recentiores antiquis Græcis aut Arabum Medicorum nonnullis antepositos?" After Rørdam, *KUH*, vol. 2, p. 331, note 3.

This tension between Galenism and Paracelsianism has been credited, among other things, with creating an atmosphere of hostility toward Tycho Brahe, which contributed to his loss of royal favor.[24] If there is any truth to the idea that Tycho's departure from Denmark was affected by anti-Paracelsian sentiment, which will be considered in the next chapter, it is likely that this hostility first arose toward the end of the century, long after Pratensis was dead. Hans Frandsen (Johannes Franciscus Ripensis), the Galenist who held the first chair in medicine from 1560 to 1584, was honored by his former student and friend, Tycho Brahe, with an epitaph that praised him as a poet. And, as is shown below, Tycho had decided Paracelsian sympathies. Pratensis was succeeded by Anders Lemvig, a Galenist described by Severinus as "a respectable youth, middling poet, and tolerably educated in physics and ancient medicine."[25] While this is not a strong endorsement, neither is it evidence for serious animosity between Galenists and Paracelsians under Frederik II's reign, some of whom were personal friends. Of much greater importance in those years was one's profession of faith, and this does not appear to have militated against Paracelsianism in Denmark before the turn of the century.[26]

24 Panum, "Vort medicinske Fakultets," p. 48, for example.

25 Quoted by Panum, Ibid., p. 45: "Juvenis honestus, poeta mediocris, physicis et antiqua medicina mediocriter institutus."

26 The advanced training in natural philosophy offered by the Jesuits was attractive to Protestant students who sought education abroad. For this reason, and because of a concern to keep to the true Lutheran faith, the University of Copenhagen was very careful to exact declarations of faith from the professors they hired, if there was doubt about their adherence to the Augsburg Confession. Once employed, a professor's private life was also subject to scrutiny for this reason. See Ibid., p. 41. The oath that was signed 9 July 1575 by Johannes Pratensis and the other professors, including Niels Hemmingsen, is printed in Rørdam, "Bidrag til de filippistiske Bevægelsers og til D. Niels Hemmingsens Historie," *[Ny] Kirkehistoriske Samlinger*, 2d ser., 4 (1867-68), pp. 300-303, and Johan Grundtvig, "Et lidet Bidrag til D. Niels Hemmingsens Historie," Ibid., pp. 744-746. The connection between Paracelsian theories and heterodox religion becomes important only in the second decade of the seventeenth century. See Jole Shackelford, "Rosicrucianism, Lutheran Orthodoxy, and the Rejection of Paracelsianism in Early Seventeenth-Century Denmark," *Bulletin of the History of Medicine* 70 (1996): 181-204.

TYCHO BRAHE

The two young medical students were not the only ones to come home to Denmark with enthusiasm for Paracelsian theories. The famous Danish astronomer and aristocrat, Tycho Brahe, had also become acquainted with Paracelsianism abroad.[27] It was probably their common interest in the new and fashionable ideology – for Paracelsianism entailed a fundamental view of the world, with ramifications for cosmology, medicine, religion, and politics, and therefore is best seen as an ideology – that brought Tycho Brahe, Severinus, and Pratensis together. The three of them formed the kernel of an informal circle of friends and correspondents who shared an interest in Paracelsian ideas.

Tycho's interest in medicine, and his friendship with Severinus and Pratensis, may well go back to the early 1560s, when all three were students at the University of Copenhagen. Tycho's textbooks from 1560 indicate that he was studying medical subjects as well as astronomy at that time, foreshadowing his later commitment to a natural philosophy that integrated the terrestrial and celestial regions into a harmonious whole.[28] In these early years Tycho studied mathematics, planetary theory, and astrology under Hans Frandsen, who was appointed professor of medicine in 1561, and perhaps also under Scavenius.[29] The ensuing years found Tycho traveling a great deal and mixing with the learned and the noble in Germany, as befitted his social rank. From 1562-68 he studied in Leipzig, Wittenberg, and Rostock, with a couple of trips back to Denmark in between. At Rostock he met Levinus Battus, a

27 There are several good biographies of Tycho Brahe, the most recent of which are John Christianson, *On Tycho's Island: Tycho Brahe and His Assistants, 1570-1601* (Cambridge: Cambridge University Press, 2000); Alex Wittendorff, *Tyge Brahe* (Copenhagen: Gad, 1994); and Thoren, *The Lord of Uraniborg*, which considers Tycho Brahe's specific scientific achievements and intellectual world. Other biographies by Dreyer (English), Norlind (Swedish), and Friis (Danish) have been consulted on particular points in this study, and are cited in context.

28 His textbooks from this period indicate his early eclectic interest: Sacrobosco's *De sphæra* is bound together with Petrus Bayrus, *De medendis humani corporis* (Basel, 1560), a medical text, and Æmilius Macer, *De herbarum virtutibus elegentissima poesis* (Basel, 1559), an herbal, and stamped "T. B. 1560." See John Christianson, "Tycho Brahe at the University of Copenhagen, 1559-1562," *Isis* 58 (1967), pp. 200-201.

29 On Frandsen, see Rørdam, *KUH*, vol. 2, pp. 543-56.

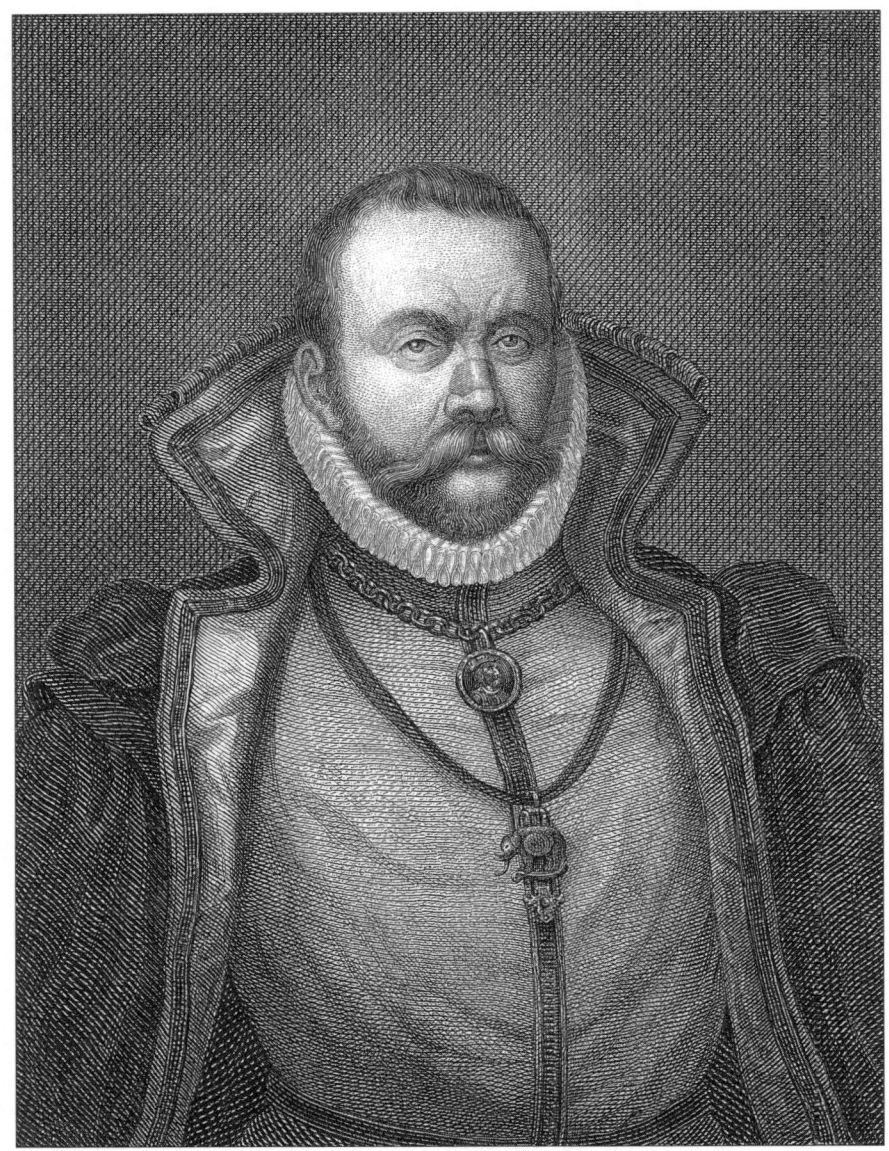

Engraved portrait of Tycho Brahe, based on a 1586 original by L.D. Gheyn. Courtesy of The Danish National Library of Science and Medicine.

Paracelsian professor of medicine with whom he struck up an enduring friendship and even resided for part of 1568.[30] It may have been Battus who first introduced Tycho to the ideas of Paracelsus. After leaving Rostock, Tycho matriculated at Basel and then settled for a while at Augsburg, where he undertook serious study of alchemy.[31] In 1570 he was called home on account of his father's illness and eventually settled at his uncle's estate at Herrevad Kloster, where both an observatory and a laboratory were built.[32]

By Tycho's own account, it was on returning to the house after a long day in the laboratory that he noted a new star in Cassiopeia; that was 11 November 1572.[33] Until this time Tycho had been devoting less time to astronomy and more time to his investigation of the chemical secrets of the terrestrial world, as he admitted in his account of the new star, published the following year.[34] This discovery, and his analysis of it in *De nova stella*, drew attention to Tycho's astronomical acumen and ultimately led to his receiving from Frederik II the island of Hven in fief and a promise of further benefices. Tycho's use of these resources enabled him to compile a corpus of astronomical observations – the positions of the "fixed" stars as well as of the known planets (including at that time the moon and sun) – which were unprecedented in terms of their number and accuracy. The new star must therefore be considered a pivotal event in Tycho's life, and *De nova stella* should be regarded as a document designed to gain him fame among the

30 F.R. Friis, *Tyge Brahe: En Historisk Fremstilling* (Copenhagen: Gyldendal, 1871), p. 23: "Tyge Brahe har rimeligvis snart sluttet sig til denne Mand, hvis Anskuelser i flere Henseender lignede hans egne."

31 Ibid., pp. 26 and 30. See also C. Doris Hellman, "Tycho Brahe," *DSB*, vol. 2, pp. 401-416.

32 On Herrevad as a possible model for Tycho's development of Hven, see John Christianson, "Cloister and Observatory: Herrevad Abbey and Tycho Brahe's Uranienborg." Ph.D. Dissertation, University of Minnesota, 1964.

33 F.R. Friis, *Tyge Brahe*, pp. 32-33.

34 Tycho recorded no astronomical observations from the end of 1570 to the end of 1572, during which period alchemy must have dominated his research effort. In his 1573 account of the new star, *De nova stella*, Tycho alluded to his preoccupation with alchemy, using a classical allusion: Urania, the muse of astronomy, complains that Tycho has been spending too much time with Vulcan, that is, at the furnace. *De nova stella*, in *TBDOO*, vol. 1, pp. 65-70.

educated elite as well as the patronage of nobles more powerful and wealthy than he was.[35]

It is interesting to note in this context that Tycho included in *De nova stella* a letter written to him 3 May 1573 by his friend Johannes Pratensis. The letter reveals an intellectual comradery between the men: "You were at our house in Copenhagen not long ago, having left behind your 'domestic studies' and pyronomic activities," Pratensis wrote to his friend, "and we freely discussed common studies, as is our custom."[36] The very printing of this letter reinforces the implication of these words, namely that Tycho held the young professor and his ideas in great esteem. Furthermore, Tycho must have wanted the readers of *De nova stella* to interpret what he wrote about the nova in light of Pratensis' ideas, which were Paracelsian. This view agrees with Victor Thoren's recent analysis concerning the publication of *De nova stella*, where he argues that Tycho solicited Pratensis' letter in order to further legitimize Tycho's putting his findings into print, a practice that might have been regarded as beneath the dignity of a great nobleman.[37] Pratensis' letter is rich in Paracelsian imagery and terminology, which we also find in Severinus' *Idea medicinæ*, and he implicitly attributes this Paracelsian view of the cosmos to Tycho when he refers to himself as "one among a few who knows your sedulous diligence in unraveling other mysteries of nature, especially in Spagyric Cabala."[38] By printing this letter in his treatise, Tycho was making public his commitment to Paracelsianism in a quiet, but noticeable way. Pratensis' use of the term Cabala in this context is also interesting. In the absence of other evidence for Tycho's interest in Cabala, we must question Pratensis' meaning – the word may mean

---

35 I discuss patronage more explicitly in Shackelford, "Paracelsianism and Patronage."

36 Letter from Pratensis to Tycho, 3 May 1573, Copenhagen, *TBDOO*, vol. 1, p. 6: "relictis domesticis Musis, et Pyronomicis tuis exercitijs, Hafniæ, apud nos esses, Tycho nobilissime: ac de communibus studij, ultro citroque, qui mos noster est, conferremus." The letter was printed and bound with *De nova stella* (1573; facsimile edition, Brussels: Culture et Civilisation, 1969). Tycho sometimes stayed with Pratensis when he visited Copenhagen, according to Rørdam, *KUH*, vol. 2, pp. 601-602.

37 Thoren, *The Lord of Uraniborg*, p. 64.

38 Pratensis to Brahe, 3 May 1573, *TBDOO*, vol. 1, p. 7: "Qui sedulam tuam, in alijs quoque Naturæ Mysterijs euoluendis, tum præcipue, in Spagyrica Cabala, diligentiam, vnus e paucis cognoscam."

"philosophical chemistry" and refer to the underlying, hidden connections between things, rather than the numerological study of Hebrew Scripture, which it generally means today. This would be in keeping with Severinus' use of the term in the title of his 1567 manuscript, "A book of exercises in which philosophical, astronomical, medical, and cabalistic questions are explained."[39]

Given Pratensis' close ties to Severinus, it is not surprising that Brahe and Severinus were also friends, although personal contact between them likely diminished over the years, as Tycho was occupied away from court circles, while Severinus, as Royal Physician, was obliged to attend the royal family. The French Ambassador to Denmark for many years, Charles Danzay, was another friend of these people.[40] When Tycho was offered Hven and the royal support to pursue his research there, he consulted his closest friends, Pratensis and Danzay, before making the momentous decision to accept.[41] When construction began on Uraniborg, Danzay provided the expensive, inscribed cornerstone and took part in the astrological ceremony consecrating the edifice to philosophy.[42]

---

39 "Exercitationum liber in quo quæstiones philosophicæ, astronomicæ, medicæ, cabalisticæ explicantur." That the term cabala refered to unraveling the mysteries of nature through alchemy and other occult sciences and natural philosophy as well as to Hebrew cabala is reinforced by a recent study of Severinus' contemporary, John Dee: Deborah Harkness, *John Dee's Conversations with Angels: Cabala, Alchemy, and the End of Nature* (Cambridge: Cambridge University Press, 1999).

40 Danzay and Pratensis were instrumental in convincing Tycho to deliver lectures at the University of Copenhagen in 1574-75. These were published by Kort Aslakssøn in 1610. Danzay died in 1589. See J. L. E. Dreyer, *Tycho Brahe: A Picture of Scientific Life and Work in the Sixteenth Century* (Edinburgh: Adam and Charles Black, 1890), pp. 73 and 131. On Danzay's general tasks and achievements at the Danish court see Rørdam, "Charles de Danzay."

41 See Tycho's letter to Pratensis, 14 February 1576, *TBDOO*, vol. 7, pp. 25-29, trans. John Christianson, "Cloister and Observatory," pp. 129-138. Pratensis consulted with Danzay and responded the following day, *TBDOO*, vol. 7, pp. 30-31, translated to Swedish in Wilhelm Norlind, *Ur Tycho Brahes Brevväxling* (Lund: Gleerup, 1926), pp. 30-32.

42 Dreyer, *Tycho Brahe*, p. 93. Tycho described the laying of the cornerstone in *Astronomiæ instauratæ mechanica*: see Hans Ræder, Elis Strömgren, and Bengt Strömgren, eds., *Tycho Brahe's Description of his Instruments and Scientific Work as given in Astronomiæ Instauratæ Mechanica* (Copenhagen: Det kongelige danske videnskabernes selskab, 1946), p. 130. A revised, more complete version of Ræder's translation of Tycho's *Mechanica* is Alena Hadravova, Petr Hadrava, and Jole R. Shackelford, eds., *Instruments of the Renewed Astronomy* (Prague: Koniasch Latin Press, 1996).

Uraniborg was more than just a nobleman's home, however, it provided protected spaces for instruments on the upper floors, from which the heavens could be observed and measured. In its basement was a laboratory, where Tycho could carry out the "pyronomic activities" that Pratensis had mentioned: the chemical nature of substances could be examined, and health-bringing elixers could be concocted. No laboratory notebooks or chemical treatises have survived to tell us what was done down there, if indeed any were ever written, but several of Tycho's recipes do exist as testimony to the iatrochemical part of his work at Uraniborg. One such remedy, "Tycho Brahe's Elixir," became sufficiently well known to merit its use (the name at any rate) into the twentieth century.[43]

Tycho's interest in the chemical arts has been long recognized but little remarked on and always dwarfed by his astronomical work.[44] The latter proved more enduring, being more easily shorn from its ideological base and applied to the task of refashioning our conception of the solar system. However, there can be little doubt that Tycho himself regarded his chemical studies as the worthy twin brother to his celestial investigation. But these twins were complementary rather than identical; As a Christian Platonist, Tycho saw the universe as a whole, a macrocosm in which astronomy (including astrology) and alchemy were companion sciences concerned with related phenomena in different regions. To

43   Karin Figala, "Tycho Brahes Elixir," *Annals of Science* 28 (1972), p. 146, has analyzed the recipe for Tycho Brahe's Elixir, a drug name surviving in Danish pharmacopoeias into the 20th century, assessed Tycho's medical prescriptions, and determined that they specified certain compounds and chemical preparations common to Paracelsian pharmacology. In particular she points to "sulphur e colchotare" and solutions of silver, gold, and antimony. These compounds are identifiable in the recipes printed in "Compositiones & Medicamentorum," *TBDOO*, vol. 9, pp. 161-169. Even a cursory perusal of Brahe's prescriptions impresses one with the careful description Tycho provided of the actual chemical preparation: the distillations, extractions, filtrations, and digestions needed to "resolve" the compounds in the tinctures. Even where traditional herbal drugs are called for, such as Theriac, they are subjected to chemical extraction in alcohol and subsequent distillation to separate the spiritual, effective tincture from the corporeal residues. Given Tycho's penchant for data collection, as is evident from his astronomical records and the extensive meteorological diary that was kept at Uraniborg, I am inclined to believe that some laboratory records must also have existed.

44   A notable exception is Carl-Johan Clemedson, "Något om Tycho Brahe och hans medicinska verksamhet," in *Sydsvenska medicinhistoriska sällskapets årsskrift 1972* (Lund: Sydsvenska medicinhistoriska sällskapet, 1972), pp. 38-59.

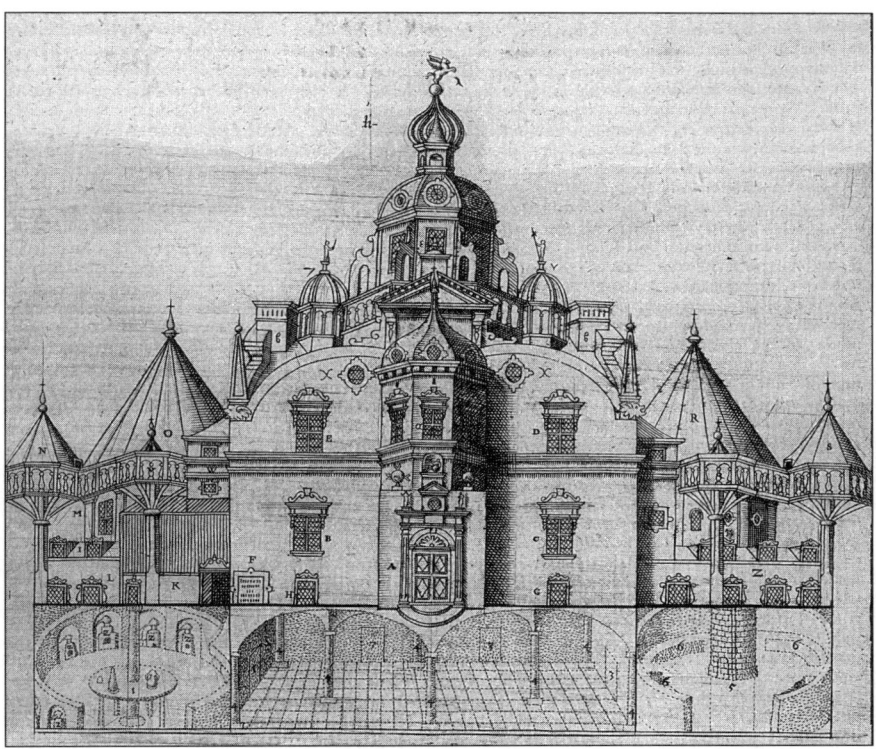

Tycho published an elevation of Uraniborg in his Mechanica instauratæ astronomiæ
*(1598) showing the location of his basement laboratory on the south end of the villa,
underneath the library. Windows shown along the top of the basement wall and in
the sloping roof of the half-round basement room permitted light into the laboratory
without sacrificing wall space along the floor. Courtesy of The Danish National
Library of Science and Medicine.*

capture this sameness he refered to the one as celestial astronomy and
the other as terrestrial astronomy.

To illustrate the integration of celestial and terrestrial sciences,
Tycho had a pair of figures cut into blocks of wood, which he used to
print emblems for use in his various publications. Apparently he sent a
set of the illustrations to his erudite friend, Falche Gøye. These came
to the attention of Christopher Rothmann, the astronomer-mathemati-
cian of Wilhelm IV of Hessen-Kassel, who recognized their symbolic
meaning:

At length I happened upon what you had sent to Falche Goye, and on the second side of the page I found a pair of images, one of astronomy, the other of that art you call spagyric. When I examined them diligently, I observed letters on both sides of them: around Astronomy, SUSPICI-ENDO DESPICIO; around the other, DESPICIENDO SUSPICIO. Considering these for a long while, again and again, at last I thought them to be hieroglyphic, and that perhaps you are indicating by these that the spagyric art encompasses the contemplation of all of nature and the world.[45]

In his reply, Tycho affirmed the message guessed by Rothmann:

You have guessed correctly that these are hieroglyphic; For they refer not only to both that superior, celestial astronomy, and that inferior ter-restrial, but also to that more divine and less commonly used theology, and what is more, to the study of all Ethics, namely the distinction of virtues and vices.[46]

This conception of an astronomy that encompasses both the terrestrial and celestial orders seems to have struck a harmonious note among those who sought knowledge of the cosmos; years later, Joachim Morsius used this same formulation in referring to Tycho's work.[47]

---

45 Letter from Rothmann to Tycho, 11 October 1587, in *TBDOO*, vol. 6, p. 118: "Incidi tandem in id, quod ad D. FALCHONEM GOYE miseras, atque ab altera paginæ parte inueni binas imagines, alteram Astronomiæ, alteram eius Artis, quam Spagyricam appellas. Quas cum diligenter intuebar, animaduerti ab vtroque earum latere literas quasdam, circa Astronomiam quidem, SVSPICIENDO DESPICIO: circa reliquam vero, DESPICIENDO SVSPICIO. Diu hæc cum admiratione etiam atque etiam considerans, cogitaui tandem Hieroglyphica esse, teque ijs forte annuere, Artem Spa-gyricam continere totius Naturæ & Mundi contemplationem."

46 Letter from Tycho to Rothmann, 17 August 1588, *TBDOO*, vol. 6, p. 144: "Hieroglyphica hæc esse recte coniectasti; Nam non saltem vtramque Astronomiam cælestem illam superiorem, & inferiorem terrestrem respiciunt, sed etiam ipsam diuiniorem minusque vulgariter vsitatam Theologiam, adeoque totius Ethices cognitionem, videlicet virtutum & vitiorum discretionem."

47 Johan Nordström, "Lejonet från Norden," *Samlaran* 15 (1934), p. 36: "Vtinam aliquis felici dextra nobis ab interitu vindicaret, eiusdem magni Paracelsi commentationes in integra Biblia, quas ante aliquot annos in itinere meo Danico Hafniæ, se vidisse olim

→

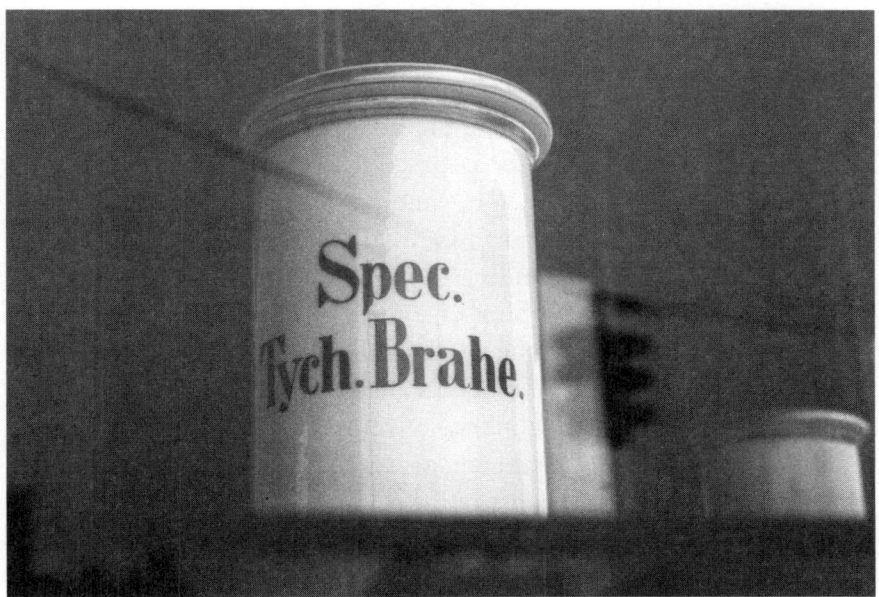

Species Tychonis Brahei was the name given to a drug that was still being sold at the beginning of the twentieth century. This jar was on display in the window of an apothecary in Copenhagen in 1985 (Christianshavns Torv Apothek). Author's photograph.

Rothmann's reference to the woodcuts as "hieroglyphic," and Tycho's affirmation of this, is in itself interesting. In the sixteenth and early seventeenth centuries it was thought in some circles that certain symbols, hieroglyphs, bore a special relationship to nature and conveyed special knowledge and power to one who understood them. John Dee's *monas*

→   apud summe peritum Uraniæ coelestis & terrestris Tychonem Braheum, vir Clarissimus & multiplicis eruditionis Conradus Aslacus, Professor Regius, mihi retulit." [Would that someone with a favorable hand would free from destruction the commentaries of that same great Paracelsus on the whole Bible, which several years ago, on my Danish trip to Copenhagen, the very illustrious man of great erudition, Kort Aslakssøn, Royal Professor, reported he had once seen in the possession of Tycho Brahe, the very great expert of celestial and terrestrial astronomy.] Note that Morsius uses the poetic "Urania" for *astronomia*.

hieroglyphica is a well known contemporary example.[48] In fact, Rothmann may have had this interpretation in mind when he wrote to Tycho, since Dee's book was well known at the Landgraf's court, and Dee himself was a visitor there in this period.[49] The emblems associated with the Rosicrucians are also of a hieroglyphic nature. These references by Rothmann and Brahe suggest that they, too, were familiar with the magical and alchemical literature of the north German Paracelsian milieu.[50]

Perhaps Tycho's understanding of the macrocosm and how it should be investigated owed something to conversation with his friends Pratensis and Severinus, or to the *Idea medicinæ* itself, or perhaps he and they drank from common Paracelsian springs. Quite likely Tycho shared Severinus' view that "stars," or centers of astral power and development, existed in all the elements, reaching their visible state only in the relative purity of the firmament. According to Severinus, the "stars" in the human body accounted for the fact that human beings and their diseases exhibit cyclical behavior, which is a conspicuous property of stars.[51] This is one of the philosophical justifications for looking to the heavens, and elsewhere in nature, to learn about the human microcosm.

Like Severinus and many others, Tycho believed that all things possessed peculiar *signaturæ* or properties, as is evident from his oration

---

48 Dee's world view is discussed in Peter J. French, *John Dee: The World of an Elizabethan Magus* (London: Routledge and Kegan Paul, 1972); and Nicholas Clulee, *John Dee's Natural Philosophy: Between Science and Religion* (London: Routledge, 1988); as well as in Harkness, *John Dee's Conversations with Angels*. The Swedish Paracelsian Johannes Bureus was also deeply immersed in symbolism of this sort. See Jole Shackelford, "Documenting the Factual and the Artifactual: Ole Worm and Public Knowledge," *Endeavour* 23 (1999), pp. 65-71.

49 Clulee, *John Dee's Natural Philosophy*, p. 226; Bruce T. Moran, "Court Authority and Chemical Medicine," p. 232.

50 Tycho purchased books on Hermetic and Paracelsian subjects and left instructions with his friends for the purchase of chemical texts. See Thoren, *The Lord of Uraniborg*, pp. 96 and 315; Tycho's letter to Joachim Camerarius, 21 November 1576, *TBDOO* vol. 7, p. 42: "Si quos alias in Mathematicis et chymicis inveneris seu novos seu veteres, quos mihi usui fore existimas, una adiungas velim." [If at another time you have found any [books] in mathematics and chemistry, whether new or old, that you think will be of use to me, please send them.]

51 Petrus Severinus, *Idea medicinæ philosophicæ fundamenta continens totius doctrinæ Paracelsicæ, Hippocraticæ et Galenicæ* (Basel: Henric Petri, 1571), p. 53.

at the University of Copenhagen in 1574.[52] He more explicitly endorsed the connectedness of the cosmos in a letter to Rothmann in 1588, where he discussed the "wonderful similitude" that connects the things of the superior and inferior worlds:

> There are seven planets in heaven, which on earth are the seven metals, and which are the seven principal organs in man, who was formed according to the idea of both and for that reason is rightly called *Microcosmus*. And all these are so excellent and mutually connected by a pleasing likeness, that they almost seem to have equal offices and the same natures and properties.[53]

This rather expansive account was in reply to Rothmann's request, a year earlier, that Tycho clarify what he meant by terrestrial astronomy.[54] Tycho explained that the sun correlated with gold in the terrestrial world and with the heart in man (*microcosmus*). A similar correspondence existed among the six remaining triples: moon-silver-brain; Jupiter-tin-blood; Venus-copper-kidneys; Saturn-lead-spleen; Mars-iron-gallbladder; Mercury-quicksilver-lung.[55] Another letter to Rothmann reveals a well developed Paracelsian cosmology that underlies Tycho's "terrestrial astronomy":

> Besides, in these seven, many [things] are mutually connected by a marvelous similitude which cannot be explained in a few words. So, too,

---

52 John Christianson, "Tycho Brahe's German Treatise on the Comet of 1577: A Study in Science and Politics," *Isis* 70 (1979), p. 112. Tycho's oration is printed in *TBDOO*, vol. 1, pp. 143-73.

53 Letter from Tycho to Rothmann, 17 August 1588, *TBDOO*, vol. 6, p. 145: "Id esse septem Planetas in Cælo, quod sunt septem Metalla in Terra, quodque in homine ad vtriusque ideam fabricato, qui ob id Microcosmus recte appellatur, septem principalia membra, atque hæc omnia tam pulcra, & concinna similitudine inuicem colligata sunt, vt paria fere videantur habere officia easdemque proprietates & naturas."

54 Letter from Rothmann to Tycho, 11 October 1587, *TBDOO*, vol. 6, p. 118: "Perquam scire cupio, quid in Arte Spagyrica appelletis Solem, quid Lunam, quid Saturnum, Iouem, Martem, Venerem, Mercurium, quid Elementa." [I would very much like to know what in the Spagyric art you would call the Sun, what the Moon, what Saturn, Jupiter, Mars, Venus, Mercury, and what the Elements.]

55 Here Tycho was repeating material presented in his oration at the University of Copenhagen in 1574. See Dreyer, *Tycho Brahe*, pp. 76-77.

the rest of the minerals of the earth, the gems, marchasites, and salts, agree with different planets by a certain law, and they are associated especially with the nature of the fixed stars, and contain powers of the planets in them, secretly as it were, just as even herbs and vegetables are assigned by a certain definite order in the terrestrial Astronomy, not only to the planets but also to the fixed stars. They emulate the nature of those same [heavenly bodies], insofar as they can.[56]

This view of the mutual connectedness of the world, a world in which celestial powers inhere in minerals and vegetables, is quite within the mainstream of Renaissance Platonism (or Hermetism), a point Tycho makes clear: "There are many authors in this more secret philosophy, among whom [are] … that famous Hermes Trismegistus, … Isaac Holland, and Theophrastus Paracelsus, whom more people attack than understand."[57] Hermes Trismegistus was the apocryphal author of a body of theological and philosophical writings from the early Christian era that in Tycho's day were thought to date back to Egypt in the age of Moses. Alchemical treatises were also attributed to him, and by the late sixteenth century, the terms "Hermetic doctor" and "Hermetic physician," or simply *Hermeticus*, were synonymous with Paracelsian theorists and chemical practitioners. Isaac Holland was, probably, a post-Paracelsian alchemical author, who was believed to have lived in the fifteenth century because of the similarities between his writings and those of Paracelsus. By listing these authors, Tycho was recreating the intellectual lineage from the ancient magi to Paracelsus, who was regarded as one of the recent receivers of the ancient Hermetic wisdom.

---

56 Letter from Tycho to Rothmann, 17 August 1588, *TBDOO*, vol. 6, p. 145: "Multa sunt præterea in his septem admiranda similitudine, quæ paucis explicari nequit, sibi inuicem colligata; Sic etiam reliqua Terræ Mineralia, Gemmæ, Marchasitæ & Salia cum diuersis Planetis certa lege consentiunt, & naturæ imprimis Affixarum Stellarum associantur, quæ Planetarum vires in se licet obscurius contineant, quemadmodum etiam herbæ & vegetabilia e certo quodam ordine, non solum Planetis sed etiam fixis Sideribus in terrestri Astronomia assignantur, eorundemque naturam, quantum in se est, æmulantur."

57 Ibid., p. 146: "Authores in hac secretiore Philosophia sunt plurimi, inter quos … Hermes ille Trismegistus … Isaacus Hollandus & Theophrastus Paracelsus, quem plures oppugnant quam intelligunt."

Severinus had similarly placed Paracelsus in this tradition in his *Epistola*, and presumably the connection was regarded as adding legitimacy to Paracelsus' work.

Thus, it is clear from Tycho's written profession of his philosophy and from the form that his research efforts took, involving chemical and astronomical studies at Herrevad, on Hven, and eventually in Bohemia, that he aimed to unravel the inner secrets of nature's workshop. Tycho's "terrestrial" astronomy reflects a commitment to a Paracelsian worldview that he had in common with Pratensis and Severinus, and it was no doubt shared with those who visited or studied on Hven.

IATROCHEMIA AT URANIBORG

Terrestrial astronomy involved more than chemical investigation. It included, for example, an attempt to correlate celestial astronomy with changes in terrestrial weather, for which Uraniborg's meteorological diary survives. But even this was chemical in the larger sense that Paracelsus had meant the term, and Tycho lavished great care on it:

> For I carefully cultivate this terrestrial Astronomy with no less effort and expense than that celestial Astronomy, by arranging to treat it properly, in suitable buildings, and with a great variety and number of furnaces, all which things the pen does not manage to convey.[58]

The layout of Tycho's facilities on Hven has fascinated students of the development of the laboratory as a location for science and also because of the laboratory's connection with the emergence of new approaches to science that characterize a scientific revolution. One recent study of Tycho's laboratory design has suggested that its placement in the basement of Uraniborg is symbolic of the dark, private nature of Tycho's Paracelsian

---

58 Ibid., p. 146: "Non enim minori conamine & sumptu Astronomiam hanc terrestrem excolo, quam illam cælestem, ordinatis ad eam rite tractandam, oportunis structuris, & fornacum magna varietate, copiaque, quæ omnia calamus referre non sustinet."

chemistry.[59] Architectural logic offers a more likely explanation for this arrangement, however, since it is hard to imagine the instruments of both Tychonic sciences combined in such a small building in any other way. Uraniborg needed to serve as the residence of a feudal lord and his research assistants as well as house the equipment and library demanded by both terrestrial and celestial astronomy.[60] Indeed, statements by visitors suggest that Tycho showed them his furnaces and retorts as readily as his sextants and quadrants. For example, Johan David Wunderer reported on his trip to the island ca. 1590:

> I have seen in an underground room devoted to the chemical art many unusual furnaces and apparatus, various large flasks of thirty measures, many amazing kettles, alembics, cucurbits and similar strange utensils, which all had been procured at great cost.[61]

Another German, one "Augustinus friherre af Mörszberg," commented on the wealth of apparatus in the laboratory:

59 See Owen Hannaway, "Laboratory Design and the Aim of Science," *Isis* 77 (1986): 585-610. Hannaway reproduces Andreas Libavius' criticism of Tycho Brahe's approach to science. It is evident from the conclusion that the author has adopted some aspects of Libavius' dialectic, which pits his open, humanist science against Tycho's Paracelsian occultism, elaborated in the secrecy of his island retreat. Ironically, Libavius may have harbored his own hidden chemical agenda, as is argued in William Newman, "Alchemical Symbolism and Concealment: The Chemical House of Libavius," in *The Architecture of Science*, ed. Peter Galison and Emily Thompson (Cambridge, MA: MIT Press, 1999), pp. 59-77.

60 There are, in fact, several factual and interpretive errors evident in Hannaway's analysis of Uraniborg. For example, we see in the sketches of Uraniborg windows to permit light into the *half* basement laboratory suggesting that Tycho was not concerned to keep chemical procedures away from the light of day. See Jole Shackelford, "Tycho Brahe, Laboratory Design, and the Aim of Science: Reading Plans in Context," *Isis* 84 (1993): 211-30.

61 "Afhandlinger om Tycho Brahe, Samlet af J. Dreyer," Kgl. Bibl. Copenhagen. Among the materials collected by Dreyer was "Et par optegnelser om Uraniborg 1894, Kjøbenhavn" by F.R. Friis. Friis copied Wunderer's letter (p. 10) from *Frankfurtisches Archiv für ältere deutsche Litteratur und Geschichte*, 1813, vol. 2, p. 174: "Demnach hab ich in einem *cubiculo etiam subterraneo, ad artem chymicam destinato* viel selzamer künst und Brenöffen, mancherlei grosze Gläszer von 30 Maszen grosz, viel wunderberlicher kessell, *Alembica, Cucurbiten* und dergleichen frembde Geschirr, die all mit grosem uncosten zu wegen bracht worden, gesehen."

Downstairs next to the wine cellar is a large vault in which Tycho's stills and furnaces are, upon which stand a large quantity of distillation flasks. A lot of them are curved at the top, made of copper, going out through some windows and in through others, in which unusual things are distilled.[62]

Tycho briefly described his laboratory at Uraniborg in his *Astronomiæ instauratæ mechanica*, which he published in 1598, after having abandoned Uraniborg and Denmark. This book highlights his facilities on Hven and contains illustrations of Uraniborg and Stjærneborg as well as Tycho's elaborate observational devices. It was an advertisement for Tycho's astronomical achievements and abilities and may well have been intended to attract foreign patronage as well as securing his place in history. Thus, when we read that Tycho devoted a great deal of time and money to the construction of an elaborate laboratory, and that he had done so with the approval and encouragement of King Frederik II, we must suspect that he intended his readers (potential patrons?) to be attracted to his chemical as well as to his astronomical expertise.[63] The following quotation from the *Mechanica*, concerning Tycho's alchemical work, illustrates this point.

I have been occupied by this subject as much as by the celestial studies from my twenty-third year, trying to gain knowledge and to prepare it, and up to now I have with much labour and at great expense made a great many findings with regard to the metals and minerals as well as

---

62 F.R. Friis, "Et par optegnelser," p. 12, quoted from *Martin Zeillers Neue Beschreibung der Königreiche Dennemarck und Norwegen* (Ulm, 1648): "Unten, neben dem Weinkeller, ist ein grosz Gewölb, in solchem sind desz *Tychonis* Diestelierwerck, und Oefen, auff welchen ein grosse Meng von Distillier Gläser stehen, etliche sind gar krumb, oben von Kupffer, so durch etliche Fenster hinausz gehen, und zum andern wieder hinein, darinnen werden sonderbare Sachen destillirt."

63 Ræder, *Tycho Brahe's Description* (*Astronomiæ instauratæ mechanica*, Wandesburg, 1598), p. 109: "When I had presented myself without delay this excellent King, who cannot be sufficiently praised, of his own accord and according to his most gracious will offered me that island in the far-famed Danish sound ... He asked me to erect buildings on the island, and to construct instruments for astronomical investigations as well as for chemical studies, and he graciously promised me that he would abundantly defray the expenses."

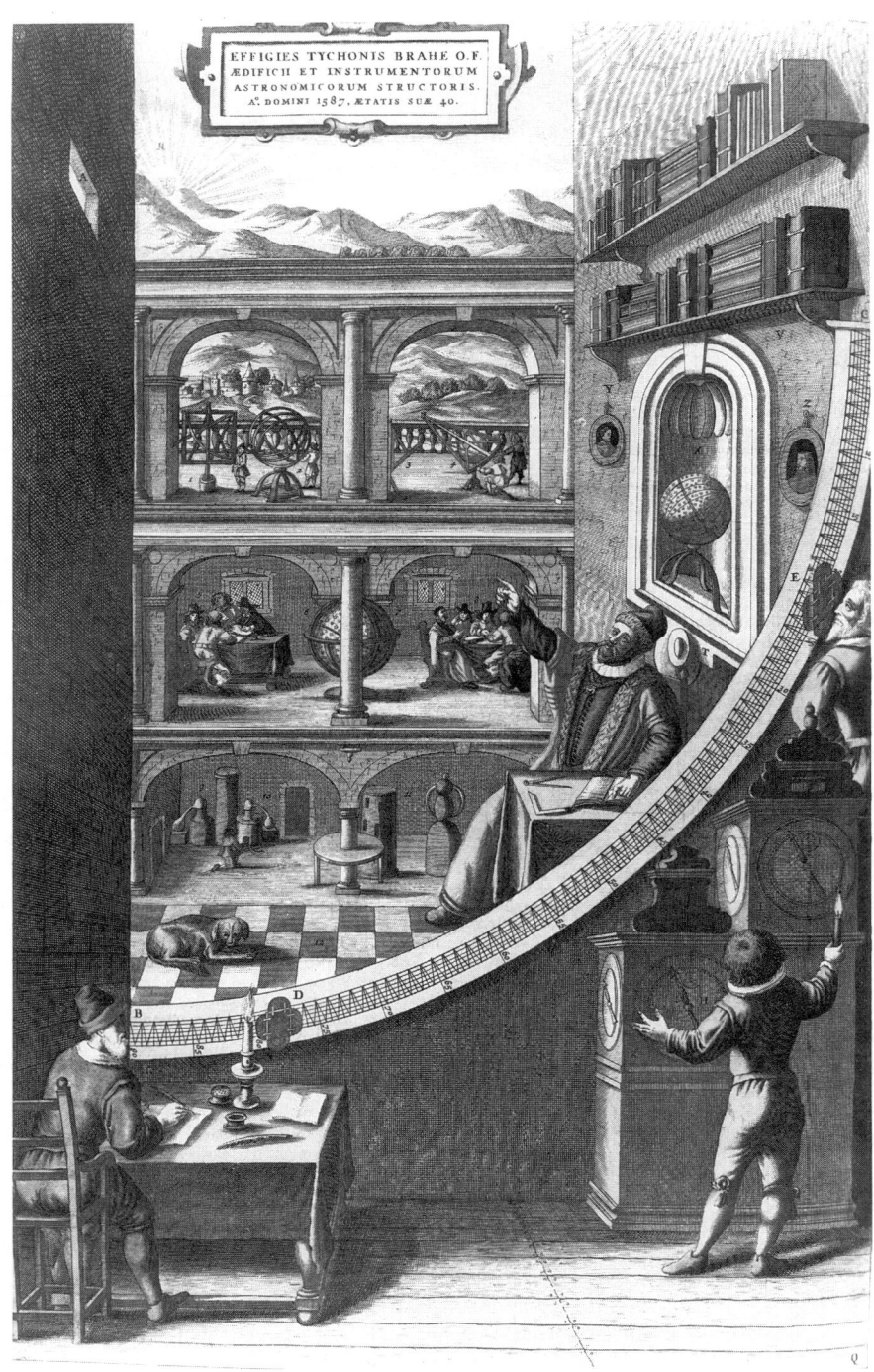

Tycho Brahe hired the Dutch painter Tobias Gemperlin to paint a mural in 1582 to decorate the wall on which he had mounted a large quadrant for accurately measuring the maximum altitude of heavenly bodies as they passed the meridian. The mural itself depicted the unity of Tycho's philosophical enterprise at Uraniborg: "Celestial astronomy," was investigated by means of sighting instruments shown on the upper story, while the mysteries of "terrestrial astronomy" (chymia) were plumbed in the laboratory located in the basement below, which was partially dug into the ground. In the library and workroom on the main floor, above the laboratory, Tycho and his assistants and perhaps visiting scholars discussed philosophy, reduced observational data, and recorded the positions of stars on the great celestial globe. The mural, quadrant, and observing team are depicted here in an illustration printed by Tycho's student Johan Blau in his Atlas major, *but copied closely from one that Tycho had printed in his* Astronomiæ instauratæ mechanica. *Courtesy of the James Ford Bell Library, University of Minnesota.*

---

the precious stones and plants, and other similar substances. I shall be willing to discuss these questions frankly with princes and noblemen, and other distinguished and learned people, who are interested in this subject and know something about it, and I shall occasionally give them information, as long as I feel sure of their good intentions and that they will keep it secret. For it serves no useful purpose, and is unreasonable, to make such things generally known.[64]

From this it is evident that Tycho regarded his knowledge of the chemistry of plants and minerals – a Paracelsian iatrochemistry – as proprietary, but to be shared with prospective patrons. Unlike his star catalogue, the publication of which would enhance his reputation, his supposed chemical secrets would be of little value unless kept exclusive. Therefore his "Pythagorean" unwillingness to open his secrets to the public seems as practical from the standpoint of securing patronage as was his willingness to share his achievements in astronomy, once his

64 Ibid., pp. 117-18.

priorities and successes were adequately credited.[65] But how private was his pursuit of chemical knowledge?

Tycho's secrecy about his various recipes has been used as a basis for generalizations about his pursuit of the contemplative life, as opposed to the active life of the responsible humanist natural philosopher and citizen. But Tycho was clearly willing to have students assist him in both celestial and terrestrial astronomy. We have his reference to the instruction he offered his students in observational astronomy "and other sciences," which from the context must have included astrology and alchemy.[66] Several of these students, young Danes who came to Hven to study for varying periods, were interested in medicine and participated in the "pyronomic activities" at Uraniborg. Among this group are Flemløse, Gellius Sascerides, and we might well include Tycho's sister Sophie, who attained a reputation for the preparation of chemical remedies.[67]

65 Thoren, *The Lord of Uraniborg*, gives a good overview of Tycho's consistent effort to assert the priority of his interpretations and techniques over those of his competitors for the sake of fame. This is most notorious in his struggle with Ursus over the "Tychonic system," but extends even down to assigning credit for accuracy to his observations in his correspondence with Landgraf Vilhelm of Hessen-Kassel and his mathematician, Rothmann. See especially pp. 271-2. For the significance of the shift from secret knowledge to public science, see William Eamon, "From the secrets of nature to public knowledge", in *Reappraisals of the Scientific Revolution*, ed. David C. Lindberg and Robert S. Westman (Cambridge: Cambridge University Press, 1990), pp. 333-365.

66 Ræder, *Tycho Brahe's Description*, p. 109: "So, in the year 1576, I began building a castle Uraniborg, suitable for the study of Astronomy ... Meanwhile I also energetically started observing, and for this work I made use of the assistance of several students who distinguished themselves by talents and a keen vision. I had such students in my house all the time, one class after another, and I taught them this and other sciences."

67 Both Flemløse and Sascerides received M.D.s from Basel after leaving Hven. On Tycho's students, see Victor Thoren, "Tycho Brahe as the Dean of a Renaissance Research Institute," in *Religion, Science, and Worldview*, ed. M. J. Osler and P. L. Farber (Cambridge: Cambridge University Press, 1985), pp. 277 and 280. On Sophie Brahe, see Frederik C. Schønau, *Samlinger af danske lærde fruentimer* (Copenhagen: N.H.M., 1753), especially pp. 198-99, 205, and 231; and F.R. Friis, *Sophie Brahe Ottesdatter* (Copenhagen: Gad, 1905), especially pp. 39-43. Sometime between 1588 and 1594 Tycho reported that his sister prepared chemical drugs, which she not only provided to friends and nobles, but also distributed to the poor. In that account he also mentioned a now-lost letter that he received from Sophie, which demonstrated that she was becoming knowledgeable in alchemy. She herself wrote to her sister, Margrete, that she was occupied with distillation. This letter is printed in Johan Ludvig Heiberg, *Johan Ludvig Heibergs Prosaiske Skrifter* (Copenhagen: Reitzel, 1861), vol. 9, pp. 325-360. Legend says that Sophie had a servant skilled in drug preparation, who was named Live Lauridsdatter and who was previously employed by Tycho at Hven and was supposed to have died in 1698 at age 123. As early as 1700, it was reported that Ole Borch, professor of chemistry at the

→

Her second husband, Erik Lange, was an old friend of Tycho. His zeal for the philosophers' stone seems to have exceeded his understanding of the proper goals of iatrochemistry, as Tycho noted in a long poem called *Urania Titani* that he composed on Sophie's behalf, in which she contrasted her own views of chemistry (or Tycho's) with Erik's:

> Ars mea (condones) celsior arte tua est.
> Ut coelum terras, sic nostra Ars Chimica vincit,
> Adde quod hæc vera est, Chimia falsa nimis.[68]

Inspection of Uraniborg was a part of the social itinerary for many of the foreign and native nobles and scholars who visited Copenhagen in Frederik II's reign, such as the two Germans whose observations about the laboratory facilities were quoted above. This comes as no surprise, since the aristocracy – Tycho's noble peers – included many besides Erik Lange who dabbled in alchemy. Frederik himself was allegedly interested in alchemy, and there are records of Queen Sophie's request of chemical glassware and materials from Tycho, implying that she also tried the art, or facilitated the efforts of another operator at court. Her father was the alchemically-inclined Duke Ulrich of Mecklenburg, who visited the island in 1586. When King James VI of Scotland came to Denmark to collect his bride, he made a trip to Hven, too. Later, as King of England,

→ University of Copenhagen in the middle of the seventeenth century, owned a large quantity of her chemical manuscripts. Her reputation persisted, and Schønau reported in the eighteenth century that she had spent considerable sums of money on "chemical distillations," but no trace of her manuscripts survives.

68 *TBDOO*, vol. 9, p. 202: "My art, you might call it, is superior to yours. As the heavens are superior to the earth, so our chemistry surpasses yours. Moreover, this is the true chemistry; yours is quite false." Heiberg's Danish translation indicates that she meant that astronomy was far superior to chemistry: "Høit som himmelen staaer over Jord, staaer over Chymien Astrologie, og er sand, hiin kun bedragerisk er." Heiberg, *Prosaiske Skrifter*, vol. 9, p. 308. I do not think this interpretation is correct. Sophie is comparing her chemical art (*nostra Ars Chimica*, i.e. Tycho's *astronomia terrestris*) to that of Erik, mundane goldmaking, which is *Chimia falsa*. This also suggests that the important social criterion in chemistry was not the avoidance of manual labor, but rather the end to which it was directed. It has been argued that Tycho actually composed this poem, but I see no reason why its content could not also reflect Sophie's message to her husband. See Peter Zeeberg, "Kemi og kærlighed: Naturvidenskab i Tycho Brahes latindigtning," in *Litteratur og Lærdom: Dansk-svenske nylatindage april 1985*, ed. Marianne Alenius and Peter Zeeberg. Renaissancestudier #1 (Copenhagen: Museum Tusculaneum, 1987), p. 150.

he became a great patron of chemical medicine.[69] The one nobleman we would most expect to have toured Tycho's laboratory and observatory and tested Tycho's hospitality was Landgraf Wilhelm of Hessen-Kassel. Wilhelm and his son, Moritz, were ardent supporters of both astronomy and chemistry, and Tycho's familiarity with the situation at the court of Hessen-Kassel may well have shaped his own aspirations for Uraniborg.[70] However, the Landgraf never came, but instead sent his mathematician, Rothmann, to confer with Tycho. Rothman and Tycho corresponded on various matters, and although we do not hear of Rothmann's interest in chemistry, he would likely have reported Tycho's activity to his superior. The meteorological diary, which Tycho had one of assistants keep, records that a certain "Johannes Rongel, noble chemist" came to Uraniborg on the evening of 28 May 1593 and apparently stayed until 18 July, and if he did not engage in chemical work with Tycho, surely he would have been at least shown the laboratory during his seven-week visit.[71] Tycho's reputation must have spread among the aristocracy, because years later, after he had left Hven, the Electress of Brandenburg (Christian IV's mother-in-law) wrote to Tycho asking him to instruct Johann Müller, their court mathematician, in the spagyric art.[72] When Müller later joined Tycho in Bohemia, he may have assisted him with alchemy as well as the mathematical computation necessary to process the astronomical data.[73]

---

69 Thoren, *The Lord of Uraniborg*, pp. 266, 334-35, and 378. Thoren does not say whether James examined Tycho's chemical laboratory, but it would surely have been part of the tour of Uraniborg for such an exalted prince.

70 John Christianson, "Cloister and Observatory," has pointed to Herrevad Cloister in Skåne as a model for the development of Hven. But Tycho had also visited Hessen-Kassel, where a great deal of money was available for these pursuits, and I suspect the Landgraf was himself, as a wealthy prince-patron of astronomy and alchemy, a model for the young Danish nobleman.

71 Frederik R. Friis, *Tyge Brahes Meteorologiske Dagbog, Holdt Paa Uraniborg for Aarene 1582-1597* (Copenhagen: H.H. Thiele, 1876), pp. 211-212: "Johannes Rongel Cymista nob." The name was unclear to the editor.

72 Letter of 14 February 1598, *TBDOO*, vol. 14, p. 135.

73 Thoren, *The Lord of Uraniborg*, p. 448. Clearly Tycho's practice of alchemy did not end with his abandonment of Uraniborg. While Tycho was moving his household to Copenhagen, he wrote to Heinrich Rantzov 22 Feb. 1597 that he intended to set up "a chemical laboratory with a printing press" there because he was "heavily occupied with all these things." Ibid., p. 370, Thoren's translation. There is also evidence that he began building a laboratory at Benatky Castle in Bohemia, too. See his letter to his sister Sophie, 21 March 1600, translated by John Christianson, Ibid., pp. 507-511.

We can see from Tycho's references to his laboratories and the chemical secrets he learned there, some of which have been mentioned above, that Tycho did indeed guard his work. But to protect knowledge and skills by not publishing them is different from keeping them totally secret and not passing them on to the worthy student. This issue, which bears most directly on the assessment of the didactic role of Paracelsian chemistry, has recently been subjected to scrutiny in the case of the Johannes Hartmann at Marburg, who was patronized by the Landgraf.[74]

The fact that Tycho published his astronomical findings and left his laboratory notes to languish, if there were any, can be explained by the proprietary nature of these data. Tycho published his work in part to secure patronage, and whereas his astronomical data was clearly unmatched anywhere, his chemical findings would not likely have attracted the sort of interest he was seeking. Even so, several of his recipes, which do survive, were circulated for this very purpose, and they were done so with the understanding that they were to be kept private.[75]

Tycho's attitude toward chemistry was in part grounded in a Paracelsian epistemology, which demanded that the physician learn of the natural world directly. He wrote that chemistry does not treat hypothetical subjects,

> but those things which are truly touched with the hands, seen with the eyes, and perceived with the external and internal senses ... Truly Paracelsus rightly said that nobody knows more in this art than [what] he has himself experienced through fire. A more than Pythagorean silence prohibits entrusting these things to other than worthy and thoroughly suited disciples.[76]

74 See Bruce T. Moran, *Chemical Pharmacy Enters the University: Johannes Hartmann and the Didactic Care of Chymiatria in the Early Seventeenth Century* (Madison, WI: The American Institute of the History of Pharmacy, 1991), an important monograph on this subject.

75 Tycho sent three recipes to Heinrich Rantzov, written in his own hand and dated 13 December 1597, as a token of his gratitude for the hospitality offered him at Wandesbeck. Another was given to Emperor Rudolf II, dated 7 September 1599, Benatky. These found their way into Thomas Bartholin's hands, and he printed them in *Cista medica*, pp. 96-109 and 89-95 respectively.

76 Letter from Tycho to Rothmann, 17 August 1588, *TBDOO*, vol. 6, pp. 145-46: "Pyronomica Schola adeunda est quæ non ea quæ plausibiliter disseruntur, sed quæ veraciter
→

Some kinds of knowledge one could only gain through laboratory experience, not by reading books.[77] This attitude, not unlike what Francis Bacon found appealing about Severinus' call for students to experience nature first hand (discussed below, in chapter five), is not quite the same as that of Baconian empiricism or the experimental philosophy of the late seventeenth century. But neither should it be confused with some kind of anti-humanist, obscurantist program. Chemistry, like medicine, involved art as well as science, and required apprenticeship as well as book-learning. As such, a degree of intellectual exchange was built into any laboratory where there were students as well as visiting *adepti*, and at Uraniborg there were both. Before we can successfully "read" the floor plans of laboratories such as Tycho Brahe's for their sociological content, we must know more about what went on there, and depend less on rhetoric composed for some specific propaganda purpose.[78] Clearly, further study of the teaching and practice of Paracelsianism in other contexts will be needed to balance the historical opinions that have been built on the rhetoric surrounding Paracelsus.

→   manibus palpantur, oculis videntur & sensibus exterioribus interioribusque percipiuntur, manifestat … Rectissime enim inquit Paracelsus, neminem plus scire in hac Arte, quam ipsemet per ignem expertus sit. Hæc etenim alijs, quam dignis & idoneis penitus concredere discipulis, silentium vetat plus quam pythagoricum."

77   This distinction between the information coded into written text and that coded directly into nature is lucidly discussed in Owen Hannaway, *the Chemists and the Word: The Didactic Origins of Chemistry* (Baltimore: Johns Hopkins, 1975). But to cast late sixteenth-century dialogue into a humanist vs. Paracelsian dichotomy forces categories on persons whose work does not acknowledge them.

78   Hannaway, "Laboratory Design," has noted that Libavius' attitude toward Tycho Brahe changed between the first and second editions of *alchemia* (1597 and 1606), the plan of Uraniborg having appeared in Tycho's *Mechanica* in between (1598). In 1595 Libavius even expressed his hope that Tycho Brahe's laboratory would contribute to the practice of chemistry (p. 598). I suspect that what happened in the meantime was less likely a reorientation in the "ideological roots" of scientific life for Libavius than a reorientation of his search for patronage. In 1595-97 Tycho was still a wealthy and well established patron of astronomy and chemistry, hoping to see Uraniborg set on some sort of institutional footing that would enable it to survive him. Tycho Brahe's Denmark was also still effectively dominated by Philippist Lutherans, who were suspected of being "crypto-Calvinists" by the Gnesiolutherans to the south. By 1606 Brahe was dead and hopes for Hven as something other than a pastoral island were vain. Uraniborg had failed, and there was little to be gained by describing it favorably. Furthermore, the struggle to rid Denmark of Philippists was just beginning, and, as Hannaway notes (p. 587), Libavius was against the crypto-Calvinist conspiracy, fearing for the humanist tradition of Melanchthonian Aristotelianism. What we learn from Hannaway (and

→

JOHANNES PRATENSIS, PROFESSOR OF MEDICINE

Little is known about Johannes Pratensis' short career as professor of medicine at the University of Copenhagen. Quite likely he resided at one of the residences provided for professors, possibly the one later occupied by his successor, Anders Lemvig. He received 200 rigsdaler annually in salary, and this was supplemented by the free housing, prebends, and the share of the university's agricultural goods that went with his chair. Anders Lemvig enjoyed the income from a vicarage at Aarhus Cathedral and a prebend at the wealthy cathedral at Roskilde, which was attached to the medical professorship, and it can be assumed that Pratensis enjoyed these benefices before him.[79]

As holder of the second chair in medicine, Pratensis was obliged to lecture on medical practice as well as on mathematical subjects that were not currently covered by the professor of mathematics. Judging from his communications with Tycho Brahe, the fact that he reported a latitude for Aarhus, and that he wrote a now-lost *Prognosticon astrologicum super revolutionibus planetarum syzygias ad annum 1566* (Copenhagen, 1566), his "mathematical" teaching may well have included the astronomical and astrological knowledge that was regarded as a part of medicine. We know there was an interest in these subjects at the university, because Tycho Brahe was asked to lecture on them. Pratensis also lectured on Pliny's *Natural History*, at least during the autumn of 1572, when Tycho first mentioned to him his observation of the new star.[80]

In addition to teaching, there were other duties attached to university professorships, including adjudicating legal cases that touched on university and ecclesiastical affairs. Some of these were of a very serious nature. In April 1572, for example, less than a year after his appointment to the medical faculty, Pratensis judged an adultery case involving one of Denmark's bishops. In the course of a dispute between a priest in Landskrone and his wife, the woman had accused the Bishop of Lund, Tyge Asmund-

---

→ Libavius) is what Libavius' ideology was for the moment, and for that moment, Libavius would reap smaller reward for praising a dead chemist – even a noble one – than by aligning himself against Paracelsian religious enthusiasts; whether or not this tells us anything about Paracelsianism and the didactic tradition is less certain.

79 Rørdam, *KUH*, vol. 2, pp. 624 and 665.

80 Ibid., p. 602.

sen, of "immoral intercourse," a charge that could not be permitted to go unchallenged. A case of this seriousness required judges of the highest standing, and the king summoned several noblemen, the highest officials in the state church, and the professors of theology, law, and medicine.[81]

Another occasion on which Pratensis' opinion was solicited concerned the university's response to King Frederik II's demand that Niels Hemmingsen, the influential professor of theology, be examined regarding several statements he had written in support of a Calvinist interpretation of the Eucharist.[82] Hemmingsen had played a major part in determining the doctrine that the Danish Church and the University of Copenhagen promulgated, and this had been generally in agreement with the precepts of Philipp Melanchthon. However, in his 1574 treatise, *Syntagma institutionum christianarum*, he favored certain doctrines that were considered to be all too Calvinist by the conservative Lutherans in Germany. Under pressure from his noble German relatives, Frederik II was forced in 1576 to demand that Hemmingsen retract or satisfactorily explain his doctrine of the Eucharist.

Pratensis was among those who, while not demanding of Hemmingsen a more concise retraction or clarification of particular points, saw the wisdom of going along with the king's demands. Hemmingsen complied, and this foreshadowed a long struggle between the Philippists in the Danish Church and the Gnesiolutheran conservatives, who finally won control of the state church in the early seventeenth century and locked it onto the path of strict Lutheran orthodoxy. This shift in the direction that the confessional wind was blowing was an essential part of the changing political context that surrounded Severinus and Tycho Brahe during his last years in Denmark and endangered the career of Tycho's student Kort Aslakssøn in the early years of the next century.[83]

81 Holger Rørdam, "Efterretninger om M. Tyge Asmundsen, Biskop i Lund," *[Ny] Kirkehistoriske Samlinger* 2d ser., 4 (1867-68), pp. 332-334.

82 Holger Rørdam, "Uddrag av Acta Consistorii 1573-80, især angaaende D. Niels Hemmingsen,"*[Ny] Kirkehistoriske Samlinger* 2d ser., 4 (1867-68), p. 279.

83 On Kort Aslakssøn and his strife with the conservative Lutherans, see Oskar Garstein, *Cort Aslakssøn: Studier over Dansk-Norsk Universitets- og Lærdomshistorie omkring År 1600* (Oslo: Lutherstiftelsen, 1953), and Jole Shackelford, "Unification and the Chemistry of the Reformation," in *Infinite Boundaries: Order, Disorder, and Reorder in Early Modern German Culture*, ed. Max Reinhart. Sixteenth Century Essays and Studies, vol. 40 (Kirksville, Missouri: Sixteenth Century Journal Publishers, Inc., 1998), pp. 291-312.

Perhaps some of the cases on which Pratensis sat in judgement required his medical expertise. On 20 October 1575 he was summoned to
decide the legality of a testament left by Herluf Trolle and Birgitte Gøye,
childless aristocrats who sought to bequeath their estate to Herlufsholm
School. Pratensis had treated Birgitte, as is noted below, and was called
to her death bed in 1574. Now that she was dead, he was one of four
professors summoned to rule on the testament.[84]

Pratensis left little written material to posterity from which a more
detailed view of his Paracelsianism can be extracted. Besides several
surviving poems, including the gratulatory poem printed with Severinus'
Idea medicinæ, Pratensis' biographers have noted two lost works, which
might have shed light on his doctrines. The first was the astrological
treatise mentioned above; the second, judging from the title, a treatment
of the history, scope, and proper subject of medicine.[85] To these must be
added a poem that was printed with two Paracelsian collections, written in Latin hexameter under the title *Theophrastus Paracelsus veritatis
amatori* and composed sometime before the autumn of 1567.[86]

Concerning Pratensis' practice of medicine there are but a couple of
references, though he must have supplemented his salary through private
practice, as was common. The published correspondence of Birgitte
Gøye reveals that Pratensis treated her during the fall and winter of
1572-73. In a letter to her he writes:

> Dear Lady Birgitte. Herein I am sending you some small papers filled
> with that powder I said you should take every fourteenth day in the
> evening, in good wine, before you sit down to dinner: each time as
> much as is in each paper, just as you usually do. For it is necessary for

---

84 Rørdam, *KUH*, vol. 2, pp. 198 and 603. His name is not listed as a judge on the following
    day, when the judgement was reversed, suggesting that the trial was controversial.

85 Ibid., p. 604, lists the surviving and lost literary output attributed to Pratensis including
    the lost *Prognosticon astrologicum super revolutionibus planetarum syzygias ad annum
    1566* (Copenhagen, 1566) and *De ortu, progressu, subjectis et partibus artis medicæ* (Co-
    penhagen, 1572).

86 Sudhoff, *Bibliographia Paracelsica*, pp. 380 and 135-6, notes the inclusion of this poem in
    Dritter Theil der Bucher ... Paracelsi genannt (Basel: Conrad Waldkirch, 1589), which I
    have not seen, and *Medici Libelli ... Theophrasti Paracelsi* (Cologne: Arnold Birckman,
    1567). The poem in the 1567 volume is attributed to "I.P. Remigius Cimb. f.," whom
    Huser had identified as Johannes Pratensis, according to Sudhoff (p. 135).

you to use this mild medicine sometimes so, that it may gradually take away the fluid that is collected in your stomach and surrounding places and thus gives you occasion for your usual illness, both in your head and elsewhere.[87]

A letter to Birgitte Gøye from Mette Rosenkrantz in February 1573 also mentions Pratensis' treatment of Birgitte. Mette sent with the letter the medicine Pratensis prescribed, along with instructions as to its use.[88] Although this correspondence does not reveal an explicitly Paracelsian diagnosis or treatment, the indications are certainly compatible with Paracelsian practice; the use of a "powder" against a fluid accumulating in the stomach suggests a non-Galenic diagnosis, but by no means is this certain. However, such "powders" were notorious as signs of alchemically-prepared drugs.[89] The localization of the fluid in the abdomen, responsible for ailments in the head and elsewhere, is compatible with Paracelsian aetiology, and administration of the drug – in this case possibly a diuretic – in well defined doses (premeasured in the papers) is another hallmark of Paracelsian cures. Nevertheless, the evidence is ambiguous. Likewise, the nature of the "Alexiterion" that Pratensis and Severinus reportedly recommended during an epidemic in 1575, which "many people used to evident advantage," is not apparent.[90]

---

87 Letter from Pratensis to Birgitte Gjøe (Gøye), 26 October, probably 1572, printed in Gustav Ludvig Wad, ed., *Breve til og fra Herluf Trolle og Birgitte Gjøe* (Copenhagen: Thaning and Appel, 1893), vol. 2, p. 213: "Kiere frue Byrgite, ieg sender ether her naagle smaa papir fulle med den puluer, som ieg sagde, ath y skulle huer xiiij dag tage tiil eder om affthenen vdj god wiin, før y ganger tiil bordtz, huergang so megitt som vdj huert papiir er, liige som y pleyer ath giøre, thj det er eder fornøden, ath y so somme tiid bruger denne lette mediciin, ath det kan efftherhanden borttagis(!) den weske, som forsamlis vdi maffuen och omliggendis ørter och giffue eder so orsage tiill eders wonlige siugdom bode vdj hoffuedit och anderstedts."

88 Ibid., p. 226.

89 Consider Holberg's comedy, *The Arabian Powder* (1727), in which a powder is sought at Copenhagen's Old Market, the place where itinerant "empirics" plied their wares. See E. C. Werlauff, *Historiske Antegnelser til L. Holbergs Lystspil* (Copenhagen: Schultz, 1838), vol. 1, p. 117.

90 Rørdam, *KUH*, vol. 2, p. 603: "Og da Pesten rasede 1575, anordnede de i Forening et 'Alexiterion', som mange Mennesker brugte med synlig Nytte mod Sygdommen."

THE DEATH OF PRATENSIS

The interest in Paracelsian cosmology and pharmacology shared by Severinus, Pratensis, Tycho, and their mutual friend and supporter Charles Danzay was no doubt sustained by personal contact as well as frequent correspondence. This intellectual fellowship, founded on their experiences as students abroad, a common commitment to reforming the sciences, and a rather liberal, Philippist Protestantism, began to come unglued in 1576.[91] Frederik II had given the use of Hven to Tycho Brahe in May of that year, and once planning and construction began, Tycho was often away from Copenhagen, where contact with his friends was most frequent. Pratensis' sudden death in June was even more detrimental to the Platonic circle, inasmuch as he was an important link in the fellowship. He, in particular, had been close to Tycho, being among the first to share in the events that moved his life – the discovery of the new star and the king's offer of Hven in fief. Pratensis was an intimate friend of Severinus from their years of travel together as medical students. He may also have been instrumental in drawing Danzay into the group. His father was French by birth, and Johannes may therefore have had a cultural affinity with the French ambassador that facilitated their friendship. Although Severinus and Tycho continued to correspond after Pratensis' death, and Tycho and Danzay remained good friends until the latter's death in 1589, contact among the members of the group probably diminished after 1576.[92]

91 Pratensis and Severinus, as Paracelsians, were *de facto* interested in broadening the scope of medicine to accommodate Paracelsian theory and practice. Tycho Brahe's wish to reform astronomy is well known in terms of his desire to put the science on a firm observational foundation and renew earth-centered cosmology, but I believe he meant this to apply to the whole of astronomy, not just the celestial part. The religious community of these four men and the role of Tycho's religious views in his alienation from Copenhagen's power hierarchy need further study. Danzay, like his successor Jacques Bongars, was a French Protestant, and his Calvinist views fit better with the Philippists' doctrine than with the growing Lutheran orthodoxy. See Rørdam, "Charles de Danzay," p. 298.

92 However, Thomas Moffet's dedication of his book *De iure et præstantia chemicorum medicamentorum dialogus apologeticus* (Frankfurt: Wechel, 1584) to Severinus included a greeting to Danzay and Tycho, which implies that an intellectual fellowship still persisted following Pratensis' death.

Pratensis' early and dramatic death was mourned by many, attesting to his popularity. Morten Pedersen noted the event in his historical calendar: "Doctor Johannes Pratensis of Århus, physician, great and learned man, died suddenly at the University of Copenhagen during his medical lecture. He suffocated in his own blood, which he spewed out."[93] Thomas Bartholin's account of Pratensis' death, taken from the memorial program given by the rector of the university, relates that Pratensis had suffered from a "very dangerous catarrh" for several years, and had been advised by a friend to stay home on the day he died, but that he insisted on lecturing as usual, since he was already prepared. As he spoke to his students, his coughing became worse, he suffered a pulmonary hemorrhage, and began expectorating large amounts of blood. He then expired in the arms of his students.[94] This report of Pratensis' sudden death in the classroom contrasts with a poem he presumably wrote to Danzay while on his deathbed, taking leave of his close friend. One explanation is that Pratensis had been severely ill for some time and composed the poem in anticipation of his death.[95]

Another friend, Isak Mouritsen, wrote a poem in fifty nine elegiac couplets to "Doctor Johannes Pratensis, learned philosopher, expert physician, exceptional poet: a good man before his death, a blessed man after."[96] In the course of the poem, Mouritsen alludes to Pratensis' many travels and achievements. A very moving account of the death itself was given by Christiern Nielsen Juel in his annal:

93   Holger Rørdam, ed., "M. Morten Pedersens historiske Kalenderantegnelser," *[Ny] Kirkehistoriske Samlinger*, 2d ser., 3 (1864-66), p. 494, entry for 1 June 1576. "Doctor Johannes Prattensis Arhusiensis, medicus, vir doctissimus et optimus, subito obiit in ipsa Academia Haphniensi in lectione sua medica, suffocatus a proprio sanguine, quem euomuit." That Pratensis was a personal friend of his is evident from a note on the latitude of Århus taken "from a most certain observation by our friend, Doctor Johannes Pratensis" (ex nostri amici doctoris Johannis Prattensis obseruatione certissima). Ibid., p. 498.

94   Bartholin, *Cista medica*, pp. 54-56.

95   If Pratensis had Tuberculosis, which is consistent with the report of his death from a severe lung hemorrhage, then he may have been mortally ill for some time and expecting to die when he wrote the undated farewell poem earlier that year. It is printed in Rørdam, "Charles de Danzay," pp. 324-326.

96   "M.D. Joannj Pratensi: Philosopho erudito: Medico perito: Poetæ eximio: Viro, ut ante mortem BONO: ita post eundem BEATO." Rørdam, *KUH*, vol. 4, #79, pp. 111-115. Rørdam reports a second memorial poem for Pratensis by the same author, along with the autograph ms. of this one, in Copenhagen, Kong. Bibl. NKS 2083g.

That same year [1576] the very learned man Doctor Johannes Pratensis, philosopher and physician at the University of Copenhagen, suddenly and against expectation, died from a cough and a very great quantity of blood, while he lectured publicly in the large auditorium. But before his spirit departed, he quickly spoke these words twice: Lord Jesus, be gracious to me, Lord Jesus, receive my spirit. Suddenly, with upraised arms, and his face turned toward heaven, and having given forth three or four gasps, he commended his soul to God, in the arms of his students, in that very place in which he had taught for nearly five years. And so he instructed his students up to the very last breath, and he migrated from the worldly school to the heavenly, on the fourth of June.[97]

Not surprisingly, this sudden death at so young an age was mourned by Pratensis' closest friends, Tycho Brahe, Danzay, and Severinus. Tycho wrote to Severinus urging him to compose a eulogy which he, Tycho, would pay to have inscribed on his friend's tomb.[98] Severinus complied with a short prose epitaph, which was evidently placed with Pratensis' corpse in The Church of Our Lady, in Copenhagen, where Severinus would eventually join him. He wrote it in the first person, as if Pratensis were speaking it, but ends with a reference to his own sadness: "If this sad, bitter fate could have been altered by tears or grief, Petrus Severinus, M.D., would not now have offered the indulgence of a dear remembrance to a friend who is without equal. He lived 32 years, 6 months,

---

97 Holger Rørdam, "Uddrag af Præsten Christiern Nielsen Juels Aarbog," *[Ny] Kirkehistoriske Samlinger*, 2d ser., 5 (1869-71), p. 367: "Eodem anno doctissimus vir Dn. Doctor Johannes Pratensis, philosophus et medicus in Academia Hafniensi, subito et præter expectationem, cum in auditorio maiore publice doceret, ex tussi quadam et ex nimia sanguinis copia extinctus est. Sed antequam emisit spiritum, *bis in hæc verba erupit: Domine Jesu, esto mihi propitius, Domine Jesu, suscipe spiritum meum. Mox sublatis manibus, et facie cælum versus conuersa, inter auditorum manus, tribus vel quatuor editis singultibus, animam Deo commendauit*, in eo ipso loco, in quo quinquennium fere docuerat. Atque ita ad extremum vsque vitæ spiritum auditores erudiebat, et e scola terrena in coelestem commigrauit die 4 Junij." The portion of the above account that I have italicized agrees verbatim with the account given in *Cista medica*.

98 Tycho's letter to Severinus, 3 September 1576, *TBDOO*, vol. 7, pp. 34-40.

and 3 days."[99] Ironically, it was Pratensis who was to have written the inscription to be cut into the cornerstone for Uraniborg that was to be sponsored by Danzay. Now Tycho was sponsoring a burial inscription composed by Severinus, and Danzay was writing to Tycho comparing the loss of their friend to the loss of half his soul.[100]

The death of his close friend at the beginning of such a massive scientific undertaking must have saddened Tycho greatly, and he wrote a poem of thirty couplets lamenting the loss of his friend:

> He died, oh woe, oh! Pratensis, has died at such a young age,
>   There was scarcely another more learned than him:
> Indeed, whatever the annals of the old sages held,
>   whatever the writings of the divine Plato held, [he knew.]
> And, Paracelsus, he practiced your arts as an expert,
>   though this astounded the empty headed lot of doctors.[101]

Once Uraniborg was fully operational as a research facility, complete with its own printing press, Tycho published this poem as a memorial to "Doctor Johannes Pratensis of Aarhus, a brilliant man possessed of virtue and education of every sort, an excellent doctor of Paracelsian and Galenic medicine," at Uraniborg in 1584.[102]

---

99   Severinus' epitaph for Pratensis is recorded in Bartholin, *Cista medica*, pp. 58-59: "Si lachrymis si moerore acerbum flecti potuisset fatum triste hoc jam caræ memoriæ obsequium incomparabili amico non detulisset Petrus Severinus Med. Doct. Vixit annos XXXII mens VI dies III obiit An. Sal. 1576 Kal. Jul. Hor. III." Note that the date of death given here is 1 July 1576.
100 Rørdam, "Charles de Danzay" p. 293. See letters from Danzay to Tycho 26 June and 14 July 1576 concerning the stone for Uraniborg.
101 *TBDOO*, vol. 9, p. 176, couplets 4-6:
     Occidit, ah dolor! ah! juvenilibus occidit annis
         Pratensis, quo vix doctior alter erat;
     Qvicqvid habent etenim veterum monumenta Sophorum,
         Divini quiquid Scripta Platonis habent,
     Et, Paracelse, tuas expertus calluit Artes,
         Doctorum licet hic vulgus inane stupet.
102 Ibid., pp. 176-77.

❀

For a short period of time in the 1570s, Paracelsian ideas must have been an important part of intellectual dialogue in Denmark. Pratensis was establishing a reputation as a good teacher at the University of Copenhagen, where he introduced something of the neoteric medical philosophy into his lectures. Severinus, whose *Idea medicinæ philosophicæ* was already beginning to attract attention abroad, brought his knowledge of Paracelsian medicine to the court of the Danish sovereign, where he would likely have engaged in conversation on these doctrines with foreign and native noblemen alike. For members of the educated aristocracy, which was a growing group in the late sixteenth century, Paracelsianism was a topic of current interest, as were other forms of Renaissance Platonism. In these years Tycho Brahe was laying the intellectual and actual foundations for what was to become perhaps Europe's first research station. At his uncle's manor at Herrevad, and later at Uraniborg, Tycho was to use Paracelsian, or at least semi-Paracelsian, cosmology as a basis for an actual research program in both celestial and terrestrial "astronomy." Tycho's quest for more and better data, painstakingly compiled by him and by those under his supervision, suggests that he took to heart Paracelsian admonitions about getting one's hands dirty.

Tycho Brahe's Hven itself became a site of iatrochemical research, drawing the curious visitor and the longer term student alike. In practice the laboratories at Uraniborg probably did more to promote interest in chemical medicine in Denmark than did the lectures of Pratensis, whose career was so brief. Several of Tycho's students were apparently drawn to Uraniborg for the opportunities he offered them as students of medicine, for which both astronomical and chemical knowledge were important.[103] These, in turn, took the precepts and practices of iatrochemistry with them into Danish society. Thus, although there were no Paracelsians in the medical faculty at the University of Copenhagen after the death of Pratensis in 1576, the concepts associated with chemical philosophy and the use of chemical medicines were sustained by those associated with Tycho Brahe and Petrus Severinus. In the last quarter of the sixteenth

103 Peder Jacobsen Flemløse was foremost among these.

century Paracelsianism enjoyed a tolerant, sometimes enthusiastic reception, but with the failure of Hven as an institution, and the failure of Paracelsianism to penetrate the official university curriculum, its influence on academic medicine was doomed to be marginal. Among the nobility, the popularity of chemical medicines seems to have run its course, as elsewhere in Europe.

Chapter Three

PETRUS SEVERINUS:
PERSONAL PHYSICIAN
TO THE KINGS OF DENMARK

ⅎROM HIS RETURN to Denmark in 1571 until his death in
1602, Petrus Severinus enjoyed the wealth and influence that accompanied his position as personal physician to the king of Denmark.
While Frederik II lived, Severinus traveled with the king as he moved
between the various royal residences and consequently had little leisure
for writing or other academic pursuits. Frederik sought to strengthen
the university and to expand the medical services available in the realm,
both of which likely involved Severinus.[1] Several new M.D.s were appointed city physicians in the regional capitals, the number of chartered
surgeons increased, and new apothecary privileges were issued by the
crown.[2] It was during these golden years that Severinus' friend Tycho
Brahe built Uraniborg on the island of Hven and established a model

---

1 As Frederik's physician, Severinus most likely would have been consulted on matters
of medical policy, such as the appointing of doctors and physicians and the regulating
of apothecaries. But the only surviving record tying Severinus to these activities is a
letter that he wrote to the Chancellor of the Realm, Arild Hvitfeld, concerning the
employment of an apothecary for Viborg (Rørdam, *KUH*, vol. 2, p. 581, note 3). I have
not seen this document.
2 According to Rørdam, *KUH*, vol. 2, p. 323, note 2, Dr. Hans Paludan was appointed
medicus in Viborg 5 Dec. 1571, Dr. Hans Lavritsen Amerinus in Ribe in 1583, and Dr.
Warwick in Malmø in 1577. In 1577 the new charter for the barber-surgeons' guild in
Copenhagen raised the number of masters from 6 to 10. During Severinus' career as
royal physician at least five new privileges for apothecaries were issued. See Sverre, *Et
studium av farmasiens historie*, pp. 81-86; Ingerslev, *Danmarks Læger*, vol. 1, pp. 209 ff.

research station there. They were years of peace and relative prosperity, and learned culture began to flourish.

A four-year regency followed Frederik's death in 1588, and during this time Severinus' life probably became more sedentary. In 1592 the new king, Christian IV, hired another personal physician, and although Severinus retained his office, he appears not to have accompanied the young king on his tours of the realm. During the last several years of the century Severinus may have become more closely associated with academic affairs and the medical community based in Copenhagen. In any case, when a chair finally became available in the medical faculty, Severinus sought to return to the academic life, where he might have continued the work begun with the publication of the *Idea medicinæ*. For thirty one years he had served the court, practiced medicine, and written, but death intervened before he managed to publish again.

Severinus was formally appointed personal physician to Frederik II by a letter of 14 October 1571, which stipulated his duties and compensation: He is required to attend the king at his pleasure, follow the court whenever and wherever he is so instructed, keep any royal matters he overhears in strict confidence, and practice medicine to the best of his ability. In particular, he is to prepare and administer medicines to the king in such a way that they do not come into the hands of strangers! In return Severinus is to receive an annual pension of 200 rigsdaler (a sum commensurate with Pratensis' salary), as well as free maintenance or a maintenance allowance and ordinary court attire for himself and an attendant. Furthermore, he is promised a free "house and dwelling" (in Copenhagen) in which he can conveniently prepare medicines. Lastly he is to be awarded a canonry at Roskilde Cathedral when one becomes vacant.[3]

In fact, Severinus received other benefices from Frederik II over the years. He was given a prebend at Viborg Cathedral in 1572 to tide him over until he could obtain the canonry at Roskilde, which he received in 1575.[4] In 1576 he was given an allowance of fodder to support two horses for as long as he lived in Copenhagen, and he also received in fief various scattered estates on Sjælland amounting to sixteen farms and

---

3 The letter is printed in Herholdt and Mansa, *Samlinger*, pp. 17-18.
4 Laursen, *Kancelliets Brevbøger*, vol. 5, pp. 98 (5 Jan. 1572) and 682 (18 oct. 1575).

two houses that had previously been held by Dr. Martinus Ædituus, who by this time had departed from Denmark.[5] Although the letter promised Severinus a house in Copenhagen in which he could prepare his medicines, and presumably this involved chemical furnaces, there is no indication that he lived independently before 1583. As a single man attached to the court, he likely spent most of his time traveling with the king and lodging in the royal residences.

On 9 June 1583 Petrus Severinus married Drude Thorsmeden, daughter of a prominent Slesvig family in Flensborg.[6] Drude was born in April 1567 and must therefore have been sixteen years old when she wed Petrus, apparently on the advice of her parents.[7] As a wedding present the university gave Severinus a silver serving piece. This sort of gift was not uncommon for professors at the time, and it indicates that Severinus, who was not a professor, was considered deserving of the gift-giving that solidified the bond between him and the university community. It may be that the medical faculty already viewed the royal physician and alumnus as a protagonist of academic affairs at the court of Frederik II, whose patronage the university needed. As a man well educated at some of Europe's best institutions, Severinus probably advised the king in matters pertaining to natural philosophy and medicine, and if so, he would have been an important ally for the university. Certainly he was fondly remembered in the university funeral program:

> He was always of great assistance to our university in many serious matters, so that for some time we expected and welcomed the idea that he would be approved as our colleague and added to the faculty, if the

---

5 Ibid., vol. 6, pp. 22 (16 March 1576) and 54 (13 May 1576); Herholdt and Mansa, *Samlinger*, p. 19.

6 Entry for 9 June 1583 in Kaae, *Almanakoptegnelser*, p. 156. Drude (Gertrude) was the daughter of councilman Reinhold Thorsmeden and Gesa Lange and was first cousin to Thomas Fincke, the great medical patriarch of seventeenth-century Copenhagen. Through this connection the leading physicians and medical professors in Copenhagen were related. Bastholm, *Petrus Severinus*, p. 33, provides a family tree.

7 Bartholin, *Cista medica*, p. 120 records her death as occurring on 21 September 1610 at age forty three years, five months, and two days, which would put her birth date at 19 April 1567. According to an account of the funeral oration delivered by the rector of the university, she married Severinus "de parentum consilio" and lived in marriage with him peacefully and blamelessly for a little over nineteen years.

kinder fates would have it, although indeed he was always very much a part of our order and council.[8]

Indeed, Severinus was consulted about university decisions despite the fact that he was not a member of the faculty. On one occasion, for example, he mediated a delay in giving a travel grant to Kort Aslakssøn, a Danish student assisting Tycho Brahe at Uraniborg, who wished to study abroad. Although Severinus may have acted on behalf of his friend Tycho, who would continue to benefit from Aslakssøn's help, it is also true that he was adhering to a previous stipulation. In his letter to the university consistory, Severinus pointed out that Aslakssøn must wait until the stipend term of another medical student is completed before he can receive the stipend.[9]

In November 1583, not many months after his marriage, Severinus was given a piece of the university's land in Copenhagen, part of the garden attached to Anders Lemvig's residence on Store Kannikestræde, northeast of The Church of Our Lady, and there he built his house. In 1592 Severinus was given some additional land adjacent to this house in exchange for building onto Anders Lemvig's residence. The site of Severinus' house is today identified with Ehlers' Collegium on Store Kannikestræde.[10] As a final note of the esteem in which Frederik II held him, Severinus was given a princely landed estate in South Jut-

8   Ibid., p. 116: "Academiæ nostræ magno semper adjumento fuit in multis rebus gravissimis, ut speraverimus & exopteraverimus ipsum aliquando Collegam nobis, si fata benigniora voluissent, adscitum & conjunctum iri, quanquam ipse quidem ordini nostro re & consilio semper fuit conjunctissimus."

9   Holger Rørdam, "Uddrag af Konsistoriets Forhandlinger 1590," *[Ny] Kirkehistoriske Samlinger*, 2d ser., 5 (1869-71), p. 64. Bjørn Kornerup, "Cort Aslaksen. I Anledning af Oskar Garsteins Disputats," *Kirkehistoriske Samlinger*, 7th ser., 2 (1954-56) pp. 360-61, argues that Severinus did not request that Aslakssøn's travel stipend be delayed on behalf of Tycho Brahe, who presumably wished to hold onto Aslakssøn awhile longer, but rather that Severinus was defending the promise made to Niels Svanning, who was a medical student and fellow Ripenser.

10 The deed of transfer is printed in Rørdam, *KUH*, vol. 4, #228, pp. 319-20. Ibid., vol. 2, p. 580 says that the land deeded to Severinus in 1583 enlarged a lot he already owned on Kannikestræde, but the deed of transfer mentions only land that belonged to Lemvig's garden; Reinhold Mejborg, *Borgerlige Huse, særlig Kjøbenhavns Professor-Residentser 1540-1630* (Copenhagen: Gad, 1881), pp. 84-85.

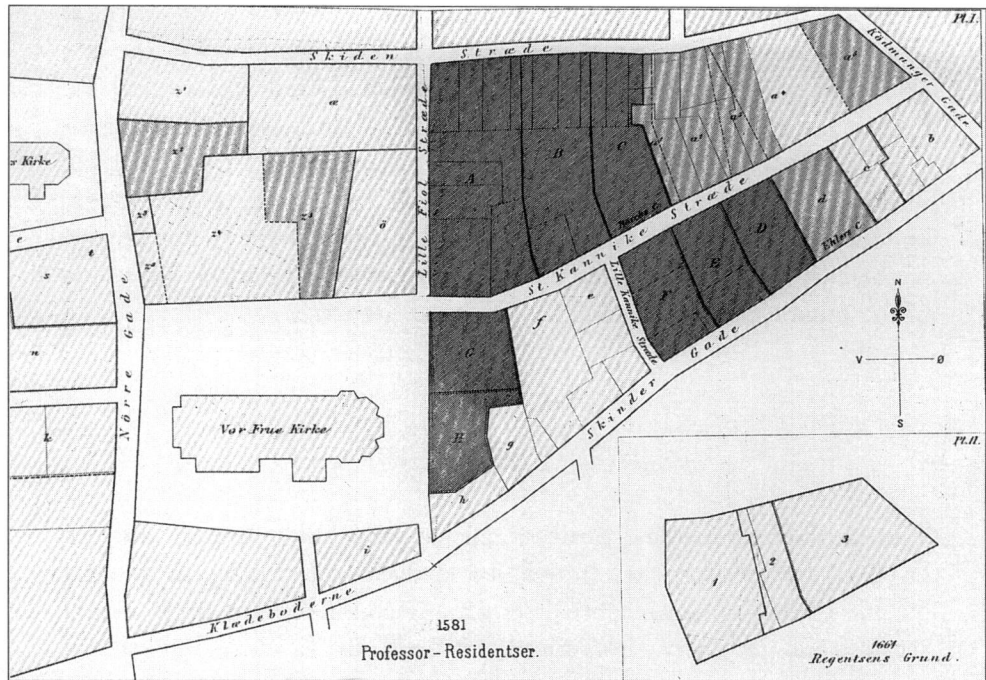

1581
Professor – Residentser.

1661
Regentsens Grund.

*Petrus Severinus' house in Copenhagen was among the residences of the professors at the University of Copenhagen, which are labeled with capital letters **A** through **H**. It is identified in this drawing as lot **d**, later Ehlers Collegium, on Skindergade, just next to Anders Lemvig's residence (lot **D**). Reproduced from R. Mejborg,* Borgerlige huse, særlig Kjøbenhavns professor-residentser *(Copenhagen: Gad, 1881), fold-out drawing at back.*

land, in 1587.[11] Frederik II died the following year, and Severinus' new patron, Christian IV, does not appear to have added to his income or properties. Nevertheless, Severinus was reckoned to be a wealthy man when he died.[12]

11 Rørdam, *KUH*, vol. 2, p. 579. Also, Laursen, *Kancelliets Brevbøger*, vol. 6, p. 728 lists a letter (dated 7 May 1587, Haderslev) giving to Severinus and his decendants a landed estate at Astrup in Brøns Parish, Hviding Herred, in South Jutland, to be held tax free, as any other privileged property of the nobility or belonging to the Duchy of Slesvig.

12 Henrik Fuiren, in his 1641-42 list of Danish students who had matriculated at Padua, recorded that Severinus had "died of plague, old and very wealthy" [obiit peste senex & ditissimus]. See Ingerslev, *Danmarks Læger*, p. 181.

Petrus and Drude had eight children, and although many of these died very young, their household was quite likely very busy in the late 1580s and 1590s. At least two of these, Anna and Frederik, would have been at home from their birth in the mid 1580s until their father's death in 1602. The high fertility and mortality characteristic of this period set its imprint on life in the Severinus household: between 1594 and 1603 six children were born, five of which died at age 3 or younger.[13] The brevity of their lives must have been a constant reminder to Petrus Severinus of the tenuousness of life and the limits of his art.

SEVERINUS AS ROYAL PHYSICIAN

The number of medical professionals resident in Denmark and the levels of service that they provided increased considerably in the last quarter of the sixteenth century, creating a complex situation in which services and authority sometimes overlapped. By the second quarter of the seventeenth century, Christian IV had access to a variety of healers, including personal physicians, court physicians, surgeons, and apothecaries. There were also medical doctors serving as court chemist and overseeing the king's botanical garden, and these, too, could be drawn on for advice. And of course the medical professors at the university were also called in for consultations as needed. But in the sixteenth century, the diversity and number of practitioners at court was more limited. Even during Frederik II's reign there seems to have been no distinction between personal physician to the king (*livmedicus*) and court physician (*hoffmedicus*), suggesting that there were fewer physicians at the top of the medical hierarchy.

Besides the royal physician or physicians, there were other healers serving Frederik's court, usually both a court apothecary and a court

---

13 The following death dates were recorded for the Severinus children in Bartholin, *Cista medica*, p. 120: Sophie, died 3 Sept. 1594 at age three years, three months, five days; Botilda, died 22 Sept. 1596 at seven months, three days; Reinholdus died 21 Oct. 1597 at nine months, thirteen days; Severinus died 11 Sept. 1602 at three years, three months; Johannes died 3 Jan. 1603 at three years, two months, five days.

barber-surgeon. Severinus would have worked with these on a regular basis, ordering *materia medica* from the court apothek and calling on the surgeon when surgical procedures were required. Severinus probably made his own chemical drugs, however, and may have let blood. Therapeutic and prophylactic bleeding was an established part of Galenic medicine, and although some Paracelsian physicians dissented, we know that Severinus was not wholly opposed to bleeding, because he performed a venesection on his friend Peder Hegelund in Germany. However, routine bleeding at court may also have been left to a barber surgeon.

In 1571, when Severinus took up his new appointment at court, Antonius Preus was the king's apothecary. It was his responsibility to procure *materia medica* from licensed apothecaries and provisioners in Copenhagen or elsewhere and to see to it that the court had on hand whatever was needed. The court apothecary was, like the royal physician, supposed to accompany the court in its peregrinations. However, Preus was permitted to open an apothek in Copenhagen, and he appointed an apprentice to travel with the king in his stead. There were complaints that Preus did not adequately supply the apprentice, requiring the purchase of drugs from other sources, and in 1580 Preus was replaced by Caspar Castorph, who remained in his post until his death in 1607. Rooms designated as "the apothek" existed at the royal castles in Copenhagen and Fredriksborg, and we can suppose that similar rooms were to be found at other residences frequented by the court as it travelled about the realm.[14] Information about court barber-surgeons (*bartskærer*) is less detailed than for apothecaries, perhaps because they were of lower rank, but two are mentioned during Frederik II's reign, Hans Bartskær and Mikkel Møller Bartskær. These men probably served the court in addition to functioning in other capacities, such as barber-surgeon to the city workhouses.[15] Christian IV hired his own personal barber-surgeon in 1591, when Daniel Hogenvald, who had been in service at

14 Ingerslev, *Danmarks Læger*, pp. 212-14; Aage Schæffer, "Studier til dansk Apothekervæsens Historie: Hofapotekere og Hofkemikere i Danmark ca. 1540-1660," *Theriaca: Samlinger til Farmaciens og Medicinens Historie*, vol. 8 (Copenhagen: Danske Farmacihistorisk Selskab, 1963), pp. 34-46.

15 Frederik Wulff, *Det Kjøbenhavnske Barberlavs Historie* (Copenhagen: Martius Truelsen, 1906), pp. 28-29.

Kronborg Castle at Helsingør, was promoted to "the king's own barber and surgeon," a position he retained until 1625.[16]

At the time that Severinus was hired there were already two doctors named as physicians to the king, Martinus Ædituus and Johan Warwick. Ædituus was hired while Severinus and Pratensis were abroad, and may have expected an appointment to the university when the salary for the chair that supported the two medical students was once more available. Recall that the king had already attempted to install Ædituus in this professorship in 1568, only to be told by the university that the money was not available. But if Ædituus had designs on the vacant chair, his hopes were dashed when the young Danes returned to Copenhagen, where one was appointed to fill the professorship and the other was hired as a royal physician. Apparently Severinus and Ædituus did not get along well as colleagues, and the latter left the king's employ already in 1571 and returned to Holland, leaving only Severinus and Warwick.[17]

Johan Warwick served as physician to Frederik II from 1564 until 1577, when he was dismissed (or quit) for some unknown reason. King Frederik II wrote to the *Lensmand* at Malmøhus, the military and administrative center for Skåne, recommending Warwick as Malmø's *medicus* and encouraging the nobility to make use of him. Clearly the king bore him no ill-will, since he sought to provide him free housing and arranged a small royal stipend some years later, when Warwick fell on hard times. It may be that Warwick, like Ædituus, found the new royal physician Petrus Severinus hard to abide.[18] For the next eleven

16 Gordon Norrie, *Kirurger og Doctores: et kritisk Bidrag til Lægeuddannelsens Historie i Danmark før 1800* (Copenhagen: Levin and Munksgaard, 1929), p. 45.

17 On Ædituus see Ingerslev, *Danmarks Læger*, pp. 174-76, and Rørdam, *KUH*, vol. 2, pp. 580-81. Johannes Paludanus' letter to Henricus Smetius, 3 June 1605, reported that Severinus and Ædituus could not happily coexist, causing Ædituus to return to Holland. See Bartholin, *Cista medica*, p. 129.

18 On Warwick see Rørdam, *KUH*, vol. 2, p. 176, note 1, and Ingerslev, *Danmarks Læger*, pp. 173-4. The royal letter recommending Warwick as Malmø's physician was dated 3 Feb. 1577. In March Warwick authored a plague tract (Rørdam, *KUH*, vol. 4, item # 195, pp. 278-80), with recommendations concerning the pestilence that was by then nearly played out for the season. It's dedication to the king, dated 9 Jan. 1577, suggests that Warwick was seeking to maintain royal favor during the early months of the year, implying that his termination as royal physician was involuntary.

years only Severinus is named in connection with king and court, and the king's care must have fallen primarily on his shoulders.

Being a man of the court and personal physician to the king, Severinus was in a position of influence. As Tycho Brahe would find out in his dealings with Christian IV, access to the king was important. At least some of Tycho's inability to patch up his relationship with the king after he had abandoned Uraniborg and Denmark can be attributed to the hostility of the royal advisors, who may have hindered Tycho's communication with Christian IV.[19] Severinus had direct contact with the king, at least when he was called on for advice or treatment, and this put him in a potentially influential position. On one occasion even Tycho Brahe himself sought Severinus' help in his dealings with Frederik II. When Tycho first observed the famous comet of 1577 on 13 November, he realized that the king would soon expect his analysis of the portent. He wrote to Severinus the very next day asking him to arrange some delay, in order to enable him to study the comet carefully, with instruments, over a long period of time.[20] It is a measure of Severinus' influence and of his friendship with Tycho that the noble astronomer and chemist would ask him, a commoner, to intercede between an aristocrat and the king.

As a member of the immediate court, Severinus was no doubt also useful to the crown as an instrument of royal policy. His close ties to the medical community in general and the university medical faculty in particular must have made him well suited as a mediator between crown and academy. The fact that the medical faculty regarded him as one of their confidants suggests this role.[21] Royal physicians were often used as political agents and as channels of communication in this period, perhaps because they were well educated and maintained contact with their peers abroad.[22] Although there is no evidence that Severinus

---

19   Thoren, *The Lord of Uraniborg*, pp. 381 and 385.

20   Fragment of a letter from Tycho Brahe to Petrus Severinus, 14 November 1577, printed in *TBDOO*, vol. 7, p. 47. This letter is discussed in John Christianson, "Tycho Brahe's German Treatise," p. 121.

21   Frederik II's support of Severinus and Pratensis can be construed as an example of what Moran, "Court Authority and Chemical Medicine," p. 246, refers to as a "court-prescribed role within the academy."

22   Hugh Trevor-Roper, "The Court Physician and Paracelsianism," in *Medicine at the Courts of Europe, 1500-1837*, ed. Vivian Nutton (London: Routledge, 1990), pp. 90-92.

was directly involved in matters of state, a brief postscript in a letter raises the possibility that he used his correspondence for more than medical purposes. The letter is from the English physician Thomas Moffet, who now urged him to continue to write in support of Paracelsian doctrine in order to counter the growing antiparacelsian rhetoric. But the postscript speaks of a "case" involving sailors commended by Severinus, which Moffet has mentioned to Sir Francis Walsingham.[23] Walsingham was one of Queen Elizabeth's most trusted ministers and was personally responsible for creating a complicated network of agents and contacts for obtaining political intelligence.[24] It is established that Moffet was Walsingham's physician by 1590, but this letter implies that he had access to him in some capacity already in 1584.[25] Whatever cause Severinus was supporting with this letter, he certainly sought help from a powerful source.

The number of letters to and from Severinus that exist today is small, but internal references point to a much larger correspondence, and this impression is strengthened by the asymmetry of the dates and kinds of correspondents. Of the more than twenty letters extant wholly or as abstracts and copies, five are addressed to Theodor Zwinger 1583-87. Most of these letters, especially those to Zwinger, deal with philosophical and medical questions, but some serve to establish contact, exchange news, or ask for personal favors. In a February 1583 letter to Zwinger, for example, Severinus praised "the talented young Thomas Fincke" and requested that Zwinger give him good advice and provide him with letters of recommendation to doctors in Padua or Bologna, where Fincke was to study. Thomas Fincke in fact matriculated at Padua in November of that year, just a few months after his first cousin, Drude

23 Letter from Moffet to Severinus, 5 May 1584. Copenhagen, Kong. Bibl. NKS 1305, letter #2; also a copy in Böllings Brevsamling D 40 1280; printed in Rørdam, *KUH* vol. 4, #229, pp. 320-322: "Quantum tua causa, Nautarum a te commendatorum causam juuerim apud honoratissimum Walsingamum, et meæ literæ et ipsorum orationes antea tibi, ni fallor, satis ostenderunt."

24 On Walsingham see Conyers Read, *Mr. Secretary Walsingham and the Policy of Queen Elizabeth*, 3 vols. (Oxford: Clarendon Press, 1925).

25 According to "Moffett," *DNB* (1967-68) vol. 13, pp. 548-550, Moffet attended Walsingham in 1590 at the latest. One wonders what behind-the-scenes diplomatic functions might have been carried out through such contacts between the personal physicians of statesmen.

Chymica studia.

Cl: Viro

Theodoro Zuingero Medico philoso
phoq Excellentiss:

Petrus Severinus.   S.P.D.

Excellens tua eruditio, vir Clariss. quam tot editis
lucubrationibus, per universam Europam patefecisti; et
virtus singularis, qua bonos omnes complecteris; ita mortalium animos vel longinquissime remotos tibi devincire
ut nemo sit qui non merito in amorem & admirationem
tui rapiatur. Cuius ni divinam professus originem, ad
radios illius Lucis non magnopere afficeretur, cuius prae-
clariss. ideam, ubiq in operibus tuis eleganter & gratiose
repraesentas. Laetabar plurimum conspectis tabulis tuis
in Hippoc. quibus obscuritatem divini illius Senis, illustras
A methodicam traditionem ut multis videtur, certa lege
componis, & fastidiosa antiquitatis taedium, grata novitate
demulces. Foreq mihi persuadebam, ut tanti Rivalis
amicitia confirmatus, aliquanto ab acerbis quorundam
censuris me sublevarem. plurimum proinde me re-
crearunt literae tuae, quibus candorem ingenii & iudicii
admirabilem dexteritatem praeclare ostendis. Anxius
certe sum, ut anticipationis in hoc officii genere, erepta
mihi palmam, literarum frequentia posthac compensem.
Amicitiae vero nostrae fundamentum a te positum, obviis
ulnis amplector, commune f: veritatis studium, quod
omnibus hominibus expetitione, philosophis vero etiam
acquisitione exoptatiss: esse debet. Neq ni aliis stimulis
impulsus ad philosophandum iuvenis accessi, nisi ut solius
veritatis & filium & haeredem me profiterer: posthabitis
omnium mortalium sectis, & a veritate non pendentibus
authoritatibus. Animadvertebam quidem difficilem me
ingressum viam, parumq tutum fore tam procelloso in mari

solitar

One of several letters Petrus Severinus wrote to Theodor Zwinger at the University of Basel. Zwinger's answers to him have not survived. Courtesy of Universitäts-Bibliothek Basel.

Thorsmeden, had married Severinus.[26] In his response to a letter from Dr. Samuel Grynæus, a professor of law at Basel, Severinus reported that he was arranging for 300 riksdaler to be paid out for the education of a young Dane under the king's protection. Grynæus may have written to Severinus because of the friendship and correspondence between Severinus and Zwinger, who was also a professor at Basel, but whatever the case, it is apparent from the letter that Severinus had the authority and responsibility to deal with this matter on the king's behalf.[27]

Four of the surviving letters to Severinus come from people connected with diplomatic service in some way. Two were written by Jacques Bongars (Bongarsius), who succeeded Charles Danzay as the French ambassador to Denmark. These letters were sent from Germany, where the Frenchman had gone for his health.[28] Jacques Bongars' friend, Cognetius de la Thuillerie, wrote to Severinus in 1588 to say that he had letters from Bongars to give to him. De la Thuillerie was a councillor to the King of Navarre, who was an important Protestant leader. The fourth letter was from Abel Berner, a German who worked for Christian IV's German Chancellory, which took care of the affairs of the duchies of Slesvig and Holstein and served as the department of state.[29] These four letters show that Severinus was in communication with diplomats and civil servants outside Denmark besides Walsingham.

Petrus Severinus was also useful to King Frederik in matters that demanded personal attention at court. This is evident from his part in the revision of the Danish Bible, which was begun during the last years of Frederik II's reign. The official Danish Church Bible, translated and published during the reign of Christian III, was printed in only 3000 copies, and by the late 1570s there was a shortage of Bibles. In 1577 a

26 Letter from Severinus to Theodor Zwinger, 23 February 1583. U.B. Basel, Fr. Gr. II 28² #338; trans. to Danish in Bastholm, *Petrus Severinus*, pp. 48-49.

27 Letter from Severinus to Samuel Grynæus, 23 February 1583. U. B. Basel, Ms G2 I. 30; trans. to Danish in Bastholm, *Petrus Severinus*, pp. 44-45.

28 Letter from Jacques Bongarsius to Severinus, 1 June 1596, printed in *Altes und Neues von Gelehrten Sachen aus Dännemark*, vol. 2, pp. 483-84; Letter from Bongarsius to Severinus, 30 March 1597, Statsbibl. Bern, MS. B. 149. Both letters trans. to Danish in Bastholm, *Petrus Severinus*, pp. 40-41.

29 Letter from Cognetius de la Thuillerie to Severinus, 14 March 1588, printed in *Altes und Neues von Gelehrten Sachen*, vol. 2, pp. 482-83; Letter from Abel Berner to Severinus, 29 June 1594, ibid., pp. 485-90.

printer in Copenhagen sought and obtained royal permission to reprint Christian III's Bible, under the condition that no changes be made. A year later, however, he suggested that Luther's marginalia be added, and the subject of a new edition of the Danish Bible came up. By 1586 no copies of the earlier edition were to be had, and the king needed to go forward with publication. But having ridden out the controversy over Niels Hemmingsen's "crypto-Calvinism" in the late 1570s, the king was concerned to proceed carefully, making no changes in the Bible that could be construed as departing from Lutheranism as it had been defined at Wittenberg and Augsburg.

The Danish Church had been reformed by Lutheran humanists trained mostly at Wittenberg, where Philipp Melanchthon had given the Christian religion a liberal arts interpretation. Philippism, as the interpretation was called, dominated Danish theology and ecclesiastical policy in the sixteenth century. It embraced classical studies, including music and drama, and was amenable to those who sought to appreciate the Creator through study of his creation – the natural world. Philippism was in this sense quite agreeable to natural philosophers like Severinus and Tycho Brahe.[30] Niels Hemmingsen was the most influential theologian in Denmark at that time and a strong supporter of Philippist views, which he had imbibed from the spring itself, at Wittenberg. He was a prolific writer and one of the few learned Danes of that century to achieve an international reputation, Severinus and Brahe being two others. This reputation, however, not only spread the Dane's ideas abroad, it also lead back to their source: when doctrinal strife erupted in Saxony between the Philippists and the rising Lutheran ultra-conservatives – the Gnesiolutherans – Hemmingsen was identified as a defender of those doctrines that now came under suspicion as Calvinist. The Gnesiolutheran party convinced the ruler of Saxony, Elector August, to exert pressure on his brother-in-law, Frederik II of Denmark, to censure Hemmingsen and his "crypto-Calvinist" teachings.[31] The resulting political

---

30 Thoren, *The Lord of Uraniborg*, pp. 11, 14, 82-84.

31 On Hemmingsen and crypto-Calvinism see Shackelford, "Paracelsianism in Denmark and Norway," pp. 232-38; Bjørn Kornerup and Hal Kock (eds.), *Den Danske Kirkes Historie* (hereafter *DDKH*), vol. 4 (Copenhagen: Gyldendal, 1959), pp. 135-220; *DBL*, 3rd ed., vol. 10, pp. 247-49. On Tycho Brahe and the reaction against Philippism, see Thoren, *Lord of Uraniborg*, pp. 100-01, 118-19, 372-73, and Christianson, *On Tycho's Island*, pp. 200-01, 204, 242.

pressure forced Frederik to order the commission on which Pratensis sat to examine Hemmingsen's publications for Calvinist interpretations in 1575. The following year Hemmingsen was forced to retract certain doctrines, which he did. But after a new edition of one of Hemmingsen's books came out in Geneva, the very home of Calvinism, Frederik II was forced to have him suspended from the faculty in 1579. This episode no doubt affected all the intellectual leaders in Denmark at that time, and certainly Tycho and Severinus. Severinus, for his part, noted in a letter to his friend Johannes Pistorius that he was tired of theologians and wished to avoid the rancor that characterized the growing controversy between the Paracelsians and their critics.[32] If Severinus' defensiveness in this letter was caused by Thomas Erastus' attacks on Paracelsian theory for being theologically unsound, a matter that would have concerned Severinus in any case, then the growing intolerance between the ultra-conservative Gnesiolutherans and the more moderate Philippists must have alarmed not only him but all those who sought freedom to speculate on the metaphysical basis of the natural world and its diseases. It was in this unstable atmosphere that the Danish Bible, the basis of religious instruction in the realm, was to be revised.

The immediate problem was that the Danish Bible had been translated from Luther's German Bible and contained what were considered to be important philological errors when compared to the Hebrew, Greek, and Latin texts. Should one follow the dictates of the humanists and check the translation against the original language wherever possible? Or would departing from Luther's translation be considered a dangerous deviation from accepted doctrine? How could one rectify the translation and still include Luther's marginalia, which were based on the incorrect German translation? These were the questions that vexed the king, and his distrust of novelty frustrated efforts to produce a corrected version called for by, among others, the chancellor and the court priest, Christoffer Knoff.

---

32 Letter from Severinus to Pistorius, printed in Rørdam, *KUH*, vol. 4, #181, pp. 260-61. This letter has been tentatively dated to 1574. The phrase that Severinus used, "Theologorum vicem hisce temporibus doluimus," can be construed to mean either that he was sorry for the theologians or that he and his friends had suffered on their account. See Shackelford, "Early Reception of Paracelsian Theory: Severinus and Erastus," *Sixteenth Century Journal* 26 (1995), p. 131.

When the king finally agreed to a new edition, with corrected text and translations of Luther's marginalia and scholia, the work was undertaken by a consortium of men at court, including Christoffer Knoff, Dr. Petrus Severinus and his brother, and two other members of the court. These five formed a contract with a printer.[33] The bishop and professors were also invited to take part in the new edition, and in order to instruct the theological faculty as to how to proceed, Severinus himself sent revisions of the first four chapters of the Bible to the university in 1588.[34] Although not trained as a theologian, Severinus was a sensible choice as a mediator between the king, the court, and the university. When the king died later that year, with both Severinus and Christoffer Knoff at his side, the new edition was still in its early stages.[35] With the king's conservative opposition to change gone, work proceeded more quickly, and the new edition was ready for the press in 1589.

Of course, Severinus' *forte* was not theology, but natural philosophy and medicine, and it was for these he was best known at court. It was likely at court that Thomas Moffet met him, when the English Paracelsian physician accompanied Lord Willoughby to Helsingør to invest Frederik II with the Order of the Garter on behalf of Queen Elizabeth. Moffet was sufficiently impressed by Severinus to dedicate to him his

33 Rørdam, *KUH*, vol. 2, pp. 240-249 describes the effort to produce a new Bible. The printed letter (25 January 1588) from Christoffer Knoff to Bishop Poul Madsen announcing the contract reads "D. Petrus cum fratre, M. Albertus, M. Johannes Michælis et ego contractum conscripsimus, quem exhibebit tibi M. Johannes Alburgensis." This is, as far as I know, the only mention of Severinus having a brother. See Holger Rørdam, "Efterretninger om Frederik den Andens Bibel," *[Ny] Kirkehistoriske Samlinger*, 2d ser., 1 (1857-59), pp. 216-17.

34 Rørdam, *KUH*, vol. 2, p. 247. Perhaps the textual corrections (allegedly by Severinus) printed in Rørdam, "Efterretninger om Frederik den Andens Bibel," pp. 220-221, were a part of this work.

35 Peder Hansen Resen, *Kong Frederichs den Andens Krønicke* (Copenhagen, 1680), pp. 355-6 records the king's death: "Docteren maatte bruge atskillige Vand oc *Confortativer* at styrcke hannem med / oc toeg hand Doctorens Haand oc lagde den paa sit Bryst / oc ragte haanden frem at hand skulde føle Pulsen." [The doctor had to use various extracts and confortatives to strengthen him. He took the doctor's hand and laid it on his breast and extended his hand so that he could feel his pulse.] Severinus is not mentioned by name, but "Docteren" must surely refer to him. Here Severinus apparently did not apply any "strong" or Paracelsian remedies, probably on account of the weakness of the patient. The use of confortatives and taking of the pulse were conventional.

next book, a defense of chemical medicines.[36] Similarly, Josias Mercer, a member of an English mission sent by Queen Elizabeth to Copenhagen after the death of Frederik II, mentioned Severinus in his diary as "a great man, who was King Frederik II's personal physician, while he lived, very skilled in chemistry and natural philosophy."[37]

Petrus Severinus' appointment as personal physician to Frederik II marked the effective end of his scientific scholarship, inasmuch as he published nothing after this date. Although he wrote much in the next thirty one years, the demands of an active life traveling with the royal court distracted him from his contemplation of medical theory and too often kept him away from the laboratory. He complained of these things in a letter to Johannes Pistorius:

> Since I returned to my fatherland and became a member of the royal court, I have been occupied the whole day with so many affairs that I can neither consult with philosophers nor carry out separations or exaltations of the properties [of substances] by the working of fire.[38]

Severinus must have similarly complained to Tycho Brahe, who commiserated with him in a letter of 3 September 1576.[39] The shortage of time to pursue both spagyric medicine and its theoretical foundations continued to plague Severinus throughout his career. Time and time

---

36 Moffet, *De jure et præstantia chemicorum medicamentorum.*

37 C. Behrend, "En Dagbog fra en Rejse i Danmark 1588," *Danske Magazin*, 6th ser., 1 (1913), p. 339: "Petrus Seuerinus uir magnus, medicus Regis Friderici II. dum uixit, peritissimus chymicæ artis, et naturalis scientiæ."

38 Letter to Pistorius. Rørdam, *KUH*, vol. 4, #181, p. 260-61: "Posteaquam in patriam reuersus aulæ Regiæ comes factus sum, tot negotiis in horas implicor, vt nec philosophos consulere, nec proprietatum separationes et exaltationes ignis adaptatione administrare possim." Rørdam believes this letter was written about 1574, just a few years after Severinus received his appointment to the court.

39 Letter from Tycho to Severinus, 3 September 1576, *TBDOO*, vol. 7, pp. 38-40: "Tu, dum necessaria Philosophiæ adminicula sectaris, libertatem Philosophicam in Aula aliquamdiu si non plane amittis, saltem in exilium abigis, unde eam revocare, ingentis, ut experiris, est difficultatis." [While you strive for the necessary conditions for philosophy, if you do not wholly lose philosophical freedom at court for some time, you at least drive it away into exile, whence it is an enormous difficulty to recover it, as you know from experience.] Brahe's preference for the relatively quiet life at Hven over a socially demanding presence at court is well known.

again he excused his failure to publish his manuscript treatise on physics.[40] To his acquaintance in Basel, Theodor Zwinger, he wrote:

> But even though I am continually occupied with other duties and con-
> siderations, and cannot free myself from court business without God's
> gracious help, I will nevertheless make every effort that you might soon
> see my compendium of physics.[41]

Half a year later he again wrote to Zwinger:

> As far as your reference to the epitome of my physics is concerned,
> I must explain that I have spent the last year and a half in continual
> travels, and I have been completely deprived of my home and the peace
> that philosophy craves.[42]

The paucity of records does not permit us to follow Severinus' movements during his career, but the dates and venues of his surviving letters
to Zwinger support his claim that he often moved around with the court
in the mid 1580s. Frederik II still ruled as the chosen representative of
the feudal aristocracy – the first among equals – and the court circulated the kingdom from castle to castle in medieval fashion. The first of
these letters was written to Zwinger in February 1583 from Kolding, an

---

40 "Physics" here refers to the subjects taught from Aristotle's books on physics, which were
preparatory to the study of medicine. The term is not a synonym for learned medicine,
"physick" as the English then used the term, although they are clearly related.

41 Letter to Zwinger, 12 August 1583. U.B. Basel, Fr. Gr. II 28² #338a: "Quamuis autem
aliis curis & cogitationibus assidue inuoluar, nec sine numinis benignitate ab aulicis
occupationibus me explicare possim, operam tamen dabo vt physicæ meæ compendium
breuj aspicies."

42 Letter to Zwinger, 18 February 1584. U.B. Basel, Fr. Gr. II 28² #339: "Quod de epitome
physices meæ scribis scias velim me toto hac sesquianno vixisse in continuis peregrinationibus, penitusque a domo mea & philosophica quiete abfuisse." Three years
later, in a letter to Zwinger 16 August 1587 (U.B. Basel, Fr. Gr. II 28² #341), he again
mentions his "burdensome tasks at court" as a cause for his failure to publish: "Fateor
sane diuturnum meum silentium a multis accusarj posse, qui curas & molestias aulicas,
quibus assidue nunc annos septemdecim implicor, non satis animadvertunt." [Indeed,
I admit that my continued silence can be blamed by many who do not sufficiently take
into consideration the burdensome tasks at court with which I have been continuously
occupied for seventeen years now.] Zwinger died in 1588.

important administrative center in Jutland. Half a year later (12 August) he wrote to Zwinger from Flensborg in Slesvig, where he had married Drude in July. Six months after that he wrote from Aarhus in northern Jutland, and the following August he wrote from Copenhagen. By this time Severinus had acquired land for a residence in Copenhagen, and his household may have become more fixed. However, his last surviving letter to Zwinger was once more written from Kolding, in 1587. Nor was travel always confined to the kingdom. In 1576 the royal family made a visit to Mecklenburg, where Queen Sophie's father was Duke. Perhaps Severinus was abroad already in June, when his friend Pratensis suddenly died. Tycho Brahe wrote to him 3 September 1576 from Copenhagen, from which we can infer that Severinus was not then in that city. In the letter Tycho states that he is responding to two he has received from Severinus, the first of which was his reaction to their friend's death. Severinus had asked Tycho to explain the three Copernican motions, which he briefly does before he closes with the hope that he will be able to find Severinus at home in Copenhagen before long.[43] That Severinus bothered to matriculate at the University of Rostock during this trip suggests that he thought he might be there for an extended period and sought to use the visit to his academic advantage.[44]

From all this correspondence it is possible to say that Severinus generally travelled with Frederik II's court, as one would expect of the king's personal physician. This situation may well have changed after Frederik's death in 1588. The new king, Christian IV, was still a minor until 1592, during which period the realm was run by a four-member regency. Johannes Bentzius (Hans Bentzen), about whom the historical record is quite vague, appears in the records as a royal physician to Christian IV in 1592. On 2 September that same year Christian IV summoned Severinus from Copenhagen to the court, which was then at Antvorskov Castle. A dangerous epidemic was feared, and the king wanted Severinus to be on hand, even though Dr. Bentzius, who is referred to as the court physician

43 Letter from Tycho Brahe to Petrus Severinus, 3 September 1576, printed in *TBDOO*, vol. 7, pp. 38-40.

44 Adolph Hofmeister, ed., *Die Matrikel Der Universität Rostock* (Rostock, 1889), p. 190 shows an entry for "Doctor Petrus Seuerinus, regis Daniæ medicus" in the month of July, 1576. There is also an entry for "Petrus Seuerini Danus" for October 1581 (p. 206), but this may have been another Danish Peder Sørensen, since he is not here identified as *Doctor*. Or, crown business may have again taken him there.

(*Hoffmedicus*), was already there. Christian's letter explained that a room at the castle had been made ready for Severinus' stay, implying that by this time Severinus did not regularly travel with the new king.[45] The following year Jacob Hasebart succeeded Bentzius and remained in this position until his death in 1607. When in 1599 Christian IV made his famous voyage over the North Cape of Norway, it was Hasebart, not Severinus, who accompanied him.[46] All this suggests that by the 1590s Severinus was much more often resident in Copenhagen than he had been under King Frederik and that he therefore functioned more as a senior medical advisor and the court's link with the university than as a personal physician. Thus, it is no surprise that when a chair opened in the medical faculty in 1602, Severinus sought it and was, apparently, not opposed by the king.

SEVERINUS AS A PRACTICING PARACELSIAN

According to seventeenth-century historians, Petrus Severinus returned to Denmark from his years of foreign study with a reputation for his successful practice of medicine in Venice and in various German cities.[47] But what sort of medicine did he practice? The only clue from his years as a student is the entry in Peder Hegelund's almanac indicating that Severinus had bled him once. Since bleeding was common therapy, this sheds little useful light on Severinus' medicine, which we must then piece together from later documents, after his appointment as royal physician.

Severinus' surviving correspondence contains several references to his medical activity, and we can ascertain from these that he practiced Paracelsian chemical medicine as well as professing it. After complaining about his lack of time for research in a letter to his friend Pistorius, Severinus spoke about his medical practice:

---

45 Bastholm, *Petrus Severinus*, pp. 10-11 reproduces the text of the letter, after Herhold and Mansa, *Samlinger*, pp. 19-20.
46 Ingerslev, *Danmarks Læger*, p. 295.
47 Bartholin, *Cista medica*, p. 115: "Quam non illic tantum & potissimum venetiis, sed & in celeberrimis Germanicæ urbibus postea ita feliciter exercuit ut magnam sui admirationem & amorem in omnium animis concitarit."

But although I frequently apply, not without success and to the honor of my art, certain specific remedies prepared by myself, yet I cannot be contented, but burn with a singular longing for that medicine that I have long foreseen, and I have faith that the result will eventually answer to my expectations. Fortune has certainly fulfilled my first hopes and has shown with the desired results that those healing methods that were introduced by Paracelsus and more distinctly explained by me far exceed Galen's loathsome methods.[48]

As is evident from this passage, Severinus' dissatisfaction with Galenism was rooted not merely in the rhetoric of medical theory, but also in the practice of medicine. "That medicine I have long foreseen" probably refers to a chemical panacea, an ideal rooted in the Paracelsian belief in a universal balsamic drug.

Severinus' disillusionment with scholastic medicine appears in various autobiographical passages, both in the *Idea medicinæ* and in his letters. He wrote to Zwinger that when confronted with perplexing theoretical contradictions, he had like many others sought explanations in "Aristotle's philosophy and Galen's medicine."

But when practice and experience seemed in conflict with theory and methods, I began to work with greater care and diligence: to look more thoroughly at the doctrines of Plato and Hippocrates, to review the theories and practices of the old chemists more frequently.[49]

It was, therefore, the disagreement between his practice of medicine and traditional humoral explanations that he credited with driving him to

48 Letter from Severinus to Pistorius, printed in Rørdam, *KUH*, vol. 4, #181, pp. 260-61: "Quamuis autem specificis quibusdam remediis a me præparatis non sine felicitate et artis honore frequenter vtar, tamen in iis animus acquiescere non potest, sed desiderio illius diu præuisæ medicinæ mirum in modum flagrat, et fore confido, vt votis nostris tandem respondeat euentus. Primas certe spes confirmauit fortuna, optatisque successibus demonstrauit, medendi indicationes a Paracelso introductas, et a nobis clarius expositas, longe superare fastidiosas Galeni methodos."

49 Letter to Zwinger 23 February 1583. U.B. Basel, Fr. Gr. II 28² #338: "... vt sub vmbra Aristotelicæ philosophiæ & Galenicæ medicinæ cum multis delitescerem. Postquam vero actiones & experimenta contemplationibus & methodis videbantur aduersarj, diligentius ingenium & industriam adhibere coepi. Decreta platonis & hippocratis penitius inspicere. Chymicorum antiquorum theoremata & praxes frequenter euoluere."

find a better theory. But what was this practice? Later in this letter he described a Paracelsian drug therapy that is based on chemical drugs administered, not according to abstract, theoretical Galenic qualities, but prepared, diluted, and prescribed according to sensible "signatures," chiefly taste and smell.

> If we look at the milder drugs, either the purgatives or those that cause changes, the spagyric, then [medicine] has taught us to reduce the dosages from a consideration of taste and smell, and to provoke the patients' senses. All pills are given, as a rule, up to one ounce, and they often work slowly, to the great disgust of those who take them.[50]

Severinus then noted that the ancients were not able to make good prescriptions because of the defective nature of their chemical knowledge. But there is hope for new spagyric drugs:

> If we can make more potent [drugs], extracted from metals and minerals, that one can easily and safely use in the treatment of the most serious diseases, [then] I ask, what age except this one will oppose our efforts?[51]

Such drugs Severinus proceeded to discuss. First he wrote of a mercurial compound that is to be very carefully processed by distillation, digestion, and oxidation, so as not to lose "its remarkable innate power, which tries to escape."[52] The result, Severinus explained, is not to be confused with the common mineral that is extensively used by those who call themselves Paracelsus' followers. Next he discussed an antimonial drug, which bears lengthy exposition here, as it tells us about Severinus' Paracelsian attitude toward the use of toxic drugs:

---

50 Ibid.: "Si leuiora spectemus remedia vel purgantia vel alterantia, spagyrica, doses diminuere, saporum & odorum gratia, sensus ægrotorum prouocare docuit. Pillulæ fere omnes dantur ad 3j, & languide sæpe operantur, magno vtentium fastidio."
51 Ibid.: "Si potentiora produxerimus ex metallis & mineralibus eruta, quibus tuto & facile in maximorum morborum curationibus vtj licet, quod quæso seculum, nisi hoc, industriæ nostræ aduersabitur."
52 Ibid.: "ob admirabilem & innatam ipsi vim, fugæ auidam."

With antimony I have conducted a very large number of experiments. In the end I drove off the toxin, but retained its diaphoretic and cathartic virtue. This [drug] can be safely offered without the accompanying worry about vomitings, a remedy appropriate to all sorts of fevers. If you like remedies of this sort, I will send you something and indicate the manner of application and dosage, so that you might actually discover by this method that the use of metallic substances is not nearly as harmful for the human body as some people foolishly claim; that the toxins really can be driven from them by art and suitable adjustment, and that the volatility that accompanies the innate heat can easily be reduced to a sweetness that is friendly in nature.[53]

This is a good indication of the fundamentally Paracelsian nature of Severinus' medicine. Finding traditional drugs ineffective or unpleasant to the patient, Severinus turned to compounds with strong manifest qualities, which are the signatures that reveal their medical power. Toxicity, one of these signatures (and a very important measure of innate power), must then be driven off or altered by the chemical art, leaving the internal curative virtue of the drug unaffected. More will be said about the theoretical justification for the use of strong, chemically prepared drugs in the next chapter.

The historian cannot easily assess the effectiveness of such preparations, nor would it be necessarily appropriate to do so. But what can be understood from physicians such as Severinus is how they believed such drugs fit into medicine. It is with some scorn or malice that critics have pictured the Paracelsian physician as freely administering toxic substances to his patients and fleeing town before they die. This image, created by early modern critics of Paracelsian medicine, has colored the historical interpretation of Paracelsus. We see in Severinus' correspond-

---

53 Ibid.: "In Antimonio plurima sum expertus, abstulj tandem venenum, diaphoretica & laxatiua ipsius virtute retenta, quæ sine anxietate vomitionum comite tuto exhiberi potest, medicam[entum] in omnium febrium generibus appropriatum. Si delectaris huiusmodi remediis, mittam ad te nonnihil & vtendi modum ac dosin indicabo, vt vel hac ratione deprehendas, vsum metallicorum, non esse humanis corporibus perniciosum vt inepte cauillantur nonnullj. Venena quoque ab iisdem arte & congrua adaptatione auferri posse, & ad dulcedinem naturæ amicam, volatilitatem innato calori obtemperantem facile reducj posse."

ence that the Paracelsian physician's judgement of the effectiveness of a drug in combating a disease was combined with his concern for side effects that were considered unpleasant by the patient. A physician in Severinus' position could hardly abandon his patient as might an itinerant practitioner, and any medical failure would be open to official criticism at the highest levels of government. The portrayal of Paracelsians as fly-by-night operators clearly does not jibe with the historical reality that many of them, like Severinus, served as court physicians.

In the next surviving letter to Zwinger, Severinus said he was sending his friend a sample of his "Turpetum," a mercurial medicament. He briefly described the chemical preparation of the drug, the twelve-fold distillation and forty-day cooking over an increasingly warm fire, and so on, until the drug is finished:

> It does not burn the tongue, nor is it caustic, but is very safely effective against most diseases, both acute and chronic. You can safely give six or seven grains. I make a pill with Theriac that is taken together with warm wine or beer. Unless the [patients'] bodies are quite polluted, I rarely observe vomitings, sometimes mild ones. [With] those who have been violently infected by plague, if the disease has its seat in the lungs and the synovia of the head and joints, it causes a moderate salivating; in other bodies [it causes] at least sweating and painless consumption of the most difficult morbid roots, which will rarely happen with other medicines.[54]

This sort of therapy is characteristic of Severinus' Paracelsian medicine. Diseases are like weeds in a garden. They have roots in the body, in one or more locations, and no medicine will rid the patient of a disease unless it tears it out by the roots. This conception of disease and accompanying

54 Letter from Severinus to Zwinger, 12 August 1583. U.B. Basel, Fr. Gr. II 28² #338a: "Nec linguam adurit nec corrosiui quicquam habet & est medica tutissime in plurimis morbis tam acutis quam chronicis. Dare potes tuto granum vj. vel vij. Conficio pillulam j. cum theriaca cum vino calido vel cerevis. deglutitur. Nisi admodum impura fuerint corpora vix vomitiones deprehendo, eas interdum lenes. Qui [?] vehementer lue infecti sunt si morbus in pulmonibus & synovia capitis ac articulorum sedem habuerit saliuam mediocrem mouet, in aliis corporibus sudores saltem & insensiles consumptiones difficillimarum radicum morbidarum quæ vix aliis remediis obtemperaturæ essent."

drug therapy is totally alien to Galenic humoral medicine, in which disease is viewed as an imbalance rather than an unwanted, growing being. Severinus was convinced of the effectiveness of this drug and realized that Galenic theory could not accommodate it:

> After the appearance of this drug (I have written a few words to you about its preparation), when in the most serious and difficult diseases I saw a surprising dissolution and expulsion of those substances that could not otherwise be dissolved or conquered by the violence of medicines, I have often asked myself to which causes Galen would, were he to come to life again, ascribe that kind of result.[55]

Still, Severinus saw room for improvement in his new drug:

> I admit that I still find traces of defective digestions and impurities, but ones which can without great trouble be easily digested and separated by the faculties of the human body. And I harbor no doubt that once all the rust and sulphurous impurity is removed, by diligence and tireless effort, I will have a mighty and useful *arcanum*.[56]

Like the Paracelsian iatrochemist he was, Severinus was not completely content with medicines that worked, but sought to attain that perfectly refined quintessence, the vital balsam and philosophers' tincture that was the ideal and universal cure.

Some of Severinus' medicine apparently survived him. "Pilulæ Severini" and his panacea are said to appear in the 1658 Danish pharmacopoeia (the *Dispensatorium hafniense*), and must therefore have attained

---

55 Letter from Severinus to Zwinger, 18 February 1584. U.B. Basel, Fr. Gr. II 28² #339: "Sæpe post exhibitionem illius remedii (de cuius præparatione pauca ad te scripsi) in grauissimis & difficillimis morbis, dum mirabiles resolutiones & dissipationes intueor, illorum corporum, quæ nulla alioquin medicamentorum violentia, vel solui vel superari valerent: mirarj soleo quibus facultatibus Galenus tales effectus ascripturus esset si reuiuisceret."

56 Ibid.: "Fateor me etiamnum deprehendere vestigia cruditatum & impuritatum, sed quæ sine magna molestia a facultatibus humani corporis facile concoqui & secerni possint. Nec dubia spe teneor quin aliquando industria & labore indefesso, sublata omni ærugine, impuritateque sulphurea, Arcanum sim habiturus Magnum & vtile."

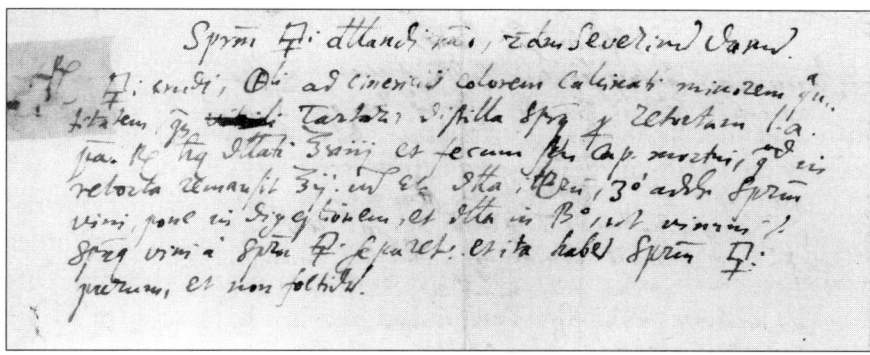

This recipe for a chemically-prepared drug, attributed to Severinus, may have been written down by Ole Worm, since it is included with a collection of his chemical manuscripts in the Royal Library in Copenhagen (Rostgaard Samling 33 8vo tillæg). Courtesy of Det Kongelige Bibliotek, Copenhagen.

some degree of official approval and recognition.[57] The famous seventeenth-century Danish anatomist Thomas Bartholin wrote in 1662 that his friend Johan Rhode had mentioned certain "highly esteemed pills of Petrus Severinus," which were subsequently replaced by Frankfurter pills of Angelica, but I have been unable to find any pills associated with Severinus' name in the *Pharmacopoea* or elsewhere.[58] At any rate, his reputation as a chemist lived on, and Holger Jacobsen (Jacobæus), describing Severinus' tomb in the late seventeenth century, referred to him as an "incomparable chemist."[59] For the sake of completeness I must

57 Herholdt and Mansa, *Samlinger*, p. 28. I have not been able to verify this claim. However, there is a reference to "Pulvis Diasenæ D.P.S." and "Pulvis Diasenæ D.P. Sever." in the 1619 (sig. G1r) and 1645 (sig. H2v) editions of the *Apotheken Taxt* respectively. D.P. Sever. is surely Doctor Petrus Severinus. There is no corresponding entry in the 1672 *Apoteker Taxt*. See the bibliography for the full bibliographical entries for these official drug lists.

58 Bartholin, *Cista medica*, p. 640: "Joh. Rhodius Not ad Scribon. Com. 128 de Ammoniaco monet, ex hoc fundo fluxisse laudatissimas P. Severini pilulas, quibus jam successerunt Francofurtenses, Angelicæ."

59 "Epitaphium Chymici incomparabilis, Petri Severini Ripensis, Archiatri 2 Regum." The account of the since destroyed tomb in The Church of Our Lady, in Copenhagen, is preserved in Vilhelm Maar, ed., *Holger Jacobæus' Rejsebog 1671-1692* (Copenhagen: Gyldendal, 1910), p. 40.

mention one other, hitherto overlooked vestige of Severinus' art. There is
a short recipe for a "method for attaining spirit of sulphur, according to
Severinus Danus" in the Royal Library in Copenhagen. It is associated
with a manuscript book that belonged to the well known seventeenth-
century physician and collector of natural artifacts, Ole Worm.[60]

Clearly, Severinus was practicing a kind of Paracelsian medicine.
Yet, this does not mean he used such drugs to the exclusion of all other
medicines and healing methods. After Severinus' death, one of his colleagues, Johannes Paludanus, mentioned him in a letter to a friend:

> I received your second letter ... in which you request that I write to
> you about the success and effect of Dr. Petrus Severinus' panacea, and
> whether it can indeed cure all those desperate and [otherwise] incurable
> diseases you name in your letter.[61]

The author goes on to say that it is true that both he and Severinus were
court physicians, but whereas Severinus was physician to the king, he,
Paludanus, was physician to the Queen Mother, who resided in Jutland.
However, on one occasion they consulted with one another with no
disagreement in diagnosis. But, Paludanus continues,

> As to what you ask about [Severinus'] miraculous and definite ability
> and success in curing intractable (and otherwise incurable) conditions,
> I must (although I do not wish to diminish a learned man, considered
> great by many) frankly admit that his reputation exceeds the facts.
>
> As far as the panacea is concerned, he tried to imitate Anwaldus'
> [panacea], and although he sought the ingredients by analyzing this
> medicament, he by no means pursued it completely. ... He used various
> drugs against various diseases. ... He did not always use Paracelsian
> medicines, and in fact often [used] the Galenic compounds. But in

---

60 The recipe is in Copenhagen, Kong. Bibl., Rostgaard 33 8vo Tillæg (Addition). Ole
    Worm and his reading of Severinus are treated in chapter 8.

61 Letter from Johannes Paludanus to Henricus Smetius, from Viborg, 3 June 1605, in
    Bartholin, *Cista medica*, p. 127: "Literas tuas secundas ... accepi, in qvibus petis, ut tibi
    de successu Panaceæ Doctoris Petri Severini, ejusdemque effectu scriberem; Et an
    omnes, qvos in literis tuis nominas morbos incurabiles nempe, ac desperatos, curare
    potuerit."

extreme diseases he applied extreme remedies. Enough said. When an epidemic disease raged in Copenhagen in 1602, he too died from the plague.[62]

This eclectic approach, a polypharmaceutical medicine that used both chemical and herbal drugs, also characterizes the therapy of Severinus' contemporary, Anders Krag (1553-1600). Anders was, like Severinus, from Ribe. He studied philosophy at Wittenberg and Basel before going to Montpellier, where he earned his doctorate in both philosophy and medicine in 1585.[63] From 1586 until his death in 1600, he held several chairs at the University of Copenhagen, first in Philosophy (*pædagogicus*), then in Mathematics, and finally in Physics. During these years he was part of Tycho Brahe's social circle, which may have then still included Severinus, and he served as personal physician to Princess Anna.[64] Despite his reputation as a keen Paracelsian chemist, only one obviously Paracelsian recipe appears in his 1586 work, *Laurea Apollinarea Monspeliensis*: a recipe for a distillate of copper vitriol, to be given in

---

62   Ibid., pp. 128-29: "Qvod inquiris de miraculosa & certa deploratorum (& incurabilium aliis) affectuum curandorum solertia & successu (qvamqvam homini docto, & apud multos magni habito, nihil detrahere volo) ingenue tamen fateor, famam factis superiorem.

Ad Panaceam qvod attinet, Anwaldinam imitari conatus est, cum per resolutionem medicamentum hoc ingredientia inqvireret, sed haud perfecte est consecutus; ... Variis medicamentis, ad morbos varios usus est ... Medicamentis Paracelsicis non semper est usus, verum & compositionibus Galenicis sæpe: Sed extremis morbis extrema adhibebat remedia. Intelligenti satis. At cum morbus epidemicus Hafniæ multum sæviret, circiter annum 1602 ipse qvoque peste extinctus fuit." Amwaldus (Georg am Wald) wrote a treatise on his panacea that appeared in several editions beginning with *Bericht und Erklerung ... wie und was Gestalt das new von jhm erfunden Terra Sigillata und universal Artzney, wider die Pestilenz und dero Zufellen ... zugebrauchen* (St. Gallen: L. Straub, 1582). His panacea was sufficiently famous in the late sixteenth century to attract the vituperation of Andreas Libavius in *Neoparacelsica* (Frankfort: Kopff, 1594), *Gegenbericht von der Panacea Amwaldina* (Frankfort: Kopff, 1595), and *Panacea Ambaldina victa et prostrata* (Frankfort: Kopff, 1596). See Kurt P. Sprengel, *Versuch einer pragmatischen Geschichte der Arzneikunde*, 3rd ed. (Halle, 1827), vol. 3, pp. 516-17.

63   Rørdam, *KUH*, vol. 3, pp. 509-11, 531. Trevor-Roper, "The Paracelsian Movement," p. 171, described Montpellier as a Huguenot institution tolerant of, and perhaps supporting, Paracelsian medicine.

64   Rørdam, *KUH*, vol. 3, p. 515. Anders' brother Niels Krag was Sophie Brahe's escort for several years, and it is reported that Tycho often stayed at the Krag residence when he was in Copenhagen.

doses up to one scruple before and after paroxysms.[65] In this book, which he dedicated to his students, Anders says he disavows adherence to any particular sect and will not allow any authority, whether old or new, to deprive him of the freedom to judge things for himself. This suggests that he thought of himself as neither Paracelsian nor Galenist, but drawing on various kinds of medicine.[66] Moreover, this eclecticism is evident from a letter he wrote to Dr. Sigismund Schnitzer, in which he says that he is glad to hear that Schnitzer values chemically prepared medicines and that "I by no means oppose these [medicines], the extraordinary fruits of which I see every day. But one should be careful to moderate and administer the Paracelsian medicines according to the Galenic method."[67] Anders Krag's friend and student, Peter Johann Viborg, later wrote to Schnitzer and said that when he had shown one of Schnitzer's letters to Anders, the latter commented that if only his old friend would come to visit, he "would immediately have four new furnaces built and show us the remarkable results of certain chemical distillations. Where there is no visible demonstration, and no untiring manual operation, there is nothing."[68] In this last comment we can see Krag's commitment to the Paracelsian ideals expressed by Severinus and Tycho Brahe, demanding first hand experience in science.[69] By his own account, Anders Krag was occupied at court in the chemical preparation of the drugs in great demand there, and if Severinus were still in attendance at this time, the two most likely would have worked

65 Ibid., vol. 3, p. 517. Anders Krag, *Laurea Apollinarea Monspeliensis* (Basel: Henric Petri, 1586), p. 109: "Ex Paracelso, libro præparationum de vitriolo."

66 Rørdam, *KUH*, vol. 3, p. 512.

67 The letter from Krag to Sigismund Schnitzer, "De chymicis quibusdam remediis," is printed in Bartholin, *Cista medica*, pp. 109-12: "Ego ab iis non prorsus abhorreo, qvorum insignes fructus qvotidie percipio. Sed cautio adhibenda est: ut Paracelsica medicamenta temperentur et propinentur methodo Galenica" (p. 110).

68 Rørdam, *KUH*, vol. 3, pp. 518-19. The letter is printed in Bartholin, *Cista medica*, p. 112-113: "Respondit si te mecum adducere possum extructurum se 4 fornaces celerrime, et demonstraturum nobis mirabilia arcana in destillationibus chymicis. Ubi non est ocularis demonstratio, et manualis operatio indefessa, nihil est" (p. 112).

69 In a similar vein Krag wrote in *Laurea Apollinaris*: "De hac re obscura, non tam ingenii acie, quam observatione, judicium faciendum est." [A judgement should be made about this obscurity not so much by a sharp mind as by observation.] See Rørdam, *KUH*, vol. 2, p. 332, n. 1.

together.[70] His death in 1600 was attributed to poisonous vapors from chemical distillation.

TYCHO BRAHE AND SEVERINUS

Sometime between the death of Pratensis and Tycho's abandonment of Hven, the relationship between Tycho and Severinus is supposed to have cooled. Historians have suspected that Severinus had a hand in facilitating the disharmony between Tycho and Christian IV that resulted in Tycho leaving Denmark and seeking patronage abroad. Unlikely as it may seem that the enmity of a one time friend could have been as important as the many other factors that tarnished Tycho's reputation at court, neither should the possibility be rejected without investigation.

Tycho had been granted Hven as a life-time fief by Frederik II, but his lifestyle and scientific work required a great deal of money, and he depended on royal patronage to supplement the considerable resources under his personal control. Now, falling increasingly out of favor with the new king – who had his own agenda of expensive projects to finance – Tycho began to feel the bite. There are many complex reasons for the withdrawal of the benefices that had enabled Tycho to support his construction, research, and printing, the loss of which injured his pride and contributed to his abandonment of Hven. Tycho had neglected his noble responsibilities for years, and the social and legal conflicts in which he was engaged during the last decade of the century increasingly alienated him from the nobles and middle-class bureaucrats who governed Denmark.[71] The key to Tycho's fortune, however, was clearly the personal support of the king: with it the efforts of antagonistic underlings to deprive him of royal patronage could be ignored, but without

---

70 Bartholin, *Cista medica*, p. 111: "Una tamen pars chymicis datur præparationibus medicamentorum nobis septentrionalibus inservientium." However, as was mentioned before, Severinus likely followed the court less and less frequently after 1592.

71 Thoren, *The Lord of Uraniborg*, reviews many of the problems Tycho was having, especially regarding the maintenance of his properties, his actions against a tenant, and his suit against his former pupil Gellius Sascerides.

it Tycho was left to his own resources. Although these, including Hven and its rents, may have been sufficient to sustain Uraniborg, the loss of the major cash-producing benefices and the uncertain status of Hven after Tycho, made staying on in Denmark somewhat unattractive to the nobleman.[72] Thus, the falling out between Tycho and King Christian IV must be considered a critical factor in Tycho's decision to seek patronage abroad.

There is a tradition, repeated by some of the leading historians of Tycho Brahe and the period, that Tycho had gained the enmity of the medical elite in Copenhagen for distributing medicines free of charge, and that Severinus was among this group.[73] According to this story, Severinus, a long and trusted advisor of the royal family, was influential in turning the king against Brahe. It seems unlikely, however, that Severinus' opinion could have been a major cause of Tycho's downfall, which seems to have been grounded in a struggle for status between two nobles – Tycho Brahe and the Christian IV. Nevertheless, Severinus ought not be dismissed as wholly without influence in this matter merely because Tycho was a noble and he was not.[74]

If contemporary rumor is to be believed, Tycho and Severinus clearly did have a falling-out. As of November 1577 they were still on good terms, and Tycho wrote to Severinus at court asking him for information concerning the comet visible at that time, which it was Tycho's duty to

---

72 Tycho wished to have his son succeed him as "Lord of Uraniborg," but Danish law did not permit his children by a commoner to be members of the nobility. See Ibid., p. 353.

73 See, for example, F.R. Friis, *Tyge Brahe*, p. 231; Panum, "Vort medicinske Fakultets," pp. 49-50; and among recent accounts, Bastholm, *Petrus Severinus*, p. 12. Wilhelm Norlind, *Tycho Brahe: Mannen och Verket* (Lund: Gleerup, 1951), p. 308, held this opinion in his commentary to his translation of Pierre Gassendi, *Tychonis Brahei vita* (Paris, 1654). Dreyer, *Tycho Brahe*, p. 232, said that tradition mentions Severinus as one of Tycho's enemies at court; that he was jealous of Tycho's medical activities and his free distribution of drugs. Gassendi, *Opera omnia*, vol. 5 (Stuttgart-Bad Canstatt, 1964), p. 444 (discussed in Norlind, *Tycho Brahe*, p. 130), wrote that Tycho had made enemies among the physicians on account of his providing free medical advice and drugs to visitors, but no source is given. If this opinion stems from one comment made by Johann Stygge, discussed below, then it is perhaps an exaggeration.

74 Thoren, *The Lord of Uraniborg*, p. 368, n. 106, writes: "It is extremely unlikely that a commoner would have had much influence in political matters," by which he means business affecting noblemen like Brahe.

interpret for the king.[75] But twenty years later, after Tycho had forsaken Hven and left Denmark for Hamburg, Henrik Ellenberg, in the employ of Moritz of Hessen-Kassel, wrote to Tycho from London. In this letter (early 1598), Ellenberg tells that word of Tycho's loss of royal favor and abandonment of Denmark had reached England, that Severinus has long borne ill-will against Tycho, and that perhaps this is the cause of Tycho's misfortune.[76] This same rumor reached the ears of Johan Stygge, who reported his conversation with some visiting Englishmen to his friend in Copenhagen, the printer and bookseller Johan Aalborg.[77] One of the Englishmen said that

> Severinus, the royal physician, quietly and long nursed a hatred of him [Tycho] (on account of his Paracelsian medicines, which he knew how to prepare so excellently and was accustomed to giving without charge, formerly to King Frederik and later to other nobles, too) ... so they say here that this man contrived against Tycho in great secrecy, so that eventually he took offense at such things and left. Thereupon I responded: how could that doctor do this, since he [Tycho] is a noble? Tycho is from a famous and great family in Denmark, and our doctors, as yours, do not have such authority. And why had he not done this before now, if he could? Then he said: even though the doctor is

75 *TBDOO*, vol. 7, p. 47.

76 *TBDOO*, vol. 8, p. 21: "Dolebam tamen, quod adversi aliquid in Dania tibi evenisse, referrent, tuæque abitionis ex Dania alij alias recensebant causas. Siquidem fuerunt hic in Anglia, qui tibi cum PETRO SEVERINO Medico litem fuisse nescio quam asseverarent, teque indignitatis adversarij puditum esse, et ideo inde discessisse. ... Verum cum in Angliam etiam delatum sit, SEVERINUM illum apud hunc novellum Cancellarium multum valere, adeo ut is ferme totus ab illo dependeat, atque obscurum non sit, Doctorem illum (ut referunt) diutina tui invidia laborasse, fortassis hoc, quod per semetipsum non potuit exequi, per hunc Cancellarium, cui Rex plurimum tribuere dicitur, effectum dedisse."

77 Thoren, *The Lord of Uraniborg*, pp. 387 and 401, regards Johan Aalborg as a former friend and preceptor (in 1566) of Tycho Brahe, who had perhaps grown more critical of Tycho toward the end of the century. This is presumably the same Johannes Alburgensis with whom Severinus had contracted to produce a new Bible in 1588 – see note 33 above. Stygge, whom Thoren describes as an "obscure Danish nobleman" (p. 386), was a critic and possibly an enemy of Tycho. It would come as no surprise if members of Denmark's lesser nobility, who saw their share of the feudal land tenure decrease dramatically in the sixteenth century for the aggrandizement of the great families (such as the Brahes), considered the crown money that was lavished on Tycho to be offensive.

not a noble, yet he holds [the confidence of] certain other nobles and even princes, who [have influence] with the king, and who listen very attentively to this doctor.

Stygge concluded the argument by saying "I have never heard any such thing [about Severinus] in Denmark, therefore how do you who are Englishmen know this?"[78]

From these letters it is clear that a rumor circulated that Severinus was responsible for Tycho's fall from power; that he had convinced the Chancellor and nobles around the king to redistribute some of the benefices supporting Tycho's extravagant lifestyle. Certainly this is a possibility, for by the 1590s Severinus was no doubt an influential advisor. As for the presumption that a commoner could not have acted effectively against a nobleman, we have the counter-argument that Tycho had felt threatened almost twenty years earlier by the success of Jørgen Dybvad in gaining the ear of Frederik II.[79] Dybvad, an ambitious and talented scholar, had (like Severinus) been supported in his studies by the salary attached to a vacant professorial chair. With this stipend he traveled abroad and returned with a reputation as a good student of mathematics and astronomy. If Dybvad, who was disliked by the leading theologians at the University of Copenhagen, can be imagined as a rival to Tycho Brahe, I see no reason to dismiss the importance of Severinus, who was apparently held in esteem by academics as well as the crown. Moreover, as nobles increasingly valued university education abroad and sought members of the educated middle class as companions and tutors for their

---

78 Letter from Johan Stygge to Johan Aalborg, 10 July 1598, *TBDOO*, vol. 14, p. 144. "Severinus, regis medicus, diutino et clandestino eius odio (ob medicamenta eius Theophrastica, quæ is tam egregie parare novit et olim regi Friderico et nobilibus postea aliis quoque gratis dare solitus est) laboravit. ... Hunc igitur apud nos dicunt multa subdole in Tychonem machinatum esse, ut tandem is talia indigne ferens discederet. Mox ego respondi: quomodo ille doctor hoc facere posset, cum [non] sit nobilis? Tycho est ex clara et magna familia in Dania, nec habent apud nos tantam autoritatem ut apud vos doctores, et quare non fecit id antea, si potuit, quam nunc? Tunc ille excepit: etiamsi doctor is non est nobilis, tamen habet alios quosdam nobiles et quidem præcipuos, qui apud regem multa possunt, qui doctori huic valde auscultant," and "nec unquam quid tale in Dania audivi; quomodo ergo vos, Angli qui estis, sciretis?"

79 Thoren, *The Lord of Uraniborg*, p. 129, does not find it unreasonable that Dybvad could have affected Tycho's reputation with the king: "Here, clearly, was a man who had won the ear of the king. This fact alone ... made him a rival."

children's travels to foreign universities, the social barrier between the university elite and aristocratic government officials narrowed.[80] There-fore, although a severe legal and social distinction between nobleman and commoner persisted, there is no reason to suppose that the advice of a trusted intellectual, such as Severinus, would be disregarded even in matters touching the aristocracy. Indeed, as was shown above, Tycho appealed to Severinus to intercede on his behalf in 1577 rather than directly asking the king for more time to study the comet.

Meanwhile, the allegation that Tycho had alienated the academic medical community by distributing medicines is not wholly unreason-able. If Tycho prepared Paracelsian medicines and gave them to noble-men, as stated by Johan Stygge, it might have upset Galenists, who would have seen this as legitimizing a rival medicine, or chemists, who derived income from the production and sale of such drugs. However, the argument that Severinus hated or envied Tycho on account of his production and free distribution of Paracelsian medicaments seems out of place.[81] Certainly Severinus would not have opposed the use of Paracelsian remedies on principle. Since he was personal physician to the king, any such drugs would likely have been administered to the king on his orders or on the orders of Johannes Bentzius, after 1592. Furthermore, even if Tycho did make and give out medicines to his peers, it was not uncommon for nobles to produce and share medicines. Even his sister, Sophie Brahe, took an active interest in alchemy and worked in the laboratory both at Uraniborg and years later at her own estate. Tycho reported that she prepared chemical drugs, which she then gave to her friends and also distributed to the poor.[82] I have, however,

---

80 This, too, is Thoren's argument. Ibid., p. 356.

81 Norlind, *Tycho Brahe*, pp. 307-8, and Thoren, *The Lord of Uraniborg*, p. 212 n. 69, were of this opinion, but I do not know what evidence it is based on, and given the incho-ate state of regulation in sixteenth-century Denmark, the argument seems to be out of place.

82 On Sophie Brahe's chemistry see Schønau, *Samlinger af danske lærde fruentimer*, pp. 198-99; F.R. Friis, *Sophie Brahe Ottesdatter*, pp. 42-43. Tycho's letter is now lost. Schønau (p. 231) reported in the eighteenth century that Sophie had spent considerable sums of money on "chemical distillations." Sophie herself wrote to her sister, Margrete, that she was occupied with distillation. This letter is printed in Heiberg, *Prosaiske skrifter*, vol. 9, pp. 325-360. As early as 1700 it was reported that Ole Borch, professor of chemistry at the University of Copenhagen in the middle of the seventeenth century, owned a large quantity of her chemical manuscripts (Schønau, p. 231).

found no evidence to indicate that Tycho gave drugs to anyone other than nobles, as mentioned in Stygge's letter, but even if he did, it would have been regarded as noblesse oblige, and can hardly have aroused justifiable anger.[83] If Tycho's medicines were a cause for envy, it would more likely be on the part of the academic physicians with influence at court, perhaps Thomas Fincke, who was an ardent Galenist and known enemy of Tycho's, or even Gellius Sascerides, who had come to serious disagreement with Tycho Brahe after nearly becoming his son-in-law.[84] Gellius' appointment as *medicus* for Malmø, in the province of Skåne, where Tycho's family was powerful, indicates that he had friends at court who were willing to support his appointment against Tycho's will, and these may have included Severinus. However, even if Severinus harbored no ill will toward his former friend, there were other reasons why he might not have supported him in this affair. After all, Severinus had married Fincke's cousin in 1583 and may not have been inclined to take Tycho's side against a relative.[85] Also, Severinus desired to obtain a professorship in medicine at the university, and he could therefore ill afford to side against the professors on that account, alone.

The intrigues and processes resulting in Tycho's loss of royal support and favor involved many factors, and opposition to Tycho's medical activity was at best one of several causes. Nevertheless, we ought not totally discount the rumors that reached Ellenberg. We are in the end left with Tycho's short and somewhat cryptic account of the matter, written for

83 Thoren, *The Lord of Uraniborg*, p. 212, n. 69, repeats the story that Tycho distributed free medicines to the poor. My guess is that Gassendi's interpretation of Stygge's comment gave rise to this claim.

84 On Fincke, see Panum, "Vort medicinske Fakultets," p. 49; Thoren, *The Lord of Uraniborg*, p. 376, n. 3. On Gellius and Tycho, see Thoren, *The Lord of Uraniborg*, pp. 356-62.

85 The family relationship is charted in Bastholm, *Petrus Severinus*, p. 33. In a larger sense one might see Fincke and Severinus as members of the middle class bureaucracy, ascending as an instrument of the consolidation and expansion of royal power, to the detriment of the entrenched aristocracy, to which Tycho was born. Tycho's position among his peers may also have been weakened by his abandonment of his hereditary estate to his brother, his rejection of the political life in favor of the intellectual life, and his attempt to secure hereditary rights for his children by marriage to a commoner. There was no doubt a conflict of social position as well as of personalities involved in Tycho's fall. One wonders, too, if his crypto-Calvinist, perhaps somewhat Paracelsian theology was not also at odds with the Danish Church's shift toward conservative Lutheran doctrine near the turn of the century.

Henrich Rantzov in December 1597. At the close of the manuscript, in which Tycho copied down in his own hand the recipes for three chemically prepared medicines, as a gift to his host, Tycho noted that Rantzov must keep these secrets to himself and his friends, "since such things have caused me to forsake my ancestral homelands; Thus, it hurts to have helped, helps to have not harmed."[86] Tycho, at least, thought that his Paracelsian medicine was an element of his current misfortunes.

PETRUS SEVERINUS' UNPUBLISHED TREATISES

As we have seen from his correspondence, Severinus occasionally complained that the demands of court life kept him from the research and writing he wished to accomplish. We must therefore suppose that he desired a professorship at the University of Copenhagen, although certainly academic life would have had its distractions, too. However, there is no mention of Severinus being considered for a medical chair when his friend Pratensis died in 1576 or when Hans Frandsen died in 1584. Pratensis was replaced by Anders Lemvig, whom Severinus had once recommended to a colleague, and who eventually became Severinus' next-door neighbor. Frandsen's chair was filled in 1585 by Anders Christensen of Ribe, who was called home from his study abroad at the recommendation of the influential Chancellor Niels Kaas.[87] Although these physicians had studied in some of the same cities as had Severinus, neither seems to have been interested in Paracelsian medicine. Anders Christensen was, if anything, a Galenist who sought in vain to bring the practice of anatomy (which Severinus would have thought to be unimportant to medicine) to Copenhagen.[88] This preference for Galen-

---

86 *TBDOO*, vol. 9, p.166. Latin elegaic couplet: "Utut
    Talia me patrias fecere relinquere sedes;
    Sic iuvisse nocet, non nocuisse iuvat."

87 Rørdam, *KUH*, vol. 2, pp. 623 and 655.

88 Ibid., p. 656. Severinus' *Idea medicinæ* (see chapter 4, below) makes it clear that Severinus devalued the cutting up of cadavers. Moran, *The Alchemical World of the German Court*, p. 55, shows that at the University of Marburg, where Paracelsian physicians advised Landgraf Moritz in the early seventeenth century, anatomy was considered secondary to Hermetic philosophy.

ists has been taken as a measure of academic opposition to Paracelsian medicine, but there is no convincing evidence for this conclusion. Both of these appointments were made during Frederik II's reign, and we can suppose that the king valued Severinus as royal physician enough not to recommend him to the university for a professorship or that Severinus preferred the power and prestige that went with his position. True, the medical faculty might have hired Anders Krag to replace Frandsen, since he was finishing both Ph.D. and M.D. at Montpellier when Anders Christensen was hired. Krag was to attain a reputation as something of a Paracelsian chemist after his return to Copenhagen, but this was after the fact and, as we have seen, he did not wholly abandon Galenism. Even so, he was appointed professor at the University of Copenhagen in 1586 and remained until his death in 1600.[89] Therefore, the university *was* patronizing a physician interested in Paracelsian medicine. And since all these appointments were made when Severinus was the king's chief medical advisor, it is difficult to believe that they were made without his approval. It is reasonable to conclude that Severinus was content with his lot as long as Frederik II lived.

When in 1602 Anders Christensen of Ribe vacated his chair in medicine, having been appointed superintendent of the aristocratic academy at Sorø, the university entered negotiations with Severinus to fill the position. Although there is no indication that Christian IV was displeased with Severinus, it is reasonable to suppose that Severinus did not have the same rapport with the young king that he had enjoyed with his father and wished to retire from the court into an academic position. Rather than signifying "a fresher wind now blowing within the university's walls," one that favored Paracelsian medicine, this offer should be viewed as a position of honor for a man of influence, who this time wished to accept it.[90] There is no evidence of active hostility between the medical professors and Severinus – who had advocated Paracelsian medicine in his *Letter to Theophrastus Paracelsus*, in the *Idea medicinæ*,

---

89 Rørdam, *KUH*, vol. 3, pp. 509-17. Krag may have studied Paracelsian chemistry at Montpellier, where Paracelsian medicine was at least tolerated and may have been supported. See Trevor-Roper, "The Paracelsian Movement," p. 171.

90 Bastholm, *Petrus Severinus*, p. 14: "En friskere vind nu blæser indenfor universitetets mure."

and in his correspondence – at any time during his career as royal physician. Certainly there could have been no serious qualms about hiring a Paracelsian to teach medicine, especially one who had distinguished himself by years of service to the kings of Denmark. Furthermore, it is clear from the funeral oration for Severinus, mentioned previously, that he was considered to be an asset to the university and already in their confidence. Unfortunately, Severinus died before he could accept the academic position that would have given him the leisure for scholarship that he had often claimed he lacked.[91]

Although Severinus failed to publish after he was appointed royal physician, he continued to write, as is clear from comments in his correspondence. There is evidence that he left several treatises in manuscript, in various stages of completion, when he died. The renowned seventeenth-century physician, medical professor, and collector, Ole Worm, recalled having seen manuscript fragments of seven works by Severinus: (1) *Astrologica commentaria*, (2) *De mixtione et rerum confluentia*, (3) *Commentaria de vita longa*, (4) *Liber de nominibus et rebus*, (5) *De generatione morborum*, (6) *Commentaria de febribus*, and (7) *Paraphrasis in libros Hippocratis de antiqua medicina*. These are mentioned in the *Idea medicinæ* and must therefore have been written during Severinus' student years.[92] Ole Worm also claimed to have seen several texts in the possession of Frederik Severinus, which he described as "written in the hand of [his] parent."[93] These were *Confessio Pucciana* in quarto; *Confessio Huberiana* in quarto; *Liber theologicus Paracelsi* in folio, *Secreta Paracelsi varia* in quarto; *Liber de præparationibus medicamentorum ex Gebro, Arnaldo Villanovano aliisque chymicis excerptus* in quarto; several fragments of a book *de generationibus et transplantationibus morborum* in quarto (which may be the same as number five above); the beginning of

91 Bartholin, *Cista medica*, gives the date of Severinus' death as 28 July on p. 116 and 29 July on p. 120, where the death dates for Drude and several of their children are also given. I think that the former date, taken from the funeral oration, is more accurate than the latter, which must have been inscribed in 1615.

92 Mention of these seven is made in the *Idea medicinæ*, pp. 130, 137, 121, 213, 234, 263, 369-70 respectively.

93 Bartholin, *Cista medica*, p. 131. *In manu parentis exaratos* could be interpreted as "written in the hand of the author," which would imply that Severinus was taken as the author of all these texts. However, as I note below, I think some were copied by Severinus from other texts.

a little book *de separatione virtutum ab invalido*, written in Frankfurt, in octavo; several reflections on Aristotle's eight books of Physics as well as on *De cælo*, etc.; a rather longwinded commentary on Synesius' book *De somniis*, in folio (reportedly the last written and most complete of the manuscripts left to Frederik Severinus); a book of dreams and letters in quarto; various fragments of Severinus' letters to his friends in quarto; and some grammatical observations.[94]

Thomas Bartholin attributed six works to Severinus: A little untitled book about the preparation and separation of metals and minerals, beginning *Duplex est humiditas vitiosa in metallis*; *De generationibus et transplantationibus morborum* (likely the same as number five above); a little book *De separatione virtutuum ab invalido* (the same as one given by Worm above); a "physics" book with the title *De principiis elementis, causis, forma, materia*; *De generatione et transmutatione mineralium et metallorum*; and a treatise beginning *Nolle in causa est, non posse prætenditur.*

Of these twenty two manuscripts attributed to Severinus, several can possibly be copies of works by other authors. In this category I would place the two *"confessiones"* as well as *Liber theologicus Paracelsi, Secreta Paracelsi varia*, and *Liber de præparationibus … ex Gebro et alia*, the last said not to be in Severinus' style or genius.[95] Nevertheless, copies of these texts in Severinus' own hand (*in manu exaratos parentis*) attests to his fascination with Paracelsian literature and may well date to his years as a student. The *Liber theologicus Paracelsi* suggests that Severinus was interested in Paracelsian theology as well as in Paracelsian medicine and cosmology. Tycho Brahe also reportedly owned a Paracelsian commentary on the Bible, and it may be that *theologia Paracelsica* was part of the intellectual world that they shared, reinforcing the argument that Paracelsianism is best thought of as an ideology that embraced religion and ethics as well as natural philosophy and medicine.[96]

---

94 Ibid., p. 130-2. It is impossible to tell from this source if, for example, "a little book *de separatione virtutum ab invalido*" refers to a manuscript with that title, or merely a book on that subject.

95 Ibid., p. 130.

96 I have made this argument in Shackelford, "Paracelsianism and Patronage," p. 85, and it has been affirmed by Pumfrey, "The Spagyric Art," pp. 50-51.

Two of the titles listed above are clearly Severinus' letters and personal notes. The manuscript *De principiis elementis, causis, forma, materia* is most likely the "physics" book that Severinus repeatedly promised in his correspondence. Finally, portions of *Commentaria de febribus* may well survive in Sloane MS 3005.[97] Oddly enough, none of all these titles corresponds to the only complete manuscript text that still exists, "*Exercitationum liber in qua questiones philosophicæ, astronomicæ, medicæ, cabalisticæ explicantur.*"[98] The authorship of the remaining texts cannot presently be verified. What became of these manuscripts (with the noted exception of *Commentaria de febribus*) is unknown. Correspondence between Ole Worm and Frederik Severinus shows that the king's chancellor, Christian Friis of Kragerup, was interested in having the manuscripts published, probably at Christian IV's request. Worm himself did not feel he could undertake the task, or any part of it, for reasons possibly linked to his negative attitude toward Paracelsianism at the time of this request.[99]

It is possible that some of the manuscripts passed from Frederik Severinus to Ambrosius Rhodius, his son-in-law. However, the fact that Rhodius' treatises only cite Severinus' published works and those letters later published by Thomas Bartholin in *Cista medica* strongly suggests that the missing manuscripts did not come into his possession, at least not before 1643, when Rhodius' last work, a defense of Severinus' *Idea medicinæ*, was published. We last hear of Severinus' manuscripts from Joachim Morsius (in 1625), who believed they were in the possession of Andreas Hoberweschelius ab Hobernfeld, a now obscure Rosicrucian political philosopher and physician. Morsius dedicated his publication of several prophetical tracts with an open letter to Hoberweschelius, which begins:

97　"Fragmentum de febribus." British Library, Sloane MS 3005, ff. 48r-54v.

98　British Library, Sloane MS 3005, ff. 1r-37v, mentioned in chapter one.

99　Letters from Ole Worm to Frederik Severinus, 25 June 1620 and 10 August 1620, in H.D. Schepelern (ed.), *Breve fra og til Ole Worm* (Copenhagen: Det danske sprog- og litteraturselskab, 1965), #73 and #74, vol. 1, pp. 46-47. On Ole Worm's change in attitude toward Paracelsian medicine, see Shackelford, "Rosicrucianism, Lutheran Orthodoxy, and the Rejection of Paracelsianism."

Very noble and excellent Hoberweschelius, Lord and singularly honored friend, I call upon you and implore you on behalf of all good men, that you not too long sit on the posthumous writings of Theophrastus Paracelsus in your possession, but at last bring them into the divine regions of light, along with your own most desired works and [those] of Petrus Severinus and others.[100]

PETRUS SEVERINUS' DESCENDANTS

On 29 July 1602 Petrus Severinus of Ribe, Doctor of Philosophy and Medicine, *Archiater* to King Frederik II and King Christian IV of Denmark and Norway, was interred in The Church of Our Lady in Copenhagen, where he joined the remains of his friend and traveling companion in life, Johannes Pratensis. Severinus' tomb, later destroyed in a severe fire that ruined the church, was ornamented with an epitaph and was sketched by Holger Jacobsen in his travel book.[101] Three of the eight children brought into the world by Petrus' wife, Drude Thorsmeden, preceded him to the grave. These were Sophie, Bothilda, and Reinhold. Two more, Severinus and Johannes, died within six months

100 Anastasius Philaretus Cosmopolita (Joachim Morsius), *Magische Propheceyung Aureoli Philippi Theophrasti Paracelsi* (Philadelphia, 1625): "Nobilissime & Excellentissime Hoberwescheli, Domine ac amice singulariter colende, communi omnium bonorum voce Te convenio & obtestor, ne diutius posthuma quæ apud te scripta Theophrasti Paracelsi premas, sed ea tandem dias in luminis oras cum Petri Severini, aliorumque: & desideratissimis tuis proprijs, proferas." The preface and part of the text are printed in Nordström, "Lejonet från Norden," pp. 36-40.

101 Bartholin, *Cista medica*, p. 116, states that Severinus was buried in the chapel of St. Roche, where his epitaph was placed, and refers to this as the "back chapel" (*in sacello postico*) on p. 117. Holger Jacobsen's travel book, however, records that the epitaph of the "incomparable chemist" was in the third part of the main section of the church (*in tertio Templi parte*). Jacobsen's next entry is for first part of St. Roche chapel (*in Sacelli Rochi … Prima Parte*), where the epitaphs for Erasmus Vinding and Thomas Bartholin were, so confusion about these locations may have been caused by their proximity. Pratensis' epitaph was in the second part of St. Roche chapel. See Maar, *Holger Jacobæus' Rejsebog*, pp. 40-41.

of their father, perhaps from the same epidemic disease, or another malady striking a weakened population on the heals of it, as part of a pandemic of the sort that often afflicted early modern peoples. On 21 September 1610 their mother died, at age forty three. The fact that the rector of the university, Johannes Erasmus (Hans Rasmussen), delivered a funeral address for her indicates that public esteem for the Severinus family continued long after Petrus Severinus' death. Epitaphs added to the tomb in 1615 noted that Petrus and Drude were entombed together with five of their children.[102]

The three children surviving to adulthood, Anna, Frederik, and Gesa, married within their parents' social class, the upper bourgeoisie. Gesa, the youngest, married the borgermester (mayor) of Copenhagen, Matthias Hansen, and died in childbirth 2 July 1613.[103] Anna (1586-1633), possibly the eldest of the children, married Jonas Charisius (1571-1619) in 1602, the year of her father's death. Jonas had studied medicine abroad, at the universities of Heidelberg and Padua, but upon his return to Denmark in 1598, he took a position in the German Chancellory, which served as the king's department of foreign affairs. He, too, was near the king, having accompanied him on his long voyage to North Norway in 1599. Eventually Jonas became one of Christian's most powerful ministers, presiding over the expansion of Copenhagen, the collection of Dutch paintings for the king, and the foundation of Danish mercantilism.[104] Anna and Jonas had a son, Peder Charisius (1608-85), who distinguished himself in service to the state. Following his father's death he was looked after by the medical professor Caspar Bartholin, who was married to a relative of his. Bartholin wrote a short tract on a recommended course of study for his sons and Peder Charisius, suggesting that Peder might pursue a M.D. as had his father, grandfather, uncle, and various relatives by marriage, but instead he followed his father's

102 Bartholin, *Cista medica*, p. 121. Bartholin printed the epitaphs, ibid., pp. 116-18. One of these was probably established by their son-in-law Jonas Charisius.

103 Ibid., p. 120; Ingerslev, *Danmarks Læger*, vol. 1, p. 179. Hansen must have been a very wealthy man, at least by 1616, when he built "Matthias Hansens Gård" at Amagertorv 6, now the sales outlet for The Royal Porcelain Factory, according to Svend Cedergreen Bech, ed., *Københavns Historie*, vol. 2 (Copenhagen: Gyldendal, 1980), p. 104.

104 Ibid., p. 41.

footsteps into diplomatic service.[105] The extended medical family that knit together the Severinuses, Bartholins, Worms, Finckes, and other families of Danish physicians, provided a certain amount of support for their scions, which included Severinus' grandchildren.

Frederik Severinus (1587-1637), the only one of Petrus Severinus' sons to survive childhood, was born the year after his sister Anna. After his father's death, Frederik looked to his brother-in-law Jonas Charisius for guidance. He refers to Jonas in an undated letter as his patron and asks him to take the place of his father, since God had taken him away at such a bad time in his life.[106] Frederik studied medicine at Wittenberg and Heidelberg, but it is not known where he was promoted to M.D. By 1616 he was practicing medicine in his mother's home town, Flensborg. In 1621 he moved back to Copenhagen, where he practiced medicine and raised a family. He must have practiced among the intellectual elite, since Thomas Bartholin published in his *Cista medica* a recipe for the drugs that Frederik had successfully used in 1631 to treat his sister Dorothea Bartholin, who was married to the astronomer Christian Longomontanus, as well as their daughter.[107] In 1635 a young Saxon student of medicine, Ambrosius Rhodius, took a room in Frederik's house and three years later married one of his daughters, Anna Frederiksdatter Severinus. Ambrosius took Anna to Norway, where he composed a commentary on her grandfather's *Idea medicinæ*, which will be discussed

---

105 Caspar Bartholin's *De studio medico inchoando, continuando, et absolvendo* (Copenhagen, 1628) is printed in Hermann Conring, *In universam artem medicam singulasque ejus partes introductio* (Helmstadt: Hammius, 1687). The advice Bartholin gives is summarized in Panum, "Vort medicinske Fakultets," pp. 58-61, and Shackelford, "Paracelsianism in Denmark and Norway," pp. 268-69. Peder Charisius had a son named Ambrosius in 1644, and it is tempting to think that he named the boy after Ambrosius Rhodius, the husband of his cousin, Anna Frederiksdatter Severinus.

106 Letter from Frederik Severinus to Jonas Charisius. Copenhagen, Kong. Bibl. NKS 1305 2°, letter # 68, pp. 366ff: "Tu mihi succede quoniam Deus patrem eripuit optimum ævo pessimo, et constituit infælici illa sede." Frederik also left a poem written as a letter to his father, in which he mourns his loss. Ibid., letter # 71, pp. 374f.

107 Bartholin, *Cista medica*, pp. 341-347. H. Ehrencron-Müller, ed., *Forfatter-lexikon omfattende Danmark, Norge og Island indtil 1814*, vol. 8 (1930), p. 143 claims that Frederik Severinus also studied at Leipzig, Leiden, and Marburg (1612) before setting up practice in Copenhagen. His matriculation at the University of Heidelberg 28 September 1609 does not indicate that he was a *magister* or *doctor* at that time. See Gustav Toepke, ed., *Die Matrikel der Universität Heidelberg von 1386- bis 1662*, vol. 2 (Heidelberg, 1886)

in detail in chapter nine.[108] Here, too, the favor of the leading medical families was at work, for Ole Worm, who was indirectly related to the Bartholins, Finckes, and therefore the Severinuses by marriage, was to look after Anna and her husband, for whom he helped to secure a royal appointment. All in all, Petrus Severinus' family enjoyed considerable success during the period of prosperity in Denmark that preceded the disastrous wars with Sweden in the 1640s and 1650s.

The correspondence of Severinus and those who knew him warrant the conclusion that he remained a Paracelsian physician in both theory and practice throughout his career. This does not mean that he wholly rejected the learned medicine that had been handed down through the centuries, but rather that he recognized the weakness of Galenic explanations and the failure of the treatments that were based on them to cope with certain diseases, particularly those that characterized the sixteenth century. Severinus was drawn to Paracelsian medicine not merely by the desire to follow a new trend, but because the ideas of Paracelsus fit better with his Platonist view of God and nature than did the Aristotelian-Galenic theory and also because they better explained what the physician saw at the bedside. Furthermore, Paracelsian-style chemical medicines held out the promise of better, more effective treatments that produced fewer unwanted side effects. In principle, Paracelsian medicine was much more optimistic than Galenic medicine, for it defined disease as a real thing that could be eliminated, expelled from the body with the proper drug. In theory, no disease was incurable if one could get at its roots chemically without killing the patient.

Truly Severinus' reputation depended not on his success in curing patients, about which we know little, as much as on his status as a royal physician and on his remarkable treatise *Idea medicinæ*, which provided a relatively coherent metaphysical basis for Paracelsian medicine. But we

108 For more about Anna and Ambrosius Rhodius and their adventures in Norway, see Shackelford, "Paracelsianism in Denmark and Norway," chapter 7, pp. 295-339, and Shackelford, "A Reappraisal of Anna Rhodius."

must not forget that as a physician Severinus tried to reconcile theory with practice, and that his observations were interpreted in the light of his theories, which were themselves probably shaped by his experiences as a student. Therefore, while Severinus seems never to have lost faith in someday obtaining the panacea, the one drug with general application and minimal side effect, he also assumed its operation would be grounded in the process of nature itself, which comprised the chemical activities that underlay the normal and pathological functioning of all creation – the true anatomy of the world. These he had put forth in the *Idea medicinæ*, and judging from the titles of his unpublished manuscripts, he must have elaborated these basic concepts in other contexts.

In the thirty one years Petrus Severinus served as royal physician to the kings of Denmark, the composition of his social network must have changed considerably, and this may partly explain his failure to publish and defend his ideas, some of which were under attack in the wave of antiparacelsian sentiment that was so forcefully expounded by Thomas Erastus and his followers, beginning in 1572. Of the generation of young intellectuals excited about the new theories and the possibilities for a republic of letters in a humanist Denmark, with its forward-looking king and growing university, many had died or otherwise departed by the end of the century. Of the immediate group of friends that had apparently eagerly discussed the ideas of Paracelsus, among other alternatives to scholastic theory – the group that had urged Tycho to transgress class boundaries and lecture at the university on a subject that transcended the traditional curriculum – only Severinus remained at the turn of the century. Pratensis had died already in 1576, Danzay in 1589, and Tycho Brahe had left Denmark for good in 1597. Younger Danish scholars took up the ideas of Severinus – of Paracelsus – from time to time, but they matured in an environment that was religiously conservative, hostile to Paracelsian ideas, and also more chemically sophisticated. In the seventeenth century it was both easier to separate chemical medicine from Paracelsian theory than it had been in Severinus' day and more expedient to do so.

It was chiefly abroad that Severinus' ideas, like the seeds they described, found fertile fields and took root. The *Idea medicinæ* proved sufficiently persuasive to elicit references to a Severinian school, a *secta Severiniana* that followed and propounded Paracelsian theory as explained by *Severinus Danus* in the *Idea medicinæ*. Like other great books, the *Idea medicinæ* was widely read, notes were taken on it, its chief ideas were applied in different contexts, it was reprinted, and commentaries were written to explain its contents. The remaining chapters of this book will describe and explain the chief doctrines of the *Idea medicinæ*, examine how they were used and by whom, and investigate the extensive commentaries that defended them and sought to explicate them to new generations of physicians.

PART TWO

A philosophical path
for Paracelsian medicine

The printer's device used by Henric Petri, who printed Petrus Severinus' Idea medicinæ philosophicæ (1571), shows divine forces at work breaking down ore. The ritual significance of the hammer or axe-head as a symbol of human mastery of divine processes in nature has a long tradition in Europe. Courtesy of The Danish National Library of Science and Medicine.

Chapter Four

THE IDEAL OF
PHILOSOPHICAL MEDICINE:
VITAL ANATOMY AND THE ANATOMY
OF DISEASE AND CURE

PETRUS SEVERINUS repeatedly promised to complete and publish a book on natural philosophy, but only two of his treatises saw print. The short and rhetorical *Epistola scripta Theophrasto Paracelso* provided an outlet for his enthusiasm for Paracelsus and the changes that he had brought to medicine. It was good propaganda for Paracelsus, which Fridericus Bitiskius no doubt recognized when he reprinted it at the beginning of the three volume Geneva edition of Paracelsus' works in 1658, but it had little theoretical content. The *Idea medicinæ*, however, expressed Severinus' interpretation of the metaphysical and physical underpinnings of medicine and, indeed, of all natural change. Aside from Severinus' personal influence and the possibility that his unpublished manuscripts may have been circulated (for which little evidence exists), the *Idea medicinæ* was his only vehicle for the dissemination of his Paracelsian medical philosophy. This theory proved sufficiently important to seventeenth-century philosophers to warrant two further editions of the *Idea medicinæ* and three extensive commentaries. Therefore, we must become familiar with the salient ideas expressed in this book if we are to understand both Severinus' theory and its importance to posterity.

The very title of the book, *Idea medicinæ philosophicæ* – *The Ideal of Philosophical Medicine* – suggests its philosophical nature, *Idea* referring to the Platonic concept of a perfect form or archetype to which actual medical practice strives to conform.[1] Platonism had attracted an enthusiastic following ever since the work of Marsilio Ficino in the late fifteenth century and forms a conceptual background against which Severinus' work was understood and assimilated. We should remind ourselves that Severinus' contemporaries and commentators saw in his *Idea medicinæ* not just Paracelsian medicine, but a Paracelsianism explained in terms of Platonist metaphysics. Medical literature such as the *Idea medicinæ* was in reality concerned not only with medicine, per se, but also with questions of a metaphysical sort, which had ideological ramifications that affected moral philosophy and religion as well. If we realize that philosophical medicine was in fact often dealing with theologically sensitive issues, then we can understand the reactions that the *Idea medicinæ* elicited, which will be treated in the remaining chapters of this book. With this in mind we turn now to explore the *Idea medicinæ*, to investigate its central doctrines, and to assess Severinus' ideas about medicine as a learned profession.

The analysis that follows is focused on two main themes: Severinus' statements about medicine and medical reform and his theory of seminal causation, upon which he built up a thorough-going biological theory. We will first assess Severinus' attitude toward medicine by looking at his summary of the history of medicine in the introductory dedication and the first chapters of the *Idea medicinæ*. There we get some idea why Severinus has written such a work, what he hopes to achieve, why he finds traditional humoral medicine wanting, and what Paracelsian medicine has to offer. The bulk of this chapter, however, will be devoted to the main doctrines expressed in the *Idea medicinæ*. If there is one central concept that dominates Severinus' philosophy, it is the idea that causation in the material world is organized around archetypal forms that intersect material existence at seedlike points called *semina*. This "*semina* doctrine" is itself an organizing principle of the *Idea medicinæ*, running through the text and lying at the basis of Severinus' conception

---

1 One might also translate "idea medicinæ philosophicæ" as "brief outline of philosophical medicine," inasmuch as the "idea" is the general form, much as a footprint provides the general form of the foot. However, I have chosen to retain the Platonic sense of form by rendering the title as *Ideal of Philosophical Medicine*. See the discussion of the seventeenth-century English translation of the title in chapter nine, below.

of all physical change, both healthy and morbid. Explication of this doctrine and related concepts of pathological and curative processes will shed some light on the attractiveness of Severinus' ideas to late sixteenth and seventeenth-century philosophers.

THE DEDICATORY EPISTLE

The *Idea medicinæ*, like many books of its time, includes a prefatory letter dedicating the work to a patron or hoped-for patron. Severinus chose to address his dedication to his king, Frederik II, for both of these reasons. The king had supported him in his studies abroad, for which the young Dane was no doubt grateful, and he also held the keys that could open the doors to fame and fortune at home. But Severinus' letter of dedication is more than a plea for patronage; it serves as a preface that introduces the reader to the author's perception of both the proper goals and methods of medicine and his contributions toward those goals. It also provides us insight into the professional and doctrinal perceptions that shaped the *Idea medicinæ* and serves as a guide to its interpretation.

The dedication contains a narrative summary of the development of medicine from ancient times up to the appearance of new diseases, which defied satisfactory classical explanations. However, its point is not primarily historical, but rather to prepare the reader to understand that the proper ends and means of medicine are found in the work of its earliest authorities. Chief among these is Hippocrates, who, in Severinus' hands, had become a symbol for an ancient medicine that was built on observation and practice and was both closer to nature and intrinsically more patient-oriented than was the later Galenic medicine.[2] The movement to find the true ancient medicine, the *prisca medicina*, and cleanse it of harmful late-classical and Arabic impurities began as part

---

2 Wesley Smith, *The Hippocratic Tradition* (Ithaca: Cornell University Press, 1979), discusses how Galen reshaped Hippocrates to suit his own purposes. See also the general introduction to *Hippocrates*, trans. W.H.S. Jones, vol. 1 (1923; reprint Cambridge, MA: Harvard University Press, 1984), pp. ix-lxix; and Owsei Temkin, *Hippocrates in a World of Pagans and Christians* (Baltimore: Johns Hopkins University Press, 1991).

of a general medical humanism, but parted ways from the humanist effort to refine classical Galenism that is evident, for example, in the work of John Caius, Johannes Guintherius of Andernach, and Andreas Vesalius. This search for ancient medicine – truly Hippocratic medicine – paralleled the search for ancient theology, sharing much of its ideology and sources as it developed from the mid fifteenth century into the Hermetic and alchemical medicine of the late sixteenth and seventeenth centuries.[3] This somewhat backward-looking reform movement, which lauded the ancient reliance on observation of nature and the search for true causes or first principles of disease and medicine, largely took shape in the latter half of the sixteenth century and forms the context for understanding Severinus' thought, which in turn made an important contribution to it.

The dedication is divided into two segments. Severinus begins with a brief survey of the natural phenomena that gave rise to the study of medicine. This is, in fact, a statement of the antiquity of human inquiry into exactly those questions that the *Idea medicinæ* addresses, questions about the causes of change in the natural world as they pertain to medicine. We can see from this preface that medicine had a much wider scope in Severinus' time than in our own; medicine, "physick" or physiology, was no less than the study of nature (*physis*) and natural change. The learned physician must therefore also be a natural philosopher, if he is to understand the principles of health and disease.[4]

According to Severinus, natural philosophy, which he defined as fundamentally an inquiry into causes and their relationship to natural

---

3 The humanist interest in ancient theology has been established by D.P. Walker, *The Ancient Theology; Studies in Christian Platonism from the Fifteenth to the Eighteenth Century* (Ithaca, NY: Cornell University Press, 1972). More recently, James Hankins, *Plato in the Italian Renaissance*, vol. 1. (Leiden: Brill, 1990), has placed early parts of this quest in the context of fifteenth-century Italian study of Platonism. The possible importance of this development, in particular the sixteenth-century fascination with Hermetic philosophy, for early modern science was raised by Yates, *Giordano Bruno*. Subsequently, controversy has arisen over claims for any role for "occult" philosophy in shaping experimental science and indeed over the very use of terms like "Hermetic," "Paracelsian," and "Rosicrucian." However, it is clear from the sixteenth and seventeenth-century texts that these terms were used then, justifying use of them here.

4 It is characteristic of Paracelsian medicine that diseases are seen as natural processes, even if the scope of the term "nature" was much wider than would be permitted today. Whether contagious, hereditary, or environmentally caused, diseases were natural.

effects, first arose out of necessity: in order to survive in a harsh environment, the ancients had to learn the rhythms of nature and use this knowledge to anticipate natural calamities. Bad weather damaged their crops, and diseases deprived them of their domestic animals and reduced their strength. By observation, the ancients discovered a regularity in nature, which Severinus calls vital astrology. This is the causal hierarchy that links things of inferior status to their superiors. The weaker are governed by the stronger and the lower by the higher.[5] Sterility and fertility, disease and health, all arise from fundamental causes that have prior existence. In this scheme, the manifest products of nature, namely animals, vegetables, and minerals – "the good gifts of the seas and lands, of the air and of the heavens" – are posterior effects arising from underlying and ontologically prior elements and principles.[6] But plagues, failed harvests, and other disasters come from these elements as surely as do beneficial gifts, and only observation will reveal which effects reliably come from which causes. Thus, observation is a cornerstone in the foundation of natural philosophy.

Learning by observation is difficult and requires great labor, and the ancients realized that they would need to divide the task. Some observed the generation and decay of plants, while others attended to animals, particularly to domestic stock. Others studied the nature of plant seeds, where they were best planted, and when, that is, under which constellations, for the stars were the measures of the seasons. By correlating the cycles of living things with the rising and setting of constellations, the ancients succeeded in predicting bad harvest years. Still others turned to the study of humans, their nourishment, the origin of diseases and their cures, and how all these depend on the season, location, and heavenly aspect. The causes of diseases and other maladies were carefully hidden in nature, and not directly evident to the senses. However, by studying the causes and effects carefully, the ancients eventually discerned the operation of the invisible seeds (*semina*) that govern them.

Severinus attributed to these early philosophers a corporate spirit. Realizing that one life was too short to acquire sufficient knowledge, they built up a tradition. They confirmed what their teachers had done

5 Severinus, *Idea medicinæ*, p. i (the first page of the dedication).
6 Ibid., p. ii: "aquarum, terrarum, aeris, & coeli fauores."

and added their own observations. They freely published their findings, illuminated the darkness of ignorance, and enlarged the scope of natural philosophy. In short, Severinus portrayed ancient medical science as a progressive, collective, and public enterprise aimed at improving human understanding of nature and consequently enhancing our ability to survive its vicissitudes. Unfortunately, "all things human are subject to errors and ruin," and medicine is no exception.[7] There were those among the ancients who failed to put forth the effort required to carefully observe and learn. Instead they sought what Severinus called "geometrical explanations of those things that only nature can measure."[8] As a consequence, medicine gradually abandoned the phenomena themselves and sought hypotheses suitable to "geometrical" demonstration. Hot, cold, moist, and dry were introduced into medicine – qualities that could be quantified by degrees and were therefore suited to mathematics. From these were deduced "convenient explanations for diseases and remedies."[9] This sophistic medicine arose already in the days of Hippocrates, but he and his students successfully opposed it, and it succumbed to the "natural and legitimate methods of medicine."[10]

In late antiquity "geometrical" medicine again gained popularity, owing to the laziness and inactivity of the age. The hypotheses of this medicine took less effort to master than did learning through experience, and they soon triumphed. Clearly Severinus had Galen in mind here, whose humoral pathology he judged better suited to pedagogy than to furthering medical enquiry.[11] The Arabic medical writers, in turn, made

7 Ibid., p. iii: "sed humana omnia, ruinis & erroribus obnoxia sunt."
8 Ibid., pp. iii–iv: "Methodos quæsiuerunt, & Geometricas Demonstrationes, earum rerum, quas sola Natura metiri potest."
9 Ibid., p. iv: "faciles Demonstrationes morborum & remediorum."
10 Ibid.: "naturales & legitimas Medicinæ Methodos." On the rejection of "hypotheses" in the Hippocratic treatise *On Ancient Medicine*, which Severinus repeatedly cited in the *Idea medicinæ*, see Jones, ed., *Hippocrates*, vol. 1, pp. 6–8.
11 Severinus dated this development to "twelve hundred years ago," or sometime in the fourth century A.D., but there can be little doubt from the content of his criticism that it is the followers of the second century Galen that he had in mind. The figure twelve hundred is also found in Jean Fernel, *De abditis rerum causis libri duo* (Venice, 1550; Frankfurt: Andreas Wechel, 1574), sig. aa3r, which Severinus may have seen: "Atque ut interim de hac nostra syncere loquar, disciplinæ & artes quæ annis prope mille ac ducentis sepultæ fuerunt, aut quæ verius extinctæ occiderant, iam plane reuixerunt, pristinum, ne dicam maiorem, splendorem adeptæ, ut nihil fere docta illi seculo debeat hæc ætas invidere."

hypotheses supreme. While it is true that they added certain experiences of their own to medicine, the results of which they displayed in their dispensatories, their investigations were not profound.[12] Yet even the Arabic physicians, who constantly strove to perfect the geometrical (Galenic) medicine, realized that there was a place in medicine for the experience of both patients and physicians, which they associated with Hippocratic medicine, and therefore they applied Hippocrates' name to their ignorance. They forced his divine utterances "to submit to strange and violent interpretations" and lambasted the "empirics" in his name.[13]

Thus, according to Severinus, what is commonly called Hippocratic medicine is not Hippocratic at all, but a kind of Galenic hypothetical medicine that was dressed up as Hippocratic by the Arabic commentators. This medicine gained widespread acceptance and reigned with "an invincible authority" (*imperium inuictum*) among his contemporaries. Greeks, Arabs, Italians, Germans, and French all followed the same path and were bound to this powerful medical monarch "by a perpetual vow of servitude."[14]

Over the course of time new diseases arose "and arise daily to this day," wrote Severinus, and these "do not correspond to the hypotheses of heat and cold."[15] As a result, the Galenic system of therapeutics that was built on these hypotheses does not work. Despite the remarkable subtleties that had been added to Galenic theory, it could not cope with the new diseases, and as a consequence occult properties quietly crept

12 Severinus, *Idea medicinæ*, p. iv-v.

13 Ibid., p. v: "peregrinis uiolentisque interpretationibus ... obtemperare coegerunt."

14 Ibid., p. v: "Nomina tam potenti Monarchiæ dederunt, seruitutis perpetua fide obligata." It is interesting to note that Severinus equates the tyranny of Galenic medicine with invariant adherence to a political superior, even in this preface to his king. This supports the contention that the Paracelsians linked medical (philosophical) reform with political reform.

15 Ibid.: "& adhuc in dies oriuntur, qui calidis & frigidis Hypothesibus non respondent." The perception that some diseases of the sixteenth and seventeenth centuries were unprecedented is the subject of Stevenson, "'New Diseases' in the Seventeenth Century." Stevenson claims that the argument that new diseases called for a renewal of medicine was typical of seventeenth-century chemical physicians, who were influenced by the Paracelsian idea that diseases are the fruits of time, that is, that new diseases unfold with the passing of time.

into it. Physicians again undertook to study the characteristics of diseases, but, remembering their oath to Galenic medicine, they gave these characteristics obscure names and "placed them under the governance of the Galenic qualities."[16] Dissenting physicians, who sought to reveal the properties of the new diseases through experience (observation) and hard work, "were called traitors, empirics, and itinerants" by those who eschewed labor and sweat.[17]

Something, Severinus pleaded, must be done. New diseases continue to multiply. Physicians either wonder at the feebleness of their remedies or they unwillingly "flee to empirical methods, eagerly taking woods from the merchants and unguents from the itinerants for the treatment of many diseases."[18] In short, medical theory is in shambles and in need of reform. But what is to be done? First of all, he wrote, we must return to the tradition of human freedom and assess the present conditions without prejudice. Then we must contemplate nature anew, consider its causes and properties, and not be frightened off by the difficulty, effort, or expense required in this holy undertaking. "We are not bound by respect to the Greeks or the Arabs," he declared; "We are servants of the sick, for whom God created medicine and committed it to our diligence."[19]

As a student of medicine Severinus "often observed that the Galenic theorems (much less the remedies) could not give satisfaction in treating the most difficult diseases."[20] But while he was in Germany he had heard scattered rumors of the success of certain Paracelsian medicines and he began to read through Paracelsus' writings with care. In this maelstrom

16 Severinus, *Idea medicinæ*, p. vi: "gubernationibus Qualitatum subiecit."
17 Ibid.: "Desertores, Empirici, & Circumforanei appellati sunt."
18 Ibid.: "Ad Experientiam, uel inuiti, confugiunt, a Mercatoribus ligna, a Circumforaneis unguenta, auide accipiunt, ad multorum morborum curationes." Severinus' opposition to the indiscriminate use of commercially available woods and unguents reflects Paracelsus' loathing for medicine's dependence on foreign *materia medica*, which were controlled by mercantile monopolies. The most notorious of these was guaiacum, a new-world wood used against Syphilis, the importation of which was regulated by the powerful Fugger family.
19 Ibid.: "Nulla uerecundia Græcis uel Arabibus obstringimur. Ægrotorum serui sumus, quibus Medicinam creauit Altissimus, & creatam, nostræ industriæ commisit."
20 Ibid., p. vii: "sæpe deprehendi Theoremata Galenica (multo minus Remedia) in difficillimorum morborum curationibus satisfacere non posse."

of difficulties, as he called it, he was presented with new and unintelligible terms, contradictions, mysterious preparations for drugs, and a new system of philosophizing. The sheer obscurity of Paracelsus' ideas piqued his interest, and he strained to overcome these difficulties through persistence, untiring work and study, much traveling, and great expense. By regularly practicing the preparation of chemical drugs, he gradually learned the natures, dwellings (sources), and compositions of things. Severinus also applied himself to the Paracelsian theories of generation and transplantation and began to read what the ancients had written on these subjects – the properties of the elements and *semina*, agriculture, astronomy, and the generation of plants, animals, and minerals. They helped explain Paracelsus' medicine – "the system of arrangement, the diversity of interpretations, and the methods of the living astrology."[21] He had begun to make sense out of Paracelsus' obscure utterances by illuminating them with the wisdom of the early philosophers.

Severinus was encouraged to rethink chemical philosophy by several unnamed philosophers, he wrote, and he set about creating a new metaphysical basis for medicine, which was built on Paracelsus' ideas: "I first established the immovable foundations of nature, and from these I deduced the causes of the effects, which are subject to nature's rule, the reasons for changes, the mechanical increases, and the orderly unfolding of causes."[22] By doing this he penetrated nature's opacity, perceived the harmony that the ancient philosophers had described, and "understood the generous providence of nature," which has provided a balsam for treating all diseases.

In keeping with what he had previously written concerning the advantages of ancient attitudes about cooperation, Severinus did not wish to keep his new understanding to himself, but sought to share what he had learned. We should imitate our ancestors, he wrote, and help mankind in its present need by working together. "What I have gained by my labors, cares, studies, and travels," he declared, "I have openly

---

21   Ibid.: "Ordinum rationem, interpretationum uarietatem, & uitalis Astrologiæ Methodos."

22   Ibid., p. viii: "Fundamenta primum Naturæ immobilia collocaui, ex quibus effectuum causas, qui Naturæ imperio subijciuntur, agendorum rationes, Mechanicos progressus, & ordinatas causarum explicationes deduxi."

communicated to others, as far as possible."[23] Severinus said he would write more, should he perceive that the *Idea medicinæ* is well received. He claimed to have trepidation on that point, since he had left the well trodden paths of philosophy and given "light to the obscure, esteem to the loathed, newness to the old, credibility to the doubtful, and names to the unknown."[24] He seemed to fear being dismissed as an ignorant neoteric and therefore sought to disarm his critics by anchoring his work in the authority of the past. Therefore, he insisted that he has offered new interpretations, but not created novelty: "I am neither a quoter nor mere transcriber," he exhorted; "I have caused streams of thought to flow from those same sources that were tapped by ancient and more recent interpreters of nature concealed."[25] Seeing the confluence of these various streams has been his reward.

GALEN, HIPPOCRATES, AND PARACELSUS

We have seen from Severinus' preface that he considered the new medicine of the sixteenth century, defined on the principles expounded by Paracelsus, to be a return to the right-minded approach of the ancient Greeks, an honest attitude toward theory and practice grounded always in observation. The professional, university medicine of intervening ages lost sight of the need for theory to be based on natural phenomena and became instead a demonstrative science from which an arbitrary therapy derived. Severinus was in the vanguard of the Paracelsian movement, which intended to reform medicine and its pedagogical basis. But the conciliatory tone that is suggested by the full title of his book, which announces a consideration of "the grounds of all the doctrines of Paracelsus, Hippocrates, and Galen," also leads us to inquire what value Severinus placed on Hippocratic and Galenic medicine.

---

23 Ibid., p. viii: "Proinde, quicquid laboribus, uigilijs, studijs, & peregrinationibus lucrifeci, quod Medicinam & Philosophiam illustrare potest, quoad licuit, alijs candide communicaui."

24 Ibid.: "Arduum certe hic fuit, obscuris lucem, fastiditis gratiam, uetustis nouitatem, dubijs fidem, ignotis nomina dare."

25 Ibid., p. ix: "Neque Recitatores, neque nudi Transcriptores fuimus. Ex fontibus ijsdem, ex quibus Antiqui, & Recentiores abditioris Naturæ Interpretes, riuos deduximus."

IDEA
MEDICINÆ
PHILOSOPHICAE,

FUNDAMENTA CONTINENS totius doctrinæ Paracelsicæ, Hippocraticæ, & Galenicæ.

AVTHORE
PETRO SEVERINO DANO
Philosopho & Medico.

AD
FRIDERICVM II. DANIÆ
& Septentrionis Regem.

Cum gratia & Priuilegio
Cæf. Maieſt.

BASILEAE, EX OFFICINA
SIXTI HENRICPETRI.
ANNO M. D. LXXI.

Title page of the first edition of Petrus Severinus' Idea medicinæ philosophicæ. Courtesy of The Danish National Library of Science and Medicine.

In the first chapter of the *Idea medicinæ* Severinus gives the reader a brief history of the development of medicine from Asclepius to Hippocrates to Galen. He praised Galen for reducing the sectarian confusion of post-Hippocratic medicine and for making a rational science from a medical art. Unfortunately, Galen chose to model the science of medicine on geometry and sought to derive all diseases and remedies from certain axiomatic qualities and elements, and in the process, he took medicine away from the phenomena and made it speculative. Health was a balance; imbalances in the mixtures of the four elements led to disease and death. Furthermore, the properties and forms of all things resulted from these mixtures. Diseases as well as *materia medica* (therapeutic materials applied to the body or taken internally) were characterized by the four qualities (hot, cold, moist, and dry), and once characterized, a disease was to be cured by the application of medicines with contrary qualities. From this theory arose a humoral pathology that aimed to achieve a mix of the four basic body fluids or humors – blood, yellow bile or choler, black bile, and phlegm – that was proper to each individual.[26] Galen was so successful in rationalizing medicine that physicians became lazy. His followers merely codified his work and continued his rational medicine; Arab physicians added some new medicines and observations unknown to Galen. It was the appearance of new diseases in the present age and the manifest inability of traditional therapy to cope with them that caused the current controversies in medicine. So many centuries have been invested in furthering Galenic medicine that there is great resistance to change. The result has been that instead of provoking a change in established medicine to meet the challenges of the times, the new diseases created new schools of thought.[27]

Paracelsus, having followed the opinions of other authorities, changed the art of medicine and explained the phenomena of nature in a far different manner, based on *vital astronomy*. Forsaking the humoral doctrine, he ascribed the generation and transplantation of diseases to mechanical causes and to minerals. He also introduced new cures, and this "filled the colleges of all the physicians, which had not expected this innovation

26 Ibid., pp. 2-3.
27 Ibid., p. 3.

of art, with disgust, regret, rage, and confusion."[28] Nevertheless, there
is much about common practice that speaks for Galenic pathology and
the Aristotelian philosophy upon which it is partly based. But in the
great new diseases, it is evident that "empirics" and even the "false and
adulterous Paracelsians" (*spurios quoque et adulterinos Theophrasteos*) are
able to cure where Galenic physicians cannot; therefore it is wise not to
limit oneself to one school, but to draw what is useful from several.[29] It
is appropriate to emphasize here that Severinus, no matter how much
an adherent to chemical medicine, was an eclectic physician and was
unwilling to throw out tried and true Galenic therapy, except where
it was proven ineffective by experience. Galenic theory, however, was
another matter.

At some point in his education Severinus adopted a basically Neoplatonist cosmology. That is, he became committed to the view that
the universe is a living thing with an underlying, spiritual basis, which
wells up or emanates material existence. Severinus' philosophy demanded
that the immaterial, rational structure of the world – form, thought,
idea, whatever the immaterial aspect of reality may be called – *cause*
the corporeal world. This strong commitment to Platonic idealism was
impossible to reconcile with the "dead" Aristotelian philosophy upon
which medieval "Galenic" medicine was based. Paracelsianism, on the
other hand, could readily be explained in terms of spiritual agents and
a transcendent formal structure that united man and universe.[30]

Severinus acknowledged that it is not easy to abandon Galenism
entirely. Those "who have now grown old with Galen" have been able
to successfully treat patients according to the old theory. Much of it
is based on common sense, and much is supported by observation.

---

28 Ibid., p. 5: "et coetus omnium medicorum, inexpectata hac artis innouatione, tædio,
poenitentia, ira & confusione repleuit."
29 Ibid., pp. 5-6.
30 One cannot rule out that there are Stoic elements in the intellectual lineage of Severinus' philosophy, but, as I argue below, these reached Severinus through Neoplatonic
intermediaries, notably St. Augustine. Paracelsian theory had appeal as a "Christian"
philosophy, an alternative to the "Pagan" philosophy of Aristotle and Galen. Moran, *The
Alchemical World of the German Court*, p. 141, tells how the Paracelsian Benedict Figulus
found Paracelsian theory preferable to Aristotelian philosophy, which he considered
too secular.

After all, doesn't one actually see blood and the other humors in the body? Furthermore, much of Galenism is rooted in the utterances of Hippocrates, whom all physicians revere, and this offers protection to the humoral doctrine.[31] It would seem from this that Severinus really did consider his medicine to be based on that of Galen and Hippocrates as well as that of Paracelsus. Indeed, although the *Idea medicinæ* offers little praise of Galen and spills much ink to explain Paracelsian doctrines, there is an unstated background of Galenic medicine that is taken for granted. The *Idea medicinæ* seems all the more Paracelsian to us because we do not see what a contemporary reader would have, namely that a core of traditional medicine remains between the lines. For example, Severinus refers to digestions taking place in the stomach, by which ingested foodstuffs are converted into chyle, which is then converted into blood by a second digestion in the liver. This much is Galenic doctrine. However, Severinus thought of these digestions as chemical processes that are governed by the spirits of salt, sulphur, and mercury that abound in the organs – a decidedly Paracelsian idea. Furthermore, he refers to a third digestion in the kidneys, and similar processes in the spleen and other organs.[32] Severinus lived in a pre-Harveyan world, before the theory of cardiovascular circulation revolutionized physiology. Nevertheless, he abandoned the linear Galenic model by which nutriments were sequentially refined into natural, vital, and psychic spirits in favor of a Paracelsian paradigm, where chemical separations were carried out locally, specific to particular organs and places in the body.

Although present, Galen is, in fact, little mentioned in the *Idea medicinæ* as compared to Hippocrates. Considering that much of medieval medicine ultimately was rooted in Hippocratic tradition, and that Galen was himself a major source of Hippocratic doctrine, we come to suspect Severinus' many recourses to Hippocrates as an authority. The fact that Severinus quoted Hippocratic texts in Greek adds to the symbolic authority vested in the ancient source. Severinus also used the name Hippocrates rhetorically, to signify what he deemed "right" about

---

31 Severinus, *Idea medicinæ*, pp. 5-6.
32 Ibid., pp. 173-75.

traditional medicine.[33] Conversely, the name Galen was used mainly in connection with the "geometrical" corruption of ancient medicine. Moreover, Severinus found that Paracelsian concepts could be read into "Hippocratic" medicine, whereas Galenism was too thoroughly infested with Aristotelian qualities. For example, although Hippocrates frequently blamed the humors for disease, we are not to suppose that he was a humoral pathologist in the same sense as Galen, who found the root of disease in a qualitative imbalance. Hippocrates did not consider bile to be a cause of disease on account of its hot and dry quality, but because of the active powers (*dynameis*), which can produce severe symptoms when they are exalted.[34] Furthermore, by giving particular credence to one Hippocratic text in particular, *On Ancient Medicine*, Severinus was consciously defining the true Hippocratic pathology as chemical, not humoral. In that treatise Hippocrates associated disease not with hot, cold, wet, and dry, but with acid, sharp, bitter, and astringent, and blamed these qualities on the active power (*dynamis*) within nature.[35] This point of view would more readily appeal to the iatrochemist than would that of Galen.

Severinus' use of Hippocrates as a symbol of what was good about the *prisci medici* grounded Paracelsian medicine in tradition, lending it the weight of ancient authority. In this way he suggested that the iatrochemists' challenge to Galenic therapy might also be based in ancient medicine. But we should also see Severinus' appeal to the authority of Hippocrates as part of a general sixteenth-century interest in seeking

33 Wesley Smith, *The Hippocratic Tradition*, p. 14, claims that Paracelsus "led the way" to disassociating the medicine of Hippocrates from Galen's corruption of it. Severinus follows his lead.

34 Severinus, *Idea medicinæ*, p. 205.

35 Pagel, *The Smiling Spleen* (Basel: Karger, 1984), p. 23. *On Ancient Medicine*, one of the most important of the Hippocratic treatises not mentioned by Galen, argues that medicine should be founded on observation and not hypotheses (like the axioms of the geometers). Severinus appears to have been strongly persuaded by the view of medicine propounded in this text. Note that one of the manuscripts reportedly in his possession at the time of his death, one also mentioned in the *Idea medicinæ*, is a paraphrase on this Hippocratic treatise, suggesting that he subjected it to particular scrutiny while still a student. See also Hippocrates, *On Ancient Medicine*, trans. W. H. S. Jones, pp. xlii, 3-64.

the historical roots of medicine, a trend that grew out of the humanists' desire to recover, edit, and publish ancient texts. This movement
culminated in the historically oriented treatment of medicine, a genre
of medical literature that takes as its starting point the origin and
progress of medicine from antiquity to the present.[36] Severinus signals
his sympathy with this view in the very first sentence of chapter one,
where he praises the healing abilities of Æsculapius, Podalirius, and
Machaon, locating medicine in the dim recollection of ancient Greece
that is manifest in the Iliad.[37] Part of this humanist medicine was an
attempt to understand the writings of Hippocrates and fit Hippocratic
medicine into a modern context. Thus, it is no more surprising to see
Severinus finding chemical philosophy rooted in Hippocratic doctrine
than it is to find another Paracelsian, Thomas Moffet, devoting a treatise specifically to Hippocratic medicine.[38] Theodor Zwinger, a near
contemporary of Severinus and mentor of Moffet, similarly believed
that Paracelsian iatrochemistry was an elaboration of principles found
in Hippocrates' works.[39]

Where are we to place the *Idea medicinæ*? It is clearly Paracelsian
and very critical of scholastic medicine and Galenic pathology. It fits
well in the general Paracelsian rhetoric of reform, but it should also
be seen as belonging immediately to a genre of compromise literature
that sought to find common ground between university medicine and
Paracelsianism, between humoral pathology and chemical cures. The
titles of treatises published about the time of the *Idea medicinæ* indicate
the appeal of such a compromise: Albertus Wimpinæus published *De*

36 The seventeenth century produced some marvelous examples of this, for instance Olaus
    Borrichius, *Dissertatio de ortu et progressu Chemiæ* (Copenhagen, 1660), and his later
    vindication of the ancient roots for chemistry against attacks by Hermann Conring, in
    *Hermetis, ægyptiorum et chemicorum sapientia ab Hermanni Conringii animadversionibus
    vindicata* (Copenhagen, 1674). See also Allen G. Debus, "The Significance of Chemical
    History," *Ambix* 32 (1985): 1-14.
37 Paracelsus wrote in the preface to *Sieben defensiones* that God had revealed medicine
    through Apollo, Machaon, Podalirius, and Hippocrates. Machaon and Podalirius were
    sons of Æsculapius. See Smith, *The Hippocratic Tradition*, p. 15.
38 Thomas Moffet, *Nosomantica Hippocratea* (Frankfurt, 1584).
39 Albrecht Burckhardt, *Geschichte der Medizinischen Fakultät zu Basel 1460-1900* (Basel:
    Universitätsdruckerei, 1917), pp. 92-3.

concordia Hippocraticorum et Paracelsistarum (On the Concord between the Hippocratics and Paracelsians) in Basel in 1569; Guinter von Andernach published his *De medicina veteri et nova* (On the Old and New Medicine) there in 1571, and of course the *Idea medicinæ* was published there in 1571. This sort of endeavor to find a compromise was in keeping with the spirit of toleration and finding common ground that captivated European intellectuals in these years, yet among some scholars it continued into the seventeenth century, as is evident, for example, in Daniel Sennert's 1619 treatise *De chymicorum cum Aristotelicis et Galenicis consensu ac dissensu* (On the Agreement and Disagreement Between the Chemists and the Aristotelians and Galenists). By that time, however, renewed interest in classical atomism was complicating the picture, and a generation of irenicism had given way to a generation of intolerance, counter-reformation, and civil war.[40]

Now that we have some sense of the general context of the *Idea medicinæ*, we turn to explore its content under three topics: general theory, pathology, and therapy. It is important to understand Severinus' medicine against the background of his general theory, to see that he thought of disease as a natural process and based his theory of curing on his pathology. Viewed in this light, it becomes clear that chemical therapy, by which I mean not just the use of mineral based distillations, but rather that all drugs are considered to operate chemically, has a dialectical relationship to chemical philosophy.

---

40 Daniel Sennert, *De chymicorum cum Aristotelicis et Galenicis consensu ac dissensu liber* (Wittenberg, 1619). Sennert is a good example of a transitional figure. One finds in his works a mixture of ideas as he attempts to synthesize observation with received theory. The influence of atomism on Sennert's changing views on transmutation is noted by Christoph Meinel, "Early Seventeenth-Century Atomism," *Isis*, vol. 79 (1988), pp. 95-8. On the failure of irenicism and the polarization of political culture in the Holy Roman Empire in the period leading up to the Thirty Years' War, see Howard Louthan, *The Quest for Compromise: Peacemakers in Counter-Reformation Vienna* (Cambridge: Cambridge University Press, 1997).

GENERAL THEORY: THE CHIEF DOCTRINES
OF THE *IDEA MEDICINÆ*

One cannot doubt Severinus' dependence on Paracelsus as a source of doctrine; one is, in fact, hard pressed to identify original doctrinal contributions. But Severinus excelled in identifying and explaining key metaphysical concepts found in Paracelsian tracts and fitting them into the much larger philosophical framework of Renaissance Platonism. The philosophical system he built earned him a prominent place in the early evolution and transmission of Paracelsian thought and made the *Idea medicinæ* a singularly valuable source for late sixteenth and early seventeenth-century students of Paracelsian philosophy. It is because of Severinus' role as codifier of Paracelsian ideas that I will not here present a full exposition of the philosophy of the *Idea medicinæ*, which would entail an extensive treatment of Paracelsian doctrine, but rather focus on its salient features and on selected key concepts that were associated with this text by later authors, concepts with which Severinus' name became attached.

THE DOCTRINE OF *SEMINA*

The one idea of central importance to the reception of the *Idea medicinæ*, one that was repeatedly taken from Severinus' book, is the doctrine of *semina*.[41] The concept of *semina morbi*, seeds of disease, had been in the medical literature since the time of Galen and came under renewed scrutiny by the early medical humanists. Notably, Fracastoro and his followers applied the idea to the pathology of certain diseases in the first half of the sixteenth century. Fracastoro's *semina*, or more usually *seminaria*, like his *fomites*, were definitely material, drawn from

---

41 Walter Pagel, *William Harvey's Biological Ideas* (New York: Hafner, 1967), pp. 239-247. In Pagel's judgement, "most of Severinus' biological ideas have influenced the subsequent generations of Paracelsists. This is particularly evident in the adoption of his concept of semina and their substitution for the elements of ancient lineage and tradition." See Pagel, *Smiling Spleen*, p. 22.

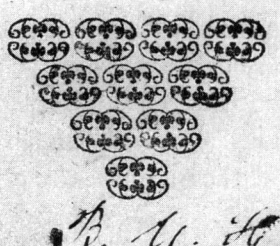

IDEA
MEDICINÆ
PHILOSOPHICÆ.

Continens Fundamenta totius Doctrinæ
Paracelsicæ, Hippocraticæ
& Galenicæ.

Authore

PETRO SEVERINO DANO
Philosophiæ & Medicinæ Doctore.

HAGÆ-COMITIS

Ex Typographia A D R I A N I V L A C Q.
Anno Domini M. DC. LX.

1660

Title page of the third edition of Severinus' Idea medicinæ philosophicæ, *published
in 1660, presumably to accompany William Davidson's preliminary commentary on
it. Few changes were made from the first edition, upon which this one must have
been based. Courtesy of The Danish National Library of Science and Medicine.*

atomistic philosophy.[42] Lucretius had used the term *semina* to mean atoms, a quite different usage from the seeds envisioned by Paracelsus and Severinus, which were dimensionless, formal in nature. *Seminaria* (seed beds) conjures up an image of a nurturing matrix rather than a seed itself, although Fracastoro does not seem to have distinguished the two terms. Paracelsus had also written of seeds of disease, and Severinus quite likely took the idea from him, although we cannot ignore the possibility that he was influenced by Fracastoro's work, or by some other sixteenth-century medical writer. However, Severinus' *semina* theory is much more general than that found in either source. It is not a concept specific to contagious or hereditary diseases, but rather a fully developed biological theory.

Semina are literally "seeds", but because Severinus uses the term in a special sense, different from any modern use of the term seeds, the Latin term is often preferable, just to remind us of this difference. *Semina* are the fundamental immaterial principles out of which material bodies arise and to which they return. They are the principles that govern the unfolding of bodies according to their foreordained, divine, ideal plans. They are therefore fundamental both to Severinus' ontology and his epistemology. Epistemologically, *semina* are an end or goal for philosophical research. Since *semina* are imperceptible to the senses, because they lack dimensions, "they can scarcely be separated [from the elements] by any subtlety of the mind."[43] The philosopher must acquire knowledge of them indirectly, through observation of their characteristics, their periodicities in individuals, and by stripping away their accidental properties through chemical analysis. This follows logically: since *semina* are supposed to operate chemically, it makes sense that one can study them chemically. Severinus attributes the chemical operation of *semina* to Hippocrates:

---

42 For a discussion of Fracastoro's use of these terms and how they affected sixteenth-century medical literature, see Vivian Nutton, "The Reception of Fracastoro's Theory of Contagion: The Seed that Fell among Thorns?" *Osiris*, 2nd ser., 6 (1990): 196-234.

43 Severinus, *Idea medicinæ*, p. 48: "Indissolubili nexu elementis conserta cohærent, uix ulla mentis subtilitate disiungi possunt."

But by what power are so many, such diverse developments of seeds perceived in nature? He [Hippocrates] teaches that this is done by virtue of separation. ... Therefore, by separation, the seeds lying peacefully in the elemental wombs are aroused at the appointed times, appear on the world stage, and with remarkable knowledge they regulate the ebbing and flowing of generation and corruption. Let him who desires a richer explanation of this separation read the *Books of the Philosophy of Theophrastus Paracelsus, Dedicated to the Athenians.*[44]

But why should the philosopher go to this effort to study *semina*?

All philosophy that, having neglected the contemplation of these seeds and stars, chases dead privations, formless matters, and dead qualities, is deaf and blind. Indeed, we cannot obtain knowledge of the elements without the seeds or stars, for they have unfolded the functions of the elements.[45]

Severinus' belief that the chemist can succeed where the Aristotelian has failed is grounded in his conception of vitality, or what he calls vital anatomy. Understanding this anatomy entails knowledge of the *semina*, the elements, and the stars.

Paracelsus used the term "anatomy" to refer to the distribution of things and the analysis of their interrelationships.[46] Whether of minerals in the macrocosm or diseases in the microcosm, "anatomy" accounted

44 Ibid., p. 86: "Sed qua potestate, tot, tam diuersæ seminum progressiones in Natura conspiciuntur? Separationis uirtute ea fieri docet. ... Separatione igitur semina in Matricibus quiete delitescentia, digestis temporibus suscitantur, in mundanam Scenam prodeunt, admirabili Scientia Generationum Corruptionumque fluxus & refluxus moderantur. Huius Separationis uberiorem explicationem qui desiderat, legat libros Philosophiæ THEOPHRASTI PARACELSI Atheniensibus dedicatos." Paracelsus' *Philosophiæ ad Athenienses drey Bücher* was published by Arnold Byrckmann, Cologne 1564.

45 Severinus, *Idea medicinæ*, p. 49: "Surda & coeca est omnis Philosophia, quæ horum contemplatione neglecta, priuationes, informes materias, & mortuas qualitates sectatur. Etenim Elementorum cognitionem, sine his adipisci non possumus. Semina enim uel Astra, officia Elementorum explicauere."

46 Our modern word "analysis" is closer in meaning to the Paracelsian *anatomia* than is the modern term "anatomy," which generally refers to cutting up bodies. Direct rendering of *anatomia* as anatomy, like translating *signaturæ* as signatures rather than characteristics or properties, gives Paracelsus' writings an unnecessarily mysterious flavor.

for why certain things were found in certain places.[47] This use of the term is somewhat baffling at times, but makes sense if one sees it against the background of medical education in the sixteenth century, when the study of human anatomy was coming into its own at transalpine universities.[48] Severinus' opinion was that one can learn only so much from the dissection of dead beings. In fact one will miss what for the physician is the crucial point, namely the vital functioning of the organism – its vital anatomy. Severinus was aware that his use of the concept of vital anatomy would meet with opposition: "Very many will complain that we are burying a manifest art in obscurity, that we are introducing a new and unheard of anatomy of causes and powers."[49] But, he says, although human dissection has its place, it is not enough:

> One [kind of anatomy] is dead, the other is living. For actions do not proceed from parts and bodies, but from powers inherent in these parts. Vital anatomy is certainly the more difficult of the two ... and therefore the physician who wishes to undertake this anatomy ought first to unravel the nature and properties of the seed.[50]

Thus, knowledge of the nature and operation of *semina* is at the root of vital anatomy, which is a *physiological* (as opposed to anatomical) understanding of how the body operates. From here it is a small jump to understanding Severinus' more general interpretation of Paracelsian anatomy. Since the world at large is filled with vitality, it too has a vital anatomy, a world anatomy. In this mindset physiological function per-

47 Pagel, *Paracelsus*, pp. 137-8.
48 Dissection had been practiced and taught at Italian universities in the Middle Ages, but it was not until the sixteenth century that anatomy was a salient part of the medieval curriculum and well enough established as a didactic tradition to generate demand for it in the northern universities. It did not become an officially sanctioned element of the curriculum at the University of Copenhagen until the seventeenth century, for example.
49 Severinus, *Idea medicinæ*, p. 32: "Conquerentur plurimi, nos obscuritate manifestam artem obruere: nouam inauditamque Facultatum & Causarum Anatomiam introducere."
50 Ibid., p. 33: "Hæc mortua est, altera uitalis. Non enim ex partibus & corporibus actiones procedunt, sed ex facultatibus partibus inhærentibus. Difficilior certe est uitalis Anatomia. ... Itaque qui hanc Anatomiam aggredi uoluerit, imprimis Seminis naturam & proprietates explicare debet."

tains to the general chemical operation of nature; as in the microcosm, so in the macrocosm, where *semina* govern chemical change. But exactly what are *semina*? How do they differ from biological seeds? Traditionally, seeds were viewed as small bodies, or particles, that carried the information or pattern necessary for the growth of organisms.[51] This was precisely the metaphor that Severinus needed, but he felt that the traditional concept of seed was too confining: "First of all the name seed comes to mind, although it has hitherto obtained an excessively narrow meaning at the hands of common philosophers. For those people consider a seed to be only that which can preserve the fecundity of its kind in a visible matter," i.e. "semen" in the modern sense.[52]

Severinus emphasized the Neoplatonist view of *semina* as formal seed-like reasons (*rationes seminales* or *logoi spermatikoi*) that are spread throughout the universe and stand as intermediaries between the creative divine ideas and their resultant creations.[53] The ontological status of *semina*, then, is something intermediate between idea (pure form) and material body. The term "spirit" has sometimes been used to denote the stuff that is neither truly form (soul) nor truly body, but somewhere in between, and we might well identify *semina* as spiritual, provided we bear in mind that the meaning of spirit varies from author to author in the sixteenth century. For Severinus, it is clear that *semina* were in actuality (i.e. as they are manifest in nature) subtly corporeal, but that this corporeality was *accidental* to the *semina*, which were essentially without dimension, and therefore not corporeal in the Aristotelian sense.[54] This should become clearer with elaboration.

---

51 See Pagel, *William Harvey's Biological Ideas*, p. 242.
52 Severinus, *Idea medicinæ*, p. 55: "Inprimis occurrit seminis appellatio: quamuis angustam nimis significationem apud uulgares Philosophos obtinuerit hactenus. Ii enim solum id semen existimant, quod uisibili materia foecunditatem sui generis conservare possit."
53 The basic idea that *semina* link the ideal and material worlds is found in Paracelsus, *Philosophia sagax*. See Walter Pagel, "Paracelsus and the Neoplatonic and Gnostic Tradition," *Ambix* 8 (1960), p. 136.
54 This is in agreement with Pagel's understanding of how Severinus used the term *semina*. See Pagel, *Smiling Spleen*, p. 20.

THE ONTOLOGICAL STATUS OF *SEMINA*

Severinus employed a variety of terms in accounting for the basic constitution of the corporeal world, many of which he inherited from Paracelsus. The relationship between these metaphysical components, the *semina*, elements, vital balsam, *matrices*, *archei*, *iliastrum*, the *tria prima principia* (salt, sulphur, mercury), and so on, is not always clearly defined; nor are their properties always distinct enough for the modern temper. At times, for example, *archei* and *semina* seem indistinguishable, and it is sometimes not clear whether they contain vital balsam, whether vital balsam contains them, or whether the question is relevant.[55] This does not mean that there is no order to Severinus' philosophy, just that it requires some patience and toleration for what has become for us, as historians looking back four hundred years, an alien frame of mind.

In brief, *semina* guide the process by which bodies are generated from spirit. This is a reification in which form, soul, or spirit emanates material being. This function, explained at greater length below, conveys a unique ontological status to *semina*. Occupying the no-man's-land between the intelligible, ideal world and the sensible world of bodies, *semina* must partake of both. They must be essentially formal, dimensionless, and without quality, but able to dress themselves in matter and take on qualities, quantity, and dimension as they evolve into bodies.[56] This is not to say that *semina* actually exist in a purely formal state, merely that they are essentially formal. For in the created world, form was joined to matter in the beginning, and the subsequent evolution of the universe is an explication or unfolding of the divine predestination.

55 Severinus may also have thought of them this way, but he does not clearly separate the roles of *semina* and *archei* in the *Idea medicinæ*. For Paracelsus, the *archei* were the agents responsible for unfolding the predestinations innate in the *semina*. See Pagel, *Paracelsus*, p. 367.

56 Paracelsus presented a case for invisible, corporeal principles that united with matter in order to clothe themselves in bodies in *De podagricis*. See Massimo L. Bianchi, "The Visible and the Invisible from Alchemy to Paracelsus," in *Alchemy and Chemistry in the 16th and 17th Centuries*, ed. Piyo Rattansi and Antonio Clericuzio, pp. 17-50, International Archives of the History of Ideas 140 (Dordrecht: Kluwer, 1994), p. 26. Ultimately the roots of this fuzzy distinction between formal and material goes back to Plotinus, who taught that both incorporeal and corporeal beings were constituted from one principle that was both form and matter. See P.O. Kristeller, *Eight Renaissance Philosophers*, p. 133.

Semina, then, lie at the origins and bases of all bodies. They are logically prior to the Aristotelian elements (earth, air, fire, water), but logically (and chronologically) posterior to the divine ideas, which existed before creation.

In this respect *semina* are much like vital balsam, or the principle of vitality. Vital balsam distinguishes living things from dead, and although it, too, shares both spiritual and corporeal characteristics, it seems to be logically posterior to *semina*. Severinus speaks of vital balsam as having *semina* within it, suggesting that it is more material or complex than *semina*, but in other respects their attributes are similar: both are responsible for the separations, digestions, nutritions, procreations, and all other faculties or functions that characterize living things. Elsewhere, he calls *semen* the intrinsic vital principle in bodies and the bearer of tinctures, implying that vital balsam (or its tinctures, at least) is also in *semina*.[57] Vital balsam, he says, has been known by many names:

> Theophrastus the Greek, student of Aristotelian philosophy, touched on this matter in his book *On the Causes of Plants*, and he called it τὸ ἔμβιον τῆς φύσεως, the vital principle in nature, by whose virtue all things live and grow: those without it are dead. But Theophrastus Paracelsus, the pride of Germany, adorned this fruitful treasury of nature with many names: he named it balsam, mummy, mercury, also quintessence, arcanum, elixir, perfected matter, Manna, etc.[58]

Vital balsam must be material, or even corporeal (having dimension), insofar as it is subject to being drawn out of its vegetable and mineral host by human art. God has placed vital balsam in animals, says Severinus, in such a way that men cannot usefully extract it. Yet, those who would call vital balsam a spirit are also right, because bodies proceed

---

57 See Pagel, *William Harvey's Biological Ideas*, p. 242; Severinus, *Idea medicinæ*, pp. 92 and 96.

58 Severinus, *Idea medicinæ*, p. 17: "Theophrastus ille Græcus, Aristotelicæ Philosophiæ alumnus, libro de Causis plantarum, hanc materiam attigit, appellauitque τὸ ἔμβιον τῆς φύσεως, uitale principium in Natura, cuius uirtute uiuunt uigentque omnia: cætera mortua sunt. Theophrastus uero Paracelsus, Germaniæ decus, multis nominibus foecundum hunc Naturæ thesaurum ornauit: Balsamum, Mumiam, Mercurium nominat: item Quintam essentiam, Arcanum, Elixir, Materiam perlatam, Mannam, &c."

from spirits.[59] Ontologically vital balsam is hardly distinguishable from *semina*; both stand at the gateway between form and body. There is, however, a marked difference in the way Severinus speaks of vital balsam and *semina*. Whereas *semina* are discrete, vital balsam is spoken of as continuous stuff. *Semina* are individual centers of actualization in the world, centers of divinely predestined activity, in other words metaphysical concepts. Vital balsam, on the other hand, is the substantial basis for medicine. It is the stuff that confers life, and thus health, and is what physicians employ in remedies.

SEMINA, ASTRA, AND THE ELEMENTS

Another distinction between vital balsam and *semina*, one likely inherited from ambiguities in the Paracelsian treatises, is that vital balsam is associated with quintessence and stellar matter, whereas *semina* may be found in each of the four Aristotelian elements. However, unlike the Aristotelian world, the Paracelsian cosmos is not plainly divided between the celestial and terrestrial, which permits stellar matter to exist among the terrestrial elements, and this further clouds the distinction between balsam and *semina*. Severinus noted that philosophers are content with earth, air, and water as elements, and that disagreement has mostly raged over fire. He recognized the essential feature of Paracelsus' rejection of fire as a mundane element, namely that by identifying fire with the elemental basis of celestial bodies, Paracelsus was breaking down the inviolable distinction between sublunary and superlunary realms. Fire as an element exists on earth, but it is celestial in origin. Severinus carried this process another step by dividing the physical world into two elemental globes or regions: fire and air occupy the upper region, earth and water the lower.[60] This makes the heavens an extension of the terrestrial world, unifying the physics of the two. Aristotelian quintessence (vital balsam), according to Severinus' system, is to be found everywhere, in accordance with the basic Platonic view that the celestial bodies, like

59 Ibid., p. 26.
60 Ibid., p. 41.

plants, animals, and minerals, are alive.

According to Paracelsus there is no direct influence of the celestial bodies on man, but man, like other terrestrial creatures, has stars (*astra*) within him.[61] The main, observable feature of the stars and the planets is that they maintain characteristic cycles. Therefore they are the very measures of time, and their motions can be correlated with the recognized periodic changes in terrestrial creatures. In this sense the *astra* in minerals, vegetables, and animals are responsible for the life-cycles that various species undergo: each individual has its times of rising and setting. Severinus defends this use of the term *astra* by Paracelsus:

> We shall teach that stars are contained in animals and plants and that the name "stars" agrees with their principles. For indeed, whether you seek the fixed periods of changes in all natural actions of herbs, animals, or minerals, or in the concoction of foodstuffs, in the separation of excrements, in all nutrition, in growth, or in procreations, you will find that the established constancy and uniformity of their changes is maintained.[62]

Severinus follows Paracelsus' lead in replacing direct astrological determinism by conceiving of *astra* that are implanted in terrestrial creatures. These terrestrial stars are coordinated with celestial *astra* through sympathy. There is no causal connection in the sense of a temporal relationship, but there is nevertheless a throughgoing harmony between what is above and what is below. This view of the cosmos is artfully captured in Tycho Brahe's definition of the two complementary sciences, terrestrial astronomy (iatrochemistry) and celestial astronomy (astronomy); the

---

61 In *Paramirum* and elsewhere Paracelsus wrote that there are terrestrial and celestial stars; that everything in the heavens is also in man (see n. 63, below). Like much about Paracelsus, this is not entirely clear or without equivocation. However, it seems that Paracelsus did not allow for a "direct" astral determinism by stellar influx. Instead there are correspondences or harmonies that associate celestial and terrestrial events. See Pagel, *Paracelsus*, pp. 67-68.

62 Severinus, *Idea medicinæ*, p. 56: "Astra in plantis et animalibus contineri docebimus, astrorumque appellationem horum principijs consentaneam esse. Etenim siue statas motuum periodos quæsiueris, in omnibus actionibus naturalibus, herbarum, animalium & mineralium, in alimentorum concoctione, excrementorum separatione, in tota nutricatione, in augmentis, in procreationibus, motuum rata constantia & æquabilitas custoditur."

philosopher learns about the heavens by studying the earth, and about the earth by studying the heavens.[63]

The relationship between *astra*, *semina*, and vital balsam is further complicated by Severinus' classification of terrestrial *astra* into two specific kinds. There is the purer sort that distinguishes individual types of animals, vegetables, and minerals: "These are those bodies, seeds, roots, balsams, vital principles, and prime matters in which, as we have now said often and will say in the future, the universal medicine is situated."[64] The other kind of astral body is tied to matter until it has fulfilled its predestination, and then it flees to a more divine, hospitable habitation, where it is no longer "exposed to any impressions of the stars."[65] One is tempted to conclude from this that *semina*, *astra*, vital balsam, etc., are all somehow made of astral matter, or matter without dimension, the prime matter that Paracelsus called *iliastrum*, and differ only in how they act in the world. Severinus sometimes uses these terms as if they were synonyms and he probably did not intend for them to denote analytically distinct essences. Words, after all, were a way of describing reality and not reality itself.

SEMINA AS RATIONES SEMINALES

Although Severinus quite likely took the basic concept of *semina* from Paracelsian tracts, he was probably aware of its origin in the ancient Greek *logoi spermatikoi*, Latinized to *rationes seminales*. *Rationes seminales* had functioned for the Neoplatonic philosophers, who took them over from the Stoics, as the intelligent agents mediating between the purely

---

63 Severinus, Ibid., p. 198, also used this term (in terrestri Astronomia). This expression of the microcosm-macrocosm correspondence may well stem from Paracelsus, who wrote in *De natura rerum* that there are both terrestrial and celestial stars and that those below were meant to govern those above, because God created man to dominate the macrocosm. See *Paracelsus: Essential Readings*, trans. Nicholas Goodrick-Clarke, (Wellingborough, Northamptonshire, England: Aquarian Press, 1990), p. 186.

64 Severinus, *Idea medicinæ*, p. 54: "Hæc sunt illa corpora, Semina, Astra, Radices, Balsama, uitalia principia, primæ materiæ, in quibus nunc sæpe diximus, & posthac dicemus, uniuersam Medicinam fundari."

65 Ibid., p. 54: "nec ullis astrorum impressionibus obnoxia."

divine *logoi* (Platonic ideas) and the materialized world.[66] Subsequently, Christian theoreticians adapted them, and they became an entrenched part of medieval Christian natural philosophy.

There is a metaphysical tension in Christianity between God's transcendence and immanence. Too much stress on God's transcendental nature, his total separation from the material world of human experience, could lead to a Manichæan view, in which evil forces were the main agents in a nature forsaken by God, or else to a Deistic materialism; Too much emphasis on divine agency in matter and God's oneness with man and creation could lead to pantheism. This was a charge frequently levied against mystical philosophies that perceived God's actual presence in the natural world or identified him with man's inner self. *Rationes seminales* provided a welcome buffer between God and nature, a cushion that permitted worldly phenomena to be the outcome of divine wisdom without requiring God to be "in" nature. Rather, matter was impregnated with his spirit, his "seed-like" reasons or plans for things becoming what they are.

Severinus may have known of the Neoplatonic interpretation of *rationes seminales* through Plotinus, an author highly esteemed among Platonists of the late sixteenth century, but since he does not often indicate his sources we can only speculate.[67] Certainly *rationes seminales* had

66 In particular, the work of Plotinus reflects unresolved tensions between Stoicism and Neoplatonism. A.H. Armstrong, *The Architecture of the Intelligible Universe in the Philosophy of Plotinus* (Cambridge: Cambridge University Press, 1940), pp. 49-64, indicates that there are two different approaches to emanation in Plotinus' philosophy: one centers on the use of light as a metaphor for the radiation of Being from the One, to *Nous*, to Soul, and to the visible world; the other emphasizes the unfolding of things by their own nature through some kind of "partless seed." The persistence of these two metaphors down through the Middle Ages reveals the continued vitality both of the Neoplatonic view that the world is really based on idea (light as generative form) and the Stoic view that spirit is merely the most subtle grade of matter (*semina* as generative matter).

67 Severinus listed Plotinus among the Platonists in his *Epistola*, probably published just before the *Idea medicinæ*. One letter-poem, at least, indicates a mutual admiration for the writings of Plotinus among the literati in Copenhagen: In a manuscript labeled "Vale pratensis ad Danzeum" (Pratensis's salutation to Danzay), Pratensis writes "Amica cape manu / Sacra PLOTINI opuscula / Qui nos vitæ immortalis avidos / cum sol noster ad occasura tenderet / dulii contemplationum flumine / suaviter & benigne recreavit." Copenhagen, Kgl. Bibl., Gramske Samling, GKS 1076 I. Zeeberg, "Science Versus Secular Life," has shown that poetry and Neoplatonic mystical expression were important to Tycho Brahe.

played the role of mediators between creator and creation in the widely read hexameral literature from St. Augustine through the Middle Ages. The hexamera, commentaries on the Biblical account of creation in the first six days, were an important source of natural philosophy in the Middle Ages. One of the features of this genre was the reconciliation of inconsistencies in *Genesis* regarding the creation of the world, and this sometimes entailed using natural philosophy to interpret the scriptural record. Augustine used *rationes seminales* to explain the two accounts of creation in the first two chapters of *Genesis*, by interpreting *Genesis I* as the creation of the *rationes seminales* for those things that were actually brought into existence in *Genesis II*. But his assignment of secondary causation to *rationes seminales* was more far-reaching, from the point of natural philosophy, because it permitted God to be the first cause of events that were carried out through the secondary causes, without his being sullied by contact with matter.

Unlike the Neoplatonists, who reduced the philosophical place of matter to near nonexistence (matter is *prope nihil*), Severinus allowed matter a limited determinative role in the generation of bodies. This is evident in the role he assigned to the elements in his philosophy. For Severinus, the "elements" serve as the *matrices* (wombs) wherein *semina* are fed the (prime) matter necessary for their seminal expression as bodies: "Elements are appropriate places for seeds, for in them the seeds are fostered and nourished, they grow and are perfected."[68] Exactly what he meant by "elements" varies somewhat, for in this context he wrote, "what we are calling elements at this point are not those bodies common to all nature – earth, water, air, and firmament – but they are rather most like receptacles for seminal matter."[69] Elsewhere, however, Severinus followed the Paracelsian idea that the elemental *matrices* limit the seminal development according to the particular element. Thus, bodies can be classified according to the elemental *matrix* that dominates them: "The first distinction of bodies is deduced from the classes of the

68 Severinus, *Idea medicinæ*, p. 79: "Convenientia loca seminibus Elementa sunt. In iis enim foventur, nutriuntur, augescunt & absolvuntur."
69 Ibid.: "Elementa hoc loco a nobis dicuntur, non communia illa totius Naturæ corpora, Terra, Aqua, Aer, Firmamentum; sed proxima receptacula seminalis materiæ."

elements – the fact that some are earthy, some aqueous, some aerial, and some are celestial – and these differ very greatly in penetration, mobility, and power for acting."[70] This conjoining of elemental *matrix* and formal *semen* provides a model for generation and corruption that is radically different from both the Aristotelian theory that bodies are built up from mixtures of elements and the atomic theory, in which different sorts of atoms combine to produce sensible bodies. Severinus agreed that the four elements do mix, but denied that the mixing and combining of the elements account for generation and growth. Instead, "each element is more than sufficient for producing and preserving its fruits, and left alone, it need not borrow even small quantities from some other place."[71]

The metaphysical system that Severinus constructed around *semina*, *astra*, and the elements provides a most satisfactory account of change and continuity. Two problems have mainly concerned natural philosophers, said Severinus: "[1] where those forms and species affecting us at defined intervals of time, which carry out the processes of this world comedy by means of generation, transplantation, and mixture, have come from and [2] where they are proceeding to."[72] Both of these problems are easily solved in this philosophy, "for we say that all those things flourish in the seed that here seem to flow and reflow in the cycle of generation and corruption, and that even the form itself of each thing is αὐτοφυὴν [self-made]."[73]

---

70 Ibid., p. 64: "Prima differentia corporum ex Elementorum ordinibus deducitur: quod alia sint terrena, alia aquea, alia aerea, alia coelestia: quæ penetratione, mobilitate, agendi potestate, plurimum discrepant."

71 Ibid., p. 46: "Vnumquodque igitur Elementum, suis fructibus producendis & conseruandis abunde sufficit, nec destitutum aliunde particulas mutuabitur."

72 Ibid., p. 81: "unde profectæ, quo pergant Formæ, Species, quæ nobiscum definitis temporum intervallis negotiaturæ, Generationum, Transplantationum & Mixtionum ministerio mundanæ Comoediæ lithurgiam peragunt."

73 Ibid.: "Dicimus enim in semine ea omnia vigere, quæ hic generationum & corruptionum vicissitudine fluere & refluere videntur, adeoque Formam ipsam uniuscuiusque, esse αὐτοφυὴν." The seventeenth-century English translation of the *Idea medicinæ* (London, British Library, Sloane MS 11, "A Mappe of Medicyne or Philosophicall Path containinge the groundes of all the doctrines of Paracelsus, Hippocrates & Galen compiled by Peter Severine a Dane, philosopher & physician to Fredericke the II King of Denmarke & the Northerne partes," f. 31r) rendered αὐτοφυὴν as "inborne."

RATIONES SEMINALES AND CHRISTIAN PLATONISM

We should miss one of the key advantages of *semina* theory if we failed to notice its appeal to the Christian Platonist. As Severinus points out, according to the *semina* doctrine the form of a body is immanent, and therefore

> does not come from without, is not infused by a giver of forms after there is an agreeable mixture of the elements, is not dispersed from a momentary arrangement of the stars onto the lower region, is not re- newed by the chance meeting of atoms, but is lying hidden in the seeds themselves: and that in various ways. These theories are Paracelsian; they are not inconsistent with Christian religion and they are close to the decrees of the Platonists.[74]

Severinus developed much of his philosophy around *semina*, allowing them responsibility for all change and continuity: "What then are gen- eration and corruption? They are the flowing and reflowing of seeds, which when they flow out are increased, and when they flow back they are diminished."[75] Thus *semina* account for cyclical behavior in nature, and, as Orpheus said, all things are circular. Just as the moon "is rightly said to be born, to be generated, to increase, decrease, and to die every month," so it is with animals; all life is a circular process of generation and corruption and regeneration.[76] Light is associated with the flowing forth of seeds in generation, and darkness with the reflowing of seeds in corruption, as the body returns to the "dark" potentiality of Orphic Night or the Hippocratic Abyss.[77]

The pivotal role of *semina* in providing natural law, as the *rationes* that govern change and the continuity of species, again points to the

---

74 Severinus, *Idea medicinæ*, p. 81: "Non extrinsecus accedere, non a datore Formarum post Elementorum consentaneam mixtionem infundi, non a stellarum momentaneo positu in inferiorem naturam derivari, non ex Atomorum fortuito congressu integrari, sed in ipsis seminibus delitescere: idque variis modis. Hæc dogmata sunt Paracelsica, a Christiana Religione non abhorrentia, Platonicorum decretis vicina."

75 Ibid., p. 89: "Quid igitur est Generatio & Corruptio? Sunt fluxus & refluxus seminum, quæ dum fluunt augentur, minuuntur vero dum refluunt."

76 Ibid., p. 89-90: "Ita Luna nasci, generari, crescere, decrescere, occidere, recte dicitur singulis mensibus."

77 Ibid.

great appeal of *semina* theory for Christian philosophy. The use of *rationes seminales* to account for divine activity in the world of nature, as intermediaries between mind and body, has had a continuous place in Christian philosophy since St. Augustine, who adapted the idea of seminal reasons to the needs of Biblical exegesis: God sowed the "waters" with *semina* at the creation of the world.[78] These same *semina* were used by natural philosophers seeking to accommodate divine activity with natural philosophy already in the Middle Ages, when they were sometimes associated with the activity of light, or else they were used to account for the seeming influence of the heavens on terrestrial affairs.[79] In the late Renaissance, *rationes seminales*, if not always identified as such, fit well with Hermetic doctrine and Florentine Platonism, and were later used to explain activity by a wide variety of natural philosophers, from Bruno to Kepler.[80] It is not

78 One of the early studies of Augustine's *rationes seminales* theory is Michael J. McKeough, *The Meaning of Rationes Seminales in St. Augustine*, Ph. D. Dissertation (Washington: Catholic University of America, 1926). For a more general treatment see Christopher J. O'Toole, *The Philosophy of Creation in the Writings of St. Augustine*, Ph. D. Dissertation (Washington: Catholic University of America, 1944). A more recent work specifically on the *rationes seminales*, drawing heavily on the above dissertations, is Jules M. Brady, "St. Augustine's Theory of Seminal Reasons," *New Scholasticism* 38 (1964): 141-58.

79 St. Bonaventure saw two possibilities by which matter is informed: either by multiplication of species, as one candle may be used to light many, or by the eduction of form already present seminally in matter. He considered both alternatives and adopted the latter view, citing St. Augustine's *De genesi ad litteram* as a source. See Fredrick Copleston, *A History of Philosophy*, vol. 2, part 1, (1950; Garden City, N.Y.: Doubleday, Image Books, 1962), pp. 305-6. On Henry of Langenstein's use of *rationes seminales* to explain causation, see Nicholas H. Steneck, *Science and Creation in the Middle Ages* (Notre Dame, 1976), pp. 34, 95, 99, and 109.

80 Although Bruno and Kepler do not treat *semina* as causal agents explicitly in their works, the idea of creative action through the unfolding of a spiritual seed can be found there, perhaps as vestiges of the parallel models of seed and light in Plotinus's writings. For example, Bruno associated *semina* with the "water" of Genesis in *De rerum principiis et elementis et causis* (1590), in *Opera Latine conscripta*, ed. F. Tocco and H. Vitelli, vol. 3 (Florence, 1841), p. 510, line 22 – p. 511, line 1: "et quia omnia rerum semina sunt humida, ideo rerum omnium semen aquam [Moises] appellat." Kepler, who elaborated on Robert Grosseteste's light metaphysics as the paradigm for creative multiplication of species in his *Ad Vitellionem paralipomena*, associated this ability of light "to communicate itself" with seeds. See Johannes Kepler, *Ad Vitellionem paralipomena*, in *Johannes Kepler Gesammelte Werke*, ed. Franz Hammer, vol. 2 (Munich, 1939), p. 31: He speaks of color multiplying in matter when excited by light, much like ginger heats up when stimulated by a fluid, "et communicare se incipit; quod idem faciunt omnia semina" [and it begins to communicate itself, the same thing that all seeds do].

surprising, then, that we find them in Paracelsian philosophy, and for the same reasons.[81]

Owing to the resurgence of interest in Platonism, philosophy in the fifteenth and sixteenth centuries had a need for a metaphysical link between soul and body, and *rationes seminales* provided a ready-made solution that also allowed divine predestination a place in cosmology. We find *rationes seminales* in the philosophy of Ficino, from which they may have entered Paracelsian doctrine.[82] Paracelsus did not state where he got his idea of *semina*, but it is clear that he, like Augustine, interpreted *semina* as the seeds of creation that provided bodies with their predestined functions and ends.[83] If Paracelsus and Severinus did not themselves connect their use of *semina* with St. Augustine, later commentators, such as Thomas Erastus (1572) certainly did.[84]

The appeal of the doctrine of *semina* to Christian Platonists who were seeking a unified theology and cosmology, a "Mosaic physics" that interpreted *Genesis* as a cosmology, can partly account for the wide use of Severinus' *Idea medicinæ*, which will be demonstrated in chapters five and six. Severinus took the incorporation of *semina* into natural philosophy further than had his predecessors, inasmuch as he gave this doctrine a central place in medicine, fusing it with chemical philosophy. The success of his synthesis is evident from the many references to him in connection with *semina* well into the seventeenth century.

How *SEMINA* FUNCTION

In order to appreciate Severinus' theory of morbidity, which can be thought of as normal physiology gone astray, we must try to understand

---

81 Paracelsus wrote in *Labyrinthus medicorum errantium* that God created seeds *ex nihilo*, and that each carries within it a predestination. See *Paracelsus: Essential Readings*, p. 102. Severinus adopted and generalized this concept.

82 Pagel, *William Harvey's Biological Ideas*, p. 241, traces the idea to Ficino's *De vita coelitus comparanda* and notes that it was taken up by later authors, such as Agrippa.

83 T. P. Sherlock, "The Chemical Work of Paracelsus," *Ambix* 3 (1948), p. 39.

84 See Thomas Erastus, *Disputationem de medicina nova Philippi Paracelsi pars prima* (Basel: Perna, 1572), pp. 6-7: "Etenim habilitatem formæ, quam rationem seminalem Augustinus nominat, simul cum forma & dispositione necessaria repente introductam fuisse oportet."

the "normal" operation of *semina* and become familiar with some of the terminology Severinus employed. The first of these terms is "tincture." Tincture is sometimes used as a synonym for *semina*, vital balsam, etc., but certain of its attributes suggest that Severinus meant tincture to be a subset or perhaps a transcendent aspect of *semina*. This interpretation agrees with his use of the term "seminal tinctures," i.e. tinctures under the guidance of *semina*. For example, Severinus said that three things are needed for harmonious generation: seminal tinctures, elements, and principles (salt, sulphur, mercury). Tinctures seem to be pure forms, species that can transfer, or be transplanted, from one body to another, affecting the *semina* of the recipient.[85] They would appear to account for the active role of imagination in nature, inasmuch as a tincture is a kind of free "impression" that can force its form onto a receiving body.[86] In its most general meaning, a tincture is something that can color another thing, in effect transferring its form. Severinus adapted this concept to explain the process that he calls "transplantation": tinctures can be favorably received by the host, in which case they are "welcome guests," or they can be received as "foreign strangers." This difference between friendly and hostile takeover of the host comprises the distinction between healthy and morbid growth.

Whether affected by external, supervening tinctures or not, the locus of generation is the seed (*semen*). *Semina* (or the tinctures "in" them) possess a "mechanical" knowledge (*scientia mechanica*) of the chemical processes that are responsible for change, which he calls the *lithurgia mechanica*. The terms warrant closer attention because of their semantic richness and oddness.

---

85 One is tempted, for the sake of illustration, to liken *semina* and tinctures to DNA and RNA: The *semina* possess the knowledge necessary for their expression as a body, whereas the tinctures may transfer that knowledge to another body, much as an invading virus can alter its host's function.

86 Severinus considered imagination an important part of the inner working of nature. Without imagination, knowledge, destiny, and predestination, he wrote, "nothing will be generated, mixed, or increased; things visible will not be made from things invisible, nor corporeals from incorporeals [non generabitur, non miscebitur, non augebitur quicquam; non fient ex inuisibilibus uisibilia, ex incorporeis corporea]." See Severinus, *Idea medicinæ*, p. 156.

SCIENTIA MECHANICA AND LITHURGIA MECHANICA

Severinus' use of the term "mechanical" to describe the innermost workings of nature gives the historian of the early modern revolution in science pause for thought. Since Severinus wrote the *Idea medicinæ* a century or so before mechanical philosophy began to supersede vitalism as an acceptable cosmological paradigm, we can but wonder if there may have been a semantic connection between his admittedly vitalist use of *mechanica* and the more familiar concept of machine that characterizes the mechanical philosophy of the seventeenth century. A thorough examination of this problem is beyond the scope and intent of this study, but a few words are called for.[87]

"Mechanical" in Severinus' terminology is less related to the modern concept of machinery than it is to the person who repairs that machinery. This "mechanic" is an active, vital agent who carries out a process. In the context of sixteenth-century Paracelsian chemistry, the mechanic is the worker, the alchemist, the smith — whoever stands between raw material and finished product. In chemical reactions it is the Paracelsian "inner Vulcan" or *archeus* that carries out the process, an operation Severinus called mechanical.[88] Thus, when he wrote of mechanical knowledge, he meant the blueprint or information (*scien-*

---

87 I have drawn attention to the "mechanical" nature of Severinus' *semina* and why this might weaken the hitherto stark distinction between the mechanical philosophy of the seventeenth century and its organic predecessors in Jole Shackelford, "Seeds with a Mechanical Purpose: Severinus' *Semina* and Seventeenth-Century Matter Theory," in *Reading the Book of Nature: The Other Side of the Scientific Revolution*, ed. Allen G. Debus and Michael T. Walton, Sixteenth Century Essays and Studies 41 (Kirksville, Missouri: Sixteenth Century Journal Publishers, Inc., 1998), pp. 15-44.

88 On one page Severinus used both the term *mechanicos processus* and *spiritus mechanicos*. The anonymous English translator rendered these terms "ordenary processes" and "workeing spirits," thus providing us with an insight into the semantics of the term, although the presence of "mechanicke" above the line in each case suggests that the meaning did not come easily. See Severinus, *Idea medicinæ*, p. 96; "Mappe," f. 35r. Quite likely Severinus took the concept of mechanical operation as a way to describe natural processes from Paracelsus, who equated "internal anatomy" (*interior anatomia*) with astral, mechanical work (*mechanica astralia opera*) and astral operation (*astralis operatio*), in *De caduco matricis*. Such mechanical skill ("Kunst *Mechanica*") was responsible for cows' conversion of grass into milk, for example. See Paracelsus, *Medici Libelli*, pp. 78, 81, 111-115.

tia), that the innate, efficient cause (*archeus*) of bodies needs in order to perform chemical change.[89]

The generative *process* that the seminal agent undertakes is variously described. For example, in the title of chapter thirteen of the *Idea medicinæ* it is plainly called a "mechanical process of generations" (*in mechanico generationum processu*).[90] In other places the much more obscure term *lithurgia* is used. The title of chapter eight, *De generatione rerum naturalium et seminum mechanica lithurgia*, was rendered into near-contemporary English as "Of the Generations of Naturall things & mechanick or vitall *proceedeinge* of Seedes."[91] A few pages later, Severinus raises the question of whether forms or species "doe by meanes of generations, transplantations, & mixtions *play their parts* in this worldely commedy" (*mundanæ comoediæ lithurgiam peragunt*). In this instance *lithurgia* was translated into seventeenth-century English as "parts."[92]

Were it not for the seventeenth-century English rendering of *lithurgia* as "proceedeinge" (process) or "part," as in the "part" an actor plays, by the anonymous translator of *Idea medicinæ*, we might be persuaded of Walter Pagel's interpretation. Pagel thought *lithurgia* must be a Latinization of a Greek word for stonemasonry.[93] This etymology has a certain logic to it. Severinus' *lithurgia mechanica* could be a creative process akin to the creation of a building from rough stone (prime matter), and the stonemason could be yet another guise for the ubiquitous *archeus*. Certainly Severinus possessed enough knowledge of Greek to figure out the proper root words. However, another possibility exists, namely that *lithurgia* is an alternate spelling for *liturgia*, and that the mechanical process Severinus writes of is to be likened to a liturgical process, and the metaphor then becomes a religious one. This interpretation is

89 Paracelsus, *Labyrinthus Errantium Medicorum*, distinguished innate knowledge, *scientia*, from knowledge that is acquired through experience, *experientia*; drugs contain *scientia*, but the physician possesses *experientia*. See *Paracelsus: Essential Readings*, p. 104.
90 Severinus, *Idea medicinæ*, p. 292.
91 Severinus, "Mappe," f. 30r, emphasis added; *Idea medicinæ*, p. 78.
92 Severinus, "Mappe," f. 31r, emphasis added; *Idea medicinæ*, p. 81: "Formæ, species … Generationum, Transplantationum & Mixtionum ministerio mundanæ comoediæ lithurgiam peragunt."
93 Pagel, *William Harvey's Biological Ideas*, p. 244. I believe that this idea may have come from William Davidson's assessment of the term in one of his commentaries. See chapter ten, below.

more persuasive than might seem the case, *prima facie*, if one recalls other terms used to describe function and means of operation, namely *officium* and *ministerium*. Phonetically, *lithurgia* and *liturgia* are equivalent in early modern Danish and German. Furthermore, we can see a similar use of these terms in the title of a 1663 treatise on the topic: *De rerum principiis et mechanica seminum liturgia*, which draws heavily on the ideas and terminology of the *Idea medicinæ*. The author of this tract clearly understood Severinus' *lithurgia* as the Latin *liturgia*.[94] Whatever Severinus' intention, it is clear that the seventeenth-century English translator took *lithurgia* to refer to a process or "role" such as an actor (or liturgist?) might perform. This interpretation is, moreover, consonant with Severinus' frequent analogy to the natural world as a world stage upon which nature plays out a predestined development.[95]

THE PROCESS OF GENERATION

No matter what semantic basis we assume for *lithurgia mechanica* and *scientia mechanica*, it is clear that for Severinus the basic metabolism of the world is chemical. It is a process predestined in the *semina* and directed by the mechanical spirits within them according to the seminal tinctures, the chemical recipes that the *archei* must follow. Although some mixing of the traditional elements is a part of this process, it should not be understood in the Aristotelian sense. To assert his theory of seminal causes for manifest qualities, Severinus had to comment on the position taken by Galenists and Aristotelians that the qualities (and the temperaments of the body) resulted from a mixing of the elements. He did not deny the importance of mixing (*mixtio*) in physics, but he believed its proper relation to qualities had been incorrectly understood in the past and that to continue in the footsteps of the Peripatetics was

---

94 Mauritus Petri Køning, *Dissertatio de rerum principiis et mechanica seminum liturgia* (Copenhagen: Godicchenius, 1663). More will be said about this work in chapter eight.

95 Severinus often refers to *semina* as having vestments and to nature as a worldly stage (*mundana scena*). This terminology reinforces the metaphor of the world as a theater, which was not uncommon in this period, as is evident from Shakespeare's observation that "all the world's a stage" (*As You Like It*, Act II, scene 7). Also wrapped up in this terminology is the idea that nature has a foreordained administrative process, which is mechanical or routine in the same way that ecclesiastical liturgy was.

vain: "I have seen philosophers whose domes were covered with snow-white hair, who consumed their whole life with this nonsense, and still they could not get the stone to the top."[96] The result of their efforts to accommodate a mixture of the four basic qualities was the doctrine of temperament, in which a temperament

> becomes diffused throughout the whole mass of the compound. Galen attributed the causes of all natural powers to this temperament, and in great error he wrote that the character of each and every thing proceeds from one or another temper of hotness, coldness, wetness, and dryness.[97]

Since mixtion is a movement, a moving cause must exist. There must be an intelligence behind this movement and coalescing.

> In sum, one should add a mover, a vital principle furnished with a knowledge, form, species, seed, star, or whatever one wishes to call it, by virtue of whose power and infallible knowledge such divine functions of mixing can be managed. This is the principle that we demonstrated before to be the foundation and root of every generation. With its knowledge and vital power, seeds coming forth from the *Iliadus* onto the world stage, from *Orcus* into light, establish the elements and native principles of bodies for themselves, and they mix according to weights and measures known only to their knowledge. And this does not happen by the mutual approach of their bodies, for they are still spiritual and are not subject to the laws of dimensions.[98]

96 Severinus, *Idea medicinæ*, p. 133: "Vidi ego Philosophos quorum tecta niue cooperiebantur, qui universam vitam in his nugis consumserant: & tamen saxum in uertice collocare non poterant." Severinus here refers to the myth of Sisyphus.

97 Ibid., p. 134: "per universam Compositi molem diffusum. Huic Temperamento omnium Facultatum naturalium causas ascripsit Galenus: & uniuscuiusque rei proprietatem, ex tali uel tali caliditatis, frigiditatis, humiditatis, siccitatis temperie proficisci."

98 Ibid., pp. 135-36: "In summa, motorem adiungere oportet, Principium uitale, Scientia instructum, Formam, Speciem, Semen, Astrum, quomodocunque appellare libuerit: cuius potestate & infallibili Scientia, tam diuina Mixtionis officia administrari possint. Hoc est illud Principium, quod antea Generationum omnium fundamentum & radicem demonstrauimus. Huius Scientia & uitali potestate semina ex Iliado in mundanam Anatomiam, ex Orco in Lucem prodeuntia, Elementa & corporum Principia domestica sibijpsis constituunt, eaque ponderibus & mensuris soli Scientiæ notis permiscent. Idque non corporum mutua appositione: spiritualia enim adhuc sunt, dimensionumque legibus non subjecta."

Therefore, mixtion is not a cause, but an effect of the vital tinctures that penetrate everything, linking it all together in composition by means of mixtion. "And he who is ignorant of these linkages has not learned the power of life, because he has only practiced the anatomy of death."[99]

Mixtion first begins when incorporeals are made spiritually corporate, and then "it is a mixing of the elements among themselves, of the elements with the principles, of the principles among themselves, and of all of them together." This mixtion attracts further nourishment, and growth ensues, "for the elements and principles of bodies are added together hourly by the vital and mechanical spirits, consequently there is need for continuous restoration, mixing, and compounding."[100] Thus, according to Severinus' philosophy, mixtion is an integral part of the growth process. It is not a root cause of physical characteristics, but rather a tool of the underlying ideal agents, the *semina*.

As mentioned before, normal generation requires three things: seminal tinctures that have the requisite knowledge (the plans), elements, which are the seminal *matrices* providing the raw materials, and Paracelsus' *tria prima*, namely salt, sulphur, and mercury.[101] The ontological status of the *tria prima* is not well defined in Severinus' work, but in this case they clearly are incorporeal principles of activity. This activity, associated by Severinus with Hippocratic *dunameis* and Paracelsian *chærionia*, is apparently another aspect of *semina*.[102] The harmonious cooperation of *semina*, elements, and principles (and tinctures, and balsam, and whatever else) results in the expression of *semina* as bodies, by a process of thickening. Incorporeal *semina*, lodged in their incorporeal *matrices* and equipped with the needed *scientia* and incorporeal salt, sulphur, and mercury, gradually *mature* into corporeal beings. The *semina* express themselves by taking on (or rather unfolding from within themselves)

---

99 Ibid., p. 136: "Haec uincula qui ignorat, Vitæ potestatem non didicit: quia Mortis Anatomiam solam exercuit."

100 Ibid., pp. 136-37: "Estque Mixtio Elementorum inter se, Elementorum cum principiis, principiis inter se, & omnium simul. ... Elementa enim ac principia corporum a spiritibus uitalibus mechanicisque, in horas consummuntur [sic] assidua proinde opus est restitutione, mixtione & compositione."

101 Ibid., p. 160.

102 Ibid., p. 114.

dimensions, number, weight, and other *signaturæ* or characteristics.[103] From beginning to end, or in the language of vital astrology, from time of rising to time of setting, this process of seminal expression is associated with the aging of the individual, which was predestined in the *rationes seminales* that gave it existence. Life, says Severinus, begins as soul and proceeds by a gradual thickening of spirits; we are born moist and we become dry and crusty and brittle before our stars set.[104]

TRANSPLANTATIONS

One of the novel aspects of Severinus' physiology is his theory of transplantation, which, like other aspects of his philosophy, seems rooted in the metaphor of horticulture and animal husbandry.[105] There are two kinds of transplantation, namely of the individual and of the species. By transplantation, individuals can be given new habits, as when a florist causes a plant to bloom in the wrong season. In this case, the transplant retains its seminal basis, its individual essence, but expresses new characteristics: "I call those transplantations in which the characteristics, such as colors, flavors, sizes, shapes, etc., have changed, while the root remains, transplantations of individuals."[106] Or, something may be so completely uprooted and moved as to seem a new species entirely:

103 The doctrine of signatures is associated with Paracelsianism and often given a mystical interpretation. In Severinus' hands, however, and in the mind of his English translator, *signaturæ* clearly meant the properties or characteristics (manifest or occult) that distinguish one thing from another, that is, they are expressed forms.

104 Ibid., p. 173. According to Severinus, mechanical spirits obtain the properties of the four elements and three principles according to their predestinations. From these are produced spiritual bodies, which "gradually departing from the spiritual anatomy, they degenerate to the corporeal family and they constitute bodies that are moist and spiritual in the beginning, but hastening to thickness and old age by the hour" [paulatim a spirituali descendentes Anatomia, in corpoream familiam degenerant: corporaque principio humida spiritualiaque constituunt, in horas crassescentia & ad senium festinantia].

105 Severinus offers examples of how man has learned to alter the natural cycles of plants by pruning and grafting. Just has he has altered the nature of his domestic plants, so can he affect the course of disease through suitable transplantations. See Ibid., p. 318.

106 Ibid, p. 140: "Indiuiduorum Transplantationes dico, in quibus manente Radice signaturæ mutantur, ut colores, sapores, magnitudines, figuræ, &c."

> But I understand the transplantation of species to be when all the
> characteristics have been changed, and the distinguishing marks of
> a new family are manifestly reproduced. Not because the vital and
> invisible principles of the seeds … are mixed up, but because the ele-
> ments and the principles of bodies subject to mixing receive foreign
> characteristics.[107]

Thus, apparently new species of things (sports) can be accounted for
as the effects of old forms transplanted to new locations, or even new
times.

If we recall how *semina* operate, we see that transplantation involves
a change of plan, either an altered tincture or a new tincture that is
received from without the organism. Transplantation can also override
the effects of environment and awaken latent signatures that were hitherto unexpressed by the *semina* because of unpropitious times (stellar
influence), place (climate), or available nutrient. Wheat, says Severinus,
has always been darnel (a wild grass occurring as a weed in cultivated
fields), and given the vast number of wheat seeds, it is no surprise if
darnel occasionally occurs by transplantation, as latent characteristics
are activated.[108] Thus, no matter how carefully a farmer selects his seed
corn, he can never raise a pure crop. When an individual receives new
knowledge, new *scientia mechanica*, it behaves differently. And if the
transplantation is radical, the metamorphosis is (relatively) permanent.
If this happens at early stages of individual growth, before seminal plans
have become too thoroughly reified, the success of transplantation is
greater than at other times.[109] Furthermore, if transplantation is made
to a receptive site (good soil, favorable conditions for nutrition), then
the transplant will succeed. We can see where this is going; Severinus'
model and terminology for generation and transplantation has a wealth
of explanatory power in it, and what works for ordinary growth will

---

107 Ibid.: "Specierum uero Transplantationes intelligo, ubi omnibus signaturis immutatis
     nouæ familiæ insignia manifeste repræsentantur. Non quod uitalia & inuisibilia semi-
     num Principia … confundantur, sed quod Elementa & corporum Principia Mixtioni
     subiecta alienas recipiant signaturas."
108 Ibid., p. 141.
109 Ibid., pp. 160-61.

work for morbid growth as well, assuming that one views pathology in biological terms, rather than as a deficiency or imbalance.

PATHOLOGY: SEEDS OF DISEASE

The Paracelsian conception of disease as a positive essence (*ens*), rather than as a privation of function owing to an imbalance of the bodily fluids, has attracted the attention of historians of medical thought in part because of its seeming modernity and in part because it was a break with Galenism. On both of these counts the perception of disease as caused by independent, exogenous agents is an important development in medical theory. Whether or not it looks forward to the nineteenth-century germ theory, however, is beside the point, and will not be considered here. The idea that a disease was caused by an *ens morbi* had profound implications for early modern medical theory and serious theological ramifications, and for this reason we must examine Severinus' description of the origin and essence of disease in some detail.[110] On the basis of this doctrine, Severinus developed a theory of therapy, which explained how strong chemical drugs acted against serious, well established diseases.

Most simply put, Severinus believed diseases, some diseases at least, to be caused by *semina morborum* or disease-seeds. The idea of seeds as agents of disease was not new with the Paracelsians, to be sure; the concept goes back to antiquity and had already experienced something of a revival in the Renaissance. It is especially evident in the work of Girolamo Fracastoro (1478-1553).[111] Fracastoro had used the idea of

---

110 It may be that the acceptance of the idea that a disease is caused by a living pathogen permitted diseases to be viewed as having a natural history. Severinus (ibid., p. 222) writes of hereditary diseases, such as podagra and leprosy, persisting for several generations and then becoming sterile. Perhaps this idea that diseases are entities with characteristic cycles contributed in some way to the idea that diseases can be studied by learning their natural histories. Natural histories as a genre of scientific discourse were becoming important in the seventeenth century – maybe there is a connection.

111 Vivian Nutton, "The Seeds of Disease: An Explanation of Contagion and Infection from the Greeks to the Renaissance," *Medical History* 27 (1983): 1-34, has shown that the idea of seeds as causes of disease goes back to the presocratics, but enjoyed no real popularity until the Renaissance.

seminaria (seed-beds) or *semina morbi* as agents of syphilis and plague earlier in the century, and by the late 1560s, when Severinus was beginning to formulate his theories, Fracastoro's work was generally known in Europe.[112] We should note, however, that Severinus does not mention Fracastoro and only rarely uses his other term for disease agents, *fomites*, and then in a different sense.[113] Severinus' *semina*, as pointed out above, were incorporeal and closely related to the *rationes seminales* of Christian Platonism, unlike Fracastoro's atomistic *seminaria* and the material bits (*fomites*) that he thought transmitted contagion. Although the writings of Fracastoro or other sixteenth-century critics of Galen, such as Giovanni Argenterio, may have influenced Severinus' pathology, it is safe to assume that he drew heavily on Paracelsus' writings, to which he refers in the *Idea medicinæ*.[114] In fact not all theories of seminal causation of disease were the same, and it is important to identify what position Severinus held on how disease came to be and what its ontological status was, if we are to understand his overall medical philosophy, its appeal to some scholars, and the opposition it engendered in others.

Severinus found contemporary pathologies wanting. The Galenists were in disagreement as to how the elements are mixed and whether all activity proceeds from the mixture or constellation of the humors and elements and their basic qualities, which was called the complexion or temperament. The newer diseases, such as venereal disease, were not adequately explained by the traditional paradigm, and this led Fernel to postulate a class of diseases that affected the whole form of the organism, which he called diseases of the substance of the whole body.[115]

---

112 See Nutton, "The Reception of Fracastoro's Theory of Contagion."

113 For example, Severinus, *Idea medicinæ*, p. 200: "Tarda enim sunt plenilunia eorum morborum, qui in circuitu astrorum, uel in habitu corporis, ut loquitur Galenus, fomites & mineras habent." [For the full moons of those diseases that have *fomites* and *mineras* in the cycle of the stars, or in the disposition of the body, as Galen says, are slow.]

114 On Argenterio and criticism of Galen in sixteenth-century Europe, see Nancy Siraisi, "Giovanni Argenterio and Sixteenth-Century Medical Innovation: Between Princely Patronage and Academic Controversy," *Osiris*, 2d ser., 6 (1990): 161-180.

115 Fernel's adoption of the idea of an occult faculty in order to explain the seeming ability of the whole substance of the human body to "concoct food and perform a range of other functions" may have influenced Severinus' philosophy. See Linda Deer Richardson, "The Generation of Disease: Occult Causes and Diseases of the Total Substance," in *The Medical Renaissance of the Sixteenth Century*, ed. Andrew Wear, Roger K. French, and Iain M. Lonie (Cambridge: Cambridge University Press, 1985), p. 182.

Besides Fernel, there were other physicians who cast aside concern for terminology and sought the truth from the phenomena themselves. They determined that a thick and mucilaginous humor in the liver, spleen, mesaraics, and elsewhere acted like cataracts act in hindering eyesight. Once these obstructions, the cause of the diseases, were removed, normal function resumed.[116]

The problem with these theories is that they all explain diseases as arising from passive causes – obstructions, excesses, and privations. Passive causes do little to account for the very active, sometimes sudden and violent nature of symptoms. One must look beyond the passive obstruction to determine what active principles are involved. There are all kinds of obstructions, and it is the chemical nature of the obstruction that *specifies* the genus of obstruction into a species of disease; "for arsenical and sulphurous mucilages are inflamed, and the aluminous are not; the arsenical are acute, the aluminous and vitriolate are chronic, and so on."[117]

The chemical activity of the obstructing material is due to the *semina* that give it its external properties. Severinus admits that previous philosophers have written about the generation of visible bodies from *semina*, but have had little success in applying their theory to disease. This is because diseases come from seeds that are better hidden than other seeds, "and their generation and transplantation are concealed in nature's laboratories and subject neither to the judgement of the senses nor the exalted principles of syllogisms." For these reasons, the explanation of diseases is quite complicated and has been comprehended by few.[118] Yet clearly some diseases, such as the hereditary diseases and those with cyclically recurring symptoms, exhibit their seminal nature. Others, such as the infectious diseases, show themselves to be transplantations. If it can be demonstrated that diseases are seminal and behave according to the principles of generation and transplantation that he has

---

116 Severinus, *Idea medicinæ*, p. 208.

117 Ibid., p. 213: "Arsenicales enim & sulphureæ inflammantur, aluminosæ non: arsenicales acutæ sunt, aluminosæ & vitriolatæ, chronicæ, &c."

118 Ibid., p. 203: "At vero morborum explicatio, quia semina occultiora obtinuerunt, & Generationes, Transplantationesque in Naturæ officina absconditas, nec sensuum arbitriis, nec syllogismorum superbis decretis subiectas, intricata plane, & a paucis comprehensa est."

already laid down, wrote Severinus, then these diseases can be cured by artificial intervention.[119]

But whence came disease? If we are to believe that diseases are seminal like other agents in nature, then were they, too, created as *rationes seminales* at the beginning of the world? Can these evil *semina* have been the creation of the divine mind? Such a position would be construed by the sixteenth-century religious thinker as hopelessly Manichæan and therefore heretical, but as we shall see, Severinus avoided this theological dilemma.[120] Severinus was not terribly clear on this point, but he did distinguish between the created *semina*, which were perfect, and the postlapsarian morbific *semina*. At first, he wrote, all "was pure, whole, perfect, and without corruption and death. But after the fall of our forefather, new tinctures supervened on those first seeds by virtue of the divine curse." The result was that "the beauty of all creation has been transplanted to a miserable fate."[121] A key point to note here is that it is new tinctures that bring in disease, not newly created *semina*. From the model of generation that we have already adduced from the *Idea medicinæ*, we can interpret Severinus to mean that the cursed tinctures (disease) impressed themselves on extant *semina* and took control of them. Logically, the new tinctures must have been an expression of God's wrath at Adam's willful disobedience, which was one explanation for the origin of disease, rather than the work of the Devil. Thus, we are still left with the problem of a "good" God creating "bad" disease, but at least the problem is not formulated in Manichæan terms of a preexistent evil disposition in matter.

From the point of view of a Paracelsian chemical interpretation of *Genesis*, impurity is intimately mixed with purity in the postlapsarian world; impure *semina* mingle with pure *semina*, with the result that "the fruits of all the elements," i.e. the corporeal expressions of the *semina*, "have death adjoined to [their] life." This is to say that morbidity and

---

119 Ibid., p. 215.
120 The importance of the theological implication of *semina* to Paracelsian critics, such as Thomas Erastus, will become evident in the next chapters.
121 Ibid., p. 216: "Fuitque hæc prima rerum facies pura, integra, perfecta, sine corruptione & morte. At uero post præuaricatione Protoplasti, primis illis seminibus, maledictione diuina, nouæ superuenerunt, Tincturæ, quarum mixtione in calamitosam sortem transplantata est totius Creaturæ pulchritudo."

mortality have become inseparable parts of living things; "the anatomy of death and disease lies hidden not only in man, but also in animals, in plants, in minerals, and in the fruits of the firmament and air."[122] Diseases, as *semina* possessing the morbific tinctures or the *scientia mechanica* of pathology, lie dormant in nature, commixed with untainted *semina*, until they are called into action. In Severinus' terms the tinctures are then "separated and exalted, [and] they cultivate enmity, the author of death and destruction."[123] Severinus did not elaborate on how this works, but it follows that either the cursed tinctures must carry their evil predestinations with them into the world, or else the disease-tinctures are activated by their host *semina* as an accident to the operation of the host's predestinations. Whichever the case, the seeds of diseases sprout and ripen as do other seeds.

By considering diseases as the "fruit" of impure *semina*, Severinus brings together Paracelsus' various ideas that diseases on the one hand come from seeds, but that on the other hand they arise from undigested impurities.[124] Such impurities are found in the "roots" of minerals, where they produce disease. When their time comes, the minerals "strive for destruction by means of rust and cuprous corruption."[125] Vegetables, too, are subject to disease. The exact form of disease depends on which principles are dominant in the impurities. Those plants with characteristic mercurial and sulphurous impurities tend to dissolve by putrefaction; those "in which mercurial impurities are not so abundant, and the nature of the salts is stronger, await ἄβαυσιν or decay, as do most trees and some

---

122 Ibid., p. 217: "Fructus omnium Elementorum, mortem uitæ adiunctam habent. ... Neque enim solum in homine, Anatomia mortis & morborum delitescit, sed etiam in animalibus, in plantis, in mineralibus, in fructibus firmamenti & aeris." The characteristically Paracelsian idea that the heavenly bodies are also mutable is evident here. This idea was "in the air" when Tycho Brahe interpreted the "new star" or nova of 1572 as a celestial mutation, just a few years after Severinus wrote this.

123 Ibid., p. 218: "Separatæ & exaltatæ, inimicitias, dissolutionum mortisque authores, exercent."

124 Paracelsus offered various causes for disease: some diseases were caused by poisons or impurities (*tartarus* taken in with food and drink, which the body has not been able to digest); others resulted from *semina* taken into the body; others were caused by sulphur in the body that was ignited by external agents. Ulcerations and other skin diseases were caused by corrosive chemicals, usually salts. See Pagel, *Paracelsus*.

125 Severinus, *Idea medicinæ*, p. 218: "rubigine & æruginosa corruptione dissolutionem moliuntur."

shrubs."[126] These same impurities are found in animals, in part because animals consume vegetables and minerals and receive their impurities. Humans are the most subject to disease of all creatures, because they are nourished from animals, minerals, and vegetables, and acquire their impurities, too.[127] Furthermore, humans deserve it: "no other creature is subject to so many misfortunes, and rightly so," because people multiply through fornication and pass their impurities on from generation to generation.[128] Thus, even hereditary diseases are in principle caused by seminal impurities.

Many factors determine the actual development of a disease. Beside its inherent seminal nature, the manifestation of a disease depends on its host. Impurities in the vegetable kingdom, for example, may behave differently when transplanted into the animal "commonwealth."[129] Other factors may affect the sprouting and growth of disease. Diet is important because it governs the types, quantities, and numbers of impurities entering the human. Weather is also a factor, because meteorological conditions affect the spreading of impurities from the superior elemental regions to the inferior, accounting for the supposed effects of winds, rains, the stars, manna from the heavens, and other macrocosmic phenomena on the development of disease. Here, too, sympathies between the macrocosm and microcosm provide explanations for the evidently seasonal diseases, although their innate, seminal predestinations can also account for this behavior.

Severinus' conception of diseases as "strangers," invasive and parasitic agents, formed the basis for a more elaborate pathology, which strikes

---

126   Ibid., 219: "In quibus uero impuritates Mercuriales non sunt ita copiosæ, & salium robustior natura, ἄβαυσιν uel cariem expectant, ut arbores plurimæ fruticesque nonnullæ.

127   That is, humans are at greatest risk because they are at the end of a food chain comprising minerals, plants, and animals and therefore are exposed to the diseases and impurities contained in all the lower forms. People also receive celestial and aerial impurities through respiration.

128   Ibid., p. 219: "Nec ulla est Creatura tot calamitatibus subiecta: & merito: fornicatione coniugia multiplicantur ac generis nobilitate inquinata, auorum delicta luunt posteri."

129   The terminology one discovers in the *Idea medicinæ* suggests a primitive understanding of ecology, namely that entities exist in an "economy" of nature, performing normal (mechanical) functions (liturgies) for the good operation of the commonwealth. Transplanted "foreign guests" upset normal function and cause disease. A political reading is perhaps warranted, but lies beyond the scope of the present work.

the reader as a modern-sounding theory of infection. We can identify five factors involved in successful disease growth. First, as strangers, or weeds in the garden of nature, morbific *semina* must successfully enter the host, if they are not congenitally present. In the case of food-borne *semina*, they must be able to survive the rigors of digestion. Medicines and poisons are alike in this respect, as they are both able to resist digestion: Foods

> are subjected to the mechanical spirits of the human body and, in favor-
> able compliance, they admit resolutions, separations, expulsions, and
> similar dispensations. But those that are rich in very powerful tinctures
> are not subject to the governance of our mechanical [spirits] and spurn
> our methods of preparation. They appear not as aliments, but as me-
> dicaments, medicinal foods, and sometimes as poisons: by the use of
> these, diseases are generated in the body suddenly.[130]

The similarity between medicines and poisons therefore lies in their possession of powerful tinctures. This perception provides theoretical support for an aspect of chemical therapy commonly associated with Paracelsianism, that of using potent toxins as a basis for pharmacological preparations.

Again, the first condition for the development of disease is the presence of disease-seeds in the host. Second, the seminal tinctures must make *repeated* impressions. Third, the tinctures or impressions must find a suitable field, place, or womb to receive them. By this Severinus could mean that the right sort of elemental matrices must be available to nurture the seminal tinctures if they are to mature into diseases, or he could mean that the region or organ that is the host must be receptive and suitable for the growth of the disease. Both interpretations are consistent with his medical thought. A fourth condition for the development of

---

130 Ibid., p. 227: "Subijciuntur enim alimenta spiritibus mechanicis humani corporis, &
facile obedientia, resolutiones, separationes, expulsiones ac similes dispensationes
admittunt. Quæ enim potentioribus tincturis pollent, neque gubernationi nostrorum
Mechanicorum subijciuntur, legesque præparationum aspernantur, non alimenta, sed
medicamenta, cibi medicamentosi, interdum uenena existunt: quorum usu, morbi subito
in corpore generantur."

manifest disease is the ability of the host to resist pernicious tinctures. If there is a debility of the innate balsam and mechanical spirit, the foreign "guests" (strangers) have little difficulty putting down roots. Lastly, if the host is not merely weak, but actually aids the morbific *semina*, then disease will surely take root, undergo transplantations within the body, and produce diverse fruits.[131]

The idea that a specific disease will develop in one or more specific organs or regions of the body is clearly taken over from the observation that organisms have their proper environments:

> But because not all seeds sprout equally in all places, but suitable ones in suitable places – for rosemary, grain, thyme, *polium*, etc. do not thrive in marshy places, and *æditis*, willows, smartweed, or pimpernel do not grow in dry places – one must therefore observe the correlation of places and seeds in the human body. For there are seeds peculiar to health as well as to diseases, which grow in the field or anatomy of the stomach and intestines and are different from those that are fostered in the liver, spleen, kidneys, bladder, blood, muscles, tissues, *synovia*, brain, heart, lungs, etc.[132]

As mentioned before, transplantations can occur, whereby *semina* are removed from one field or anatomy and implanted in another. When rooted in a new anatomy, a disease may produce new symptoms or signatures. Again, Severinus drives home a central point: just as these new signatures cannot be called disease, because they are symptoms and therefore qualities, how can Galen call "distemperature," which is a qualitative state, a disease?[133]

---

131 Ibid., p. 228. Paracelsus had written that one disease may form from another by means of transplantation. Here Severinus has generalized this principle.

132 Ibid., p. 229: "Quia uero non omnia semina omnibus locis æque nascuntur, sed consentanea consentaneis: in palustribus enim locis non prouenit rorismarinus, spica, thymus, polium, &c. neque in siccis & æditis, salices, persicariæ, anagallis: ita in corpore humano, confluentiam locorum & seminum obseruare oportet. Sunt enim propria semina tam sanitatis quam morborum, quæ in agro uel Anatomia uentriculi & intestinorum crescunt, differentia ab aliis quæ in hepate, liene, renibus, uesica, sanguine, carnibus, membranis, synouia, cerebro, corde, pulminibus, &c. fouentur."

133 Ibid., pp. 245-46.

An example of the seriousness of transplanted disease is the case of gout (podagra). Gout has its roots in the blood, but may eventually find a suitable matrix in the joints or *synovia* of the hands and feet, making itself known in the limbs on its way.[134] In this case, the joints act as "wombs" which "can admit wandering foreigners, in whom are contained the properties of the three principles cooperating with the podagrical tinctures."[135] Once well rooted, a disease sprouts and produces fruit or symptoms that signal its presence.

Inflammation is an example of a symptom wrongly interpreted by the Galenists. Severinus opposed those who he said "obstinately maintain that all inflammations are produced not from seeds, spirits, and tinctures endowed with mechanical knowledge and vital power, but only from putrifying blood."[136] Severinus' view is that inflammation is not caused by an excessive amount of blood (a humoral imbalance) which then escapes the veins and causes inflammation, but rather by those chemical impurities, *semina*, or foreign tinctures that are *in* the blood: "True infammations are not generated from such a profusion of blood, unless the seeds of pleuritises, *prunellæ*, or plague previously lay hidden in the blood which, having found the occasion and opportunity, are unseasonably excited to ebullitions and paroxysms."[137] In this case Severinus felt that personal behavior has sometimes been exaggerated as a cause of disease. It is not singing, laughing, shouting, or running about that cause these inflammations, he wrote, but rather arsenical, antimonial, sulphurous, and similar seeds that are dormant in the blood until some "slight occasion of evident causes" provokes them and the generation of plague or similar disease ensues.[138] Thus, a regimen proscribing these activities is vain.

134 Ibid., p. 271.
135 Ibid., p. 272: "Hospitem errantem admittere possint, in quibus proprietates trium Principiorum confluentes cum Tincturis podagricis continentur."
136 Ibid., p. 257: "Galenistæ ægreferentes ... obstinate contendent, non ex seminibus, spiritibus, Tincturis, scientia mechanica & uitali potestate præditis, sed ex sanguine solo putrescente, Inflammationes omnes produci."
137 Ibid., pp. 257-58: "Ex tali sanguinis profusione Inflammationes ueras non generari, nisi in sanguine, semina pleuritidum, prunellæ, pestis, antea delitescant, quæ occasionem opportunitatemque nacta, ad ebullitiones et paroxysmos intempestiue excitentur."
138 Ibid., p. 258: "In inflammationum generatione semina arsenicalia, antimonialia, sulphurea, & similia, in sanguine latitantia, maturitatique uicinia, leui occasione euidentium causarum excitata, pleuritides, pestes & prunellas produxerunt."

To sum up Severinus' conception of disease, we can say that he did not simply view diseases as autonomous entities, living outside the human body until an opportunity to invade presented itself. Although invading *semina* do play a role in disease aetiology, this is but one cause of disease, which is a much more complex thing. In the first place, he distinguished several kinds of disease: diseases can arise from external or internal *semina*, depending on whether they are taken into the body or are congenital (hereditary disease), and they can come from external physical injuries or adverse "impressions."[139] All are potentially curable. Furthermore, disease depends on many causal factors, including repeated infection and the condition of the host. To the extent that a disease may be seated in a particular part of the body, say in the blood or joints, then it can be said to be "ontological," arising from a local disease entity. This does not mean, however, that the disease itself really exists independently from the host, which is an idea rejected by Paracelsus' critics. Severinus chose not to distinguish between disease and its cause; instead he saw different states of the same phenomenon – disease in act versus disease in potency.[140]

DIAGNOSIS AND THERAPY

At the level of metaphysics, Severinus' theory of disease is based on a struggle between good tinctures and bad tinctures, as the latter attempt to overwhelm the former and interfere with their natural progressions toward their predestined ends. In theory, therapy consists of removing the disease *semina* or tinctures as well as fortifying the innate human balsam that resists them. Once well rooted in the human anatomy, having survived the body's defense, a disease must be treated, and hopefully eradicated, by externally applied medicines. Such medicines may have spirits that are stronger than those of the internal disease and they may effect a transplantation.[141]

139 Ibid., p. 340.
140 Ibid., p. 314.
141 Ibid., p. 236.

But at the level of practical therapy, we leave the realm of form and matter and enter the world of iatrochemistry. Severinus' therapy, like that of Paracelsus, is based on the understanding that the world operates on a chemical basis, and that what the chemist may see in the laboratory can reveal the hidden principles of physiology that are valid both in the microcosm and the macrocosm. Severinus was quite adamant on the methodological distinction between Galenism and Paracelsianism on this point:

> Some will say that the λογομαχίας [new terms] are pointless, that new names and principles of this sort are introduced by Paracelsus in vain, and that Galen understood the same thing when he says that fever arises from putrid bile that Paracelsus explained by a new interpretation, saying that fever is an inflamed nitrous sulphur. Thus, when Galen says that cholic is from vitreous phlegm, the same thing is explained as when Paracelsus says that cholic is from tartarous, aluminous, and styptic mucilage.[142]

But Severinus knew that Paracelsian terminology indicated a new medicine: The Galenists, who say that fever proceeds from excessive bile (choler), will not find it in the human body and they will be hard pressed to explain this disease without resorting to heat and dryness, which are mere qualities. The Paracelsian, however, will identify the cause as nitrous sulphur, perceive this chemical "in many species of the world republic," and recognize its connection with febrile symptoms.[143] The chemist can, if clever and diligent enough, prepare some of the fundamental juices and excrements of the body in the laboratory. But try as he might, he will find no melancholy, bile, or phlegm, because these are just empty names and not real things. Therefore, when Galen says that fever comes from corrupt bile, he means the same thing as

---

142 Ibid., p. 190: "Dicent nonnulli otiosas esse λογομαχίας, noua huiusmodi nomina & Principia a PARACELSO inuanum introducta: idem intelligere Galenum cum dicit febrim oriri ex bile putrida, quod PARACELSVS noua interpretatione declarauit, dicens febrim esse Sulphur nitrosum accensum: ita cum dicit Galenus Colicam esse ex pituita uitrea, idem declarari quod apud PARACELSVM dicitur, Colicam esse ex mucilagine Tartarea, aluminosa & styptica."

143 Ibid., p. 191: "in multis speciebus Mundanæ Reipublicæ."

when Paracelsus says that it comes from an inflamed nitrous sulphur, except that the latter has an objective reality.[144] Where Galen erred was in resorting to qualitative explanations because he could not find bile in the world at large. It comes down to a choice of working with real or imaginary causes. He who understands that fever comes from a nitrous sulphur can investigate the properties of this substance in the laboratory and expand his knowledge and use it to assist in determining the causes of disease symptoms, when they occur, and so on. Of course, understanding the true cause is important to proper treatment. If the Galenists had learned the anatomy of salt, they too would have recognized the saline properties in various phlegms (nitrous, aluminous, etc.).[145] Lacking this chemical understanding, they cannot perceive the true causes, and therefore their medicine is hindered.

It is because of this commitment to classifying diseases in terms of chemical causes that Severinus' therapy takes on a distinctively Paracelsian character, speaking of both diseases and cures as being antimonial or sulphureal or whatever. However, we must stand back for a moment and realize that although Severinus' medicine is Paracelsian, it is by no means true that he treated all maladies with mineral chemicals, or that he thought all diseases were responsive to chemical therapy. By being mainly attentive to the rhetoric and excitement of searching out and applying new methods, we lose sight of the fact that we are considering here only one side of his eclectic practice, and although it may be the most visible and interesting side from our point of view, his general therapy may have seemed less radical to a contemporary.[146] This caveat may well apply to Paracelsian therapy in general, where a disproportionate attention given to certain especially difficult diseases and innovative, chemical cures has perhaps caused us to ignore the fact that many traditional methods of curing remained in use. But, if we

---

144 It is not apparent why Severinus should think that bile and phlegm are less real than, say, sulphur and salt. However, he objected to the attribution of disease to accidental qualities or to matter itself. He followed Paracelsus in perceiving that it is not matter, but rather an immanent spirit, that is active in nature. Since diseases are active – increasing and decreasing – they must have spiritual causes.

145 Ibid., p. 191.

146 As it in fact seemed to Paludanus, who noted that Severinus used both Paracelsian and Galenic methods. See chapter three above.

keep that in mind, it is reasonable to focus our attention on the novel aspects of Paracelsian medicine.

Turning to a discussion of therapy, in chapter fourteen of the *Idea medicinæ*, Severinus said that expulsion of disease-producing impurities is the first method to be tried: "And so, because the impurities, roots, and seeds of all diseases are implanted in the human anatomy, either from birth or afterwards, through the use of aliments, the first and foremost suggestion for treatment or curing will be to remove such mixtures or impurities."[147] From this idea follows Severinus' emphasis on kinds of treatment that aid the expulsion of *semina*-ridden impurities: sudorifics, diaphoretics, purgatives, bleeding, etc. It is interesting to note that although the theoretical assumptions of Paracelsian medicine were quite different from those of Galenism, the goals of medical therapy remained much the same, whether viewed as an attempt to restore balance through the evacuation of a humor, or as the removal of disease-causing impurities.

This sounds simple enough, but diseases take root in different organs, and with varying degrees of tenacity. Unlike the Galenic idea that disease is countered by restoring a humoral balance to the body, a holistic and systemic therapy, Severinus' emphasis on seeds of disease rooting and growing differently in different organs requires a therapy that is specific to the disease. Expelling impurities from joints may require a method other than that used for expelling a stomach fever. Furthermore, not all diseases are curable, for some are so deeply rooted in the human anatomy that they cannot be separated "by any diligence of craftsmen or nature." These place necessary limits or predestinations on individuals: "Thus, whatever things are born immediately become subject to death."[148] The other side of this fatalism is Severinus' implicit assumption that in principle no disease is incurable unless it is predestined to

147 Ibid., p. 339: "Itaque, quia morborum omnium impuritates, radices, & semina, in humanam Anatomiam, uel ab ortu, uel postea alimentorum usu, implantantur, primum & præcipuum curationis uel sanationis consilium erit, tales impuritatum mixtiones auferre."

148 Ibid., pp. 339-40: "Nec ulla, artificum uel Naturæ industria separari possunt, sed prædestinationum terminos, immutabili necessitate constituunt. Ita, quæcunque nascuntur, morti confestim obnoxia fiunt." This idea is explicitly stated by Paracelsus in *Opus paramirum* and *De rerum natura*. See *Paracelsus: Essential Readings*, pp. 82 and 183.

be so. However, if diseases have progressed too far, they may in fact be incurable. Dead, ulcerated tissues cannot be restored "because they have lost the continuity of life."[149]

Severinus distinguished two main categories of remedies: general (perfect) cures and particular (imperfect) cures. General cures are "radical" insofar as they aim for a complete cure by "the removal of the impurities or the disease-roots, which are implanted in the human anatomy by an unnecessary mixture."[150] Such medicines have a natural balsam that is agreeable to human nature and act both by strengthening the innate balsam and by chemically separating the offending disease from its host and expelling it. Particular remedies are analgesic. They aim to take away or mitigate symptoms, but do not remove the roots of the disease. Of what use are they? Severinus believed that the general method of treating is most desirable, but realized that it is rarely discovered.[151] If a general cure is hard to find, one should resort to a particular cure. Furthermore, within the class of particulars, remedies can vary from rather gross to nearly perfect.

If there is one key to successful drug therapy it is that remedies, like the diseases they are to oppose, must be *vital*: "Thus the actions of remedies result from spirits and the vital tinctures of spirits, not from bodies or dead and Relollacean qualities."[152] It is the spirit in a drug that is its effective portion, and this spirit may vary in subtlety or vital power. Spirit, in Severinus' cosmology, is the result of a thickening of formless, prime matter, and therefore may vary from almost grossly corporeal to the thinnest ether. The ability of a spirit to be parted from the body to which it is conjoined depends on its subtlety. Consequently, a very tenuous spirit or balsam is able to penetrate well.

---

149 Severinus, *Idea medicinæ*, p. 341: "quia uitæ continuitatem amiserunt."

150 Ibid., p. 343: "Sanatio Universalis & perfecta, est ablatio impuritatum, uel Radicum morbidarum, mixtione non necessaria in humana Anatomia insitarum."

151 Ibid., p. 345: "Optanda quidem esset Vniversalis curandi ratio, sed paucis concessa fuit."

152 Ibid., p. 345: "Ita remediorum actiones ex spiritibus uitalibusque spirituum Tincturis procedunt, non ex corporibus, uel mortuis Relollaceisque qualitatibus." *Relollacean* is a Paracelsian term referring to the dead, virtueless parts of nature. See A.E. Waite, *The Hermetic and Alchemical Writings of … Paracelsus*, vol. 2 (London: James Elliott, 1894), p. 181.

Besides subtlety, spirits differ in purity and kind: "Some are pure, and others are mixed. Some reflect the properties of the salts more, others more the properties of sulphurous species, and yet others more the properties of mercurial species."[153] The key to finding the right cure is finding a material that contains a proper spirit of sufficient strength, and refining it chemically to purify it and enhance its power of penetration. Powerful medicines, be they taken from animal, mineral, or vegetable sources, will require preparation, separation, and exaltation before their latent and imprisoned virtues can be expressed.[154]

The degree of chemical preparation needed is determined by the severity of the disease and how well rooted it is. Superficial diseases do not require Paracelsian chemical remedies: "We said before that there is no need for these indications in diseases that consist of impurities that are changeable and superficial, which have not put down fixed roots, such as are most fevers, catarrhs, coughs, hoarsenesses, and similar affects."[155] These require simple purgation, mundification, etc. Even serious disease, if treated at an early stage, may respond to traditional concoctions. But, "in chronic diseases, such as epilepsies, quartan fevers, colics, podagras, and in hydropsy and leprous affects, the radical [i.e. rooted] impurities are first and foremost cured by resolution, and not by concoction," even though some concoctions may well have an analgesic effect.[156] Indeed, the traditional remedies of Hippocrates are not to be lightly abandoned, but we must remember that times have changed and not even Hippocrates' knowledge was perfect: "Surely the ages advance. Consequently, it would have been inappropriate to imitate him in all

153 Severinus, *Idea medicinæ*, p. 346: "Alij puri sunt, alij permixti: alij salium proprietates magis referunt, alij sulphurearum specierum, alij mercurialium."

154 Ibid., p. 356. Fracastoro also developed a theory that disease-causing *seminaria* must be expelled by means of a drug with a spiritual antipathy for them. See Nutton, "The Reception of Fracastoro's Theory of Contagion," p. 202.

155 Severinus, *Idea medicinæ*, pp. 372-73: "Antea diximus, in morbis qui constant ex impuritatibus, mobilibus, superficiarijs, qui non egerunt fixas radices, quales sunt febres plurimæ, catarrhi, tusses, raucedines, & similes affectus, non opus esse hisce Indicationibus."

156 Ibid., p. 374: "In morbis chronicis, ut epilepsiis, quartanis, colicis, podagris, in hydrope, & leprosis affectibus, impuritates radicales, resolutione, non concoctione, proprie & primo curantur." In general Severinus distinguishes diseases into four categories according to affinity: Leprosies, Hydropsies, Podagras, and Epilepsies. Here, however, these four appear among the chronic diseases.

things. ... He lived in a more fortunate age, one not tainted by the most difficult resolutions of the new diseases."[157]

The "chemical approach" to disease and treatment, despite our modern reaction to Paracelsian medicine as being mystical and occult, is based on a very rational epistemology. Since disease processes are beneath the threshold of sense perception, it makes sense to use *reason*, the mind's eye, to assess them.[158] Severinus' method – the method of the chemical philosopher – goes beyond pure empiricism and resorts to rational inferences based on analogies between chemistry in the laboratory and chemistry in nature. In this way the philosopher can learn from chemical analysis what cannot be learned otherwise. Severinus called this a higher analysis (*altiori Analysi*). Furthermore, the "more profound" philosopher is not content with what his senses alone can tell him, but undertakes to reveal the properties that are hidden in bodies by resolving them into their components.[159]

The physician must define diseases on the basis of evident characteristics, such as the types of symptoms, their timing, recurrence, and so on, and then cure them with chemical drugs that exhibit appropriate characteristics, which he has determined by experience. For difficult diseases, those with strong tinctures and deep roots, it makes sense to seek powerful remedies with strong "signatures" or properties. This leads us to consider one of the most controversial and historically characteristic aspects of Paracelsian medicine, namely its use of toxic materials, often poisonous minerals, as raw materials for chemically prepared drugs. "These remedies are taken alone and uncorrupt with difficulty, and they bring forth grave symptoms, unless they are rendered harmless by means of preparation, because the strengths of their mechanical spirits exceed those of the human body. Such remedies are applied in the more serious diseases." Some of these materials, continued Severinus, "are quite poisonous, such as antimony, mercury, sulphur, vitriol, and almost all minerals, hellebore, tithymal, colocynth, scammony, opium, mandrake,

---

157 Ibid., pp. 374-75: "Secula certe proficiunt. Iniquum proinde esset, in omnibus ipsum imitari. ... Feliciori seculo, nouorum morborum difficillimis resolutionibus non inquinato uixit."
158 Ibid., p. 377.
159 Ibid., pp. 70-71.

and hemlock. The use of these is necessary in the most serious diseases. ... Without preparation of this sort they can in no way be applied."[160] These especially poisonous substances must be detoxified chemically; they cannot be mitigated by compounding with milk, honey, or similar additives, and they must be used with consideration of the patient's strength, age, disease, and other case-specific circumstances. Yet there is much to commend their use, for

> the daily use of the leaves of sena, rhubarb, *agaricus, polypodium,* [and other drugs prepared from herbs] ... will not resolve, consume, or mundify those impurities that a single dose of vitrified antimony, precipitated mercury (but not the ordinary kind), crude vitriol or colcothar, tartar, and similar drugs will, [but] with great anxiety for the patient and weakening of his strength.[161]

These drugs work as follows. Once in the stomach their spirits are resolved, turned into vapors, and are thus able to "penetrate more powerfully" (*potentius penetrant*). The spirits then attack the vegetable and mineral impurities (the causes of the disease, insofar as they harbor the morbific *semina*) in the body, and by resolving and consuming them, they turn them into vapors. This chemical activity provokes the violent symptoms that the patient experiences: "palpitations of the heart, fainting, dizziness, and often convulsions that promise danger."[162] But if the patient survives, all is well: "When such difficult impurities have been

160 Ibid., pp. 381-82: "Hæc remedia, sola & sincera difficulter assumuntur & symptomata grauia adducunt, nisi præparatione innoxia reddantur, quia uires Mechanicorum humani corporis excedunt. In morbis grauioribus adhibentur talia. Nonnulla, uenenata plane sunt, ut antimonium, mercurius, sulphur, uitriolum, mineralia fere omnia, helleborum, tithymallus, colocynthis, scammonea, opium, mandragora, cicuta. Horum usus in morbis grauissimis necessarius est ... Sine præparatione hujusmodi nullo pacto adhiberi debent."

161 Ibid., p. 382: "Quotidianus usus foliorum senæ, rhabarbari, agarici, polypodij, ... impuritates illas non resoluent, consument, uel mundificabunt, quas unica exhibitio antimonij uitrificati, mercurij præcipitati, non uulgariter tamen, uitrioli crudi uel colcotharini, tartari, & similum magna ægroti anxietate, uiriumque consternatione auferet."

162 Ibid., p. 383: "palpitationes cordis, deliquia animi, uertigines, sæpe conuulsiones perniciem promittentes."

evacuated, consumed, and removed, health is unexpectedly restored," signified by an increase of the patient's strength and powers.[163]

Severinus' idea of drug therapy can best be described as polypharmacy; he did not wish physicians to abandon herbal medicines, but rather to prepare them differently and not to neglect the more potent mineral preparations. All types of drugs work fundamentally in the same way, but differ greatly in potency. Basically, drugs function as purgatives, as diuretics, anodynes, and as diaphoretics. However, elsewhere in the text he defined drugs as either "specific" ("planetary"), in which the properties of the three primary principles dominate, or "elementary," in which the elemental natures are dominant.[164]

We recall that a good indicator of the power of a material is the strength of its signatures. However, the strong smells, tastes, and caustic qualities of *materia medica* can be altered chemically *without* compromising the balsamic virtue within, which these strong signatures indicate in the crude matter. This is where chemical methods surpass traditional herbalism. Instead of diffusing the strength of herbs by decoctions, their virtues should be retained and concentrated by the chemist, and whereas the traditional compounding pharmacist will fail to hide a drug's harsh taste and smell by mixing it with sugar, egg whites, etc., the chemist can, with diligence, effectively remove the offending signatures, without harming the drug's efficacy.[165]

Take antimony, for example. "Glass of antimony is quite without taste, yet it has ended up discredited because of its dangerous vehemence for causing vomiting and purgation."[166] This sort of drug enjoyed great popularity and controversy already in the 1560s as is reflected in the *Idea medicinæ*:

Neither will those much spoken of remedies which now through all Germany are praised by some and blamed by others escape the judgement of our courts. Among them we will first bring forward glass of

---

163 Ibid.: "Inanitis uero, consumtis, & ablatis tam difficilibus impuritatibus, ex insperato, sanitas restuitur, actionum & facultatum potentiore robore insignita."
164 Ibid., p. 388.
165 Ibid., p. 394.
166 Ibid., p. 389: "Antimonij uitrum, insipidum plane est, uomitionum tamen, & purgationum suspecta uehementia, infame euasit."

antimony, which deserves accusation, because it has not received the separation of the pure from the impure; because it has not sustained the proper resolution and digestion; because it has admitted fusion to the point of forming a glass, which is to be avoided in all preparation of remedies.[167]

In short, the problem with antimonials arises from improper preparation. The same is true of all other medicines – preparation is the key, whether it be mineral turbith, crocus martis, "corrosive diaphoretic golds," tinctures of coral, oil of arsenic or lead, or other metallic drugs.[168] Imperfect preparation produces imperfect medicines: "Those that are spiritual and suitable to diseases heal: in fact those in which the corporeal impurities and crudeness still remain also heal, but not completely."[169] Thus, skill in chemical methods is a basic requirement for the good physician, who is the servant of nature.

She [nature] provided us wood, from which she wished charcoal to be made, and also flint and herbs to supply the material for glass, and potter's clay to serve for the construction of furnaces. Next she ordered us to cook, ripen the crude, separate the pure from the impure, transmute bitterness into sweetness, and soothe the irksomeness of ulcerations, hotnesses, flavors, odors, and coagulations. And she instructed us to be ministers and separators, not masters or compounders.[170]

---

167 Ibid., p. 398: "Neque censuram horum comitiorum subterfugient famosa illa remedia, quæ nunc per universam Germaniam, laudantur ab his, culpantur ab illis. Inter quæ primo Antimonij uitrum producemus: quod accusationem meretur, quia puri ab impuro separationem non recepit: quod resolutionem debitam & digestionem non sustinuit: quod fusionem uitrificatoriam admisit, in omni remediorum Præparatione fugiendam."

168 Severinus mentions these and other drugs in passing. Ibid., pp. 399-401.

169 Ibid., pp. 401-402: "Quæ spiritualia sunt & morbis consentanea, sanant: in quibus uero impuritates corporeæ & cruditates etiamnum relinquuntur, sanant quidem, sed non perfecte."

170 Ibid., p. 396: "Sed ligna coniunxit, ex quibus carbones fieri uoluit: silicem quoque, & herbas, uitri materiam subministraturas, & argillam, fornacum constructionibus obtemperaturam. Postea coquere iussit, cruda maturare, impura separare, amaritudines in dulcedinem transmutare, erosionum, calorum, saporum, odorum, coagulationum tædia mitigare: & nos Ministros esse præcepit ac Separatores, non Magistros uel Compositores."

In this flowery speech we have an explicit statement of a theme that runs through Severinus' *Idea medicinæ*; that the true physician is not a *master*, but a *minister* of nature. He does not compound drugs according to artificial classifications of quality and degree, but rather works the way nature herself does, namely through chemical separations.[171] This Paracelsian chemical philosophy unites the sense of the holiness of nature, typical of Renaissance Platonism, with medicine. Much as the *archeus* stands at the juncture of the world of ideas and the world of matter, the physician stands between the macrocosm and the microcosm, using the knowledge of the one to guide his treatment of the other.

A METAPHYSICS FOR BIOLOGY

The terminology, concepts, and chemical approach to medical treatment that Severinus advocated in the *Idea medicinæ* marks his work and philosophy as Paracelsian. Indeed, Severinus himself acknowledged the importance of Paracelsus' writings in reorienting his vision of medicine and unabashedly cited Paracelsus' texts in the *Idea medicinæ*. Contemporaries regarded him as a follower of Paracelsus, and scholars down to our own time have considered him mainly as an interpreter of Paracelsian theory. Yet the *Idea medicinæ* is more than a collation of Paracelsian concepts and a rationale for the use of chemically-prepared drugs. It is Severinus' effort to lay a foundation for a new philosophy, a biological metaphysics, using key Paracelsian concepts as building stones.

In this chapter I have focused on the chief concepts that Severinus established, namely how *semina* lie at the basis of change, how preordained changes can be altered by transplantation, how this *semina* theory can explain the generation and appearance of diseases, and how the physician can direct therapy against bad seeds and tinctures. These concepts are at the core of the *Idea medicinæ* and were what posterity found most remarkable about the book. Indeed, few readers applied *semina* theory

---

171 Beside separations, nature also makes "spiritual unions," but Severinus implies that these are beyond human capacity.

outside of chemical pathology, Edward Jorden's balneology, which will be discussed in chapter six, being a notable exception. However, we should understand that the philosophy itself was much more general, with a wider potential application. Severinus gathered support for his theory not only from medical literature, but also from what he took to be common knowledge of agricultural practice, meteorology, natural history, and Scripture. For example, his argument that generation arises from *semina* other than what are generally recognized as seeds is supported by reference to horticultural practices of asexual propagation, in which an entire organism grows from a part that, although not the seed, clearly contains the "knowledge" or mechanical science necessary for generating the whole. An entire plant, for instance, might be grown from a cutting, which is evidence that all the information needed for the whole is contained in the various parts. Likewise, Severinus' understanding of transplantation was supported by observations of grafting, forcing plants to blossom out of season, and the literal transplantation of plants to different locations. His theory agreed with what the farmer knew about agriculture and animal husbandry, such as why one could never select for a field of pure wheat (some darnel always appears by spontaneous transplantation), how hybridization worked, and the importance of soils, seasons, and climate on growth and development. Throughout, Severinus strove to create a philosophy with application to the whole macrocosm as well as to the microcosm.

Another aspect of Severinus' theory, one that did not attract the attention that his concept of *semina morborum* did, was his application of *semina* and transplantation to embryology. His treatment of sexual generation and distinction, mainly discussed in chapter ten of the *Idea medicinæ* (On human generation and transplantations arising in generation), reveals not a thoroughgoing Paracelsian, but a medical theorist sorting out the good and bad points of received Aristotelian and Galenic doctrine and knitting them together with what he has learned from Hippocrates and Paracelsus.

Severinus considered human sexual reproduction, like that of all species in which there was a "perfect" distinction between the sexes, to involve a mutual congress of seeds from both parents. Different opinions about the roles of male and female in generation had come down to the late Middle Ages from diverse ancient Greco-Roman and medieval

Arabic sources.[172] As a gross generalization, these can be grouped into "philosophical" (Aristotelian) and "medical" (Hippocratic-Galenist) points of view. The simplified extreme Aristotelian opinion was that the male contributed the form and the female the matter necessary for the development of an embryo, the sex of which was determined by heat and position within the womb. The embryo grew from this hylomorphic union, with the heart appearing first. Galen, on the other hand, followed the Hippocratic teaching that both female and male contributed seed to conceiving an embryo, in which the three basic physiological systems of the body developed from the three primitive organs, the liver, heart, and brain. Severinus adopted an intermediate position between the extremes.

Severinus believed that the knowledge to create the whole body is not just found in the reproductive organs, but in the *semina*, which are "in the mummy, balsam, or vital sulphur that is dispersed throughout the whole body."[173] This agreed with the ancient teaching that all parts are in some sense in all the parts and explained how human semen can contain the information for the whole human body, without the need to account for how this was materially possible. The testes are necessary, however, because they produce a seminal fluid that protects the spiritual tinctures of the *semina* that reside there from external injury. This is true for both sexes: "That the female sex is lacking in such a balsam, mummy, vital sulphur, or seed is absurd."[174]

Following coitus, the male and female seeds mix in the uterus. They readily embrace each other because they are drawn from the same root and have similar knowledge – they harmonize.[175] And although each parent contributes seed, the seeds themselves are not distinctly male or female. The sex of the embryo is not, therefore, simply determined by one parent, but is the result of a more complex determination of supervening tinctures and mixtures. Since humans are one species, male and

---

172 See Joan Cadden, *Meanings of Sex Difference in the Middle Ages: Medicine, Science, and Culture* (Cambridge: Cambridge Univ. Press, 1993).

173 Severinus, *Idea medicinæ*, p. 149: "in Mumia, Balsamo, uitali Sulphure, quod per uniuersum corpus dispergitur."

174 Ibid.: "Foemineum sexum tali Balsamo, Mumia, uitali sulphure, semine, destitui absurdum est."

175 Ibid., p. 150.

female are contained in one root, and the knowledge of both male and female anatomy must be contained in the *semina* of both parents. "Males often abound in female seed, and conversely, females often abound in male seed."[176] When the two mix, the resulting sex depends on a mixing and separating of the relevant tinctures, the result of which is a transplantation of some sort. It is this process, which does not depend on heat and cold, that accounts for sexual difference. If the tinctures are predominantly female, a female child will result; if predominantly male, a male child will result – if the separation is relatively complete. "But if the separation was not wholly completed and perfected, androgynes will result, that is, effeminate men and masculine women."[177] This theory can account for why individuals exhibit traits of both parents and why there is no clear distinction of humans into strictly masculine and strictly feminine individuals.

Although Severinus adopted a two-seed theory of sexual reproduction, he leaned more toward Aristotle's epigenetic account of the development of the embryo and rejected outright the Galenist opinion that the veins grew from an embryonic liver, the arteries from an embryonic heart, and nerves from an embryonic brain. "Those who have been more diligent, even in corporeal anatomy, such as Fallopius, reject this excessively material origin of the parts," he wrote.[178] However, he thought that both the Aristotelians and Galenists were missing the point in their arguments over whether the heart is the primary organ, "for they do not observe the mechanical process of generation ... and do not understand the power by which all things arise."[179]

The abundant vital spirit connected with the seed carries out the function of the heart, pulse and respiration, even before tissues are visible.[180] The faculties of the heart and arteries are immediately pres-

---

176 Ibid., p. 165: "Itaque in una radice continentur: quo fit ut sæpe mares foemineo semine abundent, & uicissim foeminæ masculino."

177 Ibid.: "Si uero separatio non fuerit prorsus absoluta, euadunt Androgyni, id est uiri effoeminati, & masculæ foeminæ."

178 Ibid., p. 164: "Qui diligentiores etiam in corporea Anatomia fuerunt, ut Fallopius, hanc nimis materialem partium originem repudiarunt."

179 Ibid., p. 162: "Non enim Generationis Mechanicam lithurgiam ... animaduertunt, nec Scientiæ potestatem, a qua omnia proficiscuntur, intelligunt.

180 Ibid., p. 164.

ent at conception. These attract nutrients, and tissues are built up and eventually form appropriately distributed rudiments of organs. Growth through nourishment continues, because the seminal knowledge in the embryo recognizes suitable aliments and attracts them, but rejects the rest as "foreigners" those that are not homogenous and do not possess harmonizing characteristics. "But natives are recognized, because their characteristics are similar, and they have common roots that are harmonious for mixing."[181] Should "foreign impressions" flow into and join with the first mixtures in generation, the harmony will be destroyed and the predestined growth will undergo transplantation. Severinus' theory of transplantation, then, accounts for defects in embryonic growth as well as the appearance of disease in previously healthy parts. The earlier such a transplantation happens, the more successful it is, and the more serious the outcome is.

We can see from Severinus' account of human generation that he extended his basic metaphysical tools – *semina*, tinctures, mechanical knowledge and process, and transplantation – to explain sexual reproduction and embryonic development. His explanation was not merely an interpretation of Paracelsian ideas, but a synthesis of Aristotelian, Galenic, and Paracelsian points of view. While he rejected the Aristotelian hylomorphic explanation in favor of a more Galenic-Hippocratic two-seed theory of reproduction, he also agreed with the Aristotelian view that the embryo grows epigenetically, by assimilating nutrients. However, he viewed his own theory as superior to both, because he understood that the real mechanism driving generation and growth was spiritual. Only by understanding this could one understand the apparent connections between natural phenomena and why the microcosm correlated with the macrocosm. While this approach can be seen as basically Paracelsian, Severinus himself sought to show that the physical manifestations of these spiritual powers might just as well be identified with the properties of plants or diseases as with mineral impurities. It was in this sense an extension of Paracelsian ideas to form a thoroughgoing chemical philosophy.

---

181 Ibid., p. 153: "Peregrina, hoc est, quæ non sunt ὁμότροπα, ab alienis sedibus pelluntur. … Domestica uero cognoscuntur, quia signaturæ sunt similes, & Radices habent communes ad Mixtionem consentientes."

PART THREE

THE INFLUENCE OF THE
IDEA MEDICINÆ PHILOSOPHICÆ

Chapter Five

THE RECEPTION OF SEVERINUS'
THEORIES IN WESTERN EUROPE

$\mathcal{S}$CHOLARS OF the Paracelsian movement have for many years identified the *Idea medicinæ* as a singularly important text for formulating and disseminating Paracelsian doctrines.[1] This opinion rests squarely on the judgements of the early historians of medical thought, who in turn relied on seventeenth-century accounts of the origin and development of medicine and on the biographical encyclopedias.[2] But it is one thing to repeat the canonized judgements of bygone generations, and quite another to understand them and document them. If indeed Severinus' work was as influential as the historians of Paracelsianism have said, then an investigation of how the *Idea medicinæ* was read and by whom should be vital to our understanding of the development of chemical philosophy.

1 For example, Trevor-Roper, "The Paracelsian Movement," p. 161: "It was thanks to [Severinus] and to his writings, above all, that Paracelsianism, in the last quarter of the sixteenth century, became internationally respectable." Debus, "Mathematics and Nature," p. 22, called Severinus "the most important Paracelsian theorist in the sixteenth century." Pagel, *The Smiling Spleen*, p. 18, labeled him "the clearest expositor and follower of Paracelsian natural philosophy."

2 For example, Kurt Polycarp Joachim Sprengel, *Versuch einer pragmatischen Geschichte der Arzneykunde*, 3rd ed., vol. 3 (Halle, 1827), p. 503: "Der berühmteste Anhänger des Paracelsischen Systems unter den ältern Schriftsteller dieses Jahrhunderts ist Peter Severin." [The most famous adherent to the Paracelsian system among the older authors of this [i.e. the sixteenth] century is Peter Severinus]. Sprengel's opinion influenced the nineteenth-century historians, e.g. Michael Benedict Lessing, *Handbuch der Geschichte der Medizin*, vol. 1 (Berlin: August Hirschwald, 1839), p. 409: "Der berühmteste Paracelsist in XVI. Jahrhundert war Peter Severin." The lasting fame of Severinus as a pioneer was undoubtedly influence by judgements of Libavius and Sennert, whose views are treated in chapter seven.

This chapter and the next three comprise a study of the reception of Severinus' ideas in the roughly one hundred year period following the publication of the *Idea medicinæ* in 1571, with special attention to those who studied Severinus' ideas carefully. A perusal of printed books from this period has revealed numerous references to Severinus and the *Idea medicinæ* as well as instances when an author's exposition of Paracelsian theory so closely resembles that of the *Idea medicinæ* that one suspects Severinus' words behind them. Some authors mentioned Severinus only in passing, perhaps just in a marginal note, while others devoted considerable space to reciting and explaining his ideas or to comparing and assimilating them into traditional medical theory. Occasionally, references to Severinus occur in non-medical contexts, and these provide us valuable clues to the penetration of Paracelsian chemical philosophy into the broader intellectual culture. Two learned physicians went so far as to publish book-length commentaries on the *Idea medicinæ*, which are treated separately in chapters nine and ten. While an examination of identifiable references to Severinus and his work can at best give only a partial understanding of his ideas, considering that early modern writers did not always credit their sources, and then did so selectively, this approach nevertheless has the methodological advantage of permitting inferences from verifiable, documented facts, rather than vague assumptions about what ideas were "in the air."

To bring some order to this examination, references to Severinus and his work have been arranged according to rough chronology, geographical context, and thematic generalization. The present chapter introduces the intellectual context in which the *Idea medicinæ* first appeared and then follows the reactions of authors writing primarily in France. In this way, we may appreciate the importance of regional dialogue or, in the case of the *Jardin du Roi* in Paris, an institutional setting. Jean Baptist van Helmont, a Belgian, is also treated in this chapter, because of his connection with French savants and tremendous influence on the reception and interpretation of Paracelsian ideas in mid-seventeenth century England, which is the subject of chapter six.

Chapter seven brings together sources appearing mainly in German-speaking areas and in those regions closely connected to German intellectual culture; Scandinavia is treated separately in chapter eight. Paracelsianism was perhaps most widespread in the German principalities of the Holy Roman Empire and it formed an important part of the ideological context of reaction and reform that underlay that stormy age. It is hoped that this detailed and carefully documented study of who read the *Idea medicinæ*, or knew of Severinus' doctrines from some other source, and *how* they interpreted or assimilated these concepts, will provide insight into what early modern readers found especially attractive (or repulsive!) about Paracelsian metaphysics.

EARLY REACTIONS TO PARACELSIANISM

The *Idea medicinæ* appeared at a time when controversy over Paracelsian doctrines and medicines was intensifying. Paracelsian incursions into traditionally Galenic territory had caused heated debate from the time Paracelsus was expelled from Basel until 1566, when the first Parisian proscription against the medical use of antimony heralded the "antimony wars." Despite this opposition, Paracelsian remedies were gaining acceptance in the 1560s.[3] The early spreading of Paracelsian medicine was mostly done by surgeons and practitioners of what might be described today as alternative medicine – itinerants proffering chemical and magical cures to patients who had not been healed by the traditional methods, which were taught in the universities and had trickled down to general practice over the centuries. The success of such alternative cures depended on reputations and promises, and they competed in the medical marketplace against "learned" medicine, so it is no surprise that educated physicians rejected chemical medicines both as a rival therapy and because they lacked foundation in rational theory. The reactions of early opponents to Paracelsian medicine indicate that it was not Paracelsus' doctrines that first awakened the pens of critics, but the use of chemically prepared drugs that were associated with his name. These often produced violent effects and violated the fundamental assumption that the patient's bodily fluids needed to be eased back into a healthful balance. But, as in any age, practice gains credibility and

---

3 On the antimony wars and the early development of Paracelsianism in France see Trevor-Roper, "The Paracelsian Movement," and Debus, *The French Paracelsians*.

professional identity through a theoretical superstructure, which Paracelsus' writings offered. The challenge that the new drugs presented to therapeutics therefore generated an interest in Paracelsus as an author of a new medical system.

Paracelsus' treatises offered a labyrinth of theoretical, even metaphysical support for chemical therapy, through which only a willing and patient student like Severinus could find his way. Since few established physicians had the inclination to abandon tradition and commit themselves to a radically different world view, assimilation of Paracelsian theory was slow. Educated physicians who found something of value in chemical medicine either attempted to abstract it from its Paracelsian context and reconcile it with Galenic theory or else they understood the need to provide an erudite defense of Paracelsian medicine.

The first learned discussions of Paracelsian chemical therapy appeared in the years immediately preceding the publication of the *Idea medicinæ*, and these gradually drew attention to Paracelsian theory. Johannes Albertus Wimpinæus published a book in 1569 that defended Paracelsian medicine and argued that chemical drugs and Paracelsian ideas are not wholly incompatible with traditional medicine.[4] The author had himself gone over to Paracelsian medicine and defended the use of antimony in treating difficult diseases, but he did not think that the old and new medicines were irreconcilable. Three years later, the well-known medical authority Johannes Guintherius Andernachus published his volumes on the old and new medicines, in the very year the *Idea medicinæ* came out and with the same printer. Guinther, who is best known today as Vesalius' teacher and for his early humanist editions of Galenic medicine, found chemical drugs to be worth incorporating into university medicine.[5] Unlike Wimpinæus, however, Guinther remained a Galenist. Thus, in 1571 Severinus' book entered

4 Johannes Albertus Wimpinæus, *De concordia Hippocraticorum et Paracelsistarum libri magni excursiones defensivæ* (Munich: Adam Berg, 1569). This is a very rare book, and I have only been able to consult a later edition, published in Strassburg, 1615.
5 Johannes Guintherius Andernachus (Guinter or Winter von Andernach), *De medicina veteri et nova tum cognoscenda, tum faciunda commentarii duo* (Basel: Henricpetri, 1571). On Wimpinæus and Guinter von Andernach, see Debus, *The French Paracelsians*, pp. 19-20.

an intellectual milieu that was already well stirred to controversy and seeking a useful reconciliation between Paracelsian and Galenic medicines. Although the *Idea medicinæ* did not offer a palm leaf to Galen, it did fill a need in the medical world for a learned exposition of Paracelsian ideas of matter, spirit, generation, transplantation, and corruption. This helped others, in turn, to find common ground between Paracelsian and peripatetic concepts. But it was conflict, not concord, that initially greeted Severinus' work.

With the augmented popularity of Paracelsian drugs and the printing of Paracelsus' manuscripts, Paracelsian doctrines came under wider scrutiny, and an anti-Paracelsian movement was launched.[6] Johannes Wier lambasted Paracelsus and his followers in his *De præstigiis dæmonum*, published at Basel in 1563 by Paracelsus' former pupil and amanuensis, Oporinus.[7] The kind of Paracelsian that Wier had in mind was not the learned sort, like Wimpinæus, but rather the itinerant and uneducated, arrogant rogues who practice magic and "have committed to memory the foul sayings of that insane man [Paracelsus]." They are content "with the confused heap of useless words with which Paracelsus filled his writings," he continued. Wier roundly criticized Paracelsus for espousing ideas about medicine and the physician that were contrary to the meaning of Scripture and he detested persons who claimed mystical talents for healing. Yet, he took care not to impugn chemical pharmacy as such: "I do not here make light of chemistry, which is an important part of medicine," he wrote.[8] Wier's book was repeatedly published, and was soon translated into German (1566) and French (1567).[9] This, along with a 1570 treatise by Bartholomæus Reussner pointing to Paracelsus' blasphemies, laid the groundwork for Thomas Erastus' attack

---

6 Allen G. Debus, "The Chemical Philosophers: Chemical Medicine from Paracelsus to Van Helmont," *History of Science* 12 (1974): 235-259, pp. 238-39, postulates the development of three basic schools of reactions to Paracelsus in the 1570s: Paracelsian (represented by Severinus), the "chemical compromise" (by Guinther von Andernach), and antiparacelsian (by Erastus).

7 Other editions soon followed: 1564, 1566, 1568, 1577, and 1583.

8 Johannes Wier, *Witches, Devils, and Doctors in the Renaissance: Johann Weyer, De præstigiis dæmonum*, trans. John Shea (Binghamton, NY: Medieval & Renaissance Texts & Studies, 1991), pp. 153-4.

9 Debus, *The French Paracelsians*, p. 26.

on Paracelsian religion and philosophy – an unequivocal rejection of Paracelsian cosmology.[10]

Thomas Erastus commenced a decade of biting criticism of Paracelsian medicine, magic, and astrology in 1572 with the first volume of his treatise on the "new medicine" of Paracelsus, *Disputationum de medicina nova Philippi Paracelsi pars prima*.[11] Erastus' religious orthodoxy had come into question after his participation in the Speyer Reichstag in 1570, where some of his closest associates were identified as antitrinitarians. To improve his image he accepted the challenge presented by the antiparacelsian physicians, chief among them Johannes Crato von Krafftheim, to undertake to discredit Paracelsus and other proponents of Hermetic medicine.[12] Erastus' *De medicina nova* was influential, both in rallying antiparacelsians and in drawing attention to Paracelsus. A number of antiparacelsian tracts soon followed, as did the apologies and vindications that they in turn induced. The very next year, for example, Bernard Dessenius Cronenburgius wrote a tract defending traditional medicine against the new medicine of the Paracelsian Georg Phædro "and the impostures of the whole Paracelsian school."[13] The antiparacelsian literature offered some readers their first exposure to the ideas of Paracelsus and was therefore important to the spread of Paracelsianism. It also created a highly charged environment in which the the *Idea medicinæ* would first be judged.

10 For a brief summary of what Erastus found objectionable in Paracelsus, see Debus, "The Chemical Philosophers," pp. 239-40, and Walter Pagel, "Erastus," *DSB*, vol. 4 (1971), pp. 386-88. Pagel, *Paracelsus*, pp. 311-333, provides a fuller account, but the most incisive recent account of Erastus' complaints about Paracelsus' ideas on creation and resurrection is Charles D. Gunnoe, Jr., "Erastus and Paracelsianism: Theological Motifs in Thomas Erastus' Rejection of Paracelsian Natural Philosophy," in *Reading the Book of Nature*, ed. Debus and Walton, pp. 45-65.

11 Thomas Erastus, *Disputationum de medicina nova Philippi Paracelsi*, parts one and two (Basel: Petrus Perna, 1572). Parts three and four followed in 1574. See Lynn Thorndike, *A History of Magic and Experimental Science* (New York: Columbia University Press, 1953-59), vol. 5, pp. 652-667.

12 Charles D. Gunnoe, Jr., "Thomas Erastus and his Circle of Anti-Paracelsians," in *Analecta Paracelsica: Studien zum Nachleben Theophrast von Hohenheims im deutschen Kulturgebiet der Frühen Neuzeit*. Heidelberger Studien zur Naturkunde der Frühen Neuzeit, vol. 4, ed. Wolf-Dieter Müller-Jahncke and Joachim Telle (Stuttgart: Franz Steiner Verlag, 1994), pp. 127-148.

13 Bernard Dessenius Cronenburgius, *Medicinæ veteris et rationalis, adversus ... Georgii Fedronis, ac universæ sectæ Paracelsicæ imposturas, defensio* (Cologne, 1573).

Despite the fact that Erastus did not launch an *ad hominem* attack on Severinus in the *De medicina nova*, there can be no doubt that he had read the *Idea medicinæ*, which had been published only a year before, and taken it as exemplary of Paracelsian thought.[14] Indeed, in summarizing the views of the Paracelsians, Erastus lifted certain passages from the *Idea medicinæ* almost verbatim, as the following comparison between the *De medicina nova* and the *Idea medicinæ* demonstrates.[15] Correlating passages have been underlined, and Erastus' gloss has been aligned, without elision, with Severinus' text in order to illustrate more clearly how he used Severinus' very words in his shortened summary of how Paracelsians view the elements.

ERASTUS

Proinde *elementa* dicunt *esse loca, matrices, domicilia, vitali validaque postestate munita: quæ semina* generationum contineant, protrudant, maturent, officioque perfunctis hospitium concedant.

    Et quia loca sunt, aiunt, *incorporea vt sint necessitas iubet*: cum aliter

      tantam corporum multitudinem recipere tam facile non possent.

        Vacua et inania sunt simili propemodum prouidentia: alioquin inæquali favore quibusdam plus obligata obscurius alia *recepissent*.

SEVERINUS

Elementa esse loca, matrices, domicilia, vitali validaque potestate munita, quæ semina generationi consecrata, foveant, digestis temporibus suscitent, ad maturitatem promoveant, emeritis receptacula concedant, immutabili quiete beata.

    Et quia loca sunt, incorporea ut sint necessitas iubet: nisi enim essent a dimensionum legibus absoluta nequaquam corporum, principiorum et seminum *tantam multitudinem tam facile reciperent*. Infinita tamen non sunt. Vitali virtute fines et terminos præscribente: quibus non solum ipsis standum est. Sed etiam seminibus, principiis, etiam corporibus, utcunque superba dimensionum explicatione triumphent. *Vacua vel inania sunt, simili propemodum providentia: alioquin inæquali favore, quibusdam* seminibus *plus obligata*, aliorum rationes *obscurius recepissent*, et minime sinceras repræsentassent.

Note 14, 15: See p. 219.

Similarly, when Erastus wrote

> Indeed in chapter five, where they talk nonsense about heaven or fire,
> air, water, and earth, they write thus: Into these four incorporeal, empty,
> and vacuous substances, the Creator placed the seminal reasons for all
> things, by an incomprehensible magic (loving piety more than wisdom,
> he said, lest he seem to support profane magic, for which Paracelsus, it
> is agreed, was most eager),

there can be no doubt that he was quoting chapter five of *Idea medicinæ*:
"Into these four incorporeal, empty, and vacuous substances, the Creator
placed light and the seminal reasons for all things, by an incomprehensible magic …." Erastus left off the rest of this sentence, in which
Severinus defined "magic" as that used by God for creating the world:
"… by the virtue of that Word and spirit that was moved over the waters, imparting the principles of bodies, in which those things about to
come forth onto the world stage were clothed."[16] The comparison of the
Latin texts below makes it clear exactly what Erastus added and deleted.
Again, correlating phrases have been underlined.

ERASTUS	SEVERINUS
Etenim cap. 5. Vbi de coelo vel igne, aere, aqua, terra, nugantur, sic scribunt. *In his quatuor naturis incorporeis, inanibus, vacuis, seminales omnium rerum rationes incomprehensibili magia* (amans pietatis dixisset potius, Sapientia: ne sceleratæ Magiæ videretur favere: cuius Paracelsum studiosissimum fuisse constat) *imposuit creator.*	*In his quatuor Naturis incorporeis, inanibus, vacuis, Lucem & seminales rerum omnium Rationes, incomprehensibili Magia*
	imposuit *Creator,* uirtute Verbi & Spiritus illius, qui super aquas ferebatur, Principia corporum adiungens, quibus induerentur in mundanam scenam proditura.

Note 16. See p. 219

It would seem that Erastus, by omitting Severinus' qualification of the term magic, prefered to color Severinus' words with a hint of the profane. This was no light matter in those times.[17]

Severinus was quite taken aback by the harsh criticism his ideas had provoked and sought to find out if there were others who agreed with his unnamed assailant, whom we can now assume was Erastus. "How, I ask, can a philosopher of words, inescapably entangled in a thousand homonyms, refute things concealed in nature's bosom, which cannot be unfolded and dug out without much philosophy and the experience of the fire?" he wrote to Johannes Pistorius. "What can he understand, so long as he applies an unreasonable mind to such contemplation and reading?"[18] Severinus thought he had succeeded in clarifying Paracelsus' doctrines and was upset by the attack:

> In the theory of the elements I have as clearly as possible shown the
> distinction between the primary and the mixed; I have set forth their

14 Erastus wrote to Bullinger on 2. November 1571 (Zurich Staatsarchiv, E II 361 fol. 74 r) that someone had dared to publish a book called the *Idea medicinæ philosophicæ*, which cloaked the absurdities and impiety of Paracelsus in beautiful prose. Erastus must have obtained and read a copy of Severinus' book soon after it came off the press. I am grateful to Charles Gunnoe for sharing this information with me.

15 Erastus, *De medicina nova*, part 2, p. 102; Severinus, *Idea medicinæ*, pp. 46-47. This analysis of Erastus' use of the *Idea medicinæ* has been published in Shackelford, "Early Reception of Paracelsian Theory," and is included here for completeness.

16 Erastus, *De medicina nova*, part two, p. 104; Severinus, *Idea medicinæ*, pp. 41-42. Erastus also quoted Severinus on p. 115 (from *Idea medicinæ*, pp. 66-67) and p. 145 (from *Idea medicinæ*, pp. 54-55, 80). Further study might well turn up other instances of quotation or even paraphrasing. In any case, it is clear that Erastus drew on Severinus' work while composing the second part of his attack on Paracelsus.

17 Not many years later, for example, Giordano Bruno satirized Christ, as Orion, in his *Spaccio de la bestia trionfante* (Paris [London?], 1584), which supported Giovanni Mocenigo's denunciation of him to the Venetian Inquisition for, among other things, regarding Christ as a magician. See, Giordano Bruno, *The Expulsion of the Triumphant Beast*, trans. Arthur D. Imerti (New Brunswick, NJ: Rutgers University Press, 1964), pp. 48, 54-55, 255-257. In northern Europe, too, religious authorities were sensitive to matters of doctrine in the post-Tridentine period.

18 Letter from Severinus to Pistorius, presumed to date to around 1574 (Copenhagen, Kgl. Bibl., Bøllings Brevsamling D 4° 1085): "Quid quæso reprehendere potest verbalis philosophus mille homonomiis inexplicabiliter implicatus in rebus naturæ gremio absconditis, quæ explicari et erui non possunt sine multa philosophia et ignis experientia, aut quid intelligere potest, dum inquinatum animum tantæ contemplationi et lectioni accommodat!"

properties and brought light to a very obscure contemplation! How often, led astray by malicious equivocation, has he inveighed against my elements – those of nature itself? What can he be thinking of, when he in so many places equivocally compares the scholastic emptinesses, dimensions, invisibilities, and incorporealities (if I may now speak thus) with my properties, which have a foundation and rationale in nature?[19]

Severinus concluded his letter to Pistorius with a request that his friend ascertain what his peers in Germany thought about this antiparacelsian polemic, "for if they find such a method of disputing pleasing, I would withdraw from this controversy without delay."[20] Almost as an afterthought he added "we have suffered on account of the theologians in these times." This cryptic comment might be an oblique reference to the Cryptocalvinist controversy, which was beginning to spread to Copenhagen in the 1570s, but it likely also refers to the theological criticism of Paracelsian doctrines that had been initiated by Wier and Erastus.[21]

    Whereas the antiparacelsians certainly aroused Thomas Moffet, who wrote to Severinus asking his help in staving off the harsh assaults, Severinus preferred to stay out of the fray. He wrote to Zwinger in 1583 saying that he was not interested in polemic and controversy, which is not in the spirit of Socratic dialogue. In 1587, fifteen years after Erastus' censure of his Paracelsian ideas, Severinus wrote to Zwinger that he continued to

19 Ibid.: "In doctrina elementorum quam clare ostendi differentiam primorum et permixtorum, proprietates exposui et obscurissimæ contemplationi lucem adhibui! Quoties æquiuocatione maligne seductus insectatus est elementa mea et ipsius naturæ! Quid illi in mentem venit, cum vacuitates scholasticas, dimensiones, inuisibilitates, incorporeitates (liceat nunc ita loqui) cum nostris proprietatibus in natura sedem ac scientiam habentibus æquiuoce tot locis contulit."

20 Ibid.: "Si enim talis disputandi ratio ipsis placuerit, receptui nobis confestim canendum est."

21 Ibid.: "Theologorum vicem hisce temporibus doluimus." This might also be rendered "I have felt sorry for the theologians in these times." The fact that Severinus used the first person singular earlier in this letter (see n. 19 above) suggests that his use of the first person plural here really means "we". Rørdam, *KUH* IV, p. 260, thought that Severinus' reference to theological trouble pertained to the charges by German Lutheran conservatives (the Gnesiolutherans) that Niels Hemmingsen was a Cryptocalvinist. Under pressure from his Saxon relatives, King Frederik II was eventually forced to dismiss Hemmingsen from his chair at the university. It is quite likely that Severinus, Pratensis, and Tycho Brahe all shared Hemmingsen's Philippist religious views, as did many academics in Denmark.

work on his treatise on "physics," but expected that some would receive it very negatively. He understood from the unanticipated and harsh reception given the *Idea medicinæ* that he could not satisfy everyone. For, even though he presented his theories in that book without referring to Aristotelian philosophy, his critics nevertheless compared it to Aristotle's teaching and condemned it from an Aristotelian perspective.[22] This comment suggests that Severinus perceived an essential incompatibility between peripatetic and chemical philosophy – that the doctrine he put forth could only be analyzed properly from the chemists' point of view and with their basic assumptions. It is as if Severinus and Erastus were not only talking past each other, in terms of semantics, but actually understood that their perspectives were incommensurable. Recent scholarship has shed considerable light on the basic communication gap between the Paracelsian Oswald Croll and his Aristotelian critic, Andreas Libavius, and has shown that even the very words that these authors used were so laden with different meanings as to render understanding between them very difficult. Yet one curiosity, at least, remains. We can easily imagine that the peripatetic philosophers, when faced with the new terms, different categories, apparent contradictions, and somewhat incoherent ideas of the Paracelsians, might well utterly fail to understand what the chemists were saying or why they rejected Aristotelian philosophy. But can it be that the generation of university-educated Paracelsian physicians that included Severinus could not understand their peripatetic critics? They were, after all, schooled in Aristotelian philosophy, and if they later rejected it in favor of "Hermetic" philosophy, they would at least have understood the sense of their opponents' words. If Severinus did not comprehend what Erastus was saying, it cannot be because he could not, but rather because he would not.[23]

22 Letter to Zwinger, 16 August 1587 (UB Basel, Fr. Gr. II).
23 Owen Hannaway analyzed the communication barrier between the Aristotelian Andreas Libavius and the Paracelsian Oswald Croll in *The Chemists and the Word*, a very fertile approach to understanding the reception of Paracelsianism. The incommensurability, if one may call it that, of the Paracelsian and Aristotelian philosophies needs further study, however, insofar as there is a troubling asymmetry: while Erastus may truly *not* have understood the chemists' language and perspective, Severinus and other university educated Paracelsians surely were schooled in Aristotelian physics, and would have understood their critics. Their rejection of Galenism and Aristotelianism, therefore, is not simply a matter of a failure to communicate.

Severinus did not elaborate on what he found intimidating about the criticisms of Erastus beyond what he stated in his letter to Pistorius, quoted above, but the incompatibility of their views is plain. Erastus was, after all, a diehard Aristotelian and a confirmed Galenist. In his 1574 *De occultis pharmacorum potestatibus* Erastus continued to condemn the "deceits of the Paracelsians" (*Fraudes Paracelsistarum*) and flatly stated that the use of fire in preparing drugs renders them more dangerous, not more safe.[24] Moreover, Erastus denied that *ideas* could be efficient causes and therefore that imagination could produce disease. Although he admitted that bodies contained an immanent incorporeal virtue, he did not accept the idea that disembodied *semina* or vital powers could exist independently and suddenly seize control of bodies.[25] In short, Erastus' philosophy wholly rejected the disease mechanism propounded by Severinus. Speaking as a theologian as well as a physician, Erastus interpreted Paracelsus' conception of disease as an evil substance introduced by God and concluded that the doctrine was heretical. Perhaps Severinus shied away from this sort of equation.[26]

Despite his thoroughgoing rejection of Severinus' Paracelsianism, Erastus considered the *Idea medicinæ* to be an erudite exception to the Paracelsian rabble, as is evident from a letter he wrote to the imperial physician, Monavius, in 1579:

> I judge the genius of Severinus the Dane to be great, and think that his *Idea* compares to the writings of Paracelsus more than any other [author]. But he is also a slave to authority, and while he promotes philosophical freedom, he also extols that garbage of Theophrastus. It is very difficult to understand [his] method. In fact he is more learned

24 Thomas Erastus, *De occultis pharmacorum potestatibus* (Basel: Perna, 1574), p. 193, margin: "Pharmaca chemica vi ignis non fiunt tutiora, sed perniciosora"; p. 194, margin: "Fraudes Paracelsicorum."

25 Pagel, *Paracelsus*, pp. 316 and 322. Few Renaissance Platonists would permit forms to actually exist in the world apart from matter. Bruno, for example, was adamant that one could discuss form as if it were separate, but that in nature it was always united with matter.

26 Ibid., p. 324. Erastus was active in the theological controversies that characterized this period. He eventually taught theology as well as philosophy and medicine at Heidelberg. According to Gunnoe, "Thomas Erastus and His Circle of Anti-Paracelsians," Erastus' attack on Paracelsian philosophy was part of his effort to demonstrate his religious orthodoxy, which had been in question.

than can be either read or understood from the disciples of Paracelsus and too severe for our people to agree with. Meanwhile, his effort to deduce Paracelsian opinions from the principles of Hippocrates is neither inept nor bad in certain respects.[27]

Others followed Erastus' lead and contributed to the antiparacelsian literature, especially in France. Jacques Aubert, for example, published an antiparacelsian tract in Lyons in 1575, which has been called "one of the more damaging Galenic polemics against Paracelsus."[28] The immediate continental reaction to this antiparacelsian onslaught was a defense of iatrochemistry (*Ad Iacobi Auberti … responsio,* also Lyons 1575) by Joseph Duchesne, known as Quercetanus. This and later works by Quercetanus were very widespread and translated into several languages. The *Responsio* itself was reprinted and translated into English by John Hester in 1591 and helped bring the controversy to England.[29] It is within this literature of contention that we first find Severinus and his *Idea medicinæ* mentioned, attacked by Erastus and other antiparacelsians and defended by Quercetanus, Claude Dariot, and other champions of the new chemical medicine.[30]

27 Letter from Erastus to Petrus Monavius, 26 March 1579, edited by Johann Crato von Krafftheim and printed in Laurentius Scholzius, *Consiliorum et epistolarum medicinalium* (Frankfurt, 1671), vol. 3, pp. 236-7: "Quæ tu ad me de Paracelsi scriptis; tanquam ad eum qui multum studii atque temporis in iis collocat, scribere videris. … Severini Dani ingenium magnum judico, & Ideam ejus ad Paracelsi scripta, plus quam ullius alterius conferre arbitror. Cæterum servit etiam ille auctoritate, & dum libertatem philosophicam præsentat, ipsas quoque Theophrasti sordes extollit. Usque adeo difficile est modum tenere. Doctior vero ille est, quam ut a Paracelsi discipulis vel legi vel intelligi possit: severior, quam ut nostri illum admittant, studium interim Theophrasteæ opinionis ex principiis Hippocrateis deducendæ nec ineptum, neque malum in quibusdam." This letter was mistakenly attributed to Theodor Zwinger by Lindroth, *Paracelsismen i Sverige,* p. 66.
28 Jacques Aubert, *Iacobi Aubertus Vindonis de metallorum ortu et causis contra chemistas breuis et dilucida explicatio* (Lyons: I. Berion, 1575). See Paul H. Kocher, "Paracelsian Medicine in England: The First Thirty Years (ca. 1570-1600)," *Journal of the History of Medicine* 2 (1947), p. 473.
29 John Hester, *A Breefe Aunswere of Iosephus Quercetanus to the Exposition of Iacobus Aubertus Vindonis concerning the Original and Causes of Metalles.* This is a translation of Quercetanus, *Ad Iacobo Auberti … responsio* (Lyons, 1575). See Kocher, "Paracelsian Medicine in England," p. 473.
30 On Dariot, who also mentioned Severinus favorably, see Debus, *The French Paracelsians,* pp. 40-44.

The violent assaults on Paracelsian theory by Erastus and his followers apparently succeeded in discouraging Severinus from any plans he
might have had for further publication – at least nothing further was
published. Severinus, as we recall from the dedicatory epistle introducing
the *Idea medicinæ*, longed for a return to the golden age when people
could publish freely and join hands to face their problems.[31] Such an
age had not yet come.

FRANCE

Joseph (Duchesne) Quercetanus (1544-1609) was one of the first to take
up the challenge of the antiparacelsians. Although French, Quercetanus
received his M.D. at Basel in 1573, just two years after the *Idea medicinæ*
was published there.[32] Spurred into action by Aubert's tract, Quercetanus
began his career in 1575 as an apologist for the use of chemical drugs
by publishing *Ad Iacobi Auberti ... responsio*, which he followed with
Sclopetarius (1576). Quercetanus returned to France in 1593 as physician
in ordinary to Henry IV, who patronized Protestant physicians and
protected them from the hostile environment of late sixteenth-century
Paris. There he continued to publish, including his *Ad veritatem Hermeticæ medicinæ responsio* (1604), the principal doctrines of which were
inspired by Severinus' work.[33] The *Ad veritatem* precipitated a conflict
between the extramural physicians, many of whom were patronized by
the aristocracy, and the Parisian medical faculty, which resulted in a
legal and polemical struggle between the local antiparacelsians and a

31 Severinus to Zwinger, 23 February 1583 (Fr. Gr. II 28² #338): "Fateor me naturæ quadam
    propensione, ad Socraticam disserendi formulam inclinarj, sæpe contemplationum oc-
    culto fluxu ad Yronias delapsum, sed quæ a Sarcasmo alienæ viderj possint benignis
    interpretibus. Feruore ætatis abreptus, liberius in seriis interdum disputationibus genio
    indulsi. Quanta vero acerbitate et quam illiberalj disputationum methodo, excepti sint a
    Critio quibusdam labores mej, norunt plurimj. Proinde silentium mihi indixj, abhorret
    animus a rixis et contumeliis."
32 On Quercetanus, see Allen G. Debus, "Joseph Duchesne," *DSB*, vol. 4, pp. 208-210;
    Idem, *The French Paracelsians*, pp. 31-35 et passim.
33 Lindroth, *Paracelsismen i Sverige*, p. 22: "Quercetanus' behandling av de naturliga tingen
    är byggd på danskens platoniserande paracelsism; de okroppsliga elementen, stjärnorna
    och de kemiska principerna lämna sitt andliga stadium och förvandlas i sinnevärldens
    kroppar."

coalition of Paracelsians, including Israel Harvet, Guillaume Baycinet, and Theodore Turquet de Mayerne.[34]

In the opinion of Andreas Libavius, who took up the defense of chemistry against both Parisian parties, Quercetanus derived part of his Paracelsian doctrine from Severinus:

> In Quercetanus' books I indeed find more from Severinus' *Idea* than from the teaching of Riolan, and indeed [it is] largely excellent; largely Hippocratic. And he is perhaps not so peculiar in deeds as in words and comparatively more an iatrochemist or Hermetist than an addict to the school of Paracelsus.[35]

Quercetanus did not cite Severinus, so we cannot be certain that the *Idea medicinæ* was one of his sources, but in many places the ideas he expounded and the words that he used to express them seem very much like those of Severinus. For example, in *Liber de priscorum philosophorum veræ medicinæ materia* (1603) he wrote that it is the physician's function (office) to eradicate, by using living and powerful remedies, those diseases that come forth from a seed and are rooted in the human body. By living (vital) remedies he means those in which vital spirit is present. Just as the corporeal can be made spiritual with the help of the alchemical art, "so, too, the spiritual can be made corporeal, or astral, or as Paracelsus says, the invisible can be made visible, and those things that once lay hidden in Hippocrates' *Orcus*, or Orpheus' night, or Democritus' well, can now be made manifest."[36] Indeed,

---

34 Trevor-Roper, "The Paracelsian Movement," pp. 173-74.

35 Andreas Libavius, *Alchymia* (second edition of *Alchemia*) (Frankfurt, 1606), sig. Aa5r: "In Quercetani codicibus invenio quidem plus de Idea Severini, quam disciplina Riolani, sed non pauca egregia: non pauca Hippocratica, & est ille fortasse non tam re, quam verbis singularis, potiusque Chymiater parabolicus seu Hermeticus, quam Paracelsi scholæ addictus." Hannaway, *The Chemist and the Word*, p. 145, notes that in the first edition (*Alchemia*, 1597), Libavius left Severinus off his list of Paracelsians. We can conjecture that he became more familiar with the *Idea medicinæ* in the intervening years. By the time he wrote the treatises published in 1615 he had become critical of Severinus.

36 Joseph Duchesne (Quercetanus), *Liber de priscorum philosophorum veræ medicinæ materia* (Geneva: Vignon, 1603), fol. iv(verso), vii(recto)-vii(verso): "Enimvero sane, ut artis beneficio corporea spiritualia reddi possunt: sic rursus etiam spiritualia corporea, vel astralia, ut vocat Paracelsus: invisibilia visibilia, & quæ modo in orco Hippocratis, vel nocte Orphei vel puteo Democriti occulta iacebant, nunc manifesta fieri possunt."

because of the similarity between the ideas expressed by Quercetanus and the *Idea medicinæ*, Libavius considered him and the other chemical philosophers to have been chiefly influenced by Severinus, rather than Paracelsus.[37]

After the assassination of Henry IV in 1610, the position of the Parisian, Huguenot Paracelsians became shaky. Quercetanus had died the year before, and under pressure to convert to Catholicism, Turquet de Mayerne emigrated to England, seemingly leaving Paris to the Galenists.[38] But if Paris was free of active Paracelsian theorists, it did not remain so for long. Working in the background, Guy de La Brosse (1586-1641) was laying the foundations for institutional support of medical chemistry outside the university, at the Jardin des Plantes.[39] Although he may not have been a "whole-hearted Paracelsian," he did respect some of the ideas of Paracelsus and Petrus Severinus, even as he criticized Croll, Quercetanus, and others for their lack of personal experience.[40] In 1628 Guy wrote that he had been testing the assertions of Severinus and Paracelsus for twenty five years, so he must be reckoned as active while Quercetanus and Mayerne were still in Paris.[41]

If we look more closely at Guy de La Brosse's medical (biological) philosophy, expressed primarily in his 1628 book *De la nature, vertu, et utilité des plantes*, we can see that Severinian doctrines are amply pres-

---

37 Andreas Libavius, *Pro defensione syntagmatis chymici contra reprehensiones Henningi Scheunemanni Paracelsistæ actio prima*, in *Appendix necessaria Syntagmatis arcanorum chymicorum* (Frankfurt, 1615), p. 54: "Sic Quercetanus, & cæteri, qui principia Chymica amplectuntur, potius sunt Petri Seuerini Dani sectatores quam Paracelsi." [Thus, Quercetanus and the others who embrace the chemical principles are followers of Petrus Severinus the Dane, rather than Paracelsus.] This is reinforced a few pages later (p. 65): "De Seuerino, iterumque Quercetano, qui in principiis Chymicis totus est Seuerinianus, quid garris homo vane?" [Why do you vainly chatter on about Severinus, and again about Quercetanus, who is wholly Severinian in [his] chemical principles?]

38 Trevor-Roper, "The Paracelsian Movement," p. 176.

39 Rio Howard, *Guy de La Brosse: The Founder of the Jardin des Plantes in Paris* (Ann Arbor, Michigan: University Microfilms International, 1981), p. 129.

40 Henry Guerlac, "Guy de La Brosse and the French Paracelsians," in *Science, Medicine, and Society in the Renaissance*, ed. Allen G. Debus (New York: Science History Publications, 1972), p. 185-6. La Brosse felt that the Paracelsians, except Severinus, accepted Paracelsus' ideas without putting them to the test.

41 Ibid., p. 186.

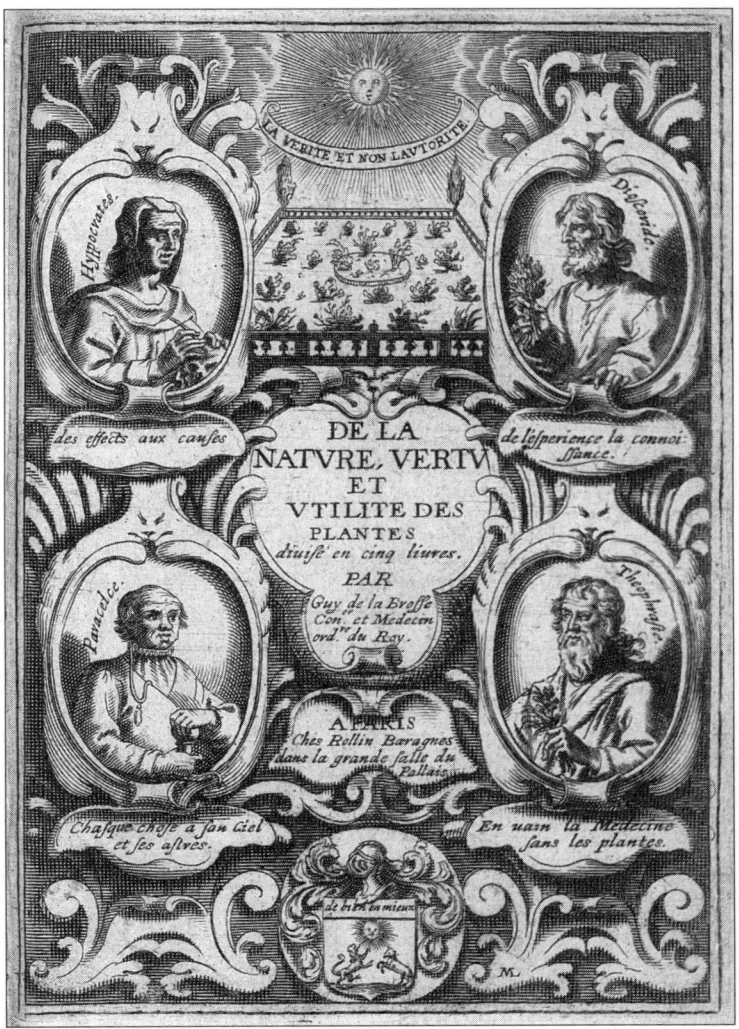

This title page from Guy de La Brosse's De la nature, vertu et utilite des plantes *illustrates the author's commitment to an eclectic medicine that draws on Paracelsian chemical theory and practice as well as the traditional pharmaceutical medicine of Hippocrates, Dioscorides, and Theophrastus. The notable absence of Galen's image suggests that La Brosse, like Severinus, whom he admired, rejected the stranglehold that Galen's teachings had on university medicine. Galenists dominated the faculty of medicine at the University of Paris, but Guy de La Brosse nurtured chemical medicine in his position as royal physician and intendant at the Jardin des Plantes, where William Davidson taught chemistry and began work on his commentaries on Severinus'Idea medicinæ philosophicæ. Courtesy of The Danish National Library of Science and Medicine.*

ent.[42] For this reason, and because the Jardin des Plantes was to become a major center for the teaching of chemistry in France, we must pause to consider La Brosse's debt to Severinus.

Guy de La Brosse, despite his criticism of some Paracelsians, accepted the basic principles of Paracelsian cosmology concerning the generation of bodies from the principles and elemental matrices; the use of fire to probe the anatomy of the world; the seminal causes, predestinations, and transplantations of diseases; and so on. Paracelsian theory, he thought, was in better accord with religion than were the precepts of other philosophical schools, including those of the Aristotelians.[43]

The similarity between Guy de La Brosse's ideas on the role of *semina* in causation and the doctrine of Severinus, whom he considered the greatest of all Paracelsians, is evident.[44] In his treatise on the nature of plants, he held that plants grow from seeds contained in the two great elemental matrices, earth and water. The seeds were placed into the world at the initial creation, and come to maturity at predestined times.[45] He considered diseases also to grow from seeds and roots, under the direction of *artisans*. Each entity is dominated by a principal artisan, but other artisans, either already present or invading from outside, can attempt to seize control.[46]

La Brosse's artisans are very much like Paracelsian *archei* and Severinian *semina*. They are invisible entities that were created in the beginning, and if new species of creatures (e.g. new diseases) have seemed to come into existence, it was because hitherto dormant artisans, upon reaching their appointed times, would spring into action.[47] These artisans, like the *semina* and *archei* upon which they were patterned, were amenable to

42 La Brosse was certainly no Galenist: On the frontispiece to his *De la nature, vertu, et utilité des plantes* (Paris, 1628) we find pictures of Hippocrates, Dioscorides, Paracelsus, and Theophrastus, but not Galen or Aristotle. See Guerlac, "Guy de La Brosse," p. 183.
43 Ibid., p. 187, and Howard, *Guy de La Brosse*, pp. 130, 140, and 146. Most of La Brosse's Paracelsian ideas are evident in the 1628 *De la nature des plantes*, but some concepts, such as the idea of disease as an exogenous *ens morborum*, are evident already in his *Traicté de la Peste*, 1623.
44 Howard, *Guy de La Brosse*, p. 169.
45 Ibid., p. 179.
46 Ibid., p. 147.
47 Ibid., pp. 137 and 152.

La Brosse's religious and methodological positions: They were capable of a degree of freedom of action not found in materialistic philosophies, and yet, as predestined *rationes seminales*, they were bound to act out the divine plan. Of course, God's will, as manifest in the operations of the artisans, could not be known with certainty by man. However, the artisans were responsible for the specific virtues of the bodies they dominated, and these virtues could be comprehended in the anatomy of the world, that is, by chemical analysis.[48]

La Brosse's belief in the attainment of knowledge through the anatomy of the world forms a bridge between Severinus' Paracelsianism and seventeenth-century attitudes toward experimentation that have traditionally been associated with Francis Bacon. Although Bacon is still commonly regarded as one of the founders of the modern scientific method and as an opponent of occult philosophy and therefore Paracelsian medicine, recent studies of his work have begun to strip off some of the historical bias that was created by the early propagandists of the Royal Society and to evaluate "Baconian" ideas in their early seventeenth-century context. Indeed, upon superficial inspection, the tangible spirits of Bacon's speculative philosophy in some sense resemble La Brosse's artisans. This is not too surprising, given that these philosophers were more or less contemporary, drew on similar sources, and had a common aim: a metaphysics that permitted divine activity in matter. The similarity between these two runs deeper, into methodology, too. Guy de La Brosse intended the Jardin des Plantes to be an alternative to the university, a practical institution for teaching and research into the chemical virtues of plants that would also supply Parisian apothecaries with pharmaceuticals.[49] This sort of institution would surely have met with Bacon's approval.

Guy de La Brosse began planning what would become the Jardin des Plantes in the period 1614-1619 and sought support for the idea in 1628, the year he published *De la nature des plantes*.[50] Political and financial backing was slow in coming, and the Jardin did not officially

48 Ibid., pp. 136, 157, and 159.
49 Ibid., pp. vi, vii, and 48.
50 Ibid., p. 44.

open until 1640, the year before La Brosse died.[51] But already La Brosse had acquired an international reputation. In that same year Ole Worm, professor of medicine at the University of Copenhagen, wrote to his young friend, Thomas Bartholin, suggesting that Bartholin meet Guy de La Brosse while he was visiting Paris, referring to him as an excellent botanist and chemist.[52] Although the institution had its ups and downs, the Jardin des Plantes fulfilled Guy's expectation as a center for the teaching of chemistry until the French Revolution.[53]

The first professor of chemistry at the Jardin, and one of the first in all of Europe, was a Scotsman named William Davidson (ca. 1593-1669).[54] Davidson came to France about 1618 and studied chemistry in the laboratory of Bishop Claude Dormy. Eventually, he began to give public lectures and demonstrations in Paris concerning chemical medicines, much as Joseph Beguin had done. Probably in connection with his teaching he wrote a textbook on iatrochemistry called *Philosophia pyrotechnica seu curriculus chymiatricus*, which was first published in Paris 1633-1635, but subsequently went through various editions in Latin and French.[55]

It is evident from the first edition of *Philosophia pyrotechnica* that William Davidson had read and incorporated Severinus' doctrines into his lectures before 1633, when parts three and four of the treatise were printed. These two parts are paginated separately from parts one and two, which bear the date 1635. The title page to part three carries the note "Excerpted from the course of W.D., Doctor of Medicine, for the

51 Guerlac, "Guy de La Brosse," p. 189.
52 Letter from Ole Worm to Thomas Bartholin in Leyden, 15 April 1640, in Worm, *Breve*, vol. 2, p. 189.
53 Guerlac, "Guy de La Brosse," p. 179: "It was here that a whole generation of chemists – Lavoisier chief among them – learned their craft from men such as G.F. Rouelle and P.J. Macquer."
54 There are various spellings of his name, the chief variants being Davidson and Davisson. The earliest chairs in chemistry are reckoned to be those at Marburg (Johann Hartmann, 1609), Jena (Werner Rolfinck, 1639), and Paris (Davidson, 1648). See John Read, "William Davidson of Aberdeen," *Ambix* 9 (1961), p. 76.
55 Ibid., pp. 80-83. William Davidson, *Philosophia pyrotechnica seu curriculus chymiatricus* (Paris: Bessin, 1633-35), was published in parts in Paris from 1635-40, and a second edition came out in 1642. A French translation by Jean Hellot, a Parisian surgeon, *Les elemens de la philosophie de l'art du feu ou chemie*, came out in Paris in 1651 and again in 1657.

use of his students only," indicating that the material presented there was included in his curriculum, as indeed is suggested by the title. Part three is prefaced by a seventeen page "Author's admonition to the curious student" (*Authoris ad curiosam ... studiosam parænesis*), in which Davidson lauded Severinus' *Idea medicinæ* for providing a theoretical basis for reconciling the true meaning of Hippocrates and Galen for use in chemical philosophy. He was so taken with Severinus' doctrine that he resolved at that time to publish a commentary on the *Idea medicinæ*.[56] However, the careers of chemical physicians, particularly foreign ones, were not yet secure in Paris.

In 1644 the antiparacelsian medical faculty succeeded in getting a parliamentary decree enacted that prohibited foreign physicians who did not belong to the medical faculty from practicing in Paris. Through influence at court, Davidson was appointed physician to the king and protected from the decree. With court patronage Davidson was able to obtain and appointment to Guy de La Brosse's former position as *intendant* at the Jardin in 1648 and he began to teach chemistry there.[57] However, in 1651 he was forced to resign his position at the Jardin in the face of political and religious unrest. In that year he dedicated the first edition of the French translation of his iatrochemical text to the King of Poland and was named *"senior archiatrus et chymicus"* to the Polish crown.

When Davidson finally published his commentary on Severinus' *Idea medicinæ* (1660), which was printed with a third edition of the Dane's work, he wrote that he had begun to compose the book while still in Paris. This commentary, which he called a *Prodromus*, or a "preliminary" for a commentary, far exceeded the *Idea medicinæ* in length – 708 pages as compared to the 212 pages of the companion third edition of the *Idea*

---

56 The *Authoris ad cvriosam iuuentutem Philosophiæ & Medicinæ Pyrotechnicæ studiosam Parænesis* is placed at the beginning of part three of the *Philosophia pyrotechnica* and is unpaginated. Davidson's references to Severinus and his determination to publish a commentary are on folia 7r-8r. Although this preface is deficient in several copies of the first edition, it is entire in the copy belonging to the National Library of Medicine. I am grateful to the staff of the History of Medicine Division for providing a photocopy for my use.

57 Ibid., p. 76.

medicinæ.[58] Perhaps Davidson really did mean the 1660 *Prodromus* to be a preliminary study, for in 1663 he issued a second commentary on the *Idea medicinæ*, this one a mere 259 pages long.[59] These commentaries take into consideration not only the main tenets of the *Idea medicinæ*, namely the doctrines of *semina*, transplantations, the nature and division of the elements, the roots of diseases, etc., but also the subsequent criticisms of these by Erastus, Sennert, and Libavius, which are mentioned below. Furthermore, Davidson sought to explain Severinus' doctrines by applying them to specific cases, to *praxis.*[60] These two commentaries will be treated in greater detail in chapter ten.

Clearly the Jardin des Plantes, under Guy de La Brosse and William Davidson, was a center of Paracelsian medical philosophy, and it is likewise evident that this Paracelsianism was in part drawn from the *Idea medicinæ*. Were others affected? Certainly both La Brosse and Davidson had many personal contacts in the intellectual community, who may have shared their zeal for chemical philosophy. The many editions of Davidson's *Philosophia pyrotechnica* attest to its popularity and suggest that his chemical lectures were of great interest. Someone must have been buying the books. We know from John Aubrey's copy of the 1641 edition of *Philosophia pyrotechnica* that Thomas Hobbes "went through a course of chymistrie" with Davidson at Paris, apparently

---

58 Ibid., pp. 78-79. William Davidson, *Commentariorum in sublimis philosophi & incomparibilis viri Petri Severini Dani Ideam Medicinæ Philosophicæ ... Prodromus* (Den Haag: Vlacq, 1660). Davidson's choice of the word *Prodromus* is interesting, inasmuch as it seems to have originated as the name for a wind that blew for eight days prior to the rising of Sirius, the harbinger of the autumnal flooding of the Nile, which was an event of importance in ancient Egypt. Compared to the 1663 commentary, the 1660 *Prodromus* is long winded indeed! The letter dedicating the book to King Casimir of Poland is dated 1653, and shows that Davidson's book was in the works a long time. In another letter published with the book, addressed to Antonius Vallot and dated 15 November 1659, Davidson wrote that this, finally, was the book that Vallot had seen in draft on the Seine some years previously, while Davidson was still "Administrator and Prefect" of the Jardin, therefore between 1648 and 1651.

59 William Davidson, *Commentaria in Idæam Medicinæ Philosophicæ Petri Severini Dani, Medici incomparabilis & Philosophi Sublimis* (Den Haag: Vlacq, 1663). This commentary builds upon the 1660 *Prodromus*.

60 The title page of Davidson's *Prodromus* (1660) tells us that after the main body of commentary he will apply Severinus' theory to fevers: "*Sub finem Authoris doctrina, febrium exemplo, in praxim reducitur.*"

along with William Petty.[61] A 1638 letter written by a Danish medical student and sent to Ole Worm reveals that Davidson attracted students of chemistry from far-off Denmark.[62] Even Isaac Newton owned a copy of Davidson's chemistry text, though it does not appear on the list of books he annotated.[63]

Besides those engaged in practical iatrochemistry and chemical education in connection with the Jardin, there were others in Paris in the 1630s and 1640s who were interested in Paracelsian medicine. C. de Sarcilly published a French translation of several Paracelsian treatises in 1631. In this book he noted that Galenist opposition to the new medicine really began in Paris after the publication of Severinus' *Idea medicinæ*, which he commended as a defense of Paracelsian doctrines.[64] Among Guy de La Brosse's friends in Paris, Severinus' doctrine was known to at least Etienne de Clave and Pierre Gassendi.[65] Although Gassendi ultimately shunned Paracelsian views of matter in favor of a mechanical atomism, it is evident that he knew of Severinus and *semina* theory,

61 Read, "William Davidson," pp. 77-78. Robert G. Frank, *Harvey and the Oxford Physiologists: Scientific Ideas and Social Interactions* (Berkeley: University of California Press, 1980), p. 102, states that Petty and Hobbes took a seven-month course with Davidson in 1645.

62 Letter from Henrik Fuiren to Ole Worm, 21 July 1638, Worm, *Breve*, vol. 2, p. 79.

63 John Harrison, *The Library of Isaac Newton* (Cambridge: Cambridge University Press, 1978), pp. 130, 271-72.

64 Debus, *The French Paracelsians*, p. 74; Paracelsus, *Les XIV Livres des Paragraphes de Ph. Theoph. Paracelse Bombast, Allemand ... Prince des Medecins Hermetiques & Spagyriques*, ed. C. de Sarcilly (Paris: Jean Guillemot, 1631), p. 20: "Quiconque voudra voir la verité de ces choses à face descouuerte, peut lire les liures du tres-docte Petrus Seuerinus Danus, en son idée Medicinale, pour la deffence de la doctrine de nostre Paracelse, apres lequel ie n'attends pas grande gloire de me rendre icy son Aduocat." I am grateful to Susan Alons for providing me a photocopy of the relevant pages of this rare book.

65 Olivier Rene Bloch, *La Philosophie de Gassendi: Nominalisme, Materialisme et Metaphysique*, International Archives of the History of Ideas 38 (Den Haag: Martinus Nijhoff, 1971), pp. 445-6: "Nous avons dit que la notion de *semina rerum*, principes des choses organisées, empruntée vers 1636 par Gassendi aux chymistes, en particulier à de Clave, et sans doute, par son intermédiaire, à Pierre Séverin le Danois." Bloch also calls Severinus "disciple de Paracelse et lui-même un des inspirateurs de de Clave." Ibid., p. 259. De Clave mentioned Severinus in the preface to book two of his *Paradoxes, ou Traittez Philosophiques des Pierres et Pierreries, contre l'opinion vulgaire* (Paris: Pierre Chevalier, 1635), p. 199. However, according to Debus, *The French Paracelsians*, p. 71, De Clave rejected both the Aristotelian elements and Paracelsus' *tria prima* as fundamental principles.

if only to modify it or reject it. Discussing matter and its qualities in *Syntagma philosophicum* he wrote:

> There is no need to anticipate here what will be brought out more fully below in due course, concerning the judgement of Severinus the Dane, admitting three principles and four elements as matrices, besides; and beyond these, he added *semina*, and in those *semina* what he calls mechanical spirits, from which would be the activity and inner economy of bodies.[66]

This view of bodies as consisting of principles, elements, and *semina* that direct their "interior economy" Gassendi called "the common opinion of the chemists ... no other can be better maintained according to sense and experience than it."[67] Such was the fame of Severinus as an exponent of Paracelsian *semina* theory that Gassendi identified this metaphysics with his name, possibly because of the attention given to Severinian doctrine at the Jardin. It is difficult to tell whether the inner principles of motion that Gassendi permitted his atoms to possess were inspired by Severinus' *semina*, but it has been argued that Gassendi used the idea of *semina* to reconcile vitalist and materialist philosophy.[68] Moreover, Gassendi's philosophy may have been the source of the Paracelsian occult qualities that persisted in the atomistic philosophy of Walter Charleton

66 Pierre Gassendi, *Opera omnia*, vol. 1 (Lyons, 1658; Facsimile reprint, Stuttgart-Bad Cannstatt: Friedrich Frommann, 1964), p. 245: "Nihil etiam necesse heic præoccupare, quod suo infra loco fusius deducetur circa opinionem *Seuerini Dani*, tria admittentis Principia, insuperque quatuor Elementa quasi matrices; ac superaddentis illis semina, inque ipsis quos dicit Mechanicos spiritus, a quibus sit actio, oeconomiaque corporum interior." I am indebted to Margaret J. Osler for bringing this passage to my attention and for her analysis of Gassendi's views. I also wish to acknowledge the useful advice provided by Faye Getz for translating this passage.

67 Ibid., p. 245: "Obseruandum proinde heic solum, opinionem illam Chymicorum communem videri eiuscemodi, qua nulla se magis tueri secundum sensum, & experientiam possit." Gassendi noted in his discussion of the relationship between temperament and the five principles (salt, sulphur, mercury, water, earth) that Severinus was foremost among those chemists who retained the four Aristotelian elements but considered them to be mere receptacles for the principles (or *semina*) and empty places. See ibid., vol. 2, p. 554.

68 See Charles Webster, *From Paracelsus to Newton: Magic and the Making of Modern Science* (Cambridge: Cambridge University Press, 1982), p. 69.

under the guise of "motive virtues."[69] If this is true, then there are historical connections between Severinus' *semina* and seventeenth-century atomism.[70]

Marin Mersenne, too, had at least heard of Severinus, since he is named several times by Mersenne's correspondents. In a letter to Mersenne in 1631, Jean Baptiste van Helmont commented that he had previously cited Severinus in connection with the doctrine that the elements are the incorporeal matrices of bodies and that bodies themselves are established by principles, not elements, as is evident from analysis. Otherwise, the principles would not be principles![71] Severinus and the *Idea medicinæ* were also mentioned in letters to Mersenne by Christophe de Villiers and Lazare Mayssonnier.[72]

Finally, it should be pointed out that not all those seventeenth-century Parisian physicians who had heard of Severinus were moving in the direction of the new science. Jean Baptiste Morin (1583-1656) practiced as a physician to various ecclesiastical and noble patrons before giving up medicine for a post as Royal Professor of Mathematics at Paris. By the time he published his *Astrologia Gallica* (1661), he had rejected the explanations that Gassendi and Descartes offered regarding the physics of mixing bodies – one of those critical areas of conflict between Aristotelian, Paracelsian, and mechanical philosophies. Although he favored the Aristotelian view, he mentioned also the opinions of the chemists, including Paracelsus and Severinus, to whom he assigned special credit for promoting the use of chemical remedies. Morin's conception of diseases as arising from seeds and possessing characteristic timings and movements that are correlated with the movements of the stars and planets sounds very much indebted to the *Idea medicinæ*. He

69 John Henry, "Occult Qualities and the Experimental Philosophy: Active Principles in Pre-Newtonian Matter Theory," *History of Science* 24 (1986), p. 340.

70 Although atomism became associated with corpuscularism and mechanical philosophy in the mid-seventeenth century, it was earlier interpreted in a more vitalistic sense by philosophers such as Bruno and Nicholas Hill. Indeed, *semina* theory owed something to Lucretius' *De rerum natura*, which was a valued source of inspiration for Bruno.

71 *Correspondance du P. Marin Mersenne Religieux Minime*, ed. Paul Tannery, vol. 3 (Paris: Presses Universitaires de France, 1946), p. 55.

72 Letters from Christophe de Villiers, 13 May 1634, ibid., vol. 4 (1955), p. 125, and December 1635, ibid., vol. 5 (1959), p. 543); Letter from Lazare Mayssonnier, 31 May 1640, ibid., vol. 9 (1965), pp. 359 and 366.

used this theory to defend the usefulness of drawing up a horoscope at
the onset of a disease.[73]

VAN HELMONT

The early seventeenth-century continental physician and author Jean
Baptiste van Helmont was an ardent proponent of chemical philosophy
and the use of chemical drugs. His work was suppressed, however, and
his ideas were most fruitful not in the low countries or France, but in
revolutionary and Restoration England. There, by mid seventeenth century, "Helmontianism" had supplanted Paracelsianism as iatrochemical
philosophy began to be blended into the other philosophical currents
of the time. For some modern scholars, such as the medical historian
Walter Pagel, Van Helmont's work marks a threshold where alchemy
and Paracelsianism began to take on modern trappings and tend toward
chemistry.[74] His use of experiment to inform hypothesis, his invention
of the word "gas," and his emphasis on the local and chemical nature
of diseases have attracted the attention of scholars looking for the
roots of modern science. However, as was the case with Quercetanus
and La Brosse, much of Van Helmont's world view was anchored in a
Paracelsian past. Indeed, the argument will be advanced here that Van
Helmont's theory of generation and to some extent his view of disease
bear a strong resemblance to Severinus' *semina* theory and pathology.
There is, however, some disagreement about Van Helmont's disease
theory, which should be clarified at the outset.

---

73 Jean Baptiste Morin, *Astrologia Gallica principiis & rationibus propriis stabilita atque in
    xxvi libros distributa* (Hague: Adrian Vlacq, 1661). I have relied on Lynn Thorndike's
    account of this book in *A History of Magic and Experimental Science*, vol. 7, pp. 477, 483,
    488-89.
74 See Pagel, *Paracelsus*, 2d ed., p. 1. Van Helmont's famous tree experiment is a canon-
    ized example of the transition between occult science and experimental, quantitative
    science in the early modern period. However, the experiment has a history going back
    to Nicholas of Cusa's *De staticis experimentiis* and before that to late antiquity. See
    Norma Emerton, "Creation in the Thought of J.B. van Helmont and Robert Fludd,"
    in *Alchemy and Chemistry in the 16th and 17th Centuries*, ed. Piyo Rattansi and Antonio
    Clericuzio, pp. 85-101, International Archives of the History of Ideas 140 (Dordrecht:
    Kluwer, 1994), p. 93.

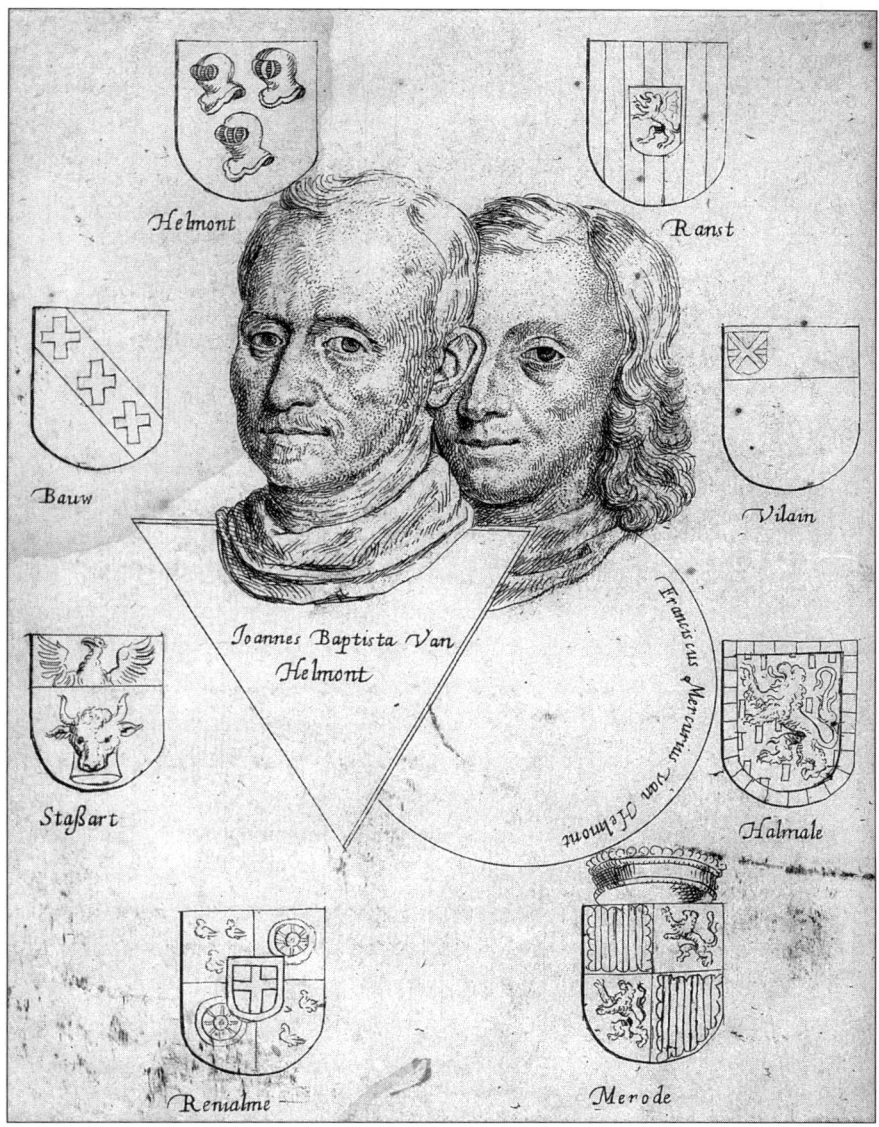

Portrait of J.B. van Helmont and his son Franciscus Mercurius van Helmont, from Ortus medicinæ *(1648). Courtesy of The Danish National Library of Science and Medicine.*

Walter Pagel has drawn attention to the origin of the "modern" definition of disease, which he terms the "ontological view," in Paracelsian doctrine as it was adapted by Van Helmont. The ontological view, whether modern or not, portrays disease as an autonomous being, a parasite that can enter and afflict the human body, rather than as a *qualitative* dysfunction of the normally healthy body. More concisely, the ontological view holds that disease is a "thing," whereas the other view, which perhaps we can call physiological, conceives of disease as a state or process.[75] However, differing definitions of "thing" as well as what is being called a disease have led to some confusion. A related concept is disease aetiology, which is the study of agents or conditions that cause disease, but are not themselves considered to be the disease.[76]

Identifying "disease" with the *cause* of illness was an important conceptual change for the Paracelsians, because it denied the Galenic emphasis on a therapy that was based on what the Paracelsians called "dead qualities." From the Paracelsian point of view, humoral pathologists were treating the effect (disease as an imbalance) rather than rooting out the cause. In order to reform therapy to treat causes rather than symptoms, Paracelsians collapsed the logical distinction between the two: disease was no longer a matter of the Aristotelian-Galenic dichotomy of causes and effects; it was a matter of seeds or roots of disease (disease in potency) and the "fruits" of these (disease in act). Both seeds and fruit were disease in an ontological sense. Thus, Severinus would not have admitted the point of view of his critics, who censured him for not distinguishing between a disease and its cause. His medical philosophy does not assign any importance to this distinction, and I suspect Pagel's lack of clear discrimination between cause and effect when discussing the Paracelsian origins of the "ontological view" arises from the blurred distinction found in the sources. Thus, in the same book, Pagel says

---

75 In particular the ontological view contrasts with the physiological humoralism maintained by the Galenists.

76 Pagel discusses the Paracelsian view of disease in many of his papers and books, including *Paracelsus*, sometimes emphasizing the identification of disease as an external parasite (the ontological view) and at other times stressing the aetiological aspects of Paracelsian medicine.

"disease is a real object and enters our body as such. ... It is a parasite, a kind of animal. ... This is the well known 'ontological' concept of disease"[77] and also that "the exogenous cause of disease is the target of Paracelsus' therapy" and "the disease entity can be defined in chemical terms. ... It is a metabolic disorder."[78] In the first instance disease is a substantial entity, but in the last it is a malfunctioning process.

Not surprisingly, Aristotelian critics of Paracelsus were offended at the Paracelsians' disregard of the distinction between disease and its cause. They sought to reformulate the process by again defining disease as the effect, a dysfunction of normal process, but they often retained the Paracelsian therapeutic emphasis on removing the cause of the disease.[79] This transition, from treating disease as qualitative imbalance, to treating it as cause, to treating the cause in order to expel the disease, happened largely between the time of the publication of the *Idea medicinæ* and the mid seventeenth century and therefore is of some importance to our understanding of Van Helmont and the reception of Severinian doctrine.

Peter Niebyl has challenged Pagel's claims for a Paracelsian origin of Van Helmont's ontological view. He argues that Van Helmont followed Daniel Sennert in criticizing Paracelsus for confusing disease as a thing (*ens morbi*) with the cause of disease (*causa morbi*).[80] This distinction, according to Niebyl, is the result of a rethinking of Paracelsian doctrine by Sennert and therefore "arose out of this Christian-Aristotelian tradition of natural philosophy, a tradition in which Paracelsus became a villain rather than a hero."[81] Niebyl's analysis of the criticism of Paracelsus by Erastus and Sennert has much to commend it, but it leads us astray

---

77 Pagel, *Paracelsus*, p. 325.
78 Ibid., p. 157.
79 Thomas Sydenham, for example, did not hold Paracelsian views on medicine, but advocated bleeding and diaphoretics as ways of ridding the body of "peccant matter," even in cases of plague. See Thomas Sydenham, *The Works of Thomas Sydenham, M.D.*, trans. R. G. Latham, vol. 1 (London: The Sydenham Society, 1848), pp. 97-115, where the author discusses treatment of fevers in London during the years 1665 and 1666.
80 Peter Niebyl, "Sennert, Van Helmont, and Medical Ontology," *Bulletin of the History of Medicine* 45 (1971): 115-37. Sennert's response to Severinus' ideas will be treated in chapter seven.
81 Ibid., p. 116.

when attributing their views to Van Helmont and also when linking Van Helmont too closely to Sennert. Admittedly, Niebyl does not claim to demonstrate that Van Helmont got his ideas on the ontology of disease from Sennert's works. But by juxtaposing the doctrines of the two, and assigning importance to theological aspects of Erastus' attack on Paracelsianism, he associates the two by implication.[82] It will be argued here that even though Van Helmont's "ontology" defines *disease* as a failure of normal function (a physiological process), the aetiological aspects of the theory strongly resemble Severinian doctrine, which is a plausible source for his ideas; that while it is true that Van Helmont abandoned the microcosm-macrocosm analogy by accepting the distinction between *ens morbi* and *causa morbi*, the difference between these two was far from clear in his work, and the theological implications cannot have been great.

The theological argument against the Paracelsian ontological view of disease can be summarized thus: Paracelsus (and Severinus) held that disease had its origin in the Biblical curse resulting from the Fall; that God sowed the seeds of disease into nature when he regretted his creation of man.[83] If, then, disease is conceived as an evil substance rather than a privation, it would be a form of Manichæan heresy to attribute the creation of disease (a positive evil) to God. Niebyl correctly attributes this line of argument to Erastus and Sennert, who, at least in part, again defined disease as a privation of health and avoided such Paracelsian heresy.[84] But how did Van Helmont view disease? First we must look at his theory of generation and then compare it with what he has to say about disease.

---

82 Ibid., p. 115: "The wealth of Sennert's references, compared with the paucity of Van Helmont's, makes it difficult to know just what, if anything, Van Helmont directly owed to Sennert. But at least Sennert's works provide an academic context within which to view Van Helmont's enthusiastic contributions."

83 Pagel, *Paracelsus*, p. 140.

84 Niebyl, "Sennert, Van Helmont, and Medical Ontology," pp. 121-22: "Instead of an ontologically existing evil as implied by Paracelsus, St. Augustine, St. Thomas, and Sennert had given a theological equivalent to the physiological concept of disease, a deviation from the normal or ideal state of being."

Van Helmont and *Semina* theory

Van Helmont's view of generation is strikingly Severinian, both in conception and terminology, and it is quite likely that his early formulation of Paracelsian theory was guided by his reading of the *Idea medicinæ*.[85] Van Helmont believed that the ontological basis of natural things was matter and immanent form; the two together constitute an efficient agent (*archeus*) that is responsible for generation.[86] Moreover, he made it clear that this efficient cause of things was not Aristotelian, by denying the peripatetic analogy of the efficient to the artist who is shaping matter from the outside: "The whole efficient cause in Nature is after another manner, it is inward and essential."[87] This inner union of matter and "seminal efficient" contains all the *information* needed to convey specificity in nature. The similarity to Severinus' inner knowledge or the *mechanica scientia* of the *semina* is manifest:

> Because that these two [matter and efficient] are abundantly sufficient to themselves, and to other things, and do contain the whole composure, order, motion, birth, sealing notions, or tokens of knowing properties:

85 Antonio Clericuzio, "From Van Helmont to Boyle: A Study in the Transmission of Helmontian Chemical and Medical Theories in Seventeenth-Century England," *British Journal for the History of Science* 26 (1993): 303-334, notes on pp. 309-10 that Van Helmont's concept of seminal principles was an elaboration of Severinus' theory, which strengthens the case that I made for similarities between the two author's views in Shackelford, "Paracelsianism in Denmark and Norway," pp. 165-177, which forms the basis for the present analysis. Clericuzio, "From Van Helmont to Boyle," p. 307 specifically identifies Van Helmont's early "Eisagoge in Artem Medicam a Paracelso Restitutam" (composed 1607) as a commentary on Severinus' *Idea medicinæ*. Fuller analysis of this text, which is published in C. Broeckx, "Le Premier Ouvrage de J.-B. van Helmont, Seigneur de Mérode, Royenborch, Oirschot, Pellines, etc., Publié pour La Première Fois," *Annales de L'Académie D'Archéologie de Belgique* 10(1853): 327-392; 11(1854): 119-191, may help clarify Van Helmont's debt to Severinus' theories.

86 J. B. van Helmont, *Oriatrike; or, Physick refined*, trans. J. C. (London: Loyd, 1662), pp. 28-29: "The Form, seeing it is the end of generation, is not merely the act of generation: but of the thing generated, and rather a power that may be attained in generation: but the matter, or subject of generation, as it is in act; so also its act, is an inward worker or Agent, the efficient, or Archeus or chief Workman." *Oriatrike* is a translation of Van Helmont's *Ortus medicinæ. Id est, initia physicæ inaudita. Progressus medicinæ novus, in morborum ultionem, ad vitam longam* (Amsterdam: Elsevier, 1648), and I have used it for convenience.

87 Van Helmont, *Oriatrike*, p. 29.

and lastly, whatsoever is required to the constituting and propogating, or increasing of a thing. For the seminal efficient cause containeth the Types or Patterns of things to be done by itself, the figure, motions, houre, respects, inclinations, fitnesses, equalizings, proportions, alienation, defect, and whatsoever falls in under the succession of dayes, as well as the business of generation, as of government.[88]

Clearly this immanent knowledge encompasses the knowledge of "whatsoever falls in under the succession of days," which Severinus called the predestination of things, "as well as the business of generation," which Severinus termed the mechanical process of generation. For Van Helmont, as for Severinus, the innate ideas or seminal forms that "inform" the *archeus* were divine creations: "For that which in the minde of the Artificer is the Being of Reason: can never obtain the weight of a cause real and natural: Because in the efficient natural cause, its own knowledge of ends and disposition, is infused naturally by God."[89]

Looked at another way, seminal forms are the *ferment* that, along with unformed matter or "water," constitute "seeds":

The Ferment is a formall created Being, which is neither substance nor accident, but a neutrall thing framed from the beginning of the World in the places of its own Monarchie, in the manner of light, fire, ... that it may prepare, stir up, and go before the Seeds.[90]

Van Helmont described this *ferment* and its function in generation, namely insuring the continuity of species, in terms reminiscent of the *Idea medicinæ*:

Therefore Ferments are gifts, and Roots stablished by the Creator the Lord, for the finishing of Ages. ... Therefore Ferments do bring forth

---

88 Ibid.
89 Ibid. It is interesting to note that whereas Severinus had likened the routine, mechanical process of organic development to the administration of holy service, liturgy, Van Helmont described it as the "business" of regulation or "government" (regiminis negotio).
90 Ibid., p. 31.

their own Seeds, not others: that is, every ones according to their own Nature and Property. … For there is in places a certain order divinely placed, a certain Reason and unchangeable Root, of producing some appointed effects, or fruits, nor indeed only of Vegetables, but also of Minerals, and Insects.[91]

Just as Severinus distinguished between *semina* as formal principles and seeds as generative bodies, so too Van Helmont distinguished between the principle, the *ferment* as a component of seeds, and the corporeal ferment, which "is not that which is one of the two original Principles; but the product of the same, and the effect of the individual Seed."[92]

Like its Severinian counterpart, the seminal form lodged in the elemental matrix, Van Helmont's ferment is "laid up in the bosoms of the Elements and suffers no change." The seed differs from the ferment in that it is the specific principle, "the scene of its Tragedy," and it "doth end in an individual conclusion."[93] Thus, the seed is the operational locus of the individual and contains *ferment* in its "storehouse": "I consider the reall beginnings of the efficient cause conceived, as the first Gifts, Roots, Treasures, and begetting Ferments."[94] And like Severinus' *semina*, the Helmontian *ferment* "is a power implanted in places, by the Lord the Creator … for ends ordained to himself in the succession of dayes."[95]

The central agent in generation is the *archeus*, which Van Helmont singles out for elaboration:

This gift hath happened to all things, which is called the *Archeus*, or chief Workman, containing the fruitfulness of generations and Seeds, as it were the internal efficient cause. I say, that Workman hath the likeness of the thing generated, unto the beginning whereof, he composeth the appointments of things to be done."[96]

91 Ibid.
92 Ibid. In the treatise *De lithiasi*, p. 41, in Jean Baptist van Helmont, *Opvscvla medica inaudita* (Amsterdam: Elsevier, 1668; reprint Brussels: Culture et Civilisation, 1966), Van Helmont identified ferments as tools or mediators of the *semina*: "Media autem organa, quibus semina materias disponunt, fermenta voco."
93 Van Helmont, *Oriatrike*, p. 31.
94 Ibid., p. 32.
95 Ibid., p. 31.
96 Ibid., p. 35.

Close attention to the *archeus*, its characteristics and its function, is warranted here because we will want to know its relationship to the disease process, the point of the present discussion.

In the human body, for example, the *archeus* directs the generation of individual, specific organs; he walks through the "retiring places of his seed" and "transforms the matter, according to the perfect act of his own Image." [97] Since corporeal act is logically limited to body, "the *Archeus*, the Workman and Governor of generation, doth cloath himself presently with a bodily cloathing," that is, he assembles bodies, specific organs, for example.[98] The ontological status occupied by the *archeus* is that of a go-between or interface between the corporeal and the incorporeal. It does not seem to be essentially material, but does have material clothing, much like Severinus' *semina*. Pagel clearly recognized the importance of this when he wrote that "the whole of van Helmont's work can be conceived as a search for the 'semina,' i.e. the active principles in beings which are responsible for their specific form and function." [99] Since Van Helmont's account of generation is so much like Severinus', we might expect that his theory of disease is also similar to that in the *Idea medicinæ*.

VAN HELMONT'S DEFINITION OF DISEASE

The crux of Niebyl's claim that Van Helmont's view of disease is significantly different from that of Severinian Paracelsianism is the ontological status that Van Helmont conferred on disease: "Van Helmont appeared to reject the Paracelsian-Manichean notion of an inherently evil "being" as a guest in man (*hospitatum ens Cacedonium*) as derived from the thorns

97 Ibid.
98 Ibid.
99 Pagel, "The Religious and Philosophical Aspects of van Helmont's Science and Medicine," *Supplements to the Bulletin of the History of Medicine* 2 (Baltimore, 1944), p. 16. This view persisted in Pagel's scholarship: e.g. *Joan Baptista van Helmont: Reformer of Science and Medicine* (Cambridge: Cambridge University Press, 1982), p. 24.

and thistles of the Biblical curse."[100] Instead, "Van Helmont believed
that the multiplicity of thorns and thistles on earth due to the curse
was the occasional cause of disease, which he also identified with 'foreign ferments'."[101] Here we again come back to the distinction between
occasional cause of disease (*ferment* divinely sown after the Fall), and
disease as a being, a physiological *effect*. But *what* is the disease? It is
an "altered Archeus," which has been altered by its "perception" of the
exogenous, occasional cause.[102] If we were to stop here with our analysis
we could argue that there is a plain distinction between Van Helmont's
conception of disease as an internal "pathophysiological" process, and
the Paracelsian-Manichæan view of disease as an exogenous, divinely
created *ens*. Closer analysis will, however, reveal that Van Helmont's view
was not that clear cut and that its difference from Severinian pathology
is more apparent than real and hinges more on changing definitions
of vitality (what is alive and what is not) than on any essential change
in ontology. This is perhaps best seen by looking at the relationship
between disease and generation.

The thrust of chapter twelve of Severinus' *Idea medicinæ* is "that diseases are produced from seeds and have seeds and roots in nature, not
separately in certain specific individuals, but they adhere to the roots
of others."[103] These "seeds" are formal (i.e. incorporeal) things, placed
into matter by God when he cursed man, and they are like any other
semina insofar as they have "received knowledge, predestinations, and
characteristics suitable to that knowledge."[104] These "seeds" of disease
are clearly exogenous causes of disease, and they can come to us in the
things we eat, because there they are joined to impurities, "the authors
of diseases." As seminal entities, diseases participate in generation and
transplantation, which is to say that diseases grow from these seeds just

---

100 Niebyl, "Sennert, Van Helmont, and Medical Ontology," p. 128. His claim is based on
     Van Helmont's *Tartar vini historia*.
101 Ibid., p. 129; based on Van Helmont's *Magnum oportet*.
102 Ibid., p. 131.
103 Severinus, *Idea medicinæ*, p. 291: "Morbos ex seminibus produci, seminaque et radices
     in natura habere, non in certis quibusdam individuis seorsim, sed aliorum radicibus
     adhærere."
104 Ibid., p. 291: "Scientias, prædestinationes et signaturas scientiis consentaneas acce-
     pisse."

as any other living thing grows from its seed. In Paracelsian terms, Severinus' diseases are creatures of the *archeus*; they grow from impurities under the direction of the *archeus*, according to the plan (predestination) inherent in the seminal image or idea. We find a strikingly similar account in Van Helmont's *Oriatrike*:

> The matter of Disease is Archeal, and its efficient cause is vital: And that I may speak more clearly, every Disease is of necessity an Ideal efficient act of the vital power, cloathing itself with a Garment of Archeal matter, and attaining a vital and substantial form, according to the difference of the slowness and swiftness of Ideal seeds.[105]

We see from this that Van Helmont viewed disease as a vital, generative process, similar to the archeal creation of organs noted above.

> Disease is a real Being, and is made in a live Creature only: Whence it follows, that although a Disease doth oppose the Life, as the forerunner of Death, yet it is bred from a vital Beginning, and the same in the Life, to wit, from the flesh of Sin.[106]

The difference between death and disease here is that "death lacks images," that is, it is not generative, whereas disease has images and grows; In Paracelsian terms, it fulfills its range of predestinations or *Iliadus* and, as Van Helmont said, "doth end in an individual conclusion."

What can be inferred here is that Van Helmont's ontology of disease is by no means a clean break from Paracelsian views, in which the distinction between cause of disease and being of disease is often not clear. Such a differentiation is certainly not important to healing, for the point of Severinus' Paracelsian therapy is that to remove the disease as a fruit, you must remove the disease as a root or seed, by using strong

---

105 Van Helmont, *Oriatrike*, p. 532. The role of the *archeus* in Van Helmont's theory of disease is briefly discussed in William R. Newman, "The Corpuscular Theory of J. B. Van Helmont and its Medieval Sources," *Vivarium* 31(1993): 161-191, pp. 188-89. In this article Newman reveals Van Helmont's matter theory to be a fusion of Paracelsian vitalism and the materialist corpuscularism of the medieval alchemists, chiefly Geber and his followers.
106 Van Helmont, *Oriatrike*, p. 537.

remedies such as diaphoretics; For Van Helmont, the disease (an enemy) is expelled by washing away the *cause* of the disease, with diaphoretics.[107] For both Severinus and Van Helmont, the ideas or images of diseases were created by God when he regretted the making of man. For both Severinus and Van Helmont these images become anchored in matter (as *semina* or *ferments*) and they alter an otherwise healthy *archeus*, the resulting activity of which becomes evident as disease. The ontology and the morbid process are much the same, and apparent differences arise only in when and where the process is defined as morbid. Therefore, if Severinus' seminal forms or the seeds of disease they constitute are subject to a Manichæan interpretation, then logically so should Van Helmont's images or ferments. In neither case is disease a privation, unless a privation can "grow." Any real difference must be owing to terminology and historical circumstance, not ontology.

Differences between the Severinian and Helmontian conceptions of disease may depend on the range of application of the term disease, which in turn is contingent on the concept of vitality. For Severinus, a true vitalist in the tradition of Renaissance Platonism, all that moves lives. Thus, the Paracelsian notion that diseases of the macrocosm are not essentially different from human diseases is quite acceptable to Severinus and renders the distinction between internal disease and external disease somewhat vague. As Niebyl points out, "the micro-macrocosmic relationship of Paracelsus makes it very difficult, if not impossible, to say whether there is anything at all that is purely internal or purely external."[108] Van Helmont's denial of the macrocosmic-microcosmic correspondence, noted by Pagel as well, would logically force this distinction between internal and external, with consequences for the ontology of disease.[109] This is the line of reasoning Niebyl follows when he places Van Helmont in the same ontological camp as Daniel Sennert.[110] But

---

107 Niebyl, "Sennert, Van Helmont, and Medical Ontology," p. 133.
108 Ibid., p. 137.
109 Pagel, *Van Helmont*, p. 48.
110 Niebyl, "Sennert, Van Helmont, and Medical Ontology," p. 137: "This barrier between the external and internal worlds as found in the vitalism of Virchow, Van Helmont, Sennert, and their predecessors has as a consequence the distinction between the cause and the disease itself."

although it may be generally true that Van Helmont was moving in this direction, it is not exclusively so. For, as has been shown above, Van Helmont considered *ferment* responsible for the orderly change that produced effects (fruits) not just in vegetables, but also in minerals and insects. Logically, diseases, as generative phenomena, should also occur in nonhuman life forms of this sort, throughout the macrocosm.

Even Van Helmont's rejection of the microcosm-macrocosm correspondence is questionable, inasmuch as some seemingly Severinian elements persist. Van Helmont may have rejected the direct action of the heavens on man, but he maintained the Severinian doctrine that the apparent analogy between sublunary and celestial things is due to the inner function of the *archeus*:

> So that sick persons do seem to carry in themselves sensible *Ephemeries*, or daily *Registers* ... Indeed in the bowels, the planetary spirits doe most shine forth, even as also, in the whole influous *Archeus*, the forces of the Firmament do appear.[III]

So, the *astra* do not causally determine the course of terrestrial events, but they mirror a common creation; each creature carries within it its own "Ephemeries" or life cycle, or what Severinus called its its predestination.

The change in conception of disease in the period between Severinus and Van Helmont is subtle. It owes less to a breakdown in microcosmic-macrocosmic thinking (although an important factor) than to the distinction between what is internal and what is external. Niebyl is quite right to emphasize this distinction, but draws the wrong historical conclusions from it, namely that Van Helmont is a Christian-Aristotelian and not a Paracelsian. For "internal" and "external" apply not to the microcosm, but to the organism. That is, there is an internal and external aspect to vegetables, insects, and minerals as well as man, and all of these can be diseased. What is new about Van Helmont's observation that disease is a function of life is the recognition that the disease, which itself is a life form and possessed of "images" (develop-

---

III Van Helmont, *Oriatrike*, p. 36.

mental potential), is acting against the interest of the host organism. In Severinian and Helmontian terms, the exogenous image or life plan (whether it be termed disease or cause of disease) imposes itself on the host's *archeus*; if successful, the supervening seminal form plays out its life cycle on the world stage and leads the host to its individual fulfill- ment and eventual death.

Van Helmont's writings had a profound influence on English chemi- cal medicine, and through the work of Robert Boyle and others, his ideas also affected the development of corpuscularian chemical theory.[112] I have argued that elements of Helmontian doctrine were plausibly influenced by the *Idea medicinæ*. If this is correct, then Helmontian medicine pro- vided a link between Severinus' formulation of Paracelsian ideas and the persistence of inner artificers and directing intelligences in the matter theory of Restoration England. However, Van Helmont's treatises be- came a salient feature of medical dialogue in England only toward the middle of the seventeenth century, before which at least one generation had already come to know of Severinus and his ideas.

112 On the reception of Van Helmont's ideas in England and their crucial role in the formation of Robert Boyle's chemical theory, see Clericuzio, "From Van Helmont to Boyle," and P. M. Rattansi, "The Helmontian-Galenist Controversy in Restoration England," *Ambix* 12 (1964): 1-23.

Chapter Six

THE RECEPTION OF SEVERINUS'
THEORIES IN ENGLAND

T HE DECADE OF the 1570s, of Severinus and Erastus, was the very time when Paracelsianism began to arouse interest in England. William Turner had mentioned Paracelsus already in 1562, but without partisan comment.[1] John Jones, another English physician, railed against Paracelsian practitioners, whom he said were as wise as geese, as reasonable as apes, and so on, in a tract on mineral baths that was published in 1572. Jones had not mentioned Paracelsus in his earlier work (1566), suggesting that Paracelsianism was not known in England, or at least was not controversial, until the very years when Severinus was writing the *Idea medicinæ*.[2] Another Paracelsian critic, George Baker, noted Erastus' attack on Paracelsus already in 1574.[3] By the time Jones published his last work, in 1579, continental antiparacelsianism had definitely come to England, and with it, a curiosity about Paracelsian medicine.[4]

After the initial reactions to Paracelsianism in the 1570s, Paracelsian tracts began to appear in English translations by John Hester, Thomas

---

1 On the early interest in Paracelsus in England, see Kocher, "Paracelsian medicine in England," and Allen G. Debus, *The English Paracelsians* (London: Oldbourne, 1965).
2 John Jones, *The Benefit of the auncient bathes of Buckstones* (London, 1572).
3 George Baker, *The Composition or making of the moste excellent and pretious oil called Oleum Magistrale* (London, 1574).
4 John Jones, *The Arte and Science of Preseruing Bodie and Soule in Healthe, Wisdome, and Catholike Religion* (London, 1579), refers to Erastus and an English antiparacelsian named Kinder. See Kocher, "Paracelsian Medicine in England," pp. 456-57. Debus, *The English Paracelsians*, p. 57, notes that most early English references to Paracelsus cite Erastus as their source, revealing the importance of the antiparacelsian movement in creating interest in Paracelsian texts.

Tymme, and others. These pieces were generally concerned with chemical drugs and offered little comment on Paracelsian doctrine and contained few references to authorities. Nevertheless, occasionally Paracelsian authors were named, and through these the English-language audience could learn the identities of the Paracelsians.

One such book is a collection of translations published by John Hester (1584) under the title *A hundred and fourtene experiments and cures of the famous Phisition Philippus Aureolus Theophrastus Paracelsus*. This book, originally published two years previously in Lyons under the title *Centum quindecim curationes experimentaque*, is a collection of Paracelsian tracts provided with introductions by B. G. a Portu Aquitano (Penotus).[5] The author's familiarity with Severinian pathology is suggested by the title of the preface, which mentions seeds of disease:

> An Apologeticall Preface of Master Barnard G. Londrada a Portu Aquitanus vnto the Booke of experiments of *Paracelsus*, wherein is prooued that sicke bodies stuffed and filled with the seeds of diseases, can hardly be cured without Metalline Medicines.[6]

This "Apologeticall Preface" was directed to the antiparacelsians, and in the conclusion Penotus challenged them to defeat the Paracelsians on the field of theory, where Severinus was their champion:

> That which we haue hytherto spoken is spoken onely vnto those that doe so deadly hate the Chymicall physicke ... Why doe you not out of those authors [Galen, Aristotle, etc.] confute those excelent men which are folowers of *Paracelsus*, amongst whome that great Doctor *Petrus Seuerinus* a Dane is chiefe, who in his *Idea* hath opened the inuincible foundation of *Paracelsian* Physick."[7]

---

5 John Hester, *A hundred and fourtene experiments and cures of the famous Phisition Philippus Aureolus Theophrastus Paracelsus ... collected by I.H.*, no date or place of publication (London, 1584?). John Ferguson, *Bibliotheca Chemica: A Catalogue of the Alchemical, Chemical and Pharmaceutical Books in the Collection of the Late James Young*, vol. 2 (Glasgow: Maclehose, 1906), p. 180, wrote that *A hundred and fourtene experiments* was first published in 1584, subsequently in 1596 and 1652.

6 Penotus, "An Apologeticall Preface," in Hester, *A hundred and fourtene experiments*.

7 Ibid., last page.

The French debate had reached England.

Hester's translation also included a treatise by Quercetanus called the "Spagerick Antidotarie for Gunshot." Here, too, the name Severinus is recommended to the English reading public: "But if authoritie be asked for, I thinke *Gesner, Guinter, Andernack, Seuerine* (to passe ouer a great many other) will be for vs great authoritie with the learned."[8] Thus, in the first Paracelsian tract to be translated for English readers, Severinus was already among those recommended as Paracelsian authors.

The first serious native defense of Paracelsianism to appear in English was *The Difference betweene the Auncient Phisicke ... and the latter Phisicke* (1585), written by Robert Bostocke.[9] Bostocke, too, mentioned Severinus as a source.[10] This was followed by another justification of Paracelsianism, *The Copie of a Letter* (1586) by I.W. Although Severinus is not mentioned by name in that tract, certain of the Paracelsian doctrines defended in it bear a strong resemblance to those of the *Idea medicinæ*, namely the analogy between the diseases of minerals and their "transplantations" in the microcosm as human diseases, that these diseases may come from consuming foodstuffs with morbid "seeds" in them, and that the physician can overcome these diseases.[11] All this

 8 "The Spagericke Antidotarie for Gunshot of Iosephus Quirsitanus," in Hester, *A hundred and fourtene experiments.*

 9 Charles Nicholl, *The Chemical Theatre* (London: Routledge and Kegan Paul, 1980), p. 65. Pagel, "The Prime Matter of Paracelsus," *Ambix* 9 (1961), p. 126, notes that R.B. was identified as Robert Bostocke as far back as 1595. Therefore, on the strength of consensus I shall refer to R.B. as Robert Bostocke. Allen Debus discusses Bostocke in *The English Paracelsians*, pp. 57-65.

10 R.B., *The Difference betweene the auntient Phisicke ... and the latter Phisicke* (London, 1585), ch. 19, sig. I2r: "There bee a great number of learned Philosophers and Phisitions ... which at this daie doe embrace, follow, and practice, the doctrine, methods, and wayes of curyng of this Chimicall Phisicke. As *D. Petrus Seuerinus* in Denmarcke Philosopher, and Phisition to the Kyng of Denmork now raigning."

11 I.W., *The copie of a letter sent by a learned Physician to his friend, wherein are detected the manifold errors used hitherto of the Apothecaries* (London, 1586), unpaginated: "Neither Apoplexia, Epilepsia, ..., or any other disease whatsoever, are the proper death or sicknesses of Microcosmi, but are the sicknesses and death of the fruit of Microcosmi, & that by transplantation they growe in Microcosmus." "Pluritis [is] the death of Antimonie. Prunella the death of Brimstone. [etc]." "They are the death of the fruites of the great world, & not of man, & that they grow not naturally in man but come in by transplantation, & therefore may be separated." "This is the cause that man dieth such sundry deaths, because hee eateth in his bread the death of all other things, which when perfect separation is not made, bringeth foorth fruit according to his kinde."

activity encouraged further translation of Paracelsian texts, especially by John Hester, with the result that England's educated elite, both those trained in Latin and those limited to the vernacular, knew something of Paracelsian philosophy before the end of the century.[12]

Although Bostocke was the first Englishman to mention Severinus or the *Idea medicinæ* in an English text, Thomas Moffet (1553-1604) took up his cause earlier in *De iure et præstantia chymicorum medicamentorum dialogus apologeticus* (1584), a Latin defense of Paracelsus and iatro-chemistry which he dedicated to Severinus. Moffet became interested in Paracelsianism while studying on the continent from 1576-1580. At Basel he wrote his doctoral thesis on pain-killing medicines (*Theses de anodinis medicamentis*, 1578) in which he openly criticized Erastus.[13] As a result the medical faculty delayed his doctorate until the thesis was amended, and with the support of professors Felix Platter and Theodor Zwinger, he was finally promoted.[14]

Although *De iure et præstantia* was published in Frankfurt, in Latin, and had no English edition, Moffet's influence on Paracelsianism in England is not disputed.[15] He was a controversial member of the College of Physicians from 1585 and a leader of a group of radical protestant physicians who were interested in Paracelsianism, including Bostocke and Peter Turner. These physicians received public preferments under Queen Elizabeth. Moffet and Bostocke both, following the lead of Severinus, hailed Hippocrates as a hero of ancient medicine and lauded Paracelsus as his modern expositor, the Hippocrates of the new age.[16]

---

12   Kocher, "Paracelsian Medicine in England," p. 475.

13   Charles Webster, "Alchemical and Paracelsian medicine," chapter 9 in Charles Webster, ed., *Health, Medicine and Mortality in the Sixteenth Century* (Cambridge: Cambridge University Press, 1979), p. 328.

14   Ibid., p. 328, and Trevor-Roper, "The Paracelsian Movement," p. 163.

15   It should be added that the *De iure* was known in Denmark. Kort Aslakssøn used it as a source (see chapter eight, below); the copy surviving at Danmarks Natur og Lægevidenskabelige Bibliotek belonged to the royal chemist and admirer of Paracelsian chemistry, Peter Payngk.

16   Charles Webster, "Alchemical and Paracelsian Medicine," in *Health, Medicine and Mortality in the Sixteenth Century*, ed. Charles Webster, pp. 302-334 (Cambridge: Cambridge University Press, 1979), pp. 329-30. The sources are Robert Bostocke, *The Difference between the Auncient Physicke ... and the latter Physicke*, sig. B1r; and Moffet, *Nosomantica Hippocratea*, sig. A5r-6v.

The implication is that Severinus' doctrines and the *Idea medicinæ* were promoted in England by this circle of Paracelsians from the mid 1580s on, accounting for the recognition given to the *Idea medicinæ* by diverse authors, as will be indicated below.

Moffet actually met Petrus Severinus and made friends with members of the informal circle around Tycho Brahe when he accompanied an English embassy to Copenhagen in 1582. His contact with Severinus and others in Denmark must have encouraged him to take up the defense of chemical medicine in 1584. The *De iure et præstantia* is an apology written as a dialogue and directed against the followers of Erastus. The two interlocutors, Chymista and Philerastus ("lover of Erastus"), represent the contrasting positions on the validity of Paracelsian ideas. Moffet wrote in the dedicatory epistle that contemplating Severinus' work had persuaded him that he will triumph over those who revile the use of chemical medicines. He claimed that his defense would have been issued sooner, had he not expected Severinus to take up the cause with a "golden reply" to the antiparacelsian attack.[17] Moffet understood that Severinus was reluctant to enter the fray for various reasons, perhaps from lost correspondence with the Dane, and he made it his responsibility to defend his beloved iatrochemistry.[18]

The dedicatory epistle to *De iure et præstantia* is dated February 1584. Scarcely three months later Moffet wrote a letter to Severinus, sending with it a copy of the new book.[19] In this letter he repeated his plea that chemistry will not be made safe until the antiparacelsian books are robbed of their authority and credibility.[20] His closing comments hint at the behind-the-scenes operation of a network of correspondents interested in iatrochemistry; Moffet referred to some business that Severinus wanted set before Walsingham, the powerful Elizabethan minister

---

17 Thomas Moffet, *De iure et præstantia chemicorum medicamentorum*, p. 7: 'Hanc autem Apologiam anno superiore accepisses, nisi tuam illam adversus Antiparacelsistam auream responsionem in dies expectassem."

18 Ibid., p. 7: "Officii mei esse duxi Misochymicos sublimes interim arripere."

19 Letter from Moffet to Severinus, 5 May 1584, Rørdam, *KUH*, vol. 4, #229, pp. 320-22: "Librum de Jure et præstantia chymicorum remediorum ad te dedicatum Francofurtum a Wecheli hæredibus imprimendum misi."

20 Ibid., p. 321.

and a patient of Moffet, and finished the letter with a note that Peter Turner will likely write to Severinus.[21]

It seems reasonable to conclude from Moffet's letter that he dedicated his book to Severinus in order to put some public pressure on him to enter into the struggle between the Paracelsians and their detractors, the followers of Erastus. Why else would these comments about Severinus' hesitancy to publish be exhibited in the dedicatory epistle? Remember that in 1584, when *De iure* was in print, Bostocke's defense of Paracelsianism was not yet published, and no one in England, at least, had stood up to the Erastians. Moffet surely hoped that Severinus, Denmark's "golden cock," would continue to crow about Paracelsian medical philosophy.[22]

Moffet's effect on English scholarly thought is difficult to assess. On the one hand, he was a member of the Royal College of Physicians and held public office, but his rapport with the established members of the College was poor. On the other hand, he was a member of the learned circle around Mary Herbert, the Countess of Pembroke, and we can suppose he expressed his Paracelsian views at Wilton House under her patronage.[23] Mary Herbert was the sister of Sir Philip Sidney, himself a patron of letters, and became an influential patron of literature and science in her own right. Writing in the late seventeenth century, John Aubrey reflected on the importance of Mary Herbert and Wilton House for late sixteenth-century English learning:

> In her time, Wilton House was like a College, there were so many learned and ingeniose persons. She was the greatest Patronesse of witt and learning of any Lady in her time. She was a great Chymist, and spent yearly a great deale in that study. She kept for her Laborator in

---

21 Ibid., p. 322: "Quantum tua causa, Nautarum a te commendatorum causam juuerim apud honoratissimum Walsingamum, et meæ litteræ et ipsorum orationes antea tibi, ni fallor, satis ostenderunt ... Salutat te ἀντάδελφος meus Turnerus, atque ipse, ni fallor, scribit." Peter Turner (1542-1614) was about the same age as Severinus. He received his M.D. at Heidelberg in 1571.

22 In the text of *De iure et præstantia* (p. 24), Moffet refers to "aureum Daniæ pullum Seuerinum."

23 Charles Webster, "Essay Review," *Isis* 70 (1979): 588-92, p. 590.

the house Adrian Gilbert ... who was a great Chymist in those dayes
... She also gave an honourable yearly Pension to Dr. Mouffet ... Also
one Boston, a good Chymist ... who did undoe himselfe by studying
the Philosophers-stone.[24]

Perhaps it was through the scholars at Wilton House that Severinus'
Idea medicinæ came to the attention of the literary world of early seventeenth-century England.

References to Severinus crop up in connection with another branch
of the Herbert family, members of which were also aristocratic patrons.
John Donne, of Welsh extraction like the Herberts, was a long-standing
friend of Lady Magdalen Herbert, the mother of George Herbert and
his brother Edward, First Lord Herbert of Cherbury. Donne included
mention of Paracelsus and Severinus in his *Ignatius his Conclave*, which
was translated and published in London in 1611: "Neither doth *Paracelsus*
truly deserue the name of an *Innouator*, whose doctrine, *Seuerinus* and
his other followers do referre to the most ancient times."[25]

Edward Herbert, not known for his love of traditional philosophy,
himself recommended Severinus as a unique source of Paracelsian doctrine: "It will not bee amisse to reade The *Idea Medecinæ Philosophicæ*
written by Severnius Danus there being many things considerable concerning the Paracelsian principles written in that booke which are not
found in former writers."[26] Edward Herbert's attention to Severinus and
Paracelsianism is an exception to the general conclusion that Paracelsian

24 John Aubrey, *Brief Lives*, ed. O.L. Dick, 3rd ed. (London: Secker and Warburg, 1958),
    pp. 138-39. Walter Sweeper left a similar description of Wilton House as "like a little
    Universitie ... [that] had in it that learned Phisitian and skilfull Mathematician M.
    Doctor *Moffet*," in *A briefe Treatise declaring the True Noble-man, and the Base Worldling*
    (1623), quoted in Gary F. Waller, *Mary Sidney, Countess of Pembroke: A Critical Study of
    Her Writings and Literary Milieu* (Salzburg: University of Salzburg, 1979), p. 60.
25 John Donne, *Ignatius his Conclave* (London, 1611), p. 29.
26 Edward Herbert, *The Life of Edward, First Lord Herbert of Cherbury, Written by Himself*,
    ed. J.M. Shuttleworth (London: Oxford University Press, 1976), p. 20. It would be
    reasonable to suppose that Edward Herbert was passing on his personal judgement of
    the *Idea medicinæ*, a copy of which he bequeathed to Jesus College Library, Oxford.
    See C.J. Fordyce and T.M. Knox, "The Library of Jesus College, Oxford; With an
    Appendix on the Books Bequeathed Thereto by Lord Herbert of Cherbury," vol. 5 in
    Oxford Bibliographical Society; Proceedings and Papers (Oxford: Oxford University Press,
    1940), p. 86.

doctrine was of little interest in England, while Paracelsian chemical drugs were. For, a few pages after Edward Herbert recommended the *Idea medicinæ*, he wrote:

> As for the Chymique or Spagerique medicines I cannot commend them to the vse of my Posterity, there being neither Emetique, Cathortique, Diaphoretique, or Diuretique, medicines extant among them which are not much more happily and safely performed by vegitable [medicines].[27]

Edward Herbert's brother, George Herbert, was a friend of Francis Bacon, and it comes as no surprise that Bacon, too, had an interest in Severinus.[28] This deserves special attention.

FRANCIS BACON

Owing to the importance that historians of science have traditionally placed on Francis Bacon as one of the founding philosophers of modern science, it is worth the effort to examine his attitude toward Paracelsian doctrine and to illuminate points of contact, both historical and philosophical, between the cosmology of Severinus and Bacon's view of nature. Bacon is widely remembered today as a champion of the inductive method for scientific research and knowledge production and for his optimistic view that state-funded, collective, and cumulative scientific investigation can be applied to solve social and technical problems and thus improve the human condition. This side of Bacon was emphasized by Thomas Spratt and the ideologues of the early Royal Society, who consciously grounded their view of what natural philosophy should entail and how it should be pursued in a tradition of English experimentalism,

---

27 Herbert, *The Life of Edward*, p. 23.
28 Bacon dedicated some translations of psalms "to his very good friend Mr. George Herbert." See Francis Bacon, *The Works of Francis Bacon*, ed. James Spedding, Robert Ellis, and Douglas Heath, vol. 7 (London, 1872; New York: Garret Press, 1968), p. 275.

in which Bacon was given a prominent place as a native son. For many historians Bacon remained well into the twentieth century a champion of progressive, rational scientific method and a critic of Renaissance magic and Paracelsian philosophy.[29] However, recent historians are aware that Spratt's construction of a legacy of Baconian science affected the subsequent reputation of Bacon and have sought to contextualize him with greater historical care.

Study of Bacon's works over the past half century have revealed him, not surprisingly, not to be a "modern," but rather a theoretician rooted in the rich world of late Renaissance natural philosophy. Bacon is still appreciated as a bold innovator of method, the author of *New Atlantis* and Baconian induction, but these are now viewed in Aristotelian, Platonic, Rosicrucian, mechanical, and even Paracelsian contexts.[30] Baconian induction, for example, under close inspection, looks less like a radical break from Aristotelian method than an elaboration of the epistemology familiar to students of Aristotle's biological works, which were being taught at Padua and other universities of the south. The *New Atlantis* and the organization and methods of Salomon's house, obviously based on the utopian tradition springing from Plato's *Republic*, is now seen in the context of the contemporary Rosicrucian-inspired *Christianopolis* (1619) and *Christianæ societatis imago* (1620), published by Johann Valentin Andreæ and Tommaso Campanella's *City of the Sun* (written ca. 1602-3). After almost four centuries, Bacon's 'great instauration' is not only viewed as one aspect of a revolution in method that engendered modern science, but as an inductionist's version of a reformed society that was promoted in radical Calvinist and Rosicrucian circles, the same circles that embraced Paracelsian philosophical and sometimes even religious

---

29 To take one example, Paulo Rossi's *Francesco Bacone: Dalla magia alla Scienza* (Laterza: Bari, 1957), which influenced a generation of English and American historians of science in its English translation, *Francis Bacon: From Magic to Science*, trans. Sacha Rabinovitch (London: Kegan Paul, 1968).

30 For a summary of current thinking about Bacon's natural philosophy, see Graham Rees, "Bacon" and "Baconianism," in *Encyclopedia of the Scientific Revolution From Copernicus to Newton*, ed. Wilbur Applebaum, (New York: Garland, 2000), pp. 65-71. William A. Sessions, "Recent Studies in Francis Bacon," *English Literary Renaissance* 17(1987): 351-71, surveys the literature on Bacon from 1945 to 1985, noting changes in scholarly emphasis.

ideas.[31] Underneath Francis Bacon's scientific instauration is a physics and metaphysics that is partly Aristotelian, but also drawn from Neoplatonist thought and sufficiently compatible with Paracelsian natural philosophy to be termed a "semi-Paracelsian cosmology" by Graham Rees, and it is here that Bacon's thought touches on Severinus' ideas.[32]

Graham Rees' analysis of Bacon's metaphysics reveals that Bacon "smuggled a version of Paracelsian chemistry into the domain of astronomy, reformulated Paracelsian ideas and brought them to bear on what he saw as the most pressing problems in that field," namely the creation of a unified theory of matter and motion.[33] But if Bacon co-opted elements of Paracelsian philosophy, he saw little to admire in Paracelsus and the Paracelsians, with the notable exception of Severinus:

> Only one of your followers do I grudge you, namely Peter Severinus, a man too good to die in the toils of such folly. You, Paracelsus, adopted son of the family of asses, owe him a heavy debt. He took over your brayings and by the tuneful modulations and pleasant inflexions of his voice made sweet harmony of them, transforming your detestable falsehoods into delectable fables. So I find it in my heart to forgive you, Peter Severinus, if wearying of the teaching of the Sophists, ... you gallantly sought a fresh foundation for our crumbling fortunes. When you came across these doctrines of Paracelsus, recommending themselves by their noisy trumpeting, the cunning of their obscurity, their religious affiliations, and other specious allures, with one impulsive

31 Recent studies of the contacts and friendships of Samuel Hartlib, called the Hartlib circle, have shown this group to be an important conduit for bringing continental reform (and also Van Helmont's ideas) to England; the Hartlibians joined the intellectual authority of Bacon's writings to the continental currents of reform often associated with Rosicrucianism and sectarian religion. See *Samuel Hartlib and Universal Reformation: Studies in Intellectual Communication*, ed. Mark Greengrass, Michael Leslie, and Timothy Raylor, (Cambridge: Cambridge University Press, 1994) and John T. Young, *Faith, Medical Alchemy and Natural Philosophy: Johann Moriaen, Reformed Intelligencer, and the Hartlib Circle* (Aldershot: Ashgate, 1998).

32 I have adopted the term from Graham Rees, "Francis Bacon's Semi-Paracelsian Cosmology," *Ambix* 22 (1975): 81-101. I rely here largely on Rees' interpretations of Bacon's philosophy. D. P. Walker, "Francis Bacon and *Spiritus*," in *Science, Medicine, and Society in the Renaissance; Essays to Honor Walter Pagel*, ed. Allen G. Debus (New York: Science History Publications, 1972), pp. 121-130.

33 Rees, "Francis Bacon's Semi-Paracelsian Cosmology," p. 95.

leap you surrendered yourself to what turned out to be not sources of true knowledge but empty delusions. You would have been well and truly advised if your revolt from ingenious paradoxes had taken you instead to nature's laws, which would have offered you a shorter path to knowledge and a longer lease on life.[34]

The first and last sentences of this passage suggests that Severinus might have lived longer but for his Paracelsianism. While there is no evidence at hand with which to illuminate this comment, Bacon may have known of Severinus' claims for a panacea and surmised that this knowledge failed to protect him from the plague that killed him. On the other hand, the allusion to dying "in the toils of such folly" may reflect the general suspicion that long hours at the alchemical hearth caused an early death.[35]

What was it that exempted Severinus from Bacon's generally dim view of "these charcoal-burners [who] on the foundation of a handful of experiments in distillation presumed to found a philosophy, dominated throughout by their grotesque idols of 'separations' and 'liberations'"?[36] Upon careful examination, certain of Bacon's ideas fit well with what Severinus wrote. As Graham Rees has pointed out, Bacon's organization of the world's matter into a bi-quaternion begs comparison to Severinus' Paracelsian account of the separation of matter at the creation of the world into a terrestrial globe (earth and water) and a celestial globe (fire and air).[37] Beyond this similarity we can see in Bacon's natural philosophy certain concepts that Severinus would have found pleasing. For example, in *Novum Organum* (1620) Bacon referred to *ideas* in the divine mind as corresponding to "the true signatures and marks set

34 Francis Bacon, *The Masculine Birth of Time*, in *The Philosophy of Francis Bacon*, ed. and trans. Benjamin Farrington (Liverpool: Liverpool University Press, 1964), pp. 66-67. Bacon's analysis of what might have attracted Severinus to Paracelsian medicine is quite astute.

35 As, for example, with the death of Anders Krag (see chapter 3).

36 Bacon, *The Masculine Birth of Time*, in Farrington, *The Philosophy of Francis Bacon*, p. 67.

37 Rees, "Francis Bacon's Semi-Paracelsian Cosmology," pp. 83-84, points to *Idea medicinæ*, chapter 8, as an "unusually clear" exposition of this theory. In this account Severinus goes on to say that God implanted "light and the seminal reasons of all things" into these four "empty natures."

upon the works of creation as they are found in nature."[38] Although Bacon rigorously denied much of Neoplatonic philosophy, some traces are still evident in his metaphysics. This is perhaps most clear in his theory of causation.

Bacon explained causation by positing that "spirit" exists in the world in three varieties or modes: imperfect (*inchoata*) spirit, spirit that is attached to matter (*devincta*), and spirit that is totally free of matter (*pura*). Bacon stopped short of equating spirit with seminal forms or reasons, referring rather to spirit as a "pneumatic matter" that is *weight-less*, highly active, and possessed of dimension and location.[39] If we put these characteristics into a Severinian or Patrizian frame, we can see that in the terms of Renaissance Platonism, Bacon's "pneumatic matter" (spirit) is like immaterial body (weightless, but extended). Furthermore, In *De augmentis scientiarum* Bacon said that this spirit springs from the wombs of the elements (*e matricibus elementorum*), a decidedly Paracel-sian and Severinian formulation.[40] So, even if Bacon cannot be classi-fied as a vital philosopher, it is clear that the metaphysical basis of his natural philosophy has roots there, and that his tangible spirits are just one step removed from form.[41] This view is not much different from that of Severinus, where material elements provide the matrices or *loci* for spiritual causation. The difference seems to be one of distinction between form and spirit. *Real* forms are ideas and have no dimensions or *loci* per se; these must be provided by *matrices* or immaterial bodies that can offer, as bodies do, spatial extension and place. Bacon's spirits, though inanimate, are in other respects similar to the Paracelsian *archei*. Bacon even refers to them as the "agents and workmen that produce all the effects in the body."[42] At one point he even hinted that vital spirit – the kind characteristic of living beings – had its origin in inanimate

---

38 Francis Bacon, *Novum Organum*, Book I, Aphorism 23, in *The Works of Francis Bacon*, vol. 4, p. 51.

39 Rees, "Francis Bacon's Semi-Paracelsian Cosmology," p. 85. In the unfinished *De viis morbis*, Bacon described spirit as tenuous, yet corporeal. See Graham Rees, *Francis Bacon's Natural Philosophy: A New Source* (Chalfont St. Giles: British Society for the History of Science, 1984), p. 51.

40 Rees, *Francis Bacon's Natural Philosophy*, p. 42.

41 Bacon's tenuous spirit is clearly corporeal; it can be broken up into very small "particles." See ibid., p. 53.

42 Bacon, *Historia vitæ et mortis*, in *The Works of Francis Bacon*, vol. 5, p. 268.

spirit, which was the kind of spirit responsible for mechanical changes in the inorganic world.[43] Such a continuity between the world of ordinary chemical processes and organic functions can be interpreted as providing the groundwork for either a thoroughgoing vitalist philosophy, in which all processes are organic, or else a reduction to a mechanical, materialist theory, in which even organic functions are at root "mechanical." We can better appreciate the points of tangency between Severinus' vitalism and Bacon's mechanism if we recall from chapter four that the anonymous seventeenth-century translation of the *Idea medicinæ* rendered *"mechanicos"* as "ordinary."[44]

According to Bacon's philosophy, change or motion in the terrestrial world is brought about by the effort that spirits trapped in matter exert to get free.[45] This theory of causation by imprisoned, innate spirits, whether gotten from Severinus or elsewhere, had epistemological implications. Bacon perceived that the problem with previous philosophies was that they stop at the limits of the senses and do not, therefore, penetrate to the roots of nature:

> Hence it is that speculation commonly ceases where sight ceases; insomuch that of things invisible there is little or no observation. Hence all the working of the spirits inclosed in tangible bodies lies hid and unobserved of men. ... And yet, unless these ... be searched out and brought to light, nothing great can be achieved in nature, as far as the production of works is concerned.[46]

In his ideas about scientific method, too, Bacon is not free of traces of Paracelsianism, although references are few. In *The Advancement of Learning*, for example, Bacon acknowledges the divine and mundane sources of knowledge: "The knowledge of man is as the waters, some

---

43 Rees, *Francis Bacon's Natural Philosophy*, p. 43.
44 See chapter four, note 88. I have suggested possible connections and overlap between Severinus' Paracelsian idea of "mechanical" and the "mechanical philosophy" of the second half of the seventeenth century, which also drew on Bacon's ideas about technology, in Shackelford, "Seeds with a Mechanical Purpose."
45 Rees, "Francis Bacon's Semi-Paracelsian Cosmology," p. 85.
46 Bacon, *Novum Organum*, Book I, Aphorism 50, in *The Works of Francis Bacon*, vol. 4, p. 58.

descending from above, and some springing from beneath; the one informed by the light of nature, the other inspired by divine revelation."[47] While the "two book" theory of creation was not limited to the Paracelsians, it was certainly widely adopted by them and compatible with their empirical approach and sense of piety about the practice of natural philosophy.

In the balance, however, it would be a mistake to see Bacon as a confirmed Paracelsian, even though traces of Paracelsian metaphysical ideas are evident in his thought, for he disavowed Paracelsus' central doctrines: the *tria prima*, the cosmogonic interpretation of Genesis, the macrocosm-microcosm correspondence, the role of human imagination in chemical processes, and so on.[48] As Bacon himself says:

> First, then, I must request men not to suppose that after the fashion of ancient Greeks, and of certain moderns, as Telesius, Patricius, Severinus, I wish to found a new sect in philosophy. For this is not what I am about.[49]

Yet, much as Bacon railed against speculative, sectarian philosophy, such "as that of Theophrastus Paracelsus, eloquently reduced into an harmony by the pen of Severinus the Dane," we must not ignore the fact that some of the roots of his own cosmology lie in Paracelsian, and probably Severinian, soil.[50] Indeed, we should not be surprised that Bacon would be attracted to the *Idea medicinæ*, for Severinus at times sounded downright Baconian:

---

47 Bacon, *Advancement of Learning*, Book II, in *The Works of Francis Bacon*, vol. 3, p. 346.

48 Ibid., pp. 370, 381, and elsewhere. Although Bacon did not directly adopt the Paracelsian *tria prima*, he did use salt, sulphur, and mercury to frame a classification of the material components of nature. See Rees, "Francis Bacon's Semi-Paracelsian Cosmology," especially pp. 88-91 and Rees, "Bacon" and "Baconianism," in *Encyclopedia of the Scientific Revolution*. Bacon is careful to keep God's word separate from his works. Hannaway, *The Chemist and the Word*, provides insight into the changing attitude toward language and Scripture in chemistry in this period, but, as recently noted by Newman, "Alchemical Symbolism and Concealment," Hannaway's results must be used judiciously.

49 Bacon, *Novum Organum*, Book I, Aphorism 116, in *The Works of Francis Bacon*, vol. 4, p. 103.

50 Bacon, *Advancement of Learning*, Book II, in *The Works of Francis Bacon*, vol. 3, p. 366.

Go, my sons, sell your fields, your houses, your clothes, and your rings. Burn your books, buy shoes, come to the mountains, investigate the valleys, the wildernesses, the shores of the sea, and the deep hollows of the earth. Observe the distinctions among the animals, the differences of the plants, the orders of the minerals, and the properties of all things and the ways they come into existence. Carefully learn the astronomy and terrestrial philosophy of the peasants, and do not be ashamed. Finally, purchase coals, build furnaces, be vigilant and tend to your preparations without weariness. For thus will you come to an understanding of bodies and their properties, and not otherwise.[51]

Bacon may have had this passage in mind when he wrote "Take Paracelsus and Severinus. When they lift up their voices and summon men to gather together in honour of Experience, then they are the right criers for me." However, he went on to doubt that experience in the service of "baseless hypothesis," by which he must have meant Paracelsian natural philosophy, could produce scientific results.[52] Even so, Bacon and Severinus clearly shared a common distrust of the written word as a final authority over matters of natural philosophy, which should properly be learned in the field. Moreover, the Paracelsian respect for the practical knowledge of the farmer, the metalworker, and the craftsman that Severinus expresses in this passage finds a clear resonance in Bacon's attitudes toward the "maker's knowledge" that such workers possess.[53] Severinus' attitude toward medicine also bore resemblances to Bacon's: Severinus despised Galen for setting medicine on a ruinous, "geometric" basis; Bacon likewise portrayed Galen as selling out experience in favor of theory.[54]

51 Severinus, *Idea medicinæ*, p. 73: "Ite filij, uendite agros, ædes, uestes, annulos, comburite libros, emite calceos, montes accedite, ualles, solitudines, littora maris, terræ profundos sinus inquirite: animalium discrimina, plantarum differentias, mineralium ordines, omnium proprietates, nascendi modos notate: rusticorum Astronomiam & terrestrem Philosophiam diligenter ediscite, nec uos pudeat: tandem carbones emite, fornaces construite, uigilate & coquite sine tædio. Ita enim peruenietis ad corporum proprietatumque cognitionem, alias non."

52 Bacon, *The Masculine Birth of Time*, in Farrington, *The Philosophy of Francis Bacon*, p. 71.

53 See Antonio Pérez-Ramos, *Francis Bacon's Idea of Science and the Maker's Knowledge Tradition* (Oxford: Clarendon, 1988).

54 Bacon, *The Masculine Birth of Time*, in Farrington, *The Philosophy of Francis Bacon*, pp. 64ff.

PHILIATROS

During the years in which Bacon was forming and refining his speculative natural philosophy, another English tract defending Paracelsian medicine appeared in print. The anonymous *Philiatros* (1615) bears witness to the influence of Severinus' ideas about the role of "balsam," here interpreted as nature, in health and disease:

> Over and besides, remember, louing Scholer, that in this worke [medicine], you apply yourselfe to Nature, or (as *Chymistes* speake) to the Balsome of Nature, whom Doctor *Seuerine* (in his *Indæa Medecinæ Philosophicæ*) tearmeth, *The Foundation of all Medecine, and of all Diseases the very sole Medicament.* Which meeting with some obstacle, is to be assisted with the Physitians Medecine, which he conscionably & cunningly is to apply, as an helper of that *Innatum calidum*, as *Hippocrates* doth stile it: for like will repaire to like, and be aydfull to the same end; that is, to sustaine health against the contrary assaultes of Corruption, too neare a Companion with the seed of Nature.[55]

Here the author used the term "seed" in connection with disease; in the next paragraph it is applied to the remedy as well:

> Now it were to be wished ... that we could finde out indeed, some one Catholique Medecine; that is, such a Medecine as in all cases might furnish that Seede or Balsum, with hability against all sorts of Diseases.[56]

Although the author seemed skeptical of finding a universal remedy, his reliance on Severinus as a source of doctrine is clear.

Philiatros also credited Severinus with one of the most striking Paracelsian ideas, namely that new diseases had appeared since ancient times and that, therefore, the methods of treatment embodied in a

---

55 *Philiatros, or The Copie of an Epistle, wherein sundry fitting Considerations are propounded to a young Student of Physicke* (London, 1615), pp. 5v-6r.
56 Ibid., p. 6r.

stagnant scholastic medicine were obsolete. This idea of new diseases and medicines is couched in the characteristically Severinian terminology of "transplantations":

> And if it be true that *Seuerine* sayth, namely, That in our age there ariseth a new troope of Diseases, upon whom the auncient Medecines will not worke, ... then let us woonder at the Lords Largesse, who for varietie of Diseases, hath created varietie of Medecines, and causeth Symples in their transplantation, to answere unto the new-tricks of olde Diseases; as if in the one and the other, there were some new Creation.[57]

Here the doctrine of the *rationes seminales* continues to offer a solution to the problem of apparently creative activity in nature. The diseases (and remedies) may appear new "by putting upon them new Tinctures," or a disease may seem new because it has been transported to a new host population, but the novelty is really just a transplantation of an old essence, which was created in the beginning, to a new situation: "If *Salomon* says, then I dare say, that, *There is no new thing vnder the Sunne*," and the Lord causes old medicines "in their transplantation, to answere unto the new-tricks of olde Diseases."[58]

Another Severinian theme evident in *Philiatros*, though not attributed to him, is the distinction between gross or corporeal anatomy and vital anatomy. The former tells of the parts of the body, the latter of the workings.

> But to slip ouer the Body with his visible parts ... what will you say to the Powers (as the *Greekes* speake) or Faculties (as the *Latines* tearme them) which act and worke upon the Body and his parts? It is one and the same Power (or Spirit) that worketh diuersely upon the parts, accordingly as the parts stand affected towards it, like as one and the selfesame Sunne acteth upon Flesh, Clay, Wax, diuersly.[59]

57 Ibid., p. 6r–6v.
58 Ibid., p. 6v.
59 Ibid., p. 7v.

This distinction between structure and function is central to the chemical philosophy of the Paracelsians. Function is dependent on structure to the extent that it limits the agent working on or in it, but structure itself is "dead" anatomy. The real changes in the world are not readily visible and are the result of the interaction of spirit and matter.

The correspondence of the microcosm and the macrocosm is also propounded in *Philiatros*, here with a comparison of diseases to weeds:

> You shall (to speake Spagirically) finde in this earth of Man, Hemlocks, Henbanes, Nettles, Mandrakes, Poppies, Wolf-banes; and what hurtfull Weede not: For the Parent-earth wee tread on, was (through the Curse) neuer more plagued with Weeds at the first hand noysome, then Mans earthly-body with varietie of noysome Diseases.[60]

Again, the doctrine in this passage is not specifically attributed to Severinus, but there can be no doubt that he was a major source for the Paracelsian ideas behind the text, as is evident from the following comment on the use of chemical medicines:

60 Ibid., p. 8r. Severinus, too, spoke of finding these individuals in the human anatomy: "And one must not search for the very forms and outward characteristics of natural things in the anatomy of the microcosm: the properties, knowledge, abilities predestinations, and the seminal tinctures, the guardians of life and power, suffice. It is pointless to look for a cow, copper, beech, wheat, grape vine, gold, or an emerald in man: but he who looks for the properties and the radical tinctures, the sources of the actions of grapes, wheat, barley, gold, emerald, roses, and violets, will find them. And not only the properties of these, but even in certain [instances] he will observe [the properties] of vitriol, sulphur, niter, mercury, arsenic, antimony, wolfsbane, nettle, arum, opium, mandrake, and hemlock." [*Idea medicinæ*, p. 319: Nec oportet formas ipsas & externas signaturas rerum naturalium, in Microcosmi Anatomia inquirere: sufficiunt proprietates, Scientiæ, Dona, prædestinationes, Tincturæ seminales, uitæ & potestatis custodes. Vanum est, bouem in homine inquirere, cupressum, fagum, triticum, uitem, aurum, smaragdum: proprietates uero & Tincturas radicales, actionum fontes, uuarum, tritici, hordei, auri, smaragdi, rosarum, uiolarum, qui quærit, inueniet. Neque horum solummodo proprietates, sed etiam in quibusdam, uitrioli, sulphuris, nitri, mercurij arsenici, antimonij, nappelli, urticæ, aronis, opij, mandragoræ, cicutæ, deprehendet.] Similar language is evident elsewhere in the *Idea medicinæ*, several places in chapter 12, for example, suggesting that the author of *Philiatros* was quite familiar with Severinus' book.

What then, must every Medecine be fetcht out of the Fornace? No, no more then all Aliament must bee fetcht out of the Oven, or from the spit, or Caldron. And this not onely *Paracelsus* teacheth the formes of Receite, layde downe in sundry of his Treatises, but *Seuerine*, *Quersitane*, and all others of iudgement, do teach it with iudgement.[61]

The general message that *Philiatros* seems to have taken from Severinus is that diseases are not intrinsic to man, but are transplantations, weeds growing in the human garden; the physician must first recognize that diseases are themselves entities and their characteristics must be known before they can effectively be treated.

EDWARD JORDEN AND BALNEOLOGY

Most instances in which Severinus is mentioned or his formulation of Paracelsian theory is used occur in the context of disease theory. Usually it is his concept of *semina morborum* and his account of the generation and transplantation of diseases that warrant repetition or citation. There is one notable exception to this generalization, however, and that is Edward Jorden's explanation of the origin of thermal springs, or baths, and the reason they confer healing virtues on those who use them. Jorden, at least, saw in Severinus' ideas a metaphysics capable of supporting a general chemical philosophy. This is plainly evident in his *Discovrse of Natvrall Bathes, and Minerall Waters*, first published in 1631, but expanded in 1632.[62]

---

61 *Philiatros*, pp. 14r-14v.
62 Edward Jorden, *Discovrse of Natvrall Bathes, and Minerall Waters* (London: Thomas Harper, 1631; reprint, Amsterdam: Theatrum Orbis Terrarum, 1971). According to Allen Debus, who has surveyed various editions of Jorden's book, subsequent editions were based on the 1632 edition, *A Discourse of Naturall Bathes, and Minerall Waters* (London: Thomas Harper, 1632). See Allen G. Debus, "Edward Jorden and the Fermentation of Metals: An Iatrochemical Study of Terrestrial Phenomena," in *Toward a History of Geology*, proceedings of the New Hampshire Inter-Disciplinary Conference on the History of Geology, September 7-12, 1967, ed. Cecil J. Schneer, (Cambridge, MA: MIT Press, 1968), pp. 100-121; and Allen G. Debus, *The Chemical Philosophy: Paracelsian Science and Medicine in the Sixteenth and Seventeenth Centuries* (New York: Science History Publications, 1977), vol. 2, pp. 344-359.

Jorden argued that the peculiar healing virtues of thermal baths arose from the generative properties specific to each spa's water and related to its particular heat. Therefore, the uniqueness of each spring hinges on the particular mixture of mineral salts dissolved in its water. Jorden identified these as "Minerall iuyces concrete: called by the Alchemists, Salts."[63] Each of these salts has its own identity and its own specific virtue, which is inherent in its species and is not the product of external conditions. The specificity of each saline form is evident when one mixes various of these salts together in one solution. Distilled, the solution will yield up its salts distinctly and simultaneously, therefore there is no mixing of forms or the creation of a separate new substantial form of the mixture.

The problem of mixtures was a weakness in Aristotelian metaphysics that the chemical philosophers frequently confronted. Jorden found an explanation for it in Severinus' *semina* theory: Minerals (and their salts) are living beings, as are plants and animals, and like them they occur in species that are distinguished by special characteristics – "euery kinde hath his owne fashion." Citing Scaliger, Jorden wrote that the reason for the differences in mineral species cannot be accounted for by the elements or their qualities (e.g. thickness, stickiness, moisture, scarcity),

> but only from the forme, *anima*, seed, &c. which frames euery species to his owne figure, order, number, quantity, colour, taste, smell, &c. according to the science, as *Seuerinus* termes it, which euery seed hath of his owne forme.[64]

Rather than fostering or causing the growth of minerals, the elements and local conditions limit the natural diversity of mineral seeds, and this can be demonstrated in the laboratory: "by artificiall preparations wee finde these distinctions."[65]

63 Jorden, *A Discourse of Naturall Bathes* (1632), p. 37.
64 Ibid., p. 39.
65 Ibid. Jorden's clear statement here that nature has generative potential, which can be made manifest artificially, along with its implication that nature may be only a partial expression of the divine powers sowed in it, ought to be of interest to those studying the appearance of new attitudes toward nature and mankind's power over nature in the scientific revolution.

Like Severinus, Jorden found a basis for the Paracelsian mineral-seed idea in *Genesis*. Moses explained that plants were not created in their mature forms, but implanted "in their Seminaries" in nature, and did not come forth until watered and nourished.[66] Likewise with minerals: "our best Philosophers, both ancient and moderne, doe acknowledge that all minerals are generated." But, Jorden added, minerals do not reproduce in the same way as plants and animals, by means of a material seed, but are perpetuated by a virtue or spirit that is analogous to a seed, "which is not resident in euery indiuiduall." These seeds are rather "in their proper wombes." "This," wrote Jorden, "is the iudgement of *Petrus Seuerinus*, howsoeuer he doth obscure it by his Platonicall grandiloquence."[67]

The metaphysics that follows from this *semina* theory is based on explanations in the *Idea medicinæ*, but elaborated and altered by the inclusion of chemical theories taken from other sources. From Erastus, for example, Jorden took the idea that minerals do not grow internally, as do plants and animals, but are augmented on their surfaces by "new matter concocted by the same vertue & spirit, into the same Species."[68] But true to Severinus' philosophy, these minerals have their generative virtues, their science, within them from the beginning. They do not depend on any direct influence from the planets, but rather on their "internall and domesticall agent, and efficient cause."[69] Jorden took care to defend the immaterial nature of this cause against the Aristotelian view of elements as the material causes for minerals. Aristotle had said that plants were nourished by various mixtures of water and earth, but Jorden refused to consider the elements to be anything other than *matrices*: "if earth and water be mixed for our nourishment, they making but mud, would make vs haue muddy braines. We will grant the Elements to be *matrices rerum naturalium*, the wombes and nurses of naturall things, but we will not grant them to be materiall causes."[70]

66 Ibid., p. 67.
67 Ibid., p. 69.
68 Ibid.
69 Ibid., pp. 70-71.
70 Ibid., pp. 77-78.

Having established the source of mineral waters' properties in the mineral salts, which owe their specificity to their *semina* and not to any material elements, Jorden developed the idea of the growth of minerals to explain the regenerative powers and heat of the baths. Here we see the Severinian metaphysics of generation and transplantation brought forth to explain why certain places produce certain waters and why these have their powers within them by necessity and do not depend on planetary influences. Jorden's goal seems to have been to support the uniqueness of each spa while at the same time denying the material causes for the effectiveness of the waters. But in refusing these material causes, he also needed to ward off the claims of astrological medicine. Severinus' theory was well suited for this. "There is a Seminarie Spirit of all minerals in the bowels of the earth," Jorden wrote, and it works on "conuenient matter," under the influence of "adiuuant causes." The spirit acts as a ferment, and the resulting generative process produces an organic heat, which aids the growth of the mineral. Therefore, the heat of baths is qualitatively different from the heat produced by fire – there are no subterranean fires creating this heat. It is, rather, akin to celestial heat, but it does not come from the celestial stars. It comes from the action of the seminary spirit on matter.[71] This matter is not the elements alone, but rather the elements as *matrices* impregnated with "subterraneall seeds," which by themselves have no independent life, but live in others. Jorden cited Moffet's *De iure et præstantia* as his source, but it is plain from his verbiage that he also used Severinus' *Idea medicinæ*: "From this confluence of seeds arise all the varieties and differences, and alterations which are obserued in the generation or nutrition of naturall things: as in their colours, tasts, numbers, proportions, distempers, &c."[72]

Jorden wrote that transplantations also occur with the expression or development of *semina*, and that these are evident in animals, vegetables, and minerals. Transplantation in animals is not common, but includes monstrous births and hybrids – "the issue which comes from Dogges

---

71 Ibid., pp. 84, 105, and 115.
72 Ibid., p. 86. I can find no specific passage in the *Idea medicinæ* corresponding to this quotation, but the language is similar to what Severinus uses throughout his book.

and Woolues, Horses and Asses, Partriges and Hens, &c."[73] Somewhat more skeptically, Jorden wrote that "some doe thinke that the destruction of sexes is a Transplantation, and that all seeds in themselues are her-maphroditicall, and neither masculine nor feminine," but become more or less masculine or feminine under the influence of "strong or weake impressions from supervenient causes," which produce masculine women and feminine men.[74] Transplantations are more frequent among insects and very frequent among the vegetables, the seeds of which sometimes produce fruits that are not proper to their species. "So likewise Wheat is changed into *Lolium*, Basil into Thyme, Musterwort into Angelica, &c." Similar transplantations occur in minerals: "Salt into Niter, Cop-perasse into Allum, Lead into Tinne, Iron into Copper, Copper into Iron, &c," all which forms the theoretical basis for the Philosophers' Stone.[75] This sounds very much like Severinus, whom Jorden did not cite

73 Ibid., p. 86. These ideas, which I presume have origins in Hippocrates and Paracelsus, are given explicit form in the *Idea medicinæ*. Compare Jorden's phrases with those of Severinus, *Idea medicinæ*: p. 139: "In genere Animalium perfecta quæ sexuum distinctione separata sunt difficulter Transplantationem admittunt: & hoc non omnia: solummodo illa in quibus magna est seminum & Naturæ affinitas, idque non nisi seminibus permix-tis, ut lupi, canes: equi, asinæ: perdices, gallinæ, &c." [In the category of animals, the perfect, which are distinguished by the distinction of their sexes, admit transplantation with difficulty, and not all of them do this; only those in which there is a great affinity between the seeds and nature, and then not unless the seeds have been mixed, such as wolves and dogs, horses and asses, partridges and hens, etc.]

74 Jorden, *A Discourse of Naturall Bathes* (1632), p. 86. Compare with *Idea medicinæ*, p. 143: "Mineralium semina quia plane hermaphroditica sunt ... æquiuocas Generationes obtinuerunt, id est, Transplantationi permixtas." [The seeds of minerals, because they are clearly hermaphroditic ... obtain equivocal generations, that is, ones mixed by transplantation]; pp. 164-65: "De sexuum distinctione ita sentimus. Contineri in una Radice, Principio vitali, Scientia, tam maris quam foeminæ exordia: supervenientibus vero Mixtionibus & Tincturis, separari: foeminamque transplantatum esse masculum, non monstrosa Transplantatione, quamadmodum Aristoteles arbitrabatur, sed naturali & necessari." [About the distinction of the sexes we think thus: that the first beginnings of both male and female are contained in one root, vital principle, and knowledge. But when mixtures and tinctures are supervening, the sexes are separated, and the mascu-line is transplanted to the feminine, not by a monstrous transplantation, as Aristotle believed, but by one that is natural and necessary.]

75 Jorden, *A Discourse of Naturall Bathes* (1632), p. 87. Compare with *Idea medicinæ*, p. 141: "Sic Sysimbrium in Mentam, Rapam in Raphanum, Imperatoriam in Angelicam, Triticum in Lolium, Ocimum in Serpyllum degenerasse & multas huiusmodi Trans-plantationes conspeximus." [Thus we have observed that *sysimbrium* has degenerated into mint, the turnip into the radish, *imperatoria* into angelica, wheat into darnel, basil

→

in this particular chapter of the more common and enlarged 1632 edition of *A Discourse of Naturall Bathes*. However, comparison of these passages with the earlier, 1631 edition, shows that the discussion of transplantation and the development of the sexes was added to the end of an account in which Severinus is explicitly mentioned as a source:

> But as *Seuerinus* affirmes of animall seedes, that they are in themsel-
> ues *Hermaphroditicall*, and neither masculine nor feminine, but as they
> meete with superuenient causes, so it is in these minerall Seedes and
> Species, which in one wombe doe beget diuers sorts of minerals, either
> according to the aptnesse of the matter, or the vigour of the Spirits.[76]

From this there can be little doubt that Jorden took his ideas about semi-nal generation and sexual differentiation from the *Idea medicinæ*.[77]

Jorden gave Severinus' *semina* and interesting twist, however. Rather than likening the seminal activity to the mechanical "science" of the ar-tisan, Jorden endowed it with the powers of an absolute monarch: "This seminary spirit of minerals hath his proper wombes where it resides, and is like a Prince or Emperor, whose prescripts both the Elements and matter must obey." Citing Hippocrates as his source, but in agreement with Severinus' idea that the *semina* are fulfilling their implanted pre-destinations, Jorden attributed fate to the seeds. It is their predestined fate, coming from the "first benediction" (*crescite et multiplicamini*), and *not* any "aduentitious" destiny coming from the planets, that guides development.[78] One is left to wonder how such a theory, which makes

---

→ into thyme, and many transplantations of this kind.]; p. 143: "Ita ex radicibus plumbi transplantatur Adamas, ex radicibus Lunæ saphyrus, ex radicibus Veneris smaragdus, ex radice Martis Berillus, &c. Individuæ uero Transplantationes Metallorum, ubique conspiciuntur in Metallis, Marchasitis, Sulphuribus, Salibus, Thermis." [Thus, steel is transplanted from the roots of lead, sapphire from the roots of silver, emerald from the roots of copper, beryl from the roots of iron, etc. But the individual transplantations of the metals are everywhere seen in metals, marchasites, sulphurs, salts, and mineral waters.]

76 Jorden, *Discovrse of Naturall Bathes* (1631), p. 59.

77 Debus, *The Chemical Philosophy*, vol. 2, pp. 344-359, places Jorden's balneology in the context of Helmontian philosophy. However, as I have shown here by examination of the first edition of Jorden's book, Jorden clearly received many of his ideas about *semina* directly from the *Idea medicinæ*, rather than through Van Helmont's interpretation.

78 Jorden, *A Discourse of Naturall Bathes* (1632), pp. 87-88.

an analogy between monarchial decrees and the unfolding of divine plans, was read in England in the 1630s.[79]

Jorden's use of Severinus' *semina* metaphysics as a foundation for a theory of mineral springs left its imprint on seventeenth-century English balneology. William Simpson, who wrote on the chemistry of baths a generation later, retained some of Jorden's ideas, but without reference to Severinus. In his *Hydrologia Chymica* he defended chemical philosophy, praised Paracelsus and Van Helmont, and, like Jorden, held the actions of mineral salts to be responsible for the heat of hot springs, but his explanations are not identifiable as Severinian, and are instead framed in Helmontian terms.[80] His *Zymologia Physica*, published six years later, carries echos of Jorden's work and Severinus' formulations in the "mechanical and efficient principles" that explain the fermentation of mineral juices, but these are now specified as *acidum* and *sulphur.* It is the "implanted principles of Acid and Sulphur" which, when suddenly excited, heat the subterranean waters.[81] When touching on similar ideas two years later, in his *Philosophical Dialogues*, the seminal spirits had become even more mechanical, and mechanical was defined in material terms.[82] By this point Simpson diverged fully from Jorden, who had used Severinus' theory to argue against a material cause for the heating of bath waters.

79 Moran, *The Alchemical World of the German Court,* claims that Hermetic philosophy supported the politics and identity of the court of Moritz of Hesse, and in so doing he implies that the patronage of Paracelsian ideas should be considered from the standpoint of political ideology, too.

80 William Simpson, *Hydrologia Chymica* (London, 1669), especially sigs. A4r, A7vff., pp. 267-69.

81 William Simpson, *Zymologia Physica* (London, 1675), pp. 19, 35-36, 66-67, 101-102.

82 William Simpson, *Philosophical Dialogues* (London: T. Hodgkin, 1677), pp. 33-35, 79. However, even though Simpson here speaks of bodies as corpuscular, having motion and collision, and extended, he still considers them to be composed from prime matter (water − "the original matrix of all concrete bodys") under the direction of seminal principles; these are "Minute Portions of the two Principles *Acid* and *Sulphur*, concentred and wound upon a very small bottom, implanted and wrapt up by the parent of Nature in small raiments of matter" and referred to as the "organical Instruments and Mechanical Agents in all those bodys vulgarly call'd Seeds" (p. 34). Clearly, even when he is generally talking the talk of what historians of science have understood as a non-vitalistic mechanical philosophy, a seed of vitalism remains. As an indication that Simpson has melded Severinus' and Helmont's descriptions, Simpson adds "By Ferments here we mean the fore-said Principles (being seminal sparks hidden in matter)."

Severinus and the English Chemists

By the middle of the seventeenth century, English chemical speculations were strongly affected by the medical ideas of Van Helmont and
the Paracelsians, as well as by the older alchemical sources that had
come down from the Middle Ages. It has been shown above that the
English understanding of Paracelsian philosophy owed a great debt to
Severinus' interpretations, espoused in the *Idea medicinæ*, but it is also
true that this text attained a place in the corpus of literature used to
illuminate the obscure writings of the alchemists, and therefore bears
directly, if only slightly, on the development of English chemistry in
the age of Robert Boyle and the Royal Society. We see Severinus mentioned in one such compendium of alchemical thought, Elias Ashmole's
Theatrum Chemicum Britannicum (1652). Among the tracts that Ashmole
reprinted is that English favorite, Norton's *Ordinall of Alchemy*. In the
gloss to Norton's phrase "And for the *Red Stone* is preservative, Most
precious thinge to length my Life," Ashmole referred to chapter twelve
of Severinus' *Idea medicinæ*:

> It is apparent that our *Diseases proceed chiefly from Transplantation* ... for,
> by what we *Eate* or *Drinke* as *Nourishment*; the corrupt and harmfull,
> nay deathfull qualities ... is removed from them into our *Bodyes*, and
> there grow up and multiply till (having heightened the *Sal, Sulphur,* and
> *Mercury,* into an irreconcileable *Contestation,* through the impurities
> wherewith they are loaded and burthened) they introduce a miserable
> *decay,* which consequently become a *Death.*[83]

From this late reference we can infer that Severinus' most lasting contribution to English medical thought was his clarification and elaboration of the idea that many diseases are transplantations of exogenous,
autonomous disease agents, and not merely an imbalance of the body's
humors. Furthermore, that Ashmole was reading the medieval alchemists through a Paracelsian filter indicates the difficulty of attempting

---

83 Elias Ashmole, *Theatrum Chemicum Britannicum* (1652; New York: Johnson Reprint,
1967), pp. 88 and 448. The reference to the *Idea medicinæ* is in the margin adjacent to
the text here quoted.

to sort out the many streams of chemical thought that flowed together into the chemistry of the scientific revolution.

Several library lists surviving from the seventeenth century include the *Idea medicinæ* and indicate that the book was available to a wider circle of educated Englishmen than can be documented from citations. The English alchemist Robert Child, for example, owned a copy of the *Idea medicinæ*, as is evident from a list of his books that he sent to his friend John Winthrop, Jr., whom he had visited at the Massachusetts Bay Colony.[84] Winthrop also owned the *Idea medicinæ*, which may have been the same copy, since Child is known to have provided books to his friend. This book was thought to have belonged to John Dee and to be inscribed with his marginalia, which will be evaluated below in chapter nine.[85] Not surprisingly, John Webster also owned a copy of Severinus' book, although in the somewhat corrupt Erfurt edition. Webster was a strong proponent of including Paracelsian chemistry in the university curriculum, as he made clear in his running debate with Seth Ward and others.[86] In *The Displaying of Supposed Witchcraft* (1677), he mentioned Severinus along with several other "most strong and invincible Champions," who have defended Paracelsus against "the malevolent Pen of *Erastus*" and others who have laid "horrid and abominable false scandals" on Paracelsus.[87] However, the only reference to Severinus in Webster's *Metallographia* (1671) occurs in a seven page quotation from Jorden's treatise on baths, discussed above.[88] In this book Webster drew heavily on Jorden's theory of the generation of metals, which was strongly influ-

84 William Jerome Wilson, "Robert Child's Chemical Book List of 1641," *Journal of Chemical Education* 20 (1943): 123-29. "Severini *Idea*" is entry 63, p. 127.

85 Ronald Stearne Wilkinson, "The Alchemical Library of John Winthrop, Jr. (1606-1676) and His Descendants in Colonial America," *Ambix* 11 (1963): 33-51; and 13 (1965): 139-186. Entry no. 251 for Severinus is on p. 182.

86 Peter Elmer, *The Library of Dr John Webster: The Making of a Seventeenth-Century Radical*, Supplement no. 6 to *Medical History* (London: Wellcome Institute for the History of Medicine, 1986). Entry no. 608, p. 94 indicates the 1616 (Erfurt) edition. On the debate between John Webster and Seth Ward, see Allen G. Debus, *Science and Education in the Seventeenth Century. The Webster Ward Debate* (London: Macdonald; New York: American Elsevier, 1970).

87 John Webster, *The Displaying of Supposed Witchcraft* (London: J.M., 1677), p. 9.

88 John Webster, *Metallographia: Or, An History of Metals* (London: A.C., 1671), pp. 61-68.

ence by Severinus' *semina* doctrine. This evidence suggests that Webster's knowledge of the *Idea medicinæ* was indirect and not profound.

Walter Charleton, who was responsible for introducing Gassendi's atomism to the English reader, also mentioned Severinus' theories in the context of the chemical virtues of mineral baths.[89] In his Latin book on stones in the human body, *Spiritus Gorgonicus* (1650), Charleton first referred to Severinus in connection with explanations for the formation of stones from solutions, noting that this can be accounted for by heat and cold or by some stone-forming seminal power, as Van Helmont would have it. He said that some such explanation must exist for the concretion of minerals from liquids, but thought that it was madness to hope to determine whether such a concretion is caused by the qualities or, as Severinus said, by the action of a seminal form constructing a corporeal shelter for itself.[90]

Although he was quite enthusiastic about Helmontianism before mid century, Charleton came to reject such theories as phantasms and idle speculations of the Paracelsians, which are sometimes based on fantastic suppositions. Already in his *Spiritus Gorgonicus* he referred to the "wholly ridiculous hypothesis" that terrestrial virtues come from celestial powers and that the stars above have engendered stars below as "Severinus' dream" (*Severini insomnium*). This even warranted a marginal rubric to draw the reader's attention to the passage: "Severinus' nonsense about the stars, or Olympic craftsmen, bringing forth

---

89 Walter Charleton helped introduce Gassendi's molecular hypothesis to the English reader in his *Physiologia Epicuro-Gassendo-Charletoniana* (London: Thomas Newcomb, 1654). Charleton's translation of Van Helmont's work, *Ternary of Paradoxes, Of the Magnetick Cure of Wounds, Nativity of Tartar in Wine, Image of God in Man* (London: James Flesher, 1650) was also an important source to the vernacular public. There he mentions Severinus as a source in the preface (sig. D4r) and in his supplement to Van Helmont's text (p. 101). Charleton's early interest in chemical philosophy is discussed in Nina Rattner Gelbart, "The Intellectual Development of Walter Charleton," *Ambix* 18 (1971): 149-68.

90 Walter Charleton, *Spiritus Gorgonicus* (Leiden: Elsevir, 1650), p. 33: "Si quis vero harum concretionum potius quam materiæ terrestreitatem, succo caussam efficientem exploraturus, calorem vel frigus, lapiscente, seu, ut loquitur *Severinus*, forma domicilium sibi fabricante, prægnantem amplectatur, ad Anticyras digne est ablegandus." [But if anyone who is to explore the efficient cause of these concretions embraces heat or cold, rather than embracing the matter's earthiness, [which is] full of a petrifying juice, or, as Severinus says, a form making itself a dwelling, he should be sent off to Anticyra.]

similar stars in the lower world."[91] Charleton's attitude here is skeptical
of Severinus' ideas, even scornful perhaps. However, it is clear that he
had read the *Idea medicinæ* and at least found worth repeating Severinus'
idea that stones generated in the human body arise from foreign seeds
or rudiments of diseases that are lodged in the human anatomy. This
serves as at least one example that the Dane's ideas were being read and
taken seriously in England in the transition from vitalism to mechanism
as the dominant philosophical framework for understanding nature.[92]
Furthermore, it is now apparent that this transition was anything but
clean, inasmuch as Severinus' "mechanical spirits" were still protean in
this period when seminal virtues were being attributed to corpuscles,
giving rise to a vitalistic corpuscularism, in which the inner efficient
of Paracelsian matter theory was assigned directly as an instrument of
God's immediate will (voluntarism).[93] In his 1654 *Physiologia* Charleton
still spoke of "specificall seminaries" that are contained within the basic
moleculæ of his version of Gassendi's mechanical philosophy, by which
time he had supposedly turned his back on Paracelsian and Helmontian
theory and adopted the new mechanical paradigm.[94]

91 Ibid., p. 45: "Diliramentum Severini, de astris, seu fabris Olympicis similia astra in
   mundo inferiore parientibus."
92 Charleton, *Spiritus Gorgonicus*, p. 78, cites chapter twelve of the *Idea medicinæ*.
93 See Shackelford, "Seeds with a Mechanical Purpose." Newman, "The Corpuscular
   Theory of J. B. Van Helmont," uses the term "vitalistic corpuscularism" to describe
   Van Helmont's synthesis of Paracelsian *semina* theory and the *minima naturalia* theory
   of medieval Aristotelian alchemy, and the term seems apt for Robert Boyle's matter
   theory as well. On the importance of voluntarism in the natural philosophy of Gassendi,
   Boyle and their contemporaries, see Margaret Osler, "The Intellectual Sources of Robert
   Boyle's Philosophy of Nature: Gassendi's Voluntarism, and Boyle's Physico-Theo-
   logical Project," in *Philosophy, Science, and Religion in England 1640-1700*, ed. Richard
   Kroll, Richard Ashcraft, and Perez Zagorin (Cambridge: Cambridge University Press,
   1992), pp. 178-98; and "Providence and Divine Will in Gassendi's Views on Scientific
   Knowledge," *Journal of the History of Ideas* 44(1983): 549-560.
94 Antonio Clericuzio, "A Redefinition of Boyle's Chemistry and Corpuscular Philcsophy,"
   Annals of Science 47 (1990): 561-589, p. 580. Gelbart, "The Intellectual Development of
   Walter Charleton," pp. 151-54, claims that Charleton's disenchantment with Paracelsian
   philosophy occurred sometime between the *Spiritus Gorgonicus* (1650) and the *Physiologia* (1654), probably between the writing of the *Spiritus Gorgonicus* and the *Ternary
   of Paradoxes*, also published in 1650, but the example above (n. 91) shows that he was
   hostile to some Paracelsian ideas already in the *Spiritus Gorgonicus*. The transition from
   vitalism to clockwork mechanism cannot have been abrupt or decisive in many cases.

ROBERT BOYLE

Given Charleton's prominence among mid-century English natural philosophers, it is perhaps not surprising that Robert Boyle, arguably the single most influential figure in setting chemistry on the road to becoming a respectable discipline in England, had heard of Severinus. He went so far as to refer to Severinus as one of the "innovators" of natural philosophy in his *The Excellency of Theology Compared with Natural Philosophy* (1674), where Boyle contrasted the fame of theologians with the relative obscurity of natural philosophers:

> And accordingly we see, that the writings of *Socinus Calvin, Bellarmine, Padre Paulo, Arminius,* & cet. are more famous, and more studied, than those of *Telesius, Campanella, Severinus Danus, Magnenus,* and diverse other innovators in natural philosophy. And *Erastus,* though a very learned physician, is much less famous for all his elaborate disputations against *Paracelsus,* than for the little tract against particular forms of church government.[95]

Clearly Boyle had some familiarity with the *Idea medicinæ* when he ranked Severinus with other leading authors who challenged Aristotelian philosophy. Despite this, he did not cite Severinus in his published medical and chemical treatises, although the plausibility of Severinus' indirect influence on Boyle's ideas will be argued below.[96]

Boyle is one of those transitional figures in the history of ideas, like Charleton, who sit astride several intellectual traditions and are therefore difficult to place into any one of them. He was once seen mainly as the "skeptical chemist," one of the founders of modern science, who

95 Robert Boyle, *The Excellency of Theology Compared with Natural Philosophy*, in *The Works of the Honourable Robert Boyle, in Six Volumes*, ed. Thomas Birch, vol. 4 (London, 1772), p. 63. I wish to thank Rose-Mary Sargent for bringing this passage to my attention.

96 That Boyle did not cite Severinus is by itself little sign that he had not read him. Boyle gave sparse recognition to Daniel Sennert, whose work Bill Newman has shown to have been an important source for his matter theory. See William R. Newman, "The Alchemical Sources of Robert Boyle's Corpuscular Philosophy," *Annals of Science* 53(1996): 567-585.

eschewed metaphysical speculation and enabled chemistry to be pursued as a Baconian science rather than as an occult art. However, a more historically nuanced view of Boyle has emerged from recent research, which suggests that Boyle was in fact more diffident than skeptical; that he was not willing to openly commit himself to metaphysical propositions that could not be demonstrated, but which he nevertheless entertained in private.[97]

In the balance, history has shown Boyle to have publicly rejected sectarian religion and the occult, Paracelsian philosophy with which it was linked. But it is apparent that at an early stage of his development as a chemist he was strongly influenced by the mid-century resurgence of interest in Van Helmont and other Paracelsians, much as Charleton had been.[98] Furthermore, although the mature Boyle ostensibly despised the notion that chemical changes came about by means of spiritual agents acting from within matter and preferred a physical theory based on the mechanical action of material corpuscles, he did not succeed in entirely banishing vitalism from his philosophy. He built his matter theory on the medieval Aristotelian tradition of *minima naturalia* and on the somewhat materialized atomism of Gassendi, which, as we have seen, probably grew out of the Frenchman's efforts to reconcile classical atomism and chemical philosophy within a Christian framework. Boyle took Gassendi's molecular hypothesis and made from it what

97 Rose-Mary Sargent promotes this view of Boyle in *The Diffident Naturalist: Robert Boyle and the Philosophy of Experiment* (Chicago: University of Chicago Press, 1995). Other recent studies that pertain to Boyle and his metaphysics include Barbara Beigun Kaplan, *"Divulging of Useful Truths in Physick": The Medical Agenda of Robert Boyle* (Baltimore: Johns Hopkins University Press, 1993); Clericuzio, "A Redefinition of Boyle's Chemistry"; and Antonio Clericuzio, "Robert Boyle and the English Helmontians," in *Alchemy Revisited*, Proceedings of the international conference on the history of alchemy at the University of Groningen 17-19 April 1989, ed. Z.R.W.M. van Martels (Leiden: Brill, 1990), pp. 192-199.
98 Recent examination of Boyle's treatises and papers and those of his social and intellectual contacts, especially George Starkey, Benjamin Worsley, and others of the Hartlib Circle, are revealing Boyle to have been very interested in astrology and intimately engaged in the alchemical pursuit of the philosopher's stone. On Boyle's transmutational chemistry, see Lawrence M. Principe, *The Aspiring Adept: Robert Boyle and His Alchemical Quest* (Princeton, N J: Princeton University Press, 1998).

he called the "corpuscular hypothesis."[99] Corpuscles, regardless of the metaphysics that might explain their inner being, could be treated as material, mechanical units that were driven by external agents only. In part, the debate over whether Boyle articulated a resolutely mechanical philosophy or did, in fact, retain the vestiges of occult qualities or active principles depends on whether one asks what Boyle thought about the inner nature of these corpuscles.[100] Boyle's point, however, was that at the phenomenological level, chemistry could proceed as a mechanized, experimental philosophy regardless of this inner nature. I think that Boyle would like to have been a mechanical philosopher for various social and intellectual reasons, but could not in good conscience extend mechanism to include the finest workings of nature, which could not be measured or tested in any way, and which seemed to show evidence of self organization.[101]

Despite his opposition to vitalism, Boyle was not able to reconcile fundamental aspects of life with a purely mechanical scheme. His unpublished treatises show that he considered it possible that generation was produced by seminal agents or plastic principles. Indeed, certain elements of his medical philosophy bear a resemblance to Severinus'

---

99 Kaplan, *"Divulging of Useful Truths"*, pp. 27-9, 57-8. Gelbart, "The Intellectual Development of Walter Charleton," p. 156, distinguishes three main streams of corpuscular thought in this period: an animistic monadism, the *minima naturalia* of Aristotelianism, and the strictly mechanical atomism of Epicurus. According to this classification, Severinus' *semina* theory would fall into the first category, while Gassendi's molecular hypothesis would be a mixture of monadism and atomism. Newman, "The Alchemical Sources of Robert Boyle's Corpuscular Philosophy" and "Boyle's Debt to Corpuscular Alchemy," in *Robert Boyle Reconsidered*, ed. Michael Hunter (Cambridge: Cambridge University Press, 1994), pp. 107-117, emphasizes the medieval roots of Boyle's corpuscularism in Geberian alchemy, which is materialist, not vitalist, and therefore not Paracelsian.

100 In this regard any difference between John Henry's opinion that Boyle admitted a divinely inspired "active principle" or "seminal principle" to matter and Antonio Clericuzio's claim that Boyle did not believe in active matter but rather "active corpuscles" or "seminal principles" is subtle indeed. See Henry, "Occult Qualities and the Experimental Philosophy," pp. 345, 368, and Clericuzio, "A Redefinition of Boyle's Chemistry," pp. 561, 583.

101 Gelbart, "The Intellectual Development of Walter Charleton," p. 166, said much the same thing about Charleton, namely that his sensitivity to the complexity of life indicated a craftsmanship that is difficult to account for purely by mechanism.

semina theory, which may have been one of his sources either directly, via Van Helmont's interpretation, or as mediated by Gassendi's molecular hypothesis. This invites examination, because it again demonstrates that the distinctions between mechanical and occult philosophies in the seventeenth century were in important cases quite fuzzy.[102]

Boyle believed that human bodies in a state of health have a certain texture or material constitution, and that disease is an alteration of this texture. This is almost a mechanized form of Galenism, inasmuch as a state of health can be viewed as a textural complexion or temperament. A healthy complexion possesses a kind of inertia, which explains the body's resistance to disease and natural ability to heal. Boyle thought that the body's texture could be altered by the action of material *simulacra* or effluvia given off by external bodies. Moreover, such effluvia could be of animal, vegetable, mineral, or even celestial origin.[103] There were precedents for this kind of thinking. Terrestrial exhalations and miasmas had figured into previous explanations for how environmental changes could occur on a large enough scale to account for epidemic diseases, which are otherwise difficult for Galenic theory to explain. Boyle considered that mines could be sources of such mineral effluvia, a theory that is reminiscent of Paracelsus and is probably reflected in Severinus' use of the term *minera*. Boyle noted that the symptoms of arsenic poisoning, caused by exposure to orpiment, resembled those of plague, which supported the hypothesis that epidemic plague was caused by mineral exhalations or effluvia.[104] If we compare Boyle's effluvia with Severinus' *semina*, we see certain similarities that might account for interest in the Dane's work among the proponents of corpuscular theories.

When Boyle descended from the aloofness of the experimental philosopher to hypothesize about the nature of life, he speculated that vitality resulted from preordained combinations of corpuscles. Spontaneous generation could then be explained by seminal particles that

---

102 Clericuzio, "A Redefinition of Boyle's Chemistry," p. 583, claims that Severinus was one of Boyle's sources. The fuzziness of the distinction between mechanical and occult philosophies, specifically regarding Severinus' idea of "mechanical," is the subject of Shackelford, "Seeds with a Mechanical Purpose."

103 Kaplan, *"Divulging of Useful Truths"*, pp. 72, 107.

104 Ibid., pp. 112-13.

were programmed by God to create a specific texture.[105] As a model of generation, there are apparent similarities between this view and Severinus' conception of generation as the action of *semina* creating corporeal bodies on the basis of their divine science – their predestinations.

Boyle's effluvia, although they are mechanical, can leave an "either friendly or hostile impression" on bodies that admit them. Such hostile impressions can cause disease to develop in the host, depending on the numbers of effluvial particles involved and the length of their contact with the host body.[106] Again, this is similar to Severinus' theory, which specifies that foreign *semina* inflict their hostile impressions on a body and can overcome it if the numbers of impressions, repetition of contact, and debility in the body's innate balsam are sufficient. Moreover, much as Severinus had noted that a disease agent could affect different organs in different ways, with the result that the manifestation of the disease depended on the local anatomies, Boyle thought that a morbific effluvium could affect different parts of the body variously, an idea that has been viewed as a forerunner of the eighteenth-century doctrine of metastasis.[107]

One can see that some aspects of Severinus' pathology could be applied in a context that was otherwise antithetical to the Paracelsian conception of nature, and this overlap of explanations illustrates the difficulty in assessing paradigm shifts in early modern medical thought. Yet, despite these similarities, Boyle's chemical theory was more elaborate, perhaps more sophisticated, and certainly easier to visualize, than was that offered in the *Idea medicinæ*. Where Severinus wrote rather imprecisely about the ability of one seminal tincture to overcome another, by

---

105 Kaplan, *"Divulging of Useful Truths"*, pp. 62 and 67; also Clericuzio, "A Redefinition of Boyle's Chemistry", pp. 585-86. About the initial creation of things Boyle wrote: "And when he made the Protoplasts or first Individuals of each kind of lieving creatures and lodgd the seminall Principles he thought fit in certain portions of matter he did fforesee & Designe that when such an Animall should have made an end of acting its part on the scene of the Universe, these parts ..." ("A Fragment of the Essay De Spontaneo Viventium Ortu," Boyle Papers II, f. 141v). The imagery here is very like Severinus' *Idea medicinæ*.

106 Ibid., pp. 107-108. The quotation is cited by Kaplan from Boyle's *Essay of the ... determinate nature of Effluvia*, in *Works*, vol. 3, p. 678.

107 Kaplan, *"Divulging of Useful Truths"*, pp. 111 and 169, argues that *metastasis* presupposes a corpuscular pathology similar to what Boyle constructed.

inflicting a stronger impression on its weaker adversary, and focused his therapy on introducing drugs that possessed even stronger impressions, which could then overcome the morbific *semina* and their tinctures, Boyle viewed the process in terms that were more physically mechanical and therefore could be more readily visualized. Boyle thought of drugs as specific chemicals, corpuscular aggregations, which could either expel the pathogenic effluvia or chemically (mechanically) dismantle them on location. Some of these drugs were prepared from toxic minerals – a pharmacology associated with the Paracelsians. But by using a mechanical model, Boyle succeeded in making the therapeutic connection between specific chemical drug and specific chemical pathogen – an idea that was central to Severinus' medicine – acceptable in terms that suited late seventeenth-century interpretations of mechanism.[108]

From the evidence presented above it is apparent that Severinus was known by many scholars in seventeenth-century England, and that the *Idea medicinæ* was therefore quite likely an important source of Paracelsian theory for English physicians and philosophers alike, especially before chemical philosophers and physicians began to be styled as Helmontians, rather than Paracelsians. Even so, Severinus was still being read by a generation of natural philosophers like Boyle, who cut their teeth on Van Helmont before moving on to less vitalistic explanations for nature's phenomena that were *prima facie* more mechanical in the clockwork sense of mechanism. Even then, though, vestiges of divinely-sown, seminal virtues were still at work behind the scenes. The success of this materialist version of mechanical philosophy in satisfying the religious and methodological needs of Restoration England and the early Enlightenment helped to erase most traces of the vitalist heritage of Baconian experimentalism and mid-century corpuscular philosophy, a heritage in which Severinus played an important role.

108 Ibid., pp. 126 and 134.

Severinus' synthesis of Paracelsian medical ideas and his elaboration of a compatible, general theory of generation and corruption had a profound influence on the development of chemical philosophy in England and France in the late sixteenth and seventeenth centuries, as is clear from our examination of the contexts in which Severinus and the *Idea medicinæ* were cited, paraphrased, and quoted. In many instances it is apparent that the readers were chiefly interested in his explanation of fundamental aspects of Paracelsianism, such as the relationship between the four elements and three principles. Severinus was among those authors who brought these ideas to the attention of the scholarly world, as is clear from the wide range of educated people who mentioned him, from La Brosse and Gassendi in France, to Bacon, Donne, and Boyle in England.

Severinus' most enduring contribution, however, was his account of the generation and corruption of living beings from dimensionless, divinely created *semina*. Medical writers and natural philosophers used this metaphysical apparatus as he had used it, that is, as a biological explanation for growth and decay, sexual mixing, the unfolding of apparently new forms, and the spreading, generation, mutation, and destruction of diseases. But the power of this metaphysics is perhaps seen most clearly in how, on the one hand, it was adapted by Jorden to explain subterranean heat and the restorative powers of mineral waters and how, on the other hand, it was extended by Van Helmont. Van Helmont did not cite Severinus as a forerunner or authority upon which his biological theories rested, but the similarity of his ideas and terminology to those of Severinus makes an organic connection between the *Idea medicinæ* and the *Ortus medicinæ/Oriatrike* quite plausible. Further, we know from Van Helmont's letter to Marin Mersenne that he was familiar with Severinus' book, on which he presumably drew heavily for his early work, the "Eisagoge." Through Van Helmont's *ferments* and *archei*, Severinus' ideas lived on, dressed in new terminology. In the next chapters it will be shown that Severinus' ideas were also influential in the Germanic world of central Europe and Scandinavia, where the number of medical philosophers following Severinus' basic ideas was sufficient to warrant the creation of the term *secta Severiana* to describe their dependence on the *Idea medicinæ*.

Chapter Seven

THE "SEVERINIAN SCHOOL" IN CENTRAL EUROPE

ARACELSIAN IDEAS found the fields of the German-speaking regions of Europe to be the most fertile of all. Paracelsian chemical remedies for difficult diseases, which had sparked such a controversy in Paris, were taken up by alchemists throughout Europe, and Paracelsian theory crept into the philosophical tracts of many Western European scholars, medical and non-medical. But in the German lands these ideas really took root and produced a varied harvest of pharmaceutical, surgical, cosmological, political, and religious fruits – the latter being a part of a general and widespread unease that characterized the Holy Roman Empire and its neighbors through much of the period.

The courts and universities of the German Emperor and princes, from Prague to Marburg to Heidelberg, became foci for much of the political intrigue and ideological alignments and realignments that preceded the Thirty Years' War. Paracelsians were drawn to the courts for patronage and protection, and their ideas, which were hotly contested by entrenched academics, became a part of the court culture. Thus the environment in which Severinus' ideas were weighed often reflected political and religious concerns more directly than was the case in Paris or London. In France and England the reception of Paracelsian theories was also influenced by issues relating to the nature and authority of Protestant doctrine and political power, but in the German regions, which produced many radical protestant sectarian movements and suffered the associated political turmoil, Paracelsian ideas were evaluated in an especially highly charged context. In this furnace of central Europe, Paracelsian themes were fused with the mystical, sometimes separatist religious doctrines of Valentin Weigel and Jacob Boehme and given symbolic shape by Michael Maier. The result was an amalgam in which the intellectual contents of Paracelsian theory were tightly bound with the social conditions.

Political and religious concerns do not often reach, in an obvious and documentable way, to the level of medical abstraction that typifies much of what Severinus wrote in the *Idea medicinæ*. But, as we have seen in the case of Erastus' criticism, issues pertaining to religious doctrine did impinge on chemical philosophy. They helped create a tension within the medical community that is perhaps most clearly seen in Andreas Libavius' attacks on the Paracelsians and Rosicrucians, but also in the acceptance and rejection of "vital philosophy" in Scandinavia, as Lutheran orthodoxy struggled for control of the Danish and Swedish state churches. How this charged atmosphere affected the reception of Severinus' doctrines by German and Scandinavian authors is the subject of this and the next chapter.

Debate over Paracelsianism in Switzerland and Germany intensified in the decade after the publication of the *Idea medicinæ* in 1571 and the first parts of Erastus' *De medicina nova Philippi Paracelsi* in 1572. Erastus was not alone in his views that Paracelsus' ideas were antithetical to medicine and religion. He represented a strongly anti-Paracelsian faction, which intervened against Thomas Moffet, as was noted in the previous chapter. But Moffet eventually overcame opposition to his promotion at Basel with the help of Theodor Zwinger, which suggests that discussion of Paracelsian medicine was not entirely one-sided at the university.

Zwinger had opposed Paracelsianism in the 1560s, but by the late 1570s he had come to appreciate certain aspects of it, and although he never became a thoroughgoing adherent, he began to teach Paracelsian ideas and publish Paracelsian books. Under his guidance, Paracelsian ideas diffused into the university curriculum.[1] Exactly what Zwinger thought about Paracelsus' metaphysical ideas and what his relationship to Conrad Gesner and other early critics of Paracelsus may have been must await further study. However, it is evident from Severinus' letters

---

1 Trevor-Roper, "The Paracelsian Movement," p. 164. Sennert, *De chymicorum*, p. 34, listed Zwinger among the Galenists who cultivated chemistry ("Chymiam coluerunt Galenici").

to Zwinger that they were in regular contact in the mid 1580s and held each other in some esteem, but to what extent Zwinger agreed with Severinus' Paracelsian doctrines is not clear.[2] Nevertheless, sources both favorable and hostile to Paracelsian medicine indicate that Severinus' interpretation profoundly affected the subsequent development of Paracelsian thought in the German-speaking world.

Three widely read and prolific writers, Andreas Libavius, Gregor Horst, and Daniel Sennert, bear witness to the seminal importance of the *Idea medicinæ* in the late sixteenth and early seventeenth-century formulation of chemical philosophy. All three sought to repudiate certain Paracelsian concepts while defending the value of iatrochemistry. Their comments indicate that the *Idea medicinæ* was an influential text and that Severinus' philosophical opinions were incorporated into the teachings of several medical instructors and writers.

Andreas Libavius shares with Thomas Erastus the distinction of being the earliest and most vehement critics of Paracelsian theory on both medical and religious grounds. Libavius began a life-long verbal crusade against the Paracelsians in 1594 with the publication of his *Neoparacelsica*.[3] By December 1597, at the latest, Libavius knew Severinus' work well enough to cite it as an example of the Paracelsians' total destruction of the Aristotelian philosophical tradition. In a letter to Jacob Zwinger, dated 14 December 1597 but published in 1599, Libavius rants about Paracelsian chemists who appropriated a chemical interpretation

---

2   Only the letters from Severinus to Zwinger have survived, but we know from Theodor's son, Jacob Zwinger, that Theodor shared his knowledge of chemical drug preparation with Severinus. Jacob Zwinger, *Principiorum chymicorum examen ad Generalem Hippocratis, Galeni cæterorumque Græcorum & Arabum consensum institutum* (Basel, 1606), p. 79: "Adscribam ea paucis, quæ Theodorus Zuingerus parens noster, cum Petro Seuerino Ideæ medicinæ philosophicæ scriptore communicauit: Recipe partes æquales Stibij & Meteori vel sublimati: per retortam educ glaciem ..." [Let me add, in a few words, those things that my father, Theodor Zwinger, shared with Petrus Severinus, the author of the *Idea medicinæ philosophicæ*: "Take equal parts of antimony and meteor or sublimate. Make a solid in a retort ..."]

3   I have not examined this book to see if Libavius knew of Severinus at that time. For an account of Libavius and his role in the early seventeenth-century Parisian debate over chemical medicine, see Debus, *The French Paracelsians*, pp. 59-62. Bruce T. Moran, "Libavius the Paracelsian? Monstrous Novelties, Institutions, and the Norms of Social Value," in *Reading the Book of Nature*, ed. Debus and Walton, pp. 67-79, further explores Libavius' opposition to Paracelsian medicine and his concern with properly defining chemical discourse.

of Genesis, death, and resurrection; they apparently wanted a theology that was compatible with their philosophy, in order to give it a credibility that it lacked on its own merits. He scorns their account of the elements, the creation of the world, the creation of man, and the role that they have assigned to salt, sulphur, and mercury. He also rejects the notion of spiritual agents dwelling within the elemental wombs:

> [The Paracelsians] establish empty spaces in the little chests of the elements, penetrate the dimensions by means of spirits, and place an actual infinite space between bodies; for the essences concealed in the corporeal enclosures do not have number nor finite size. How much do they differ [from the Aristotelians] regarding what is produced and changed? Just consider Severinus' *Idea*. You will learn that the nature of things has been changed and accordingly that the theory of the Aristotelians is obsolete.[4]

Libavius goes on to say that the Paracelsians laugh at the temperaments, sensible qualities, and the humors. They do not call urine urine, but rather dissolved salt. Bile is no longer bile, but an arsenical fluid. They consider everything pertaining to humans to correspond to minerals and stars; stones form in the human body in the same way as in rivers, and the heart is no longer merely the heart, but the sun, the lion, and gold. Libavius' disgust for the basic natural philosophy of the Paracelsians knows few bounds in this letter, the bottom line of which is his demand that chemistry not overturn the "solid and genuine doctrines of the other arts," but work within a traditional philosophical framework.[5]

---

4 Letter from Andreas Libavius to Jacob Zwinger, pp. 41-49 in Andreas Libavius, *Rervm chymicarum epistolica forma ad philosophos et medicos qvosdam in Germania*, vol. 3 (Frankfurt: Petrus Kopffius, 1599), p. 47: "Vacuitates in capsulis elementorum statuunt dimensiones penetrant spiritibus, infinitum actuale inter corpora ponunt, cum essentiarum claustris corporeis occultatarum non sit numerus, nec finita magnitudo. De generabilibus transmutabilibusque quantum variant? Libeat tibi intueri Ideam Severini. Rerum naturam mutatam cognosces, pro ut est Aristotelicorum obsoleta doctrina." Severinus' name also appears in the margin of the printed version of a previous letter, written to Orontius Aretæus and dated 13 December 1597. Ibid., p. 22.
5 Ibid., p. 49: "Semel dico non est Chymiæ evertere aliarum artium solida & genuina decreta, non est." On early modern perceptions of the Paracelsians' confusion of analogies and identities, see Brian Vickers, "Analogy Versus Identity: The Rejection of Occult Symbolism, 1580-1680," in Brian Vickers, *Occult and Scientific Mentalities in the Renaissance* (Cambridge: Cambridge University Press, 1984), pp. 95-163.

He did not quote Severinus in this letter, nor did he explicitly blame him for all the wicked ideas of the Paracelsians, but the *Idea medicinæ* is manifestly the only source cited in the context of the above-mentioned violations of accepted philosophy. Severinus and his book must at least have been on Libavius' mind as 1597 drew to a close.

In the years that followed, Libavius became an even more outspoken proponent of an Aristotelian, humanist chemistry, which he believed could benefit both medicine and manufacturing. Part of this task required severing the connection that he perceived between chemical practice and Paracelsian metaphysics. To do this he embarked upon a campaign to discredit the major Paracelsian theorists, including Severinus.[6]

The sheer intensity of his criticism of the Paracelsians Johann Hartmann, Oswald Croll, Henning Scheunemann, and others points to the success of Paracelsian ideas among German academics and the alarm they had raised in some, notably in Libavius! Clearly he saw the growth of Paracelsianism in the early seventeenth century as a real threat to both medicine and religion, and he made a career of attacking Paracelsian and Rosicrucian ideas in print.[7] In Libavius' general invective against Paracelsianism, Croll and Hartmann became targets of specific tracts that were grouped together under the title *Prodromus vitalis philosophiæ Paracelsistarum Examen philosophiæ novæ, quæ veteri abrogandæ opponitur* (hereafter, *Examen philosophiæ novæ*) and published in 1615.[8] In these

6 Extensive references to Severinus are also made in Libavius, *Lapis philosophicus dogmaticorum* (Paris: Doulceur, 1608), which I have not been able to examine carefully.
7 This is the interpretation of Hannaway, *The Chemists and the Word*, p. 97, who has compared the philosophical outlooks of Croll and Libavius. There can be no doubt that both Libavius and Sennert regarded *religio Paracelsica*, the sectarian views of Weigel and the Rosicrucians, as a threat.
8 Andreas Libavius, *Prodromus vitalis philosophiæ Paracelsistarum Examen philosophiæ novæ, quæ veteri abrogandæ opponitur: in quo agitur de modo discendi novo: De veterum autoritate; De magia Paracelsi ex Crollio; De philosophia vivente ex Seuerino per Johannem Hartmannum; De philosophia harmonica magica Fraternitatis de Rosea Cruce* (Frankfurt, 1615), hereafter cited as *Examen philosophicæ novæ*, in *Syntagmatis selectorum undiquaque et perspicue traditorum alchymiæ arcanorum, tomus primus* (Frankfurt, 1615). Libavius' treatises present bibliographical problems, so as much information as possible has been provided here to aid the reader in locating these works. They are paginated separately, but seem to have been bound together by the publisher. I do not know if they circulated independently.

treatises we find Severinus mentioned as a specific source of the Paracelsian doctrines that Libavius opposed.

Croll's *Basilica chemica* (1609), a very influential chemical textbook, was an attempt to pull together various aspects of Paracelsian teaching, medical and theological, and to forge them into a coherent philosophy.[9] In the process, Croll presented the fundamentals of Severinus' theory of the elements, *astra*, and *semina* in the "Admonitory Preface," which served as an introduction to the theory behind the chemical medicines specified in the body of the *Basilica*. In a one and a half-page passage attributed to Severinus he described how the elements were empty wombs, "receptacles for all creation," which nourish the seeds. Into them, the divine spirit that moved upon the face of the waters, according to *Genesis*, planted light and the seminal reasons for all things. These seeds and *astra* bind the visible to the invisible and lay hidden in the invisible treasuries of the elements from the beginning of Creation, springing up at their appointed times, and so on. The three Paracelsian principles are inseparably attached to the *semina*, which strive to imitate the economy of the world. Johann Hartmann, who edited Croll's *Basilica* for publication, indicated that Croll had taken this passage from the *Idea medicinæ* by marking it with quotation marks running along the inside margin, the only passage so distinguished in the entire preface.[10] However, the "quotation" was not actually lifted intact from Severinus' book, but rather is a collage of paraphrases and verbatim or near verbatim passages extracted from various chapters of the *Idea medicinæ*, resulting in a summary of several of Severinus' key concepts.

9 Oswald Croll, *Basilica chymica* (Frankfurt: Godofridi, 1609). *Basilica* includes a section on chemical preparation preceded by a lengthy preface in which theory is presented. The *Admonitoria præfatio* was not included in the English translation of the *Basilica*, which was published under the title *Royal Chymistry*, in Oswald Croll and Johann Hartmann, *Bazilica Chymica, & Praxis chymiatricæ, or Royal and Practical Chymistry in Three Treatises* (London, 1670). However, an English translation was published by H. Pinnell as *Admonitory Preface*, in *Philosophy Reformed and Improved in Four Profound Tracts* (London, 1657).

10 Oswald Croll, *Admonitory Preface*, pp. 33-36; *Basilica*, pp. 19-20.

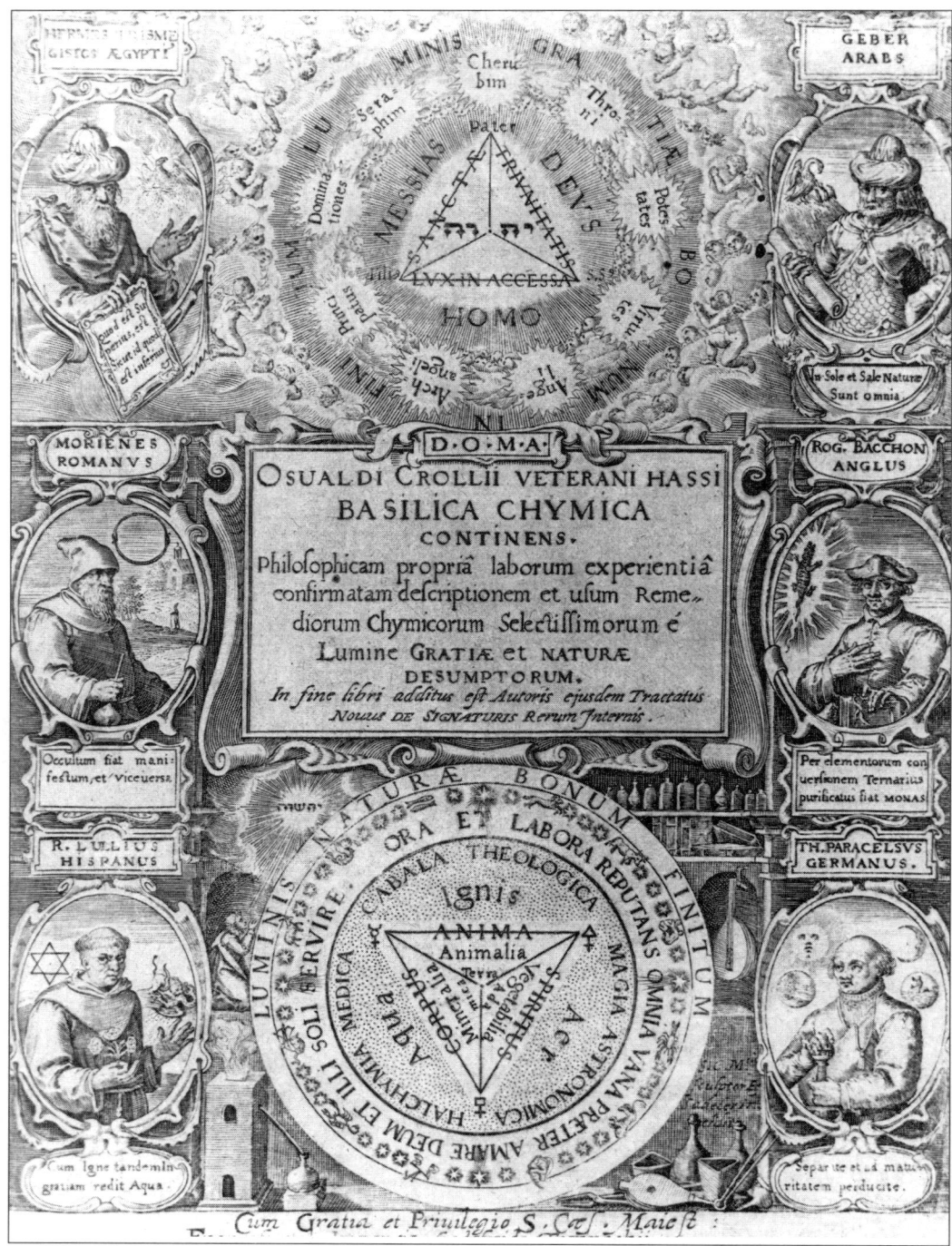

This title page of Oswald Croll's Basilica Chymica *(1608) illustrates the alchemical tradition which formed the interpretive framework for Severinus' Paracelsian ideas in the years preceding the outbreak of the Thirty Years' War. The portraits of Geber, Morienus Romanus, and Roger Bacon indicate Croll's debt to the European medieval alchemical tradition; the images of Hermes Trismegistus and Ramon Lull denote the religious and cabalistic context of Renaissance* chymia; *and Paracelsus' image represents the medical and perhaps religious background to Croll's chemistry. The conflation of mystical religion, laboratory alchemy, medicine, cabala, and astrology that is indicated by these images and the emblems at the top and bottom center of the page amply demonstrates the fusion of occult sciences and religion that characterized Paracelsian and Rosicrucian ideology and alarmed early seventeenth-century religious leaders. Courtesy of The Danish National Library of Science and Medicine.*

Croll attempted to elucidate Severinus' ideas by incorporating them into Paracelsian explanations drawn from other texts.[11] It must be pointed out, however, that he did not wholly grasp an essential, metaphysical characteristic of Severinus' *semina*, namely that they are knowledge-filled loci, where bodies come into being and where they retreat into incorporality when their functions are exhausted and their predestinations are completed. For, Croll equated Severinus' *semina* with the more general concept of a seed that must rot in the process of renewal.[12] Nevertheless,

---

11 Hannaway, *The Chemists and the Word*, p. 35, writes that Croll attempted to clarify Severinus' opinion on the elements and principles, but abandoned the effort after a few pages and set out his own intepretation. However, since Croll repeatedly used ideas and phrases that are also found in the *Idea medicinæ*, which he highly praised, it does not seem plausible that he rejected Severinus' explanations.

12 Croll, *Admonitory Preface*, p. 42; *Basilica*, p. 23: "Omnia crescentia, herbæ, arbores, pisces, aves, animalia, possunt se augmentare beneficio corporis hoc modo (semen enim vel Astrum sine corpore nil facere potest) quamprimum ubi Semen vel Astrum moritur, & putrescit in sua matrice, tunc Astrum progreditur in novum corpus, & multiplicat se, ut Christus similitudine & exemplo Naturæ ipse utitur …" [All growing things, herbs, trees, fish, birds, and animals, are able to become larger by means of body in this way (for the seed or *astrum* cannot do anything without a body): when the seed or *astrum* dies, and decomposes in its matrix, then as soon as possible the *astrum* develops into a new body, and multiplies itself, as Christ himself makes use of nature's likeness and example …]

Croll praised Severinus and the *Idea medicinæ* for laying a solid foundation for Paracelsian theory:

> It is of greatest concernment that all Chymists should be well acquainted with this true Fundamentall of the occult Phylosophycal Physick, because of the Harmonicall concord and conspiration between the superiour and inferiour things of the greater and lesser world, in clearing which (Foundation) next to *Paracelsus, Petrus Severinus* the Dane, together with *Pratensis* that faithfull *Achates,* deserveth to be numbred among the Ancient wise men, having got perpetuall praise by discovering to the Children of Art and Truth, this firme and unmovable Foundation with much solid and unshaken verity in his Idæa of Paracelsean Physick.[13]

Croll was apparently cognizant of controversy over Severinus' ideas and, although he did not name individual detractors, he judged that their criticisms had been sufficiently answered by his friend Quercetanus, by Thomas Bovius of Verona, and by Thomas Moffet, "the best Hermetick Physitians of this age."[14] Perhaps this is an echo of the criticism that Severinus had found unsettling, which Moffet had mentioned.

Both Hartmann and Libavius noticed the operational similarity between Croll's metaphysics and Severinus' *semina* theory and his explicit use of the *Idea medicinæ* as a source. Indeed, the text of the *Basilica* proper opens with a quotation from Severinus: "The method of healing for all diseases (if I may use the distinct words of P. Severinus here, as they are very appropriate) is twofold,"[15] which the English translator correctly

---

13 Croll, *Admonitory Preface,* pp. 74-75; *Basilica,* pp. 39-40: "Maximopere interest, ut hoc verum occultæ Medicinæ Philosophicæ Fundamentum Chymiæ studiosis innotescat, propter Harmonicam concordantiam & conspirationem superiorum & infericrum, majoris & minoris mundi, in quo manifestando, post Paracelsum *Petrus Severinus* Danus, una cum *Pratensi* fideli Achate, merito in numerum Antiquorum sapientum referendus, perpetuam sui nominis gloriam assecutus est, quod in sua Idæa Paracelsicæ Medicinæ invictissimum hoc solida & inconcussa veritate stabilitum Fundamentum Filiis artis & veritatis patefecerit."

14 Croll, *Admonitory Preface,* p. 75; *Basilica,* p. 40: "a præstantissimis nostri sæculi Hermeticis Medicis."

15 Croll, *Basilica,* p. III: "Sanationes omnium Morborum (ut hic etiam convenientissime significantibus P. Severini verbis utar) sunt duplices."

identified as coming from chapter fourteen of the *Idea medicinæ*, but admitted that "many think *Peter Severinus* not to be the Author of the *Idea*, but rather *Pratenses*, whose Verse annexed to the end thereof, being compared with the whole Writing, seems to declare the same."[16] Passages identified with marginal quotation marks in the first three pages of the *Basilica* introduce Severinus' definitions of general and particular cures, but, as in the preface, these are not always verbatim quotations. Nevertheless, for anyone reading both the Admonitory Preface and the *Basilica* proper, Croll's dependence on Severinus as a source would be plain. So it was for Libavius. In the second tract of his *Examen philosophiæ novæ*, named *"De magia Paracelsi ex Crollio,"* Libavius attacked Croll, whom he labeled "a disciple of Paracelsus and P. Severinus and such men."[17] In another tract published in 1615, this one directed primarily against Henning Scheunemann, Libavius went further and claimed that Croll was influenced to a greater extent by Severinus and others than by Paracelsus himself.[18]

Libavius directed the third tract of his *Examen philosophiæ novæ* at Johann Hartmann, a prominent Paracelsian who is best known today as the first professor of chemistry at Marburg.[19] That Libavius saw Hartmann as a Severinian is clear from the title of this treatise: "On the living or vital philosophy of Paracelsus, according to P. Severinus Danus, from the repetition of I. Hartmann, Iatrochemist at Marburg."[20] Indeed, Hartmann was greatly influenced by the *Idea medicinæ*, as is

16 Croll, *Bazilica* (1670), p. 3, note b.
17 Libavius, *Examen philosophiæ novæ (Syntagmatis)*, p. 16 marginalia: "Crollius discipulus Paracelsi, & P. Severini, & sic hominum."
18 Andreas Libavius, *Pro defensione syntagmatis chymici contra reprehensiones Henningi Scheunemanni Paracelsistæ actio prima*, in *Appendix necessaria*, p. 54: "Ipse [Crollius] Hermetem, Agrippam, Seuerinum & alios magis sequitur quam Paracelsum." [Croll himself follows Hermes, Agrippa, Severinus, and others, more than Paracelsus.]
19 On Hartmann and the establishment of the first chair in chemistry see Bruce T. Moran, "Privilege, Communication, and Chemistry: the Hermetic-Alchemical Circle of Moritz of Hessen-Kassel," *Ambix* 32 (1985): 110-126; Idem, "Court Authority and Chemical Medicine"; *Chemical Pharmacy Enters the University*; and *The Alchemical World of the German Court*.
20 Libavius, *De philosophia vivente seu vitali Paracelsi iuxta P. Severinum danum ex repetitione I. Hartmanni Chymiatri Marburgensis*, in *Examen philosophiæ novæ* (in *Syntagmatis*), p. 88.

especially apparent in his exposition of vital philosophy.[21] Hartmann, like Severinus, was interested in combining Paracelsian chemical pharmacy with what he perceived as the true Hippocratic medicine. To succeed, he argued, one must learn the laws of generation and transplantation that govern the chemical basis of life, and this must be learned from experience.[22]

Although directed to Hartmann, Libavius' criticisms were aimed squarely at the fundamental Paracelsian idea of vital philosophy, which he found obnoxious. "Consider your vital philosophy," he wrote in the preface to Hartmann. "Consider how you would offend not only most living philosophers, but also the dead, ancient ones, men very highly praised in all liberal schools the world over – just so that you might force your Paracelsianism and Severinianism upon your students."[23] He subsequently criticized the central doctrines, one by one, upon which Severinus' philosophy was built, beginning with the elements.[24] Behind Hartmann's account of the elements, Libavius wrote, "I hear Severinus dreaming the visions of a sick man and telling stories about empty elements, whose nature is suited to these *semina* ... [These are] the remarkable dreams of the infernal god Morpheus."[25] However, he traced Hartmann's failure to grasp the truth of natural philosophy to his origins as a mathematician, which meant that Hartmann was a late comer to the subtleties of philosophy: "From the mathematicians you have insinuated yourself into Paracelsian kitchens, in which you have thus far lingered and have consumed a good part of your studies on Severinian foolish-

21 Johannes Hartmann, *Introductio in vitalem philosophiam*, in *Opera omnia medico-chymica*, ed. Conrad Johrenius, vol. 7 (Frankfurt am Main: Balthas. Christophori Wursti, 1684), pp. 1-61. See Moran, *Chemical Pharmacy*, p. 20.

22 Hartmann, *Opera omnia*, vol. 4, p. 9, col. 1. See Moran, *Chemical Pharmacy*, pp. 17-18, 20.

23 Libavius, *De philosophia vivente* (in *Examen philosophiæ novæ*, in *Syntagmatis*), p. 89: "Inspice Philosophiam tuam vitalem, & perpende quam tu offenderis non viuentes tantum plurimos, sed & priscos mortuos, viros toto orbe per omnes scholas liberales laudatissimos, vt tuum Paracelsismum & Seuerianismum studiosis obtrudas."

24 Ibid., p. 92. Libavius criticized Hartmann's theory of the elements as empty places and receptacles, which he identified in a marginal note as taken from chapter five of the *Idea medicinæ* and from Croll, who also learned it from Severinus.

25 Ibid., p. 160: "Audio Seuerinum instar ægri somniantem, & fabulas narrantem de vacuis elementis, quorum natura sit ornata seminibus istis cohærentibus indissolubili nexu ... Mira somnia dei infernalis Morphei."

ness."[26] Libavius severely criticized Severinus' conception of *semina*, *astra* (which he found to be nothing other than *semina*), and the entire metaphysics based on them, which he judged to be impious:

> Your Severinus very acutely mocks the Creator and his creatures and he insults the principles of theology and philosophy and the common sense and judgement of all men, when he babbles on about the elements; that the elements (heaven, air, water, earth) are incorporeal natures, empty, void, in which God placed light and the seminal reasons of things by an incomprehensible magic (so that even God's most holy majesty is defiled by a foul term), adjoining the principles of bodies, in which they were clothed for coming forth onto the world stage.[27]

Libavius' total rejection of Severinus' doctrines should be viewed as a part of his opposition to Paracelsian theory and the Calvinist and Rosicrucian beliefs that it supported. There is a rhetorical force behind his writing that suggests a more than academic disagreement about philosophy, and the targets of his venomous pen were often supporters of Calvinist or Crypto-Calvinist doctrine, such as Tycho Brahe, Croll, Hartmann, and probably Severinus, too. In general Libavius faulted Severinus for giving too much credence to Paracelsian ideas and blamed him for being a major source for the errors of Quercetanus, Croll, Hartmann, and other Paracelsians.[28] Thus, when he described

26 Ibid., p. 93: "Nam ex Mathematicis irrepsisti in culinam Paracelsicam, in qua adhuc hæres, & bonam partem studiorum tuorum consumsisti fatuitatibus Seuerianis."

27 Ibid., p. 157: "*Seuerinus* tuus *valde nasute illudit creatori*, & creaturis, insultatque Theologiæ & Philosophiæ principiis, communique omnium hominum sensui & iudicio, dum de elementis garrit *elementa* (coelum, aerem, aquam, terram,) *esse naturas incorporeas, inanes, vacuas, in quas Deus Magia incomprehensibili*, (vt Dei sanctissima Maiestas etiam polluto vocabulo inquinetur) *imposuerit lucem & seminales rerum rationes, adiungens corporum principia, quibus induerentur in mundanam scenam prodituræ.*"

28 Libavius, *Pro defensione syntagmatis chymici contra ... Scheunemanni* (in *Appendix necessaria*), p. 50, writes under the marginal rubric, "Cur Paracelsista potius velit Hippocraticus esse, quam Galenicus" [Why the Paracelsian wishes to be Hippocratic rather than Galenic]: "Seuerinus in Idea mirifice sententias Hippocratis vt videantur paracelsicæ esse deprauat. Eum sequuntur Crollius, Hartmannus, & alii Hermetici simul & dogmatici." [Severinus, in the *Idea medicinæ*, astonishingly misrepresents the opinions of Hippocrates, so that they seem to be Paracelsian. Croll, Hartmann, together with the other Hermetics and dogmatics, follow him.]

the author of the *Idea medicinæ* as Hartmann's god, it was not a benign attribution.[29]

Severinus and the *Idea medicinæ* are most commonly cited by proponents of chemical philosophy or by its detractors, such as Libavius. Therefore, it is perhaps to be expected that our view of the assimilation and reaction to his chief ideas is colored by the rhetorical context in which these concepts were evaluated. However, Severinus' book was read and used by a generation of medical students in the early seventeenth century who sought to understand the differences between the Paracelsian point of view, which they sometimes called Hermetic medicine, and the Galenic-Peripatetic medicine that was taught in the universities.[30] In the dissertations and medical treatises of many of the medical men of this period we find an eclectic attitude prevailing. There is no strong desire to abandon the hard-won wisdom of Galen and the Arabic authors, but rather a willingness to assay the writings of the chemical philosophers, in order to help fill in gaps or weak points in traditional medicine and to find some way to incorporate the seemingly successful chemical therapy into learned medicine. This was not quite the same as an "Elizabethan compromise," in which recipes for chemical drugs were plucked from their Paracelsian contexts and placed into Galenic foster homes, but rather an attempt to evaluate the Paracelsian doctrines that supported the preparation and use of these drugs and to accommodate parts of them to humoral pathology.[31] Some authors went to considerable lengths to elucidate similarities between basic Paracelsian ideas and the Aristotelian metaphysics that underlies Galenic medical theory. The *Idea medicinæ* was used by these authors as one of several sources of Paracelsian (Hermetic) doctrine. Gregor Horst and Daniel Sennert

29 Ibid., p. 161: "Tuus Deus *Seuerinus*."

30 Historians today prefer to distinguish Hermetic philosophy from other forms of Renaissance Platonism and occult philosophy, including Paracelsian theory, and seek to restrict the term "Hermetic" to the narrow meaning of 'connected with the doctrines and traditions of the Hermetic Corpus.' This is understandable, given the claims that have been made for Hermetism in recent years, but we must not overlook the fact that the term was used much more generally in the late sixteenth and seventeenth centuries.

31 Debus, *The English Paracelsians*, p. 80 claims that the English reception of Paracelsianism differed from that on the continent, where Paracelsian theory was more readily accepted. See also, Allen G. Debus, "The Paracelsian Compromise in Elizabethan England," *Ambix* 10 (1962): 108-18.

are two examples of this new generation of eclectic physicians. Both were influential educators and writers, Horst at Giessen and Sennert at Wittenberg, and both commented on certain ideas treated by Severinus, permitting us another view of how the *Idea medicinæ* was read in the years immediately preceding the Thirty Years' War.

GREGOR HORST

Gregor Horst (1578-1636) was educated at Wittenberg and Basel, where he received his M.D. in 1606. The Landgrav of Hesse appointed him to the University of Giessen in 1608 and made him chief physician or *archiater* the following year. His reputation as a healer became so great that he was remembered as "The Asculapius of Germany."[32] In a dissertation on the distinctions and causes of diseases, published at Giessen in 1612, Horst considered one of the questions that fundamentally divided Galenists and Paracelsians: whether diseases arise from an imbalance in the body's material (humoral) constitution, that is, from an "affect" or disposition of the parts, or are caused by spiritual agents as the Paracelsians maintained. He offered several points in favor of the Paracelsian position, the fifth of which was: "Because according to the school of the Hermetic philosophers, spirits perform all actions, as is evident from chapter two of Petrus Severinus' *Idea*."[33] After considering the Galenists' positions, Horst responded:

> To the fifth point, the opinion of the Hermetic philosophers can be conceded, so long as they understand "spirit" to be nothing other than τό θερμὸν ἔμφυτον [the innate heat] proper to each part of the body, for which reason they agree with the Galenists, who do not under-

---

32 On Gregor Horst and his sons, see *Biographie Universelle, Ancienne et Moderne*, vol. 20 (Paris: Michaud, 1817), pp. 579-80. Gregor Horst, Jr., *Operum medicorum* (Nuremberg, 1660), included a biographical *Oratio funebris* for his father.

33 Gregor Horst, *De morborum differentiis et causis, exercitatio I* (Geissen: Caspar Chemlinus, 1612), p. 7: "5. Quia secundum Hermeticorum scholam spiritus omnes actionis [sic] perficiunt, ut patet ex *Idæa P. Severini c. II*."

stand "parts" to be dead parts, but living ones, that is, endowed with innate vital spirits of this kind, which are inherent in the original moisture. So it is true when Severinus says that the stomach concocts because it possesses spiritual bodies abounding in the properties and knowledge of salt, sulphur, and mercury, which can resolve, separate, and arrange the ingested aliments and equip them with appropriate characteristics, because he means here nothing other than that the stomach has τό θερμὸν ἔμφυτον of this kind, an innate heat that is proper to it and suited to performing this function.[34]

Thus, Horst agreed that spirits are involved in the causing of disease, if spirit is the same as innate heat. But if this is true, he wrote, then neither health nor disease can be attributed to *matrices* or other parts of the body. What is important here is that although Horst in the end adhered to the Galenist position, he carefully considered the Paracelsian or Hermetic doctrines and tried to accommodate them to Galenism on key points of contention; he did not seek to condemn "Hermetic" medicine *per se*, but rather sought to make use of the attention it drew to chemical processes and enrich medicine by joining the Paracelsian idea of vital anatomy to the traditional Galenic concept. He examined this topic explicitly in the preface to his much larger treatise *De natura humana libri duo*, also published in 1612.[35]

Horst understood that medicine must address man's corporeal and spiritual natures, since man is both body and soul. To this end, book one of *De natura humana* treats the structure of the body, and book two the soul. The "Preface to the candid reader about the living and dead

---

34 Ibid., p. 8: "Ad 5. Concedi potest Hermeticorum sententia, quando per spiritus nihil aliud intelligunt, quam τό θερμὸν ἔμφυτον cuique parti proprium, qua ratione idem dicunt cum Galenicis, qui per partes non intelligunt mortuas, sed viventes, h.e. ejusmodi spiritibus vitalibus insitis, humidoque primogenio inhærentibus præditas. Ita verum est, quando Severinus ait, ventriculum concoquere, quia spiritualia obtinet corpora, proprietatibus & scientiis, salis, sulphuris & mercurii vigentia, quæ alimenta ingesta resolvere, separare, digerere, & signaturis consentaneis vestire possunt: quia nihil aliud hic intelligitur, quam quod ventriculus habeat ejusmodi τό θερμὸν ἔμφυτον, innatum calidum, sibi solum proprium & ad hanc operationem perficiendam accommodatum."

35 Gregor Horst, *De natura humana libri duo … Cum præfatione de Anatomia vitali & mortua pro conciliatione Spagyricorum & Galenicorum plurimum inseruiente* (Frankfurt am Main: Erasmus Kempfer, 1612).

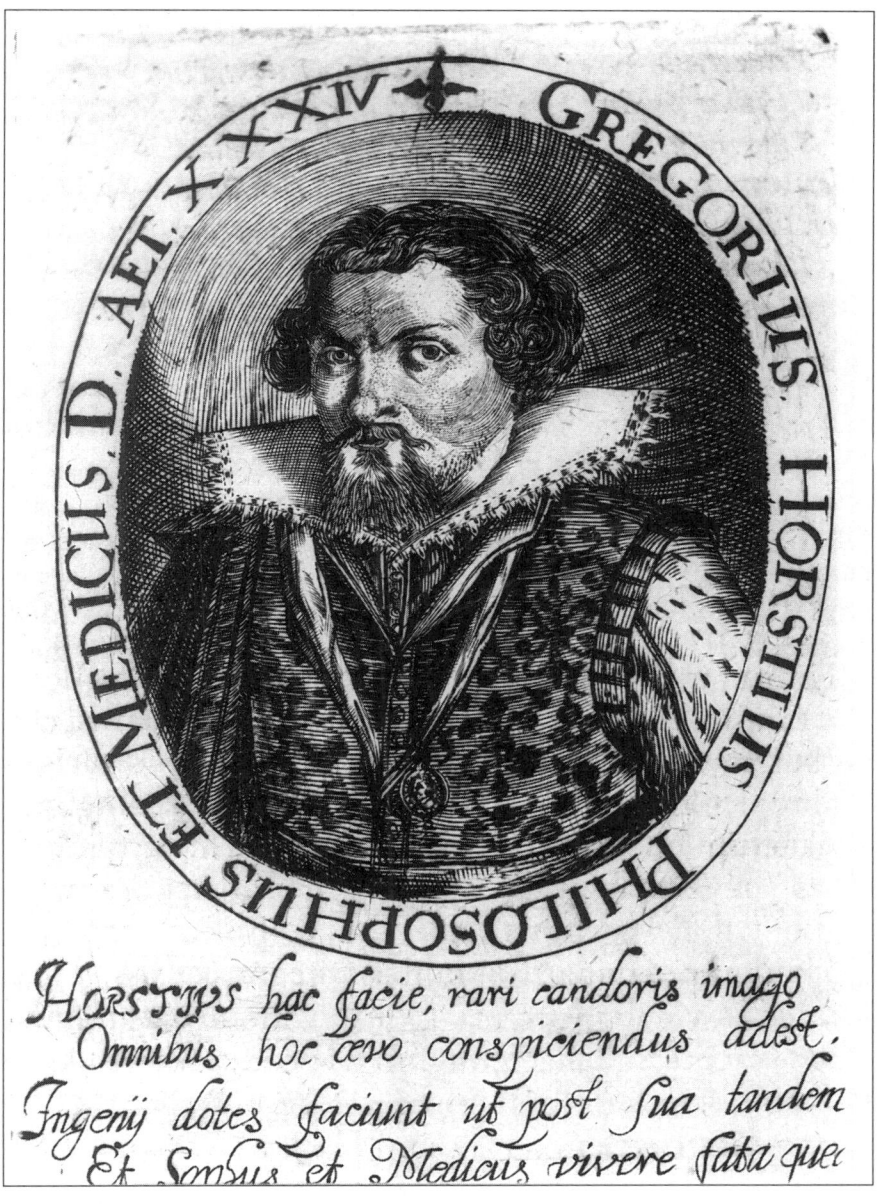

Portrait of Gregor Horst, from his De natura humana *(1612). Courtesy of the Health Sciences Library, Rare Books and Special Collections, University of Wisconsin at Madison.*

anatomy" serves to define the scope of the work and clarifies the general meaning of anatomy as the knowledge or

> cognition of both body and soul at the same time: Anatomy is largely devoted to this cognition, not so much that kind by which the body is skillfully cut up into the least parts, the utility of which we shall consider later, but that other kind, which is rightly called vital, where we are not so much concerned with the body, as with the essence, principles, faculties, and functions of the body.[36]

Horst gave metaphysical priority to vital anatomy over the anatomy of cadavers, because form is more noble than matter, but he considered "dead" anatomy to be prior in the order of cognition, since vital anatomy is very difficult to observe. Physicians are not content to study the shape, composition, position, and comparisons of the body's parts, he wrote, but must go farther and examine its innermost principles and the various properties proceeding from them.[37] The marginal note adjacent to this portion of the text directs the reader to see chapter three of Severinus' *Idea medicinæ.*

Clearly, Horst did not object to the idea of vital anatomy, which comprises study of both the metaphysical bases for life and its chemical physiology, but neither did he wish to give it a prominent place in medical education, which properly considers the manifest before the occult. He felt that those who criticized university physicians for neglecting vital anatomy misunderstood the importance of the dead anatomy for physicians, surgeons, lawyers, and theologians. Furthermore, they were wrong in assuming that his contemporaries had failed to take vital anatomy into consideration.[38] "Moreover," he wrote, "since vital anatomy consists of the investigation and perfect understanding of nature, according to the Hermetic physicians, it is necessary that we first understand the

---

36 Ibid., p. 2: "Huic cognitioni plurimum inseruit Anatomia, non ea tantum, qua corpus in partes minimas artificiose secatur, cuius vtilitatem postea considerabimus, sed & illa, quæ merito vitalis dicitur, vbi non tam de corpore, quam ipsius corporis essentia, principiis, facultatibus atque functionibus solliciti sumus."
37 Ibid., pp. 2-3
38 Ibid., pp. 3-4. On pp. 21-24 Horst defended the necessity of having traditional "dead" anatomy in the university curriculum.

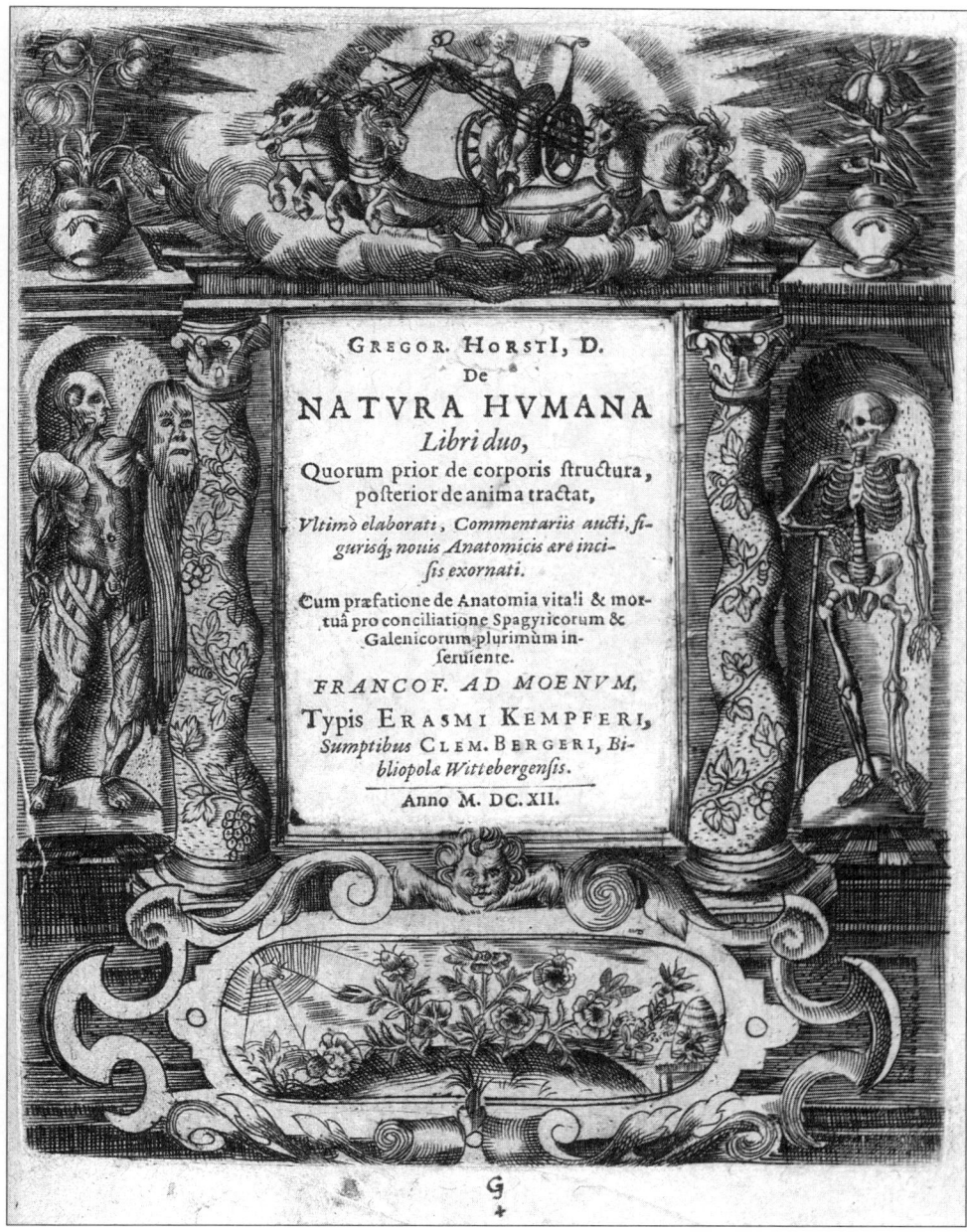

GREGOR. HORSTI, D.

De

NATVRA HVMANA

Libri duo,

Quorum prior de corporis ſtructura,
poſterior de anima tractat,

*Vltimò elaborati, Commentariis aucti, fi-
guriſq́; nouis Anatomicis ære inci-
ſis exornati.*

Cum præfatione de Anatomia vitali & mor-
tuâ pro conciliatione Spagyricorum &
Galenicorum plurimùm in-
ſeruiente.

FRANCOF. AD MOENVM,

Typis ERASMI KEMPFERI,
Sumptibus CLEM. BERGERI, *Bi-
bliopolæ Wittebergenſis.*

Anno M. DC. XII.

Title page of Gregor Horst's De natura humana *(1612). Courtesy of The Danish
National Library of Science and Medicine.*

doctrine of generation and transplantation."[39] What follows is a rather lengthy introduction to *semina* theory that was largely taken from the *Idea medicinæ*, but also from Quercetanus and Reusner. As he had done in *De morborum differentiis & causis*, Horst cited Severinus and quoted the *Idea medicinæ* in this preface as an example of Hermetic medical doctrines. It is apparent from his quotations, paraphrases, and analyses that he had read the *Idea medicinæ* carefully, and these indicate which aspects of Severinus' philosophy he found most interesting and useful, providing us yet another clue to how the *Idea medicinæ* was read in this period.

First he defined "generation according to the Hermetic physicians," citing chapter eight of the *Idea*:

> Generation according to Hermetic medicine seems to be a progression of *semina* previously lying hidden in Orpheus' night, in Hippocrates' underworld [*Orcus*], in Theophrastus' *iliaster*, or in the blessed recesses of the elements, which occurs when, at the appointed times, they are visibly brought forth from the elements into act, with all their properties, with the help of the previously mentioned principles [salt, sulphur, and mercury].[40]

Horst noted that this doctrine rested on three hypotheses. First, that the Hermetic philosophers consider the principles of things not as abstracts, but as real things in nature, because they arrange the elements necessary for the generation of mixtures. The elements, by themselves, do not suffice to account for generation, but seem to be nothing other than receptacles and places for the hypostatic principles and *semina*, from which natural entities are produced.[41] Horst claimed that this idea

---

39 Ibid., p. 4: "Cum autem Anatomia vitalis secundum Hermeticos consistat in inquisitione & perfecta cognitione naturæ, necetssarium est, vt primo generationis atque transplantationis doctrinam cognoscamus."

40 Ibid., p. 4: "Hinc ergo generatio iuxta Medicinam Hermeticam videtur esse progressio seminum antea in nocte Orphei, in orco Hippocratis, in iliastro Theophrasti, seu in elementorum beatis recessibus latitantium, quæ fit, quando determinatis temporibus ex elementis, ope principiorum dictorum visibiliter cum omnibus suis proprietatibus actu producuntur." The marginal notes to this read "Vide Petr. Seuer. in Idea Med. Philos. cap. 8," and "Generatio secundum Hermeticos."

41 Ibid., p. 4.

was not entirely foreign to Peripatetic philosophy, especially since it is agreed that according to Aristotle, too, the pure and simple elements exist more in the conception of a thing than in the thing itself. Things are not made by the elements, since their forms are educed from the potencies of the prime matter, according to its aptitude. The Hermetic philosophers do not overturn this Peripatetic assertion, but rather attempt to proclaim that in the generation of things, before anything else, there are *semina* concealed in the recesses of the elements, and these possess all the parts, faculties, and properties of each species that should be generated, not by mass or quantity, but by a variety of gifts and by the power of the mechanical spirits.[42]

From this, Horst educed a second hypothesis underlying the Hermetic doctrine, namely that the forms and essences of things in act lie hidden in their principles, an idea that he said was taken from Hippocrates' *On Diet*, but is also found in Parmenides, in the Stoics' "containing cause," in Anaxagoras' mingling of atoms, and in the works of Scaliger, Quercetanus, Petrus Severinus, and others.[43] Horst reconciled this idea with Peripatetic doctrine, by equating the forms and essences that are internal to the *semina* with the Aristotelian concept of potency. For example, the Aristotelian philosopher says that a chicken will come from a chicken egg because the egg has in it a potency with an aptitude (*habilitas subjecti*) for generating the chicken.

> But if you should ask further, what is that aptitude, by reason of which a chicken and not a dog is generated from an egg, the Hermetic philosophers will respond in keeping with the present hypothesis, that the form of the chicken [is] in the egg invisibly and indeterminately, and it will come forth onto the world stage, once it has been given the necessary prerequisites: "For such is the strength of the mechanical spirits in the seed," Reusnerus says, in exercise six of *De Scorbuto*, "that if they possess the knowledge of the brain, they will form a brain from the attracted nutriment – if they possess the knowledge of the kidney, they will form a kidney from that same nutriment – with the arrangement, proportion,

42 Ibid., pp. 4–5.
43 Ibid., p. 5. Horst cited Scaliger's *De subtilitate*, exercise 8, Quercetanus' *Defensiones*, bk. 1, ch. 14, and Severinus' *Idea medicinæ*, ch. 8.

quality, quantity, shape, mercury, sulphur, salt, location, concord, and predestinations of timings defined by nature's process [*lithurgia*]."[44]

Therefore, Horst considered these mechanical spirits, which had come to him by way of Reusner, to be nothing but the faculty of the hidden form or potency, as Aristotle called it. Thus, Horst used Severinus' *semina* doctrine to elaborate further an essentially Aristotelian theory of epigenesis.

Horst's third basic hypothesis is that there are three constituent principles, namely salt, sulphur, and mercury. He recognized that the Paracelsians did not mean everyday salt, sulphur, and mercury, but rather abstract principles that are most fully manifested in these three visible materials. Yet he did not find compelling reasons for accepting them over the three Peripatetic abstracts, namely matter, form, and privation. Therefore, Horst concluded that the Aristotelian doctrine of generation should be adopted, with the understanding that the "complete privation of a natural thing," which is in the elements before that thing is generated, along with its aptitude or form, be determined by what the Hermetic philosophers call the properties of the *semina* and principles. However, these properties are not to be those of the Paracelsian salt, sulphur, and mercury.

Horst next considered the efficient cause of generation and whether the stars had any part in determining the proper mixtures or temperaments of things on earth. Here, too, he quoted Severinus' explanation of the timings of generation, maturation, fruiting, and so on in terms of the half moons, full moons, and other phases that all stars manifest.

---

44 Ibid., pp. 5-6: "At quæras ulterius, quid sit illa subiecti habilitas, cuius ratione pullus & non canis ex ovo generatur? Hic iuxta præsentem hypothesin Hermetici respondent, formam pulli invisibiliter & indeterminate in ovo [esse], quæ datis necessariis requisitis in mundanam scenam prodeat: *tantum enim est robur spirituum mechanicorum in semine*, inquit Reuserus lib. de Scorb. exerc. 6. *ut si scientiam habuerint cerebri, ex alimento attracto cerebrum, si hepatis, ex eodem alimento hepar forment, ordine, proportione, qualitate, quantitate, figura, mercurio, sulphure, sale, situ, consensu, temporumque prædestinationibus a lithurgia naturæ definitis.*" The terminology and ideas in the source that Horst mentions here, Hieronymus Reusnerus, *Diexodicarum exercitationum liber de scorbuto* (Frankfurt: Patheniana, 1600), sound familiar to the reader of the *Idea medicinæ*, but I have not found Severinus explicitly quoted or cited. On the basis of these similarities, I suspect Reusner was one of the "Severinians" that Libavius and Sennert mentioned.

But, he noted, this "assertion of the chemists" is not new and is easily reconciled with both Hippocrates and Aristotle, who recognized that the heavens were the cause of all change and generation in the sublunary world.[45]

Horst also cited Severinus as his source for the "Hermetic" understanding of mixture, transplantation, and human generation, all which came about as the unfolding of seminary potencies under the guidance of mechanical spirits.[46] As before, he extracted several key hypotheses underlying these doctrines and interpreted them in Aristotelian and Galenic terms, either showing them to be nothing new, or reconciling them with Peripatetic theory. For example, about the mechanical spirits he wrote: "Therefore, insofar as we concede definite properties and powers for acting to nature, we cannot deny that knowledge to the mechanical spirits."[47] Regarding the statement that these spirits formed all parts of the fetus from suitable elements and principles drawn from the nutriment, he wrote that "this assertion coincides with the idea common to all philosophers and physicians," namely that a formative virtue makes the rudiments of the parts from the seminal matter, which are then fed by the mother's blood.[48]

Like Severinus, Horst considered not just the living anatomy of "normal" generation, but applied *semina* theory and the ideas of transplantation to disease. Humans would attain their full development, he wrote, "if certain impurities had not supervened on the first and pure *semina* by virtue of the divine curse, for which reason the generation of disease follows."[49] Diseases also have seeds in nature, but these are not independent. Rather, they adhere to other *semina* and principles, for

45 Horst, *De natura humana*, pp. 8-9.
46 Ibid., pp. 9-10.
47 Ibid., p. 11: "Quatenus igitur certas proprietates & agendi virtutes naturæ concedimus, eatenus scientiam illam spiritibus mechanicis denegare non possumus."
48 Ibid.: "Hæc assertio coincidit cum illa Philosophorum & Medicorum communi, quod fiat quidem prima partium delineatio ex seminali materia per virtutem formatricem, quæ tamen non sufficit, nisi sanguis maternus affluat, quo tanquam alimento partes incrementum suscipiunt & generationem suam absoluunt."
49 Ibid., p. 12: "Hæc humana generatio finem suum perfecte assequeretur, nisi primis, purisque seminibus impuritates quædam diuina maledictione superuenissent, qua ratione morborum generatio suboritur."

which reason Horst considered the origin of disease to be metaphysical (*præter naturam*). Horst regarded this doctrine as "not absurd," since there are diseases that have internal antecedent causes:

> For unless the seeds of such diseases were either contained within us or communicated to us, mixed with our food and air, they would never occur. Hence it is established in general that some causes of diseases are internal, born with us, but others are external, communicated by the air and foods. In the second place, add to this the idea that seeds of disease supervened on the principles of our generation by virtue of the divine curse. This agrees very well with holy scripture, where it is evident that every kind of disease eventually arose after the Fall, because at that time new tinctures supervened on the first seeds, placed in the invisible treasuries of the elements, and by the mixture of these tinctures, the beauty of all creation was transplanted into a miserable fate, as Petrus Severinus says in chapter twelve of the *Idea*.[50]

From this statement it is apparent that Horst also adopted Severinus' account of the origin and generation of diseases from *semina* that were stained by tinctures, rather than heeding Erastus' opinion that attributing diseases to original *semina* was a Manichæan heresy. Severinus' theory explained that the morbific nature of the seeds was not created in the beginning, but rather imposed as tinctures on already extant seeds, a point repeated by Horst: "In the third place, it is to be added that morbific seeds are not found separately, but that they adhere to other seeds and principles."[51] This agrees well with the Galenic conception of disease as something that does not exist by itself, *per se*, but rather happens to

---

50 Ibid., p. 12: "Nisi enim talium morborum semina vel nobis inessent, vel alimentorum, aerisque medio nobis communicarentur, nunquam acciderent. Hinc in communi alias morborum causas internas nobiscum nasci, alias vero extrinsecas ab aere, alimentisque communicari statuitur. Additur secundo loco, quod semina morborum diuina maledictione superuenerint principiis generationis nostræ, quod maxime conuenit cum scriptura sacra, qua patet omne morborum genus post lapsum tandem aduenisse, quia tum demum primis seminibus in thesauris elementorum inuisibilibus collocatis nouæ tincturæ superuenerunt, quarum mixtione in sortem calamitosam totius creaturæ pulchritudo transplantata est, *vt inquit Pet. Seuer. in Idea cap. 12*."

51 Ibid., p. 12: "Tertio loco subiicitur, quod semina morbosa non seorsim inueniantur, sed quod aliis seminibus atque principiis adhæreant."

another body – ours![52] Here Horst had put his finger on a sore spot, a fundamental difference between the Galenists and the Paracelsians regarding the ontology of disease, and he attempted a reconciliation by interpreting Severinus' doctrine of tinctures and *semina* in Galenic terms. However, he fully understood the frustration that Galenists had expressed over the imprecise Paracelsian definition of disease, noting that "Hermetic" physicians use the term "disease" to denote not only the ailment, but also its cause and symptom, and that, unlike the Galenists, they prefer to think of all these as aspects of one thing.

After considering inflammation and the generation of fevers from both the spagyric and Galenist points of view, citing Quercetanus as a source, Horst concluded that the chemical theory, which held that these were caused by some kind of inflamed sulphur, had some merit:

> Hence, fevers are generated from corrupt beans, meats, fish, oils, grain, and wine that are polluted with febrile tinctures, according to Severinus, because resolved, sulphurous impurities are contained in impure foods of this sort.[53]

Horst did not find this assertion at variance with Galenic doctrine, because it is evident that some sort of flammable exhalation is present in "the impure and foetid excrements of the first coction," which inflame when brought near a burning candle.[54]

Horst continued in this same vein, considering the origin of catarrhs, the generation of calculus, how diseases can mix, how hereditary diseases arise, and where diseases arise, from both Paracelsian and Galenist perspectives. In general he gave Galenic readings to "Hermetic" doctrines, but clearly he was seeking to construct a better, reconciled medical philosophy rather than merely to refute or deny the Paracelsian successes.

---

52 Ibid.: "Hoc optime conuenit cum essentia morbi, quæ per se non subsistit, sed alteri nimirum corpori nostro accidit."

53 Ibid., p. 16: "Hinc igitur ex leguminibus corruptis, carnibus, piscibus, oleribus, frumentis, vino impuritatibus febrilibus inquinatis febres generantur, teste Seuerino, quia in eiusmodi alimentis impuritates sulphureæ resolutæ continentur."

54 Ibid.: "Videmus enim, sensu teste quod impuri & foetidi primæ coctionis excrementi fuligines & vapores instar sulphuris accendantur, vbi flatus emissi candelis ardentibus inflammantur."

One of these successes was *semina* theory, which proved useful to explain the metaphysical origins of diseases, how they enter the body (or are in it at birth), and how occult entities give rise to manifest diseases:

> It should be noted that the roots and rudiments of most diseases are hidden, so that although their mature fruits are perceived, the beginnings of their courses and their developments are not at all observed. For this reason, the origins of the fruits are very often sought from other directions than in those places where their impressed tinctures are apprehended. But the Galenists can in no way deny this, since frequently it happens that an "affect" is present whose root is elsewhere than in the affected part.[55]

Severinus would have approved.

DANIEL SENNERT AND OTHERS

The widespread interest in and adoption of Severinian Paracelsianism did not escape the attention of Daniel Sennert, the prolific critic of Paracelsus. He gave Severinus' doctrines special attention in his *De chymicorum cum Aristotelicis et Galenicis consensu ac dissensu Liber* (1619). This book is a defense of chemistry, to which end Sennert offered an account of its origins and critically evaluated Paracelsian contributions to the art. Here he singled out Severinus as an important Paracelsian exponent:

> In the year 1493, in Switzerland, Philippus Theophrastus Paracelsus was born ... whom Alexander of Suchten, Dorn, Phædrus, Thurneisser, and P. Severinus Danus have followed. Yet even these do not quite

---

55 Ibid., p. 19: "Notandum tamen, quod radices & primordia morborum plerumque occulta sint, ita vt quamuis illorum maturi fructus percipiantur, exordia tamen itinerum & progressiones nequaquam perspectæ sint, quam ob causam sæpius aliunde fructuum origines petuntur, quam iis in locis, vbi impressæ eorundem tincturæ deprehenduntur. Quod ipsum Galenici nullo modo negare queunt, cum frequenter accidat, vt affectus adsit, cuius radix alibi, quam in affecta parte quæritur."

agree, either with Paracelsus or among themselves. Nevertheless, most of those who today would be called iatrochemists follow Petrus Severinus, who has undertaken to bring the doctrines thrown out here and there by Paracelsus into a learned form, better than Paracelsus himself. For this reason, today a new school, as it were, has been born, which can be called Severinian.[56]

We have seen in the previous chapters that the Severinian *semina* theory was known in England and had a definite presence at the Parisian *Jardin*; we can therefore surmise that the identification of a "Severinian" school of thought by Libavius and Sennert refers especially to the widespread adoption of the concept of *semina* regulating the "inner economy" of bodies, as is evident in the work of Horst and of Reusner before him. Sennert's recognition of Severinus as a prominent Paracelsian accounts for why he directed his criticism of Paracelsianism to Severinus.[57] One by one, Sennert critically examined the Paracelsian terms to which Severinus had given special meaning – anatomy, tincture, *archeus*, etc. – sometimes quoting at length from the *Idea medicinæ* and taking note of the opinions of Libavius and Erastus where relevant.[58] And although he recognized Severinus' efforts to correct some of the doctrines of Paracelsus,[59] in the end he regarded many of the Paracelsian terms that

---

56 Sennert, *De chymicorum*, p. 57: "Natus est tandem anno Christi 1493 in Helvetia Philippus Theophrastus Paracelsus ... Quem secuti sunt Alexander Suchtenius, Dornæus, Phædro, Dornheiserus, P. Severinus Danus; qui ipsi tamen nec cum Paracelso, nec inter se plane consentiunt. Plerique tamen, qui hodie Chymiatri audire volunt, Petrum Severinum, qui dogmata a Paracelso hinc inde disjecta in artis formam redigere conatus est, potius, quam ipsum Paracelsum, sequuntur. Hinc hodie nova quasi secta nata est, quæ Severiana dici potest."

57 Ibid., p. 106: "Quantæ auctoritatis apud multos sit P. Severinus quondam Regis Daniæ Medicus, omnibus notum est." [How great an authority P. Severinus, former physician to the King of Denmark, is for many is known to all.]

58 Ibid., pp. 111ff.

59 For example, Sennert understood that Severinus gave a subtle interpretation to the microcosm-macrocosm correspondence, which was apparently rather grossly stated by Paracelsus; that the various stones, trees, gems, and herbs of the world are not literally in man, but rather that the same principles active in these, their properties, are also at work in man. This was a proposition Sennert did not deny. Ibid., p. 135: "Atque hoc si voluit P. Severinus, dum *pag 319.* in homine non bovem, non cupressum, sed proprietates horum quærere jubet; ipsi non plane adversamur, imo summe necessarium esse putamus,
→

Severinus had used as merely new words for old concepts and thought that much of Severinus' metaphysics was but a recent version of "a common doctrine about forms, especially of living things, which are called souls."[60]

No doubt Sennert and Libavius were correct in their judgement of the great influence of the *Idea medicinæ* on their contemporaries. Despite their criticisms, Severinus' doctrines, particularly his *semina* theory, continued to offer medical writers a cogent explanation for the generation of diseases which was compatible with a Paracelsian reading of Genesis and therefore was religiously satisfying. The success of this metaphysics is evident in a book on vital anatomy written by Johann Sophron Kozak (1602-1685) and dedicated to the town councilmen of Bremen. This tract is distinctly Paracelsian, and Kozak frequently cited both Paracelsus and his followers, including Severinus and Thomas Moffet.[61] Kozak held to the Paracelsian interpretation of Genesis as an account of the world's creation through chemical processes that are guided by a vital *spiritus mechanicus*, which pervades all.[62] Generation subsequent to the initial creation is the development of a mixture of celestial and elemental seeds located in *matrices*.[63] Man, the microcosm, has all sorts of seeds in his elemental body, and these are the authors of all changes, generations, and transplantations. It is for this reason that the human body is a domicile

→ ut Medicus inquirat, quæ gemmæ, mineralia & metalla, plantæ ac animalia, imo si fieri posset, stellæ cum homine & singulis ejus partibus consensum & dissensum habeant." [And if Severinus wished this, when he demanded on page 319 [of *Idea medicinæ*] that not cattle, nor cypress, be sought in man, but the properties of these, then we ourselves clearly do not disagree. Indeed, we judge it wholly necessary that the physician inquire which gems, minerals and metals, plants and animals, indeed if it can be done, which stars, have agreement and disagreement with man and his individual parts.]

60 Under the marginal rubric "Semina & astra Severini sunt formæ rer. nat." [The *semina* and *astra* of Severinus are the forms of natural things], Sennert wrote "Ista autem omnia quæ de Seminibus & Astris a Severino & alijs Chymicis ex eo traduntur, si in genere spectes, nova non sunt, sed vulgatam de formis, inprimis viventium, quæ Animæ dicuntur, doctrinam continent." [Moreover, all those things which are said about *semina* and *astra* by Severinus, and other chemists from him, if you contemplate them in general, they are not new, but comprise a common doctrine about forms, especially of living things, which are called souls.] Ibid., p. 181.

61 Johann Sophron Kozak, *Anatomia vitalis microcosmi in qua naturæ humanæ proprietates ... explicantur* (Bremen: Berthold Villerian, 1636), p. 268.

62 Ibid., pp. 104-7.

63 Ibid., pp. 67-68.

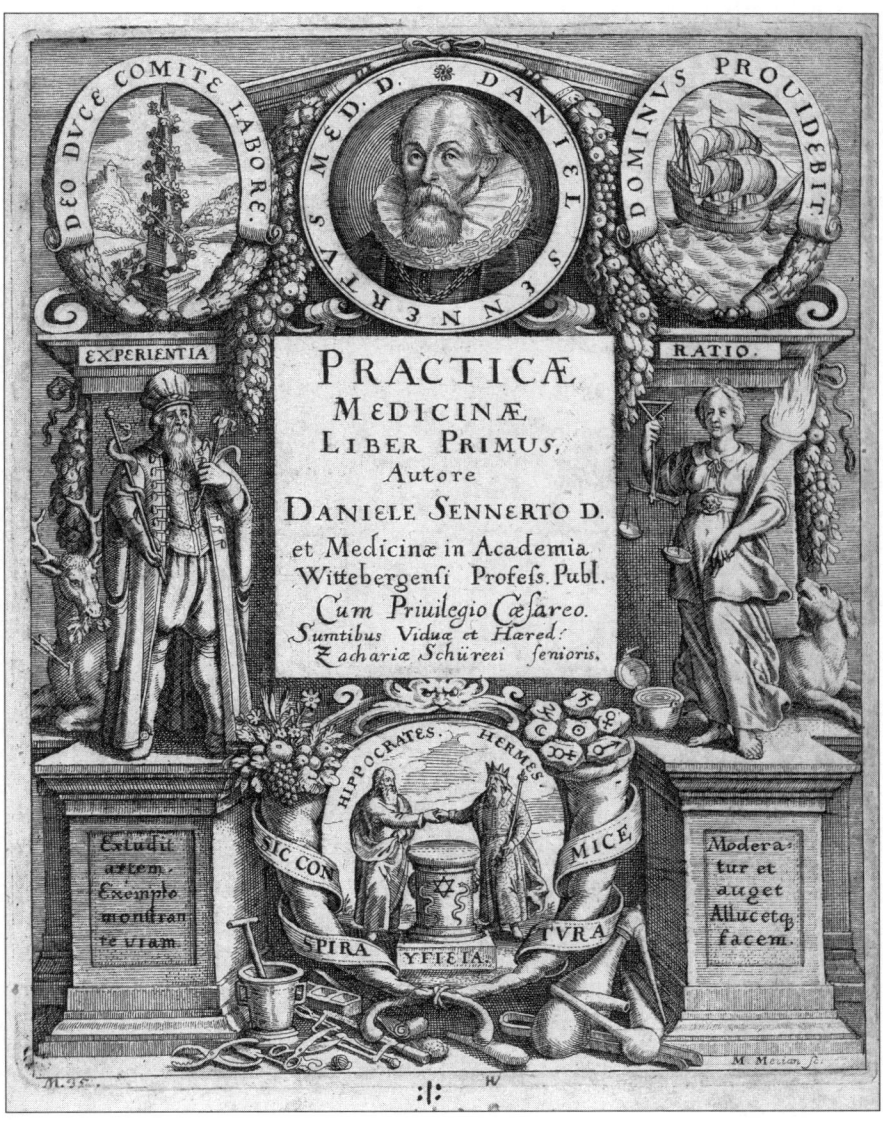

This title page from Daniel Sennert's Practicæ medicæ liber quartus *(1628)* illustrates his commitment to bringing chemical medicine (symbolized by Hermes and
the metalic/planetary symbols) into agreement with traditional medical therapeutics
(symbolized by Hippocrates and plants), which is emblematized by the two figures
shown shaking hands over "health" (Hygieia). Courtesy of The Danish National
Library of Science and Medicine.

of life and death.[64] The meeting and cooperation of these *semina*, their power and way of generating and transplanting, are prominent parts of Kozak's book, as he explained in the introductory dedication.[65]

According to Kozak's view, people possess within them both health-giving and morbific *semina*. The resolutions of the latter cause diseases, despite Sennert's criticism of Severinus' opinion that diseases come from seeds.[66] For Sennert, diseases have no substantial existence, but remain as qualities (accidents) of beings; To consider diseases as things is to mix categories. But, as Kozak wrote,

> In so doing I do not confuse the highest families of things, as [Sennert] himself feared, for I imitate not logic, by abstracting terms for things, but physics, by investigating the natures of things, as is fitting for a physician. The method of teaching pertains to logic, but that of know-ing pertains to physics. The very talented Dane, Severinus, preferred a single bread-making to all the meager arrangements [*digestionibus*] of the predicaments [i.e. categories].[67]

Kozak, taking his methodological lead from the Paracelsians, argued that the senses are better friends to the physician than are Aristotle and Plato, and he prefered a medical theory based on chemical principles to one based on didactic logic, which Severinus had called the method of the geometers. *Semina* theory provided what Kozak needed: explanations for the timings of diseases, their chemical operation, their transplanta-tion, and their curing. For the art of medicine is intended not to await

---

64 Ibid., p. 54.

65 Kozak (Ibid., p. 136) regarded the "chaos" that was the Paracelsian, quality-less matter from which the *semina* fashioned bodies, as a vapor. This is interesting in light of the transformation of "chaos" from prime matter to a concept of "gas," which has been credited to Van Helmont. See Pagel, *Paracelsus*, 2d ed., p. 358.

66 Kozak, *Anatomia vitalis*, pp. 156-57.

67 Ibid., p. 157: "Idque agendo summa rerum genera non confundo, ut ipse metuit, nam modo non Logicum, voces a rebus abstrahendo, sed Physicum rerum naturas indagando, ut Medicum decet imitor. Modus docendi ad Logicum, Sciendi autem ad Physicum pertinet. Ingeniosissimus Severinus Danus, unum Panificium omnibus jejunis prædicamentorum digestionibus anteponit." Severinus made such a claim in *Idea medicinæ*, p. 31: "Ego certe unicum Panificium, omnibus Modalium subtilitatibus & ieiunis Prædicamentorum digestionibus antepono."

or bring on the maturation of disease, but rather to speed, impede, or transplant its development.[68] And this meant attempting to alter the disease-causing *semina*, expel them, or deprive them of the conditions they require for development. Like Paracelsus and Severinus, Kozak believed that no disease was incurable, if only one understood its nature and knew how to affect it:

> For that reason Severinus the Dane said that whether the impurities and roots of diseases are introduced into the human anatomy by the hereditary seed of the parents, through the fault of foodstuffs, or from the harm caused by external impressions, they have a medicine in nature, with whose help they can be separated, resolved, and removed, leaving the first root of human nature unharmed and unaltered.[69]

Thus, Kozak's medicine illustrates that although the Paracelsians maintained a theory of disease and treatment that differed considerably from the Galenic doctrine, the core of traditional therapy, namely diet, purgation, and venesection, retained a place in their medicine. But whereas these three previously were used to restore a deficiency or remove a surfeit of the body's four basic constituent humors, now they were employed to control the intake or expel noxious *semina* or the harmful impurities that they produced; besides evacuating them through the urine, stools, vomit, and "insensible transpirations," one could also rid the body of them through bleeding.[70]

That medical writers continued to rely on Severinus as a major source of Paracelsian theory in the mid seventeenth century is also evident from *Gemma magica oder magisches Edelgestein* (1688) by Abraham von Franckenberg. In the preface to the reader, dated 1641, the author directs us to examine the secrets of nature according to the true judgements

---

68 Kozak, *Anatomia vitalis*, p. 189.
69 Ibid., p. 222: "Ideo inquit Severinus Danus, sive hæreditario parentum semine, sive alimentorum culpa, sive externarum impressionum iniuria, impuritates & radices morborum in humanam anatomiam introducuntur, medicinam in natura habent, cujus beneficio, separari, resolvi & aboleri possunt, illæsa & constante manente radice prima humanæ naturæ."
70 Ibid., pp. 245-6.

of Paracelsus, Sendivogius, and Severinus.[71] In the text itself Abraham von Franckenberg singled out "the *Idea medicinæ* of the famous Doctor Severinus Danus" as a supplement to Paracelsus' *Philosophy to the Athenians* and *Great Astronomy* for understanding Paracelsus' interpretation of *Genesis* and also concerning the astral virtues in *semina*, namely the faculties that form matter.[72]

The concept of a *secta Severiana*, as indentified by Libavius and Sennert, persisted in seventeenth and eighteenth-century medical literature and may even have helped draw the attention of those interested in Paracelsian doctrine to the *Idea medicinæ*. When, for example, Johann Gabriel Drechssler mentioned Paracelsus and his followers in his 1673 treatise on the transmutation of metals, he wrote that "a large number of today's [chemical physicians] follow P. Severinus, who brought the doctrines thrown out here and there by Paracelsus into a learned form, whence a Severinian school originated."[73] The verbal similarity between this assessment and that given by Sennert strongly suggests that Drechssler paraphrased Sennert's 1619 treatise and may not have actually read the *Idea medicinæ*. On the other hand, since William Davidson and his editor judged there to be sufficient demand for the book to warrant a third edition in 1660, somebody must have been reading it. Indeed, references to Severinus and his work continued to appear in medical books that took a large view of the subject and sketched the historical development of the field.

Hermann Conring's *In universam artem medicam ... introductio* (1687) and Johann Conrad Barchusen's *De medicinæ origine et progressu dissertationes* (1723) provide additional examples of Severinus' persistence in the medical literature of both antagonists and defenders of "Hermetic" medical doctrines.[74] Conring was an outspoken critic of Paracelsian medicine,

---

71 Abraham von Franckenberg, *Gemma magica oder magisches Edelgestein* (Amsterdam, 1688), sig. A 3r: "Drauff wird uns dem wahren Urtheil *Theophrasti, Sendivogii*, und *Severini Dani* nach das Licht der Nature welches sonsten unsern Augen nicht durchsichtig jederzeit richtige Unterweisung verleyhen die Geheimnissen zuerforschen."

72 Ibid., pp. 25-6, and 58.

73 Johann Gabriel Drechssler, *Disputatio I, De metallorum transmutatione* (Leipzig: Wittigau, 1673) f. 6v: "Plerique tamen P. Severinum ex hodiernis, qvi dogmata a Paracelso hinc inde disjecta in artis formam redegit, seqvuntur, unde *secta Severina* nata est."

74 Conring, *In universam artem medicam*; Johann Conrad Barchusen, *De medicinæ origine et progressu dissertationes* (Trajecti ad Rhenum: Paddenburg and Croon, 1723).

which he assailed in his 1648 treatise on the "new" Hermetic medicine of the Paracelsians, and again in subsequent tracts that he wrote as part of an ongoing debate with the Danish chemical physician, Ole Borch, who will be mentioned again in the next chapter.[75] Barchusen's book was a revision of his earlier *Historia medicinæ* (1710), which was written in dialogue format. After devoting the nineteenth dissertation of this book to Paracelsus, Barchusen surveyed the hypotheses of Severinus, Croll, Scheunemann, and Van Helmont in the twentieth. It begins:

> Paracelsus had several disciples [*sectatores*], who followed him blindly and swore by the words of the master. Yet, there were others, who, if they rejected his doctrines that seemed to be absurd and inharmonious beyond measure, at least they organized them and made them less harsh. I consider Petrus Severinus to be among their number, a man exceedingly well versed in the study of the literature, and from him Paracelsus' theory was first handed down to posterity.[76]

Like Libavius, Barchusen considered Croll and Scheunemann to be followers of Severinus.[77] However, unlike Libavius and Conring, Barchusen was somewhat sympathetic to "Hermetic" medicine.[78]

---

75 Hermann Conring, *De hermetica Ægyptiorum vetere et Paracelsicorum nova medicina liber unus* (Helmstedt: Henningius Mullerius, 1648).

76 Barchusen, *De medicinæ origine*, p. 397: "Sectatores quidem Paracelsus habuit nonnullos, qui eum cæco impetu secuti sunt, & in verba magistri jurarunt; fuerunt tamen alii, qui ejus dogmata, quæ extra modum absona & absurda videbantur, sin rejecerint, saltem compta & mitiora redderent. Horum in numero habeo Petrum Severinum, virum oppido in studio literarum multum versatum, abs quo doctrina Paracelsi primum posteritati propagata est."

77 Ibid., p. 404: "Crollius ... est, ut ex ejus scriptis liquet, in numero sectatorum Severini," and p. 410: "Scheunemannus, quamvis pleraque Severini placita amplexus, cumulavit tamen ea variis dictionibus obscuris."

78 Barchusen summarized the chief points of Severinus' doctrine, ibid., pp. 397-404. A commemorative poem affixed to his earlier *Historia medicinæ* (Amsterdam: Jansonius-Wæsbergii, 1710) reads: "Who does not know that there is no one more accomplished in the Hermetic art than you, Barchusen"? [Barchusi Hermetica quam sis perfectus in arte, / Est nemo, qui non noverit.]

Chapter Eight

THE "SEVERINIAN SCHOOL" IN SCANDINAVIA

𝕬LTHOUGH SEVERINUS lived and worked in Denmark for thirty two years after he completed the *Idea medicinæ*, the reception given his theories in Scandinavia was muted when compared with what the German authors had to say. This is quite likely owing to the correspondingly smaller interest in Paracelsianism in general that was exhibited by the seventeenth-century Danish, Norwegian, and Swedish authors.[1] Nevertheless, there were several who read and commented on the *Idea medicinæ* and used its doctrines, and there continued to be an influx of Paracelsian impulses from Germany, which kept interest in the Dane's ideas alive.

The *Idea medicinæ* and Severinus himself were no doubt sources of Paracelsian doctrine for his contemporaries in Denmark, for example Tycho Brahe and Tycho's Norwegian student, Kort Aslakssøn. Even if Severinus and Brahe eventually became estranged, toward the end of the century, they shared common philosophical interests and made up a part of the circle of "Renaissance" intellectuals patronized by Frederik II. Both were close friends of Pratensis, and we can suppose they came into contact at the latter's house in Copenhagen (until Pratensis' death in 1576) whenever the great astronomer visited town. Or, conceivably they met at court, where Brahe's presence was occasionally required, and

---

1 In the early modern period Norway and Iceland were ruled by the King of Denmark, and Finland was a province of Sweden. An Icelandic manuscript, "Ex Paracelso Plinio et alijs de magnete" (University of Copenhagen, Arnamagnæanske Samling, A.M. 191a 8vo), shows that Paracelsus was known even in Iceland. I know of no Icelandic reference to Severinus.

where Severinus was royal physician. Brahe did not write anything that unambiguously reflects Severinus' ideas, although he evidently shared a similar Paracelsian view of the world, as was established earlier. Kort Aslakssøn, however, incorporated Paracelsian doctrines into his cosmology, some of which were clearly drawn from Severinus. Aslakssøn became a leading theologian in the first decade of the century, making his interest in chemical philosophy of importance to understanding the interaction of Lutheranism and Paracelsianism in Denmark during the years prior to the outbreak of the Thirty Years' War.[2]

KORT ASLAKSSØN

The earliest indication we have that the *Idea medicinæ* was being read in Denmark occurs in a treatise written by Kort Aslakssøn (Cunradus Aslacus Bergensis, 1564-1624). Born in Bergen, Norway, as his Latin name indicates, Aslakssøn was admitted to the University of Copenhagen, where he studied philosophy and theology, in 1584.[3] From 1590 to 1593 he assisted Tycho Brahe at Hven and then returned to Copenhagen to take a master's degree under the direction of Severinus' colleague, Anders Krag. Aslakssøn received his doctorate in theology, was appointed professor in 1607, and is best known to historians as a theologian.[4] Nevertheless,

2 Up until about 1615, the Philippists in Denmark were struggling to keep the much more conservative Gnesiolutherans, or Lutheran hardliners, from gaining control of the state church. The Philippists, or followers of the teachings of Philip Melanchthon, were connected with the renaissance in education begun by Frederik II and were somewhat more sympathetic to Paracelsianism than were the Saxon Gnesiolutherans, who sought to weed out Calvinist-sounding doctrines from the Lutheran church. Tycho Brahe can certainly be numbered among the Philippists, as was Kort Aslakssøn and quite probably Petrus Severinus. The success of the hardliners in silencing the hitherto dominant Philippist theologians in Denmark and Kort Aslakssøn's involvement in this are treated in Shackelford, *Paracelsianism in Denmark and Norway*, chs. 5 and 6; and idem, "Unification and the Chemistry of the Reformation."

3 Francis Bull, "Aslakssøn," *NBL*, vol. 1, p. 294.

4 Ibid., p. 295; Rørdam, *KUH*, vol. 3, pp. 521 and 587. For a general biography of Aslakssøn, see Garstein, *Cort Aslakssøn*. A portion of my analysis of Aslakssøn's cosmology and Ole Worm's subsequent reaction is printed in Shackelford, "Rosicrucianism, Lutheran Orthodoxy, and the Rejection of Paracelsianism."

he was a prolific writer, treating strictly theological issues as well as more generally expounding a Christian cosmology.[5] His first significant text, begun the year after his departure from Hven, was a lengthy tract dedicated to Tycho Brahe and titled *Three Books on the Nature of the Threefold Heaven* (*De natura cæli triplicis libelli tres*, 1597).[6] The three aspects of "heaven" noted in the title, the aerial, sidereal, and eternal, are reminiscent of the threefold division of the world into terrestrial, celestial, and supercelestial regions, which was common to Renaissance Platonism. The world view described in this text agrees with Paracelsian cosmology in fundamental aspects and indicates a familiarity with the arguments of chemical philosophy. It is in this respect much what one might expect from a student of Tycho Brahe and Anders Krag.

Aslakssøn portrayed nature as a living thing that is composed of corporeal and incorporeal beings knit together by a pervasive world soul – a psycho-physical principle or spirit that radiates through the cosmos and is the form of the world, which sustains all Creation.[7] He compared this spirit to that described by chemical philosophy:

> In chemistry, too, a very subtle essence, drawn out of minerals, herbs, and other natural things by the spagyric art, is also called spirit; not because it is entirely spiritual and incorporeal, since clearly it makes itself evident to the senses, but because with respect to the rest of the principles and bodies it is of a certain more divine, noble, and subtle essence.[8]

5 Aslakssøn was one of several writers of the late sixteenth and early seventeenth centuries who were attempting to create a "Mosaic physics" or natural philosophy that was compatible with their interpretation of *Genesis*. See Ann Blair, "Mosaic Physics and the Search for a Pious Natural Philosophy in the Late Renaissance," *Isis* 91(2000): 32-58.

6 Kort Aslakssøn (Cunradus Aslacus Bergensis), *De natura cæli triplicis libelli tres* (Siegen, 1597). A list of Aslakssøn's literary output can be found in Rørdam, *KUH*, vol. 3, pp. 595-99.

7 Garstein, *Cort Aslakssøn*, pp. 179 and 190.

8 Aslakssøn, *De natura cæli triplicis*, pp. 93-94: "In Chymia quoque, essentia subtilior, quæ e mineralibus, herbis, aliisque naturis Spagyrica arte elicitur, Spiritus quoque nominatur; non quod omnino spiritualis & incorporea sit: quippe cum sensibus sese obviam præbeat: sed quod reliquorum principiorum & corporum respectu, divinioris, nobilioris ac subtilioris cujusdam essentiæ sit."

Turning to the nature of heaven, Aslakssøn considered it plausible that heaven is also living, since "it is endowed with a certain *energetic* faculty" and an *energetic* soul; "For what is life, taken in a broad sense, other than an *activity* implanted in created things by God?"[9] To support this view, Aslakssøn quoted Severinus' criticism of Peripatetic philosophy, of the inability of disputations to teach us about nature: "What, he asks, is the use of words? Which ones are endowed with a strong faculty of savors and smells? Who will claim that things endowed with a strong faculty of savors and smells are dead? There are distinctions and degrees of life, as of vital Balsam; and not all things are manifestly living."[10] Severinus' ideas agreed with what Aslakssøn had learned from Hermes Trismegistus, namely that movement denoted life, and that even the earth was alive with generation and alteration.[11]

Aslakssøn proceeded to discuss the vital activity of animals and vegetables, and, turning to minerals he again depended on Severinus' authority:

> About this matter Doctor Petrus Severinus, in his *Idea medicinæ*, said very clearly "minerals also live. However, entangled in the shackles of bodies, they cannot produce vital actions. Nevertheless, if they are reduced to act, they demonstrate vital qualities by the extraordinary virtue of their actions." And after that he said, "by most they are considered to be wholly lacking life. But certainly those who have more diligently

9 Ibid., p. 100: "Plausibilior multo eorum sententia, qui cælum propterea animatum esse dixerunt, quod ἐνεργητικῇ quadam facultate præditum sit. Siquidem quicquid virtute aliqua imbutum, id anima quoque ἐνεργητικῇ donatum esse non dubitarunt. Quid enim vita lato modo sumpta, aliud, quam ἐνέργεια rebus creatis a Deo insita?"

10 Ibid.: "Quid, inquit, verbis opus? Quæcunque saporum & odorum valida facultate præditæ sunt, ea quis mortua pronuntiabit? Vitarum discrimina sunt & gradus, ut balsami vitalis; nec omnia manifeste vivunt." This quotation is almost verbatim from Severinus, *Idea medicinæ*, p. 25.

11 Aslakssøn, *De natura cæli triplicis*, p. 101: "Totum, inquit, quod in Mundo est, aut crescendo aut decrescendo movetur. Quod autem movetur, id propterea vivit: & cum omnia moveantur, etiam Terra, maxime motu generativo & alterativo, ipsa quoque vivit." This is likely a paraphrase of Ficino's translation of the Hermetic Corpus. See Marsilio Ficino, *Opera omnia* (Torino: Bottega d' Erasmo, 1959), p. 1854: "Quod est in mundo, aut crescendo aut decrescendo, movetur. Quod vero movetur, id præterea vivit."

investigated the workshops of those [minerals] have often demonstrated manifest signs of life in them. For they grow, have their times of maturity, are nourished, and produce excrement, which they often cast off in powerful paroxysms, to the miners' great fear; they leave other [excrements] behind on the surface a little at a time."[12]

Aslakssøn's reading of Severinus is not just a peripheral reference, but fits in well with his basic metaphysics, his theory about the generation of beings from prime matter, which is plainly Paracelsian. He wrote in *De natura cæli triplicis* that the differences between beings arise through

the diverse operation of the Archeus and occult Nature, by which some things are more perfectly separated, elaborated, and brought to the desired end that he [Archeus] intended; others develop less perfectly, abandoned at intermediate stages, before reaching their highest end, whence also imperfect and less enduring [metals] result. Come out onto this worldly stage and assess the wonderful economy of nature. You will discover such a diversity in almost every single class of creatures, by which some are more perfect and enduring than others. Therefore, what prevents a similar diversity from occurring in that celestial workshop of nature from one and the same mass, but digested and exalted differently?[13]

---

12 Ibid., pp. 103-104: "De qua re etiam Doctor Petrus Severinus præclare in Idea Medicinæ: Vivunt quoque, ait, Mineralia, quamvis corporum compedibus implicata vitales actiones depromere non possunt: Nihilominus si in actum reducentur, mira actionum virtute vitales qualitates demonstrant. Et idem postea: A plurimis vita penitus carere existimantur. At certe vitæ manifesta indicia illis sæpe demonstrarunt qui illorum officinas diligentius scrutati sunt. Crescunt enim, maturitatis tempora habent, nutriuntur, excrementa pariunt, quæ potentibus paroxysmis sæpe rejiciunt magno Metallicorum pavore: alia paulatim in superficie relinquunt." The quotations are nearly verbatim from *Idea medicinæ*, pp. 24-25.

13 Aslakssøn, *De natura cæli triplicis*, pp. 150-51: "Metalla (si Metallographis & Chymicis credimus) ex una & eadem omnia materia proveniunt? Unde igitur tanta in his discrepantia & dissimilitudo, qua alia aliis præstantiora, perfectiora, diuturniora? Respondent tibi; ex diversa Archei & Naturæ occultæ operatione id fieri; qua alia perfectius digeruntur, elaborantur, & ad optatum, quem intendit finem perducuntur: Alia minus perfecte: quæ relinquuntur in intermediis, antequam ad summam metam perveniatur, spatiis; unde etiam imperfecta, & minus diuturna evadunt. Egredere in hanc mundanam scenam, & mirandam Naturæ oeconomiam expende. Reperies in singulis ferme Creaturarum generibus talem diversitatem, qua alia aliis perfectiora & diuturniora sunt. Quid igitur impedit, quo minus in cælesti illa Naturæ officina, ex una & eadem mole sed diversimode digesta & exaltata, similis contingat varietas?"

Aslakssøn's extension of the chemical process of creation to include the celestial realm, evident in the above passage, is characteristically Paracelsian but also reflects his own circumstances. As a student assistant at Uraniborg, he certainly knew that Tycho had proven that change occurs in the heavens, too, so that even stars and comets must be in some sense living. Another of Tycho's students, the astronomer Christian Sørensen from Longberg, known as Longomontanus, maintained that new stars and comets appearing in the heavens have seminal origins, a view clearly related to the Severinian *semina* theory.[14]

It is plausible, then, that Severinus' ideas were a part of intellectual discussion among the students of the celestial and terrestrial astronomies at Tycho Brahe's Uraniborg. It is apparent that Aslakssøn's cosmology was deeply affected by Paracelsian theory. He used Paracelsian terminology, describing the diversity in the material world as a product of chemical processes (digestion, separation, elaboration, exaltation), which are the function of the *archeus* or inner workman in nature. This view is consistent with Severinus' medical terminology and conception of the vital balsam as a vital principle providing food and medicine to the living organism, and Aslakssøn cites both Severinus and Thomas Moffet as sources. There is no hint that he abandoned this cosmology as he became more and more occupied with theology. In his 1605 oration at the university he again spoke of the world soul (*anima mundi*) that sustains the world, and he cited a series of Renaissance Platonists to support this assertion: Hieronymus Wolf, Sebastian Fox, Paracelsus, Patrizi, and Fernel.[15] It is evident from his 1613 work, *Physica et ethica Mosaica*, that he sought to fuse this Renaissance Platonist natural philosophy with the account of Creation in *Genesis* – a cosmological synthesis wholly in the spirit of the seventeenth-century Paracelsians.[16]

---

14 Christian Sørensen Longomontanus, *Disputatio prima astronomica* (Copenhagen, 1611). I have not seen this tract and rely on the account of it given in Kristian Moesgaard, "Cosmology in the Wake of Tycho Brahe's Astronomy," in *Cosmology, History, and Theology*, ed. Wolfgang Yourgrau and Allen D. Breck (New York: Plenum, 1977), pp. 293-305. The discussion of Longomontanus' *semina*-theory is on p. 299.

15 Garstein, *Cort Aslakssøn*, p. 179.

16 Ibid., p. 197. Kort Aslakssøn, *Physica et ethica Mosaica, ut antiquissima, ita vere christiania, duobus libris comprehensa* (Copenhagen, 1613). There is a continuity of approach and even text between Aslakssøn's 1597 *De natura cæli triplicis* and this 1613 book.

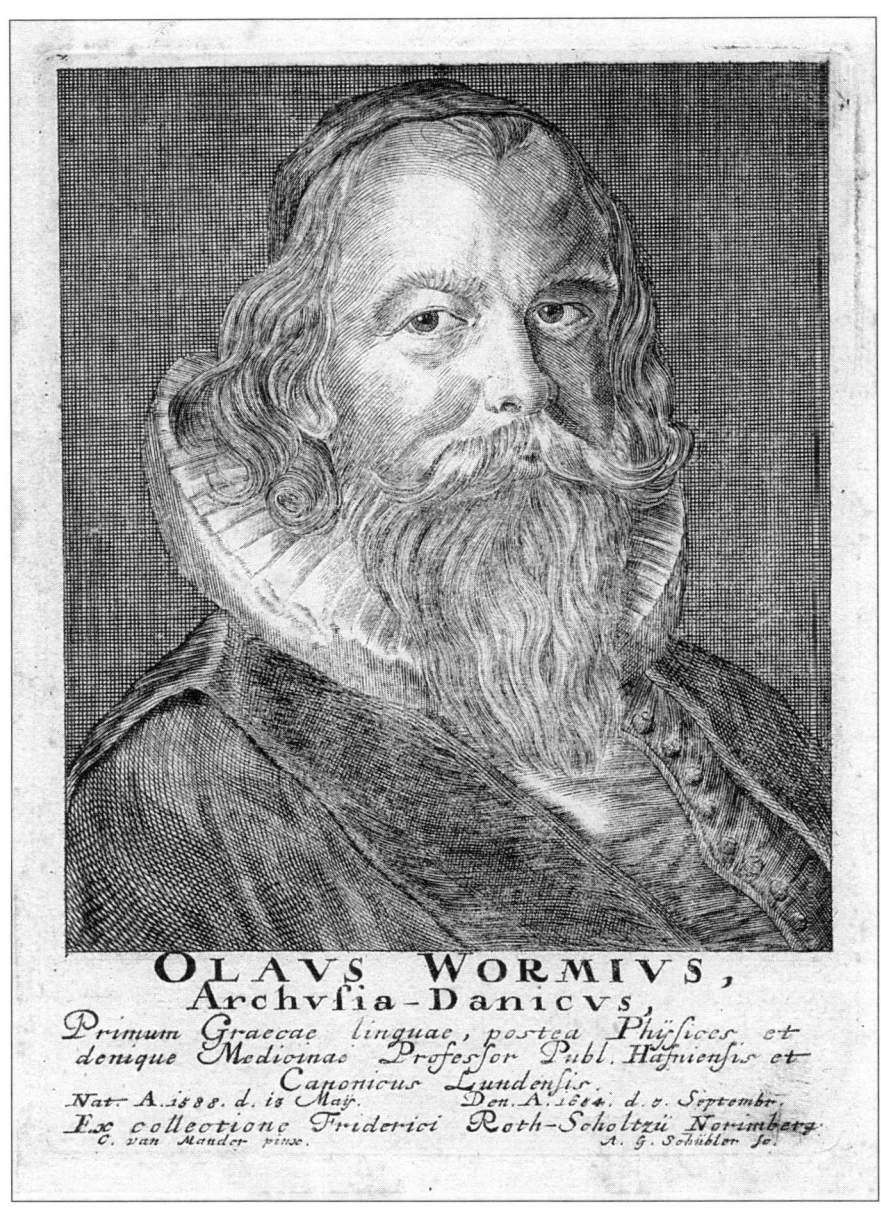

OLAVS WORMIVS,
Archvfia-Danicvs,
Primum Graecae linguae, postea Phisices et denique Medicinae Profesfor Publ. Hafniensis et Canonicus Lundensis.
Nat. A.1588. d. 13 May. Den. A.1654. d. 5 Septembr.
Ex collectione Friderici Roth-Scholtzü Norimberg.
C. van Mander pinx. *A. G. Schübler sc.*

Danish physician, professor, and collector of natural and artificial objects, Ole Worm. Courtesy of The Danish National Library of Science and Medicine.

ACADEMIC MEDICINE

After Severinus' death there were no prominent physicians in the academic medical community in Denmark who were receptive to Paracelsian ideas – Anders Krag had already died, and the two medical professors were Galenists. Therefore, when Ole Worm, as a young student of medicine, wished to study iatrochemistry, he went south. The fact that this man, who was later renowned as a medical professor, royal physician, and collector of *naturalia*, was eager to learn from the Paracelsians is little known and merits digression.[17]

In 1607 Ole Worm and his attendant, Michael Döring, were matriculated at Basel. Döring was keenly interested in the spagyric art and may have encouraged the young Worm's study in this direction.[18] At Basel, Worm came under the influence of the iatrochemist Jacob Zwinger, who, like his father Theodor Zwinger, sought to find and extract the valuable elements of Paracelsian doctrine, although without embracing Paracelsian cosmology. There, too, Worm made contact with the Paracelsian critics, Caspar Bauhin the elder and Felix Platter.[19] From Basel he traveled to Padua, from which place he wrote to Zwinger in 1609, telling him of his plans to travel to France in pursuit of the chemical

17 A version of the account of Ole Worm's interest in and rejection of Paracelsianism given here also appears in Shackelford, "Rosicrucianism, Lutheran Orthodoxy, and the Rejection of Paracelsianism." Worm's correspondence has been collected and rendered into modern Danish in *Breve fra og til Ole Worm*, an essential source for the history of science and medicine in seventeenth-century Denmark. H. D. Schepelern, *Museum Wormianum, dets forudsætninger og tilblivelse* (Aarhus: Wormianum, 1971), takes as its main subject the collecting activity for which Worm is best known today. One should not be fooled by the title, however, as the book is really an insightful biography of Ole Worm and his context. Ejnar Hovesen, *Lægen Ole Worm 1588-1654: En medicinhistorisk undersøgelse og vurdering* (Aarhus: Aarhus Universitetsforlag, 1987) contains some useful information and Danish translations.

18 Schepelern, *Museum Wormianum*, p. 57. Sprengel, *Versuch einer pragmatischen Geschichte der Arzneikunde*, 2d ed., vol. 3, pp. 423-24, identified Döring as a conciliator. He was a Hippocratic physician who rejected Paracelsian mysticism but defended the use of Paracelsian medicines and parts of Paracelsus' philosophical system, even against Erastus: "Auch *Michael Döring* aus Breslau, Professor in Giessen, gehört zu diesen Conciliatoren. Er war eigentlich ein Hippocratischer Arzt; aber die Arzneymittel des *Paracelsus*, und verschiedene Theile seines Systems vertheidigte er sogar gegen den *Erastus*."

19 Schepelern, *Museum Wormianum*, pp. 60-61.

art. He hoped Zwinger would commend him to Quercetanus and Turquet de Mayerne, two Paracelsian royal physicians whom he desired to
meet.[20] After returning to Copenhagen in 1610, Worm again set off in
search of iatrochemical enlightenment (in 1611), this time to Marburg,
with the intention of studying under the widely known Paracelsian
Johan Hartmann, who had recently become Europe's first professor of
chemistry. En route he visited Conrad Khunrath and Frederik Severinus
(Petrus Severinus' son) in Heidelberg.[21]

Marburg had become a major center of scientific activity under the
landgrafs Wilhelm and Moritz of Hessen-Kassel in the late sixteenth
and early seventeenth centuries. Chemical research was encouraged by
the patronage and active guidance of Moritz, whose intellectual network
drew Paracelsians to the principality. While much of this may have been
philosophical chemistry of an inward looking, Hermetic sort, there was
also an emphasis on iatrochemistry and a synthesis between medical
theory and chemical therapy, and many students came to Marburg to
learn chemical techniques from Hartmann.[22]

Worm's contact with Hartmann was fairly brief and not entirely
happy. He evidently found that the fees Hartmann demanded exceeded
the value of his teaching and he became disaffected.[23] But there were
others to choose from. Heinrich Petræus, with whom he had earlier
travelled to Italy, was now a professor of medicine at Marburg. He
was a devoted iatrochemist and interested in bridging the gap between

---

20 Ibid., pp. 66-67.
21 Ibid., pp. 46, 72-74. It should also be noted that Hartmann and Worm corresponded.
    A letter from Hartmann to Worm survives in Copenhagen, Kgl. Bibl., Rostgaard 33
    8vo Tillæg.
22 Moran, "Privilege, Communication, and Chemiatry," especially pp. 112, 116, and 120.
    On Hartmann's teaching of chemistry see Moran, *Chemical Pharmacy*, and idem., *The
    Alchemical World of the German Court*.
23 Several years later (26 February 1616), Ole Worm wrote to Niels Christensen Foss,
    who was then studying with Hartmann in Marburg. He warned him against having
    anything to do with Hartmann without first signing a contract, saying "Probably he is
    now selling to you what I bought from him earlier at a high price." [Maaske sælger han
    nu til Jer, hvad jeg tidligere for en høj Pris har afkøpt ham.] Worm advised Niels Foss
    to seek out instead an apothecary and to learn what he has to teach. Worm, *Breve*, vol.
    I, p. 9. In 1623 Worm again advised a student not to pay much for chemical enlighten-
    ment, citing his "own bitter experience" with Hartmann (Letter to Hans Andersen
    Skovgaard, ibid., p. 77: "Av egen bitter Erfaring kender jeg Hartmann."

Galenism and Paracelsianism.[24] Worm's dissatisfaction with Hartmann and subsequent attraction to Petræus' more conciliatory approach foreshadowed his later rejection of the extravagant philosophical claims of the Paracelsians.

Although Ole Worm probably intended to take his doctorate at Marburg, he left town because of plague and went to Kassel, where he met Gregor Horst. By this time Worm seems to have been won over to an eclecticism like that of Petræus and Horst, adopting a Galenism modified to accept Paracelsian therapeutic agents. Both Hartmann and Horst were conversant with Severinus' ideas, as was shown earlier, but Horst was less enthusiastic about Paracelsian medicine than was Hartmann. In any case, when responding to Ambrosius Rhodius' enquiry about Severinus' Paracelsianism many years later, Worm stated that he agreed with the opinions of Horst on such matters, indicating his familiarity with Horst's work.[25] From Kassel, Worm returned to Basel, where he quickly wrote his thesis, *Selecta controversiarum medicarum centuria*, and received his M.D. In the *prooemium* to this work, Worm declared himself to be the adherent of no single school, but dedicated to truth alone.[26] This is rhetoric, to be sure, but in Worm's case it is consistent with the attitude he maintained throughout his life.

As direct evidence for Worm's interest in Paracelsianism we have a rather long manuscript book attributed to Ole Worm and affirmed by the Danish scholar H.D. Schepelern to be for the most part written in his hand.[27] This book contains several short tracts, a number of which seem to be copies of Paracelsian writings or extracts from them. If the many references to Paracelsus and the Paracelsians are any indication,

24 Ibid., p. 75. Petræus' attempt to accommodate Galenism and Paracelsianism found written expression in Heinrich Petræus, *Nosologia harmonica* (Marburg, 1614-16).

25 Schepelern, *Museum Wormianum*, pp. 75-78. Although Worm's letter does not survive, Ambrosius Rhodius repeated in his reply to him 21 March 1641 that Worm said he held to Horstius' opinion on the elements. See Worm, *Breve*, vol. 2, p. 238. Rhodius had been Worm's student for a short time. He will be discussed at length in chapter nine.

26 Schepelern, *Museum Wormianum*, p. 80.

27 Copenhagen, Kgl. Bibl., Rostgaard 33 8vo. I am grateful to Dr. Schepelern, the foremost authority on Ole Worm, for personally affirming that most of this manuscript was written in Ole Worm's hand. I have listed its contents in the following note.

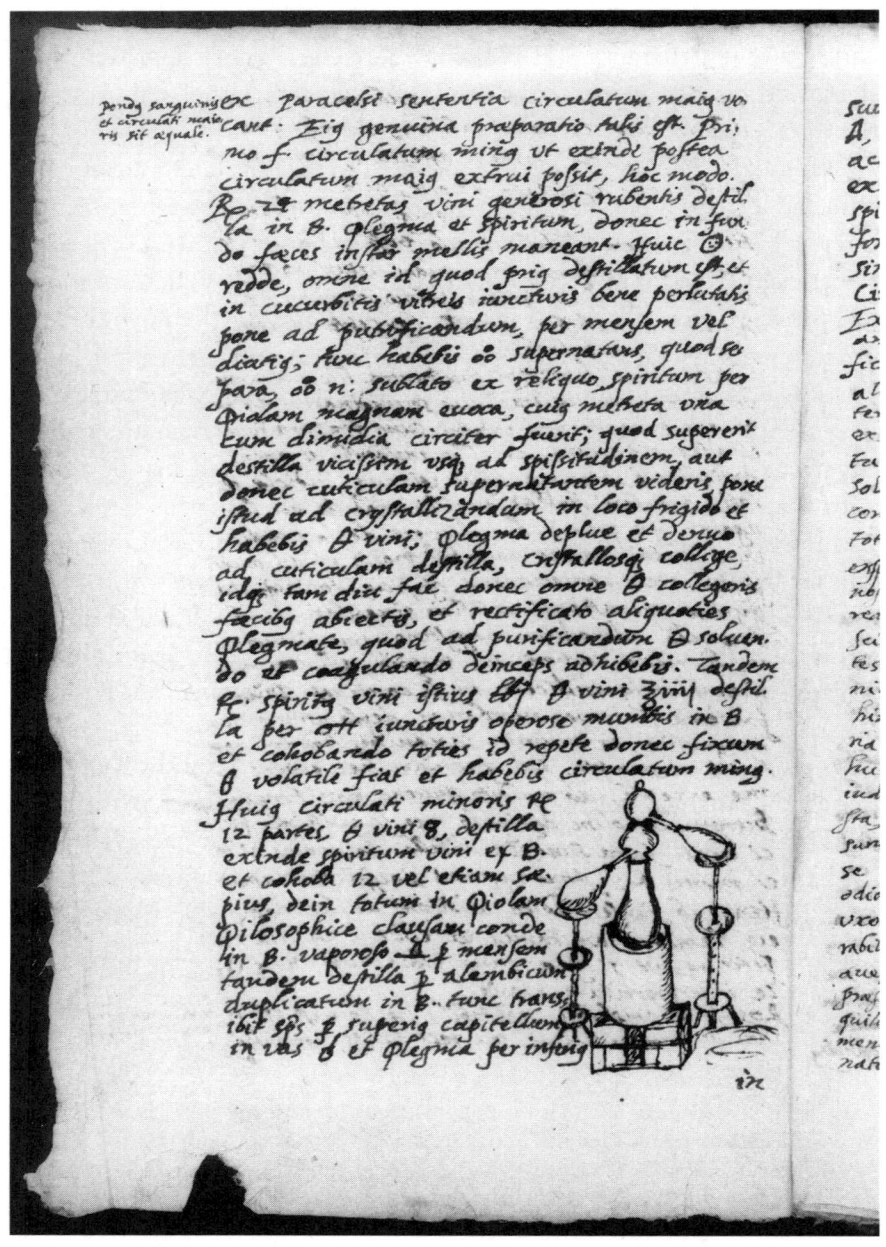

This page from Ole Worm's chemical notebook, part of the Rostgaard Collection at the Royal Library in Copenhagen, reveals his early interest in Paracelsian chemical medicine. Courtesy of Det Kongelige Bibliotek.

Worm had read quite a bit of the Paracelsian literature as a student, including Severinus' *Idea medicinæ.*[28]

From what has been said above, it is clear that Ole Worm actively sought iatrochemical knowledge and instruction while he was abroad during the years 1607-1612. After that he returned to Copenhagen to practice medicine and begin his climb up the academic ladder in 1613.[29] Although the teaching and practice of Paracelsian medicine had been established by Severinus and Johannes Pratensis in the 1570s, the attitude toward Paracelsianism exhibited by the University of Copenhagen's medical faculty in the early seventeenth century was mixed. After Severinus died (1602) no professorship of medicine was offered to a Paracelsian. Instead, Thomas Fincke and Gellius Sascerides promoted Galenism at the university. Despite this, the prevailing attitude in the sciences can best be described as eclectic.

A short tract from the 1620s on the proper course of study for medical students illustrates this broad eclecticism. This treatise, *De studio medico inchoando, continuando, et absolvendo,* was written by Caspar Bartholin, who was a professor of medicine at the University

28 Rostgaard 33 refers to Severinus frequently in the tract titled "De morbis eorumque causis secundum Medicinam Hermeticam." It is possible that this treatise was either copied from or inspired by one of Hartmann's texts.

   Tracts found in Rostgaard 33 8vo

   1. De generatione, mixtione, et transplantatione.
   2. Omnium morborum astralium et materialium acutorum et chronicorum vera et philosophica explicatio.
   3. De morbis eorumque causis secundum medicinam Hermeticam.
   4. Tractatus de tartaro.
   5. Diatribe iatrochymica de microcosmi usu medico.
   6. De fructibus terræ.
   7. De fructibus aquæ.
   8. De metallis.
   9. De præparatione et compositione medicamentorum chymicorum artificiosa Duncani Bornetti Scoti (Duncan Burnett, the only attributed text in Rostgaard 33).

   The rest of the manuscript contains miscellaneous medical and chemical notes, as well as notations concerning the history of Denmark, apparently written later and bound with the iatrochemical extracts.

29 Worm was initially hired as Professor of Pedagogy in 1613 and was promoted to professorships in Greek (1615) and Physics (1621) before finally achieving the desired chair in the medical faculty in 1624.

This page from Ole Worm's chemical notebook illustrates his familiarity with the ideas in Severinus' Idea medicinæ philosophicæ. *Courtesy of Det Kongelige Bibliotek.*

of Copenhagen from 1613 to 1624, when he took a chair in theology.[30] Ostensibly written as advice for the education of his sons and Peter Charisius, Severinus' grandson, it recommends that the student of medicine read from the Christian Bible every day, be well grounded in Latin and Greek logic, and study physics and mathematics, which he considered necessary to medical education. Astrology is included, too, since it was considered an important part of medicine. The medical student should read the leading authors on the natural history of metals, minerals, and stones (including Libavius), on Botany, and so on. When it comes to the study of medicine itself, he first mentioned Galen and Hippocrates, followed by Fernel and Sennert (especially for fevers), and for pharmacology, Cordus, Wecker, Quercetanus, etc. *Chemical pharmacology* is to be studied with care, and not only from whatever books might be currently available; one must seek arcana from learned men, even princes. Bartholin especially recommended the arcana that Tycho Brahe and Petrus Severinus had invented, the recipes for which can be found in Severinus' bookshelves or Caspar's own chemical library. Further, Severinus is mentioned as a source of Paracelsian doctrine. But even as Galen noted long ago, one must travel to learn, and for spagyrical pharmacology Caspar advised studying under Sennert at Wittenberg and Fabricius at Rostock.[31]

Caspar Bartholin's recommendations should be taken as a summary of the scholar's ideas over many years. They are above all a strong statement of his commitment to a wide range of authorities, and not adherence only to Aristotle and Galen: the list of authors reflects the most modern scholarship available to the student at that time. Caspar Bartholin's endorsement of chemical drugs and his recommendation of Severinus' *Idea medicinæ* as a source for these doctrines should not be construed as an acceptance of Paracelsian philosophy in general. During the second decade Bartholin was an advocate of Aristotelian natural philosophy, as was Ole Worm, and they considered Paracelsian ideas within an Aristotelian frame. Moreover, in 1620s Denmark, select Paracelsian ideas

---

30 Panum, "Vort medicinske Fakultets," p. 58. Panum highlights Bartholin's advice on pp. 58-61.
31 Ibid., p. 60.

were blended into a larger concept of iatrochemistry, and Bartholin's recommendations should not be interpreted as a general enthusiasm for Paracelsianism, which had by that time come under suspicion.[32]

If Paracelsian medical ideas were tolerated in Denmark in the years before Bartholin's *De studio medico*, the political and religious views associated with them were not. After the turn of the century Paracelsian ideas were linked with Rosicrucian calls for a broad-based renewal, which were regarded as dangerous by the authorities. Paracelsian chemical philosophy was part of a larger ideological matrix that encompassed Rosicrucian political aims and radical, sometimes mystical religion. Once given a public face, through the printed manifestos of the Rosicrucian Brotherhood and the open letters from would-be Rosicrucians that soon followed, the "Rosicrucian furor" evoked a strong reaction from those who feared radical socio-political and religious changes. Although the brunt of this storm broke on France and the Holy Roman Empire, where the struggle for control was greatest, it also affected Scandinavia, which sought the shelter of strengthened, orthodox Lutheran state churches. Whatever interest Worm may have had in Paracelsian doctrines as a student gave way in this environment to a general rejection of Paracelsus' basic cosmology and the religious views it presupposed.[33]

32 On the place of Aristotelian natural philosophy in the early seventeenth-century Danish conservative reaction against religious heterodoxy and on Bartholin's and Worm's attitudes toward Paracelsian theory, see Jole Shackelford, "To Be or Not to Be a Paracelsian: Something Spagyric in the State of Denmark," in *The Paracelsian Moment: Science, Medicine, and Astrology in Early Modern Europe*, ed. Gerhild Williams and Charles Gunnoe, Jr. Sixteenth Century Essays and Studies 64 (Kirksville, MO: Truman State University Press, 2002), pp. 35-69. Religious aspects of their rejection of Paracelsian ideas are elaborated in Idem, "Paracelsianism and the Orthodox Lutheran Rejection of Vital Philosophy in Early Seventeenth Century Denmark", *Early Science and Medicine* 8 (2003), pp. 210-52.

33 The existence and nature of the actual Rosicrucian Brotherhood has been the subject of controversy. However, there is no doubt that people in the early seventeenth century believed Rosicrucians to exist. Rosicrucianism, as an abstract, captures the religious and political dissatisfaction of a generation, perhaps two generations of N. European intellectuals in the period leading up to and including the Thirty Years' War.

ROSICRUCIANISM AND OLE WORM'S
REJECTION OF PARACELSIANISM

In 1619, in a long address written for the promotion of fifteen students of philosophy to the master's degree at Copenhagen, Ole Worm spoke out against the Rosicrucian attempt to reform philosophy. Worm noted his initial contact with Rosicrucian ideas when he was a student in Germany. He described the subsequent publications of the Rosicrucian tracts that marked the public declaration of the Rosicrucian call for reform, as well as various tracts written afterwards in support of the Rosicrucian Brotherhood.[34] Given that Worm was speaking at such a formal academic occasion and had the address published that same year, it is plausible that he was expressing not only his own convictions about the Rosicrucian movement, but also a view consistent with the opinion of the medical faculty and closely allied theological faculty. In effect Worm, as dean of the philosophy faculty, was proclaiming the official attitude of an increasingly conservative university toward heterodox Rosicrucian dissent.

Worm's attack was directed specifically at the brotherhood and its opposition to Galenic medicine and Aristotelian philosophy, but it implicitly struck at the Paracelsian world view that supported Rosicrucianism as well.[35] Why did Worm, who not many years before had been an eager student of Paracelsian chemical medicine, speak out so vehemently in defense of Peripatetic philosophy and Galenic medicine at this time? Worm alludes to his own early reaction to Rosicrucianism:

> In the hands of those who have given an oath to Hermetic medicine, this *Fama* was famous for several years before it was published; and indeed, a version of this extraordinary secret was given to me in the year 1611 by a certain celebrated iatrochemist of a certain German university. At that time he caused me, considering these to be pure fantasies or

---

34　Ole Worm, "Oratio Inauguralis de Fratrum R.C. philosophiam reformandi conatu," *Laurea philosophica summa* (Copenhagen: Henrik Waldkirch, 1619).

35　Ibid. "Si hisce missis ex harmonia majoris & minoris Mundi a Paracelso & aliis tentata Philosophiam suam eruere tentent, quo successu id sint facturi videant."

else riddles hiding something more secret, to change my mind, and for reasons that were not unimportant.[36]

This passage at once illuminates two important aspects of Rosicrucianism. First, although the publication of the *Fama* (1614) has been considered the beginning of the "Rosicrucian furor," it is clear that the *Fama*, and no doubt other Rosicrucian tracts, were circulating among Paracelsians years before their publication.[37] Second, these tracts were taken seriously by chemical *adepti* in northern Germany, while Worm was a student there. Worm did not identify the "celebrated iatrochemist" and "German university," but Hartmann and Marburg seem likely candidates. Marburg was a hotbed of Rosicrucian (and Paracelsian) activity at this time, and although Hartmann's religious views remain obscure, Worm certainly found something about him disagreeable.[38]

Ole Worm continued to have a passing interest in news of the Rosicrucians after returning to Denmark, as his correspondence from the following years reveals. He wrote to Jacob Fincke in Giessen looking for information about the supposed brotherhood in August 1616.[39] The

36 Ibid. "In manibus quorundam qui Medicinæ Hermeticæ sacramentum dixerunt, antequam publice typis divulgaretur, annis aliquot erat famosa hæc de Fratribus *Fama*; ac mihi quidem anno 1611 singularis secreti instar, communicata est a celebri quodam cujusdam Academiæ Germaniæ Chymiatro; qui me, mera hæc esse phantasmata aut ænigmata secretius quid occultantia reputantem, rationibus haud levibus tunc temporis a sententia dimovit."

37 Sprengel, *Versuch einer pragmatischen Geschichte*, vol. 3, p. 426, found the first trace of Rosicrucianism in Adam Haslmeyer's admission that he had read the *Fama* in manuscript in 1610. A.E. Waite, *The Brotherhood of the Rosy Cross* (New York: University Books, 1961), pp. 115-16, concluded that Haslmeyer was drawn to the brotherhood because he believed it to be a school of Paracelsian thought. See also the recent work on Haslmeyer by Carlos Gilly, "*'Theophrastia Sancta'* – Paracelsianism as a Religion, in Conflict with the Established Churches," in *Paracelsus. The Man and His Reputation, His ideas and Their Transformation* (Leiden: Brill, 1998), pp. 187-206.

38 On Marburg as a center of Rosicrucian interest, see Moran, *The Alchemical World of the German Court*, chapters three and six.

39 *Olai Wormii et ad eum Doctorum Virorum Epistolæ*, ed. Hans Gram (Copenhagen, 1751), p. 8: "Si quid de *Fratribus Roseæ Crucis* certo perceperis, indica, ubi sint, qui sint, an ex eorum ordine (ut narrant) Princeps Vester, & siquid, quod publicis scriptis (quæ ad nos pervenerunt) non innotuit, habeas, expedi." [If you have learned anything reliable about the Rosicrucian Brothers please enlighten me about where they are, who they are, or – as one says – whether your prince belongs to their order; and if you have anything about them that does not appear in the published writings (those we have), please send it to me.] I have consulted Schepelern's Danish edition (Worm, *Breve*) in translating Worm's correspondence.

following spring he inquired about it in a letter to a correspondent in Strassburg, saying that he could not completely dismiss Rosicrucianism as fiction because of the attention it had aroused among serious scholars.[40] In January 1618 he again wrote to Jacob Fincke in Giessen, wanting to hear any news concerning the Rosicrucians.[41] Two months later he wrote to Lauritz Scavenius in Strassburg; he was intrigued by Scavenius' report on the Rosicrucian Ardeiius and would like further news of the sect.[42] A few months later Worm again wrote to Scavenius, saying that he doubted that the Rosicrucians would attract many followers, because they had failed to produce any worthwhile literature to support their claims:

> I now hardly doubt that the society of these lunatic Rosicrucians will finally incite even its proponents against it, since they have for so long a time led the credulous on with an empty hope. For, what have they provided us after so many bragging promises, so many boastings about reforms in language and sciences, beyond some empty stories and some pages smeared with sweet dream-visions? If they do not keep to what

40 Letter from Worm to Niels Christensen Foss, 1. March or 1. May 1617, *Olai Wormii Epistolæ*, p. 13: "Si quid de *Roseæ crucis fratribus* certo perceperis, indica, quæso. Varia de iis video hominum judicia; Sed relatio illa *Moltheri*, nundinis præcedentibus edita, facit, ut non meram esse fabulam existimem." [I ask you to tell me whether you have heard anything definite regarding the Rosicrucian Brotherhood. I see that people judge them very differently. But the account by Molther [*Antwort, Brüderschafft dess Rosenkreutzes auf etzlicher an sie ergangen Schreiben* (place unknown: 1617, 8°)], which came out at the last fair, requires that I cannot dismiss it as pure invention.]

41 Ibid., p. 9: "Si quid de *Fratribus Roseæ Crucis* apud vos novi, illud data occasione indicatum cuperem; Mira enim de iis, hic apud Nos, tam scriptis publicatis, quam fama, perferuntur." [If there is anything new about the Rosicrucian Brothers down your way, I would very gladly know it, should the opportunity arise. Here many remarkable things are said about them, both in print and by rumor.]

42 Ibid., p. 39: "Cæterum illæ, quibus historiam dedisti illius Ardelionis, qui se asseclam Societatis R. C. proclamavit, adeo me affecerunt, ut magni beneficii loco reputem, si crebrius de talibus, quæ apud vos geruntur, erudiar. Si quid posthac de eo reliquisque hujus sectæ complicibus perceperis, id ne me celes rogo." [Moreover, that letter, wherein you report on your Ardelius {Mr. Busybody}, who declared himself a follower of the Rosicrucian Society, has agitated my mind to such a degree that I would consider it a great kindness if I can be informed quite regularly about what is going on down your way. If you henceforth discover anything about him and the others in that sect, please do not keep it from me.]

they have promised in such gaudy manners of speaking, all their efforts will go up in smoke.[43]

His use of the terms "Crucigeri" and "Cruciferi" (cross-bearers) in this and subsequent letters, instead of the more dignified "Fratres Roseæ Crucis" used earlier, suggests that his attitude toward the Rosicrucians shifted from curiosity to disdain in the spring of 1618.

By summer 1618 Worm had decided that the Rosicrucians were a suitable topic for a speech to the university that he was considering for May 1619, the results of which are noted above.[44] Finally, in a letter to Andreas Jacobsen Langebeck in Jena (12 August 1620), Worm summed up his opinion of the Rosicrucians:

I have seen this little book by "The Brothers" about whether *the host is the real bread*; I own it and judge therefrom that the whole Rosicrucian Society, if it is in fact anything at all, is an amalgamation of all sects. Although they, in other tracts, declare themselves to be Lutherans, there

43 Letter of May/August 1618, ibid., p. 40: "Delirum illud *Crucigerorum* genus spe inani cum jam tanto temporis tractu credulos lactaverit, quin proprios patronos tandem in se sint concitaturi, vix dubito. Quid enim, post tot magnicrepa promissa, tot linguarum & scientiarum reformationes jactatas, præter inanes quasdam fabellas, & svavibus quibusdam insomniis commaculatas chartas, nobis obtulerant? Ni præstiterint, quod verbis pomposis polliciti sunt, in auras omnes illorum evanescent conatus."

44 Letter from Worm to Jacob Fincke in Giessen, ibid., pp. 9-10: "Jucunda admodum mihi fuit relatio tua de deliro illo *Hierosolymitano Rege*, quem si pro Antesignano agnoscant fraterculi illi *Crucigeri*, ex eo, quid de reliquis sentiendum, abunde colligitur. Interim, quid de eo factum, quidve apud Vos molitus sit, expeterem: an ubi terrarum reperiatur novum Collegium indicaverit, an quosdam in suam societatem pertrahere conatus fuerit, quæso proximis indica, vel, si visum fuerit, coram expone. Mihi munus Decanatus cum imposuerit Facultas Philosophica, decrevi, ad proximum Pascha, solennem Magistrorum promotionem adornare." [I have greatly enjoyed your description of this crazy King of Jerusalem; if these Rosicrucians regard him as their standard bearer one can fully conclude from him what one ought to think of the rest. Meanwhile I would surely like to know what has happened to him, and what he has done down your way. I beseech you to mention in your next letter (or, if you prefer, tell me personally) whether he has said where in the world the new college is located, and if he has tried to entice certain persons into his Society. Since the philosophy faculty has promoted me to a deanship, I have decided to arrange a formal Master's promotion next Easter.]

is still a part of their account that smacks of heresy or Anabaptistry mixed together with Paracelsus.[45]

Here, in one sentence, Worm came to the core of the matter: Rosicrucianism is to be opposed because it is religiously heterodox, and it is linked with Paracelsianism. Why was this to be shunned? Religious heterodoxy was perceived as a danger to religious and political stability. On the one hand, reformers who were interested in a religion based on close adherence to Scripture found sectarian emphasis on the establishment of paradise on earth to be in direct conflict with Scriptural teaching about the Day of Judgement. Libavius, on this account, associated the Rosicrucians with the Anabaptist heresy.[46] Paracelsian detractors from Erastus to Libavius had commented on the heresy in Paracelsian doctrines, and this extended to the Rosicrucian ideas they fueled. On the other hand, for the German theologians who were intent on bringing a political unity to Protestantism, in order to help face the threat of a papal counter-reformation, Rosicrucianism was a disruptive movement upon which no Lutheran religion could be based.[47]

Libavius' opposition to Paracelsianism was no doubt grounded in a fundamental disagreement about epistemology, but it is also true that he was a strict Lutheran opponent of Calvinism, and the sectarian discord among Protestants was another facet of the ideological disquiet that produced Rosicrucianism. Libavius had begun an extended diatribe against the Paracelsians already before the turn of the century, and this led to a series of treatises published together in 1615. In the opinion of Owen Hannaway, who has studied Libavius' rhetoric, Libavius' outburst against Paracelsianism in 1615 was probably inspired "by what Libavius perceived as an unholy alliance between Calvinism and Hermetic-Paracelsianism," which he felt was responsible for generating the early Rosicrucian

45 Ibid., pp. 54: "Libellum illum *Fratrum*, disquirentem, an *Hostia sit verus cibarius?* vidi & habeo, atque ex eo colligo, totam illam *Societatem Cruciferorum*, si modo quæ sit, omnium sectarum esse conflugem; cum in aliis scriptis profiteantur, se esse Lutheranos, in discursibus vero Enthusiasmum aut Anabaptisticum quid, Paracelsico mistum, redoleant."

46 Waite, *Brotherhood*, p. 238, note 1.

47 This was an objection voiced already in the anonymous *Fama remissa ad Fratres Roseæ Crucis*, 1616. See Waite, *Brotherhood*, pp. 240-41.

tracts.[48] That Libavius and his contemporaries readily linked Rosicrucianism to the Calvinists is evident from Robert Fludd's declaration to
King James I regarding Fludd's published defense of the Rosicrucians
against Libavius' attacks. "This School of Philosophers is acknowledged
even by the Germans, Catholics as well as Lutherans (among whom
the Brothers are said to live), to embrace firmly the Calvinist Religion,"
Fludd explained.[49] Thus, one axis of the dispute between Paracelsians
and their harshest critics seems to have been the fundamental confessional controversy between Lutherans and Calvinists.[50]

Andreas Libavius' concerns may well have affected Ole Worm. In
his 1619 attack on the Rosicrucians, Worm mentioned one exception to
the early support for the Brotherhood's aims:

> But as far as I know, only one man has come forward, the very renowned
> theologian and physician, Andreas Libavius, who has undertaken, as it
> were, to hammer back the first onslaught of the brothers.[51]

It is plausible that Worm's sources of information included two tracts
published at Frankfurt in 1615 by Andreas Libavius. The first of these
(*Examen philosophiæ novæ*) is a critique of the "new philosophy" as it is
presented in 1) ancient authors, 2) Croll's "Paracelsian magic", 3) the
vital philosophy of Severinus, as presented by Johan Hartmann, and 4)
the magic, harmonic philosophy of the Rosicrucian Brotherhood.[52] The

---

48 Hannaway, *The Chemists and the Word*, p. 94, n. 7.

49 Robert Fludd, "Declaratio Brevis," trans. Robert A. Seelinger, Jr., in William H. Huffman and Robert A. Seelinger, Jr., "Robert Fludd's 'Declaratio Brevis' to James I," *Ambix*
25 (1978): 69-92, p. 81.

50 One cannot, of course, push the denominational alliance between Calvinism and Paracelsianism too far, but it is true that controversy over Paracelsian ideology in France
was generally between Catholics and Huguenots, who were influenced by Calvinism,
and in England between Puritans (Calvinists) and Anglicans.

51 Worm, *Laurea philosophica summa*: "Sed unicus, quod sciam, tum extitit *Andreas Libavius Theologus & Medicus celeberrimus* qui primum fratrum impetum retundere quasi
aggressus est."

52 Libavius, *Prodromus vitalis philosophiæ Paracelsistarum … in examen philosophiæ novæ quæ
veteri abrogandæ opponitur: 1) De veterum autoritate; 2) De magia Paracelsi ex Crollio: 3) De
philosophia vivente ex Severino per Johannem Hartmannum; 4) De philosophia harmonica
magica Fraternitatis de Rosea Cruce* (in *Syntagmatis*). Libavius also wrote *Wolmeinendes
Bedencken von der Fama und Confession der Bruderschafft dess Rosen Creutzes* (Frankfurt,
1616), in which Severinus is repeatedly mentioned.

second treatise is much shorter but devoted specifically to an analysis of the Rosicrucian *Confessio.*[53]

Although Libavius did not single out Severinus for direct attack, as he did Croll, he mentioned him frequently as a source of Paracelsian doctrine, especially when it came to the harmonic "magic" working between the macrocosm and the microcosm and the function of the spiritual *semina* in that regard. This he ridiculed as non-science.[54] The effect of Libavius' 1615 treatises was to show that Paracelsianism underlies Rosicrucian cosmology, and in the course of criticizing it, he clearly implicated Severinus' ideas. As noted above, a major section of *Examen philosophiæ novæ* (173 pages in 2°) was wholly devoted to a critique of Severinian vital philosophy as echoed by Hartmann, in which, among other things, Libavius dismissed the "Archeus and mechanic Vulcan of Paracelsus" as "dreams of the delirious," in this case specifically referring to Severinus.[55]

In an anti-Rosicrucian treatise published the following year, Andreas Libavius noted that whereas some saw the Rosicrucian tracts as documents contrived by Paracelsians to strengthen their attack on Galenists and Aristotelians, others viewed the Rosicrucian demand for reformation of all the arts and politics as a "war horn of sedition"

---

53 Andreas Libavius, *Analysis Confessionis Fraternitatis de Rosea Cruce* (Frankfurt am Main, 1615).

54 In *Examen philosophiæ novæ* (in *Syntagmatis*), p. 285, for example, Libavius writes: "Quo modo fit coctio & nutritio in homine? Respondet *Severinus*, non per canales distributis humoribus, sed spiritibus invisibilibus invisibiliter per meatus arcanos penetrantibus, qui corporascunt in partibus, & in substantiam earum cedunt. Qua fide? Harmonica. Sicut enim magni mundi spiritus, & spiritualia semina sine canalibus per elementa feruntur, omniaque constituunt & nutriunt ex incorporeis corporea facta: ita est in minore mundo. Rideo hanc rationem. Cur? Quia argumentum concordantiæ fallit ... Essentia effecti & causæ longe sunt alia. Hinc scientia est, non inde." [How do coction and nutrition occur in man? Severinus responds that it is not by means of humors that are distributed through channels, but by means of invisible spirits, invisibly penetrating hidden passages, which become incarnate in the parts and give them substance. By what means? Harmonic. For just as the spirits of the great world and the spiritual seeds are carried through the elements without channels, and establish and nourish all things, having become bodies from non-bodies, so it is in the lesser world. I laugh at this reasoning. Why? Because the argument of concordance deceives. ... Causes and effects are quite different in essence. This, not that former [theory], is knowledge].

55 Ibid., p. 156: "Archæus & mechanicus Paracelsi Vulcanus sunt delirantis somnia."

calling for rebellion, such as had happened in the Peasants' Rebellion and the rebellion at Muenster.[56] Many people, some of them important, are suspected, continued Libavius, and Paracelsians in particular must be careful, since the *Fama* and *Confessio* come from their camp.[57] The end result was that for Worm and his colleagues, Paracelsianism was linked with Rosicrucian beliefs at the very time that the Rosicrucians were coming under scrutiny for their religious and political views, and commitment to one could be interpreted as commitment to the other.[58]

Ole Worm's abandonment of Paracelsian vital philosophy is evident in a collection of "questions" he addressed in a 1622 publication, *Questiones Miscellarum Decas*.[59] Of particular interest are the third, fourth and ninth questions. The third question, *"An Philosophia alia vitalis, alia mortua?"* (Is there a living philosophy and a dead one?), reaches the conclusion that there is no useful distinction between a living and dead philosophy, and that "vital philosophy" was in fact invented by the chemists in order to exaggerate their discoveries.[60] Severinus was the primary source of the view Worm is criticizing here:

> 2) Hence, that chapter 6, page 94 of Petrus Severinus' *Idea medicinæ* [says]: "All philosophy that pursues privations, formless matters, and dead qualities is deaf and blind." 3) But if you ask what they might mean by vital philosophy, they respond that that philosophy is vital

---

56 Libavius, *Wolmeinendes Bedencken*, p. 13: "Andern bedünckt es eine *Tuba* zu einer Sedition / oder Auffruhr zuseyn / weil von einer allgemeinen Reformation in allen Künsten / auch in der Policey nach Art der Magen / in Arabia geredt/ ... wird." See also Will-Erich Peuckert, *Die Rosenkreutzer* (Jena: Eugen Diderich, 1928), p. 102.

57 Libavius, *Wolmeinendes Bedencken*, pp. 13-14: "Es sey nun ein kurtzweilig Gedicht / oder Ernstes wercke / dabey man vermeint auch ansehnliche Personen sich finden sollen / ists nicht ohn Verdacht bey vielen / unnd hetten sich die Paracelsisten sonderlich fürzusehen / auss welcher Gründe die *Fama* und Confession gehet."

58 Concern for the religious heterodoxy inherent in Paracelsian ideas is discussed in Siegfried Wollgast, "Zur Wirkungsgeschichte des Paracelsus im 16. und 17. Jahrhundert," in *Resultate und Desiderate der Paracelsus-Forschung*, ed. Peter Dilg and Hartmut Rudolph, *Sudhoffs Archiv*, Beihefte 31 (Stuttgart: Franz Steiner Verlag, 1993), pp. 113-144.

59 Ole Worm, *Questiones Miscellarum Decas* (Copenhagen, 1622).

60 Ibid., f. 2v, question 3, point 1: "A Chymicis non ita pridem excogitata hæc est distinctio, ad sua inventa exaggeranda, hactenus vero receptam philosophandi rationem extenuandam."

which is engaged in explanation of the vital principles, *semina*, and powers.[61]

It may sound as if Worm approves of Severinus here, but in fact he had completely undercut vital philosophy, which was axiomatic to Paracelsianism, by denying one of its basic premises, that everything that 'moves', using the term broadly, is alive.[62]

In the fourth question, *"An rebus non novis nova & inusitate imponenda nomina?"* (Should new and useless names be imposed on things that are not new?), Worm accused Paracelsus and his followers of introducing new names for known things, with the result that philosophy is obscured. Worm had all along objected to the obscurantist nature of Paracelsianism; now he took Croll to task for defending Paracelsus' use of "magical style" to preserve doctrine from the common people.[63] This intentional occultation of philosophy, Worm thought, is not suitable for teachers, whose object it is to make things more understandable, not less so. And if Paracelsus intended to keep his ideas from the uneducated rabble, why did he publish in German?[64]

Worm more directly addressed Paracelsian theory in the ninth question, *"An tria chymicorum principia locum in physicis obtineant?"* (Do the chemists' *tria prima* have a place in physics?), again drawing on the *Idea medicinæ* as the main source of Paracelsian teaching on the subject. Of the eighteen paragraphs or points constituting the ninth question, Severinus is quoted in seven, and is the only Paracelsian specifically cited. Worm first defined the Paracelsian *tria prima*, acknowledging that these appellations do not refer to the observed compounds salt, sulphur, and mercury, but rather to consistencies of matter:

61 Ibid., f. 2v, question 3, points 2 and 3: "(2) Hinc illud P. Severini Ideæ medicinæ cap. 6 p. 94. *Surda & cæca est omnis Philosophia quæ privationes, informes materias, & mortuas qualitates sectatur.* (3) Si autem, quid per vitalem Philosophiam intelligant, quæras; respondent Philosophiam vitalem esse, quæ circa explicationem principiorum vitalium, seminum, & potestatum versatur."

62 Ibid., f. 3r, question 3, point 6.

63 Ibid., f. 4r, question 4, point 8. Worm cited the preface of Croll's *Basilica*: "Paracelsum expertis stylo magico scripsisse, non vulgo, sed sibi & intelligentibus, in Schola magica educatis Sapientiæ filiis."

64 Ibid., f. 4r, question 4, point 9. These criticisms sound suspiciously Libavian.

These things are described one by one by Severinus, in chapter eight. He says that "salt gives consistency, solidity, and coagulation to things; sulphur, by its fatty and oily substance, tempers the coagulation of salt. And mercury, by continually moistening, bathes the two former [principles], which are hastening by the abundance of their actions, by the hour, to drought and decay, and it makes the mixing of all things easier by means of its fluid and smooth substance."[65]

Worm was quite ready to concede that immaterial principles underlie the elements, and quoted Hippocrates and Galen on this. But by the end of the question he had reduced these to agreement with Aristotelian philosophy, by using Severinus' own words:

We should by no means eliminate these [Paracelsian] principles from the field of physics, especially since they do not demolish the Peripatetic ones, but confirm, presuppose, and explain them. Severinus himself attests to these in chapter seven of the *Idea medicinæ*: "Paracelsus, when he said that all bodies are composed of salt, sulphur, and mercury, was not opposed to Aristotle, who appointed matter, form, and privation as the principles of things, nor to Plato, who called them God, exemplar, and matter."[66]

Worm then likened the *tria prima* to simple material bodies (elements), and their "powers and properties" to forms, saying that salt, sulphur, and mercury can be seen in Aristotelian terms as passive, material principles with active, formal principles connected. Using (or abusing) Severinus' statements, Worm allowed Philosophy to retain the idea of salt, sulphur, and mercury as philosophical descriptions,

65 Ibid., f. 8r, question 9, point 6: "Hæc autem sigillatim varie describuntur, Severinus cap. 8. *Salis esse ait, consistentiam dare rebus, soliditatem & coagulationem. Sulphuris pingui oleosaque, sua Substantia Salis coagulationem temperare. Mercurij assidua irrigatione duo priora, actionum frequentia ad siccitatem & senium in horas festinantia fovere, fluidaque & labili Substantia mistionem omnium faciliorem reddere.*"

66 Ibid., f. 9r, question 9, point 14: "Neutiquam ex agro Physico hæc principia eliminabimus, præsertim cum Peripatetica non evertant, sed confirment, præsupponant & declarent. Quod & ipsemet Severin[us] cap. 7 Ideæ hisce testatur: *Paracelsus cum dicit corpora omnia constare ex Sale, Sulphure & Mercurio non repugnat Aristoteli, qui rerum principia statuit materiam, formam & privationem, nec Platoni dicenti Deum, exemplar & materiam.*"

but stripped them of the meaning Severinus had given them within a vital philosophy.

> And neither are [the principles] confused with the elements themselves. For indeed, although salt might seem to correspond to earth, yet the former dissolves in moisture, the latter by no means. Oil or sulphur burns and catches fire, but air does not. Mercury is strong in various properties which water lacks. Let me use the words of Severinus, chapter eight, p. 118: "The principles of bodies are distinguished from those common elements in this way. The functions of the former are more common and maintain the order of matter, but those of the latter are fixed by properties and rules; they flourish by the marvelous power of the properties. Nevertheless, the principles of bodies so cohere to the elements by an indissoluble link that never by the laws of nature, scarcely by any diligence of art (and then not perfectly), can they be separated."[67]

For Worm it was only reasonable that active forms drive passive matter, and to assign special vitality to these forms was utter nonsense. He could, however, accept Severinian (Paracelsian) language insofar as it was reducible to an Aristotelian ontology.

Eventually even this concession seems to have been devalued. When his protegé, Ambrosius Rhodius, wrote to him 7 December 1640 and asked his opinion on Paracelsianism and the merits of the *Idea medicinæ*, Worm replied 24 December 1640 that he had indeed read the book, but did not comment further, offering instead to send his own theories. Ole Worm's unwillingness to engage in discussion with Rhodius, who was married to Severinus' granddaughter, tells us that Worm, at least, considered the topic closed.[68]

---

67 Ibid., ff. 9r-9v, question 9, point 18: "Nec cum ipsis confundantur elementis. Sal etenim licet Terræ videatur respondere, tamen in humido liquescit illud, hæc neutiquam. Oleum seu Sulphur ardet & flammam concipit, aer neutiquam. Mercurius variis proprietatibus pollet, quibus aqua destituitur. Utar verbis P. Severini cap. 8 pag. 118. *Ab Elementis illis communibus hoc pacto distinguuntur corporum principia. Illorum officia communiora sunt, & materiæ rationem obtinent, horum vero proprietatibus & rationibus destinata, mirabili proprietatum potestate vigent. Nihilominus indissolubili nexu ita elementis corporum principia cohærent, ut naturæ legibus nunquam, vix ulla artis industria, idque non perfecte separari possint.*"

68 Rhodius wrote to Ole Worm 7 December 1640 requesting his opinion of Severinus' theory of the elements. See Worm, *Breve*, vol. 2, pp. 215 and 222.

Ole Borch

The teaching of chemistry and chemical medicine, as a course of study in its own right, began in the early seventeenth century. It was kindled by the patronage of princes and kings and fueled by an increasing demand for practical skills in preparing chemical drugs. Moritz of Hesse-Kassel established the first chair of chemiatry (chemical medicine) at the University of Marburg in 1609, to which he appointed Johann Hartmann. The French crown supported the teaching of chemistry by Guy de la Brosse and William Davidson at the *Jardin*, laying the foundation for a tradition of didactic chemistry at Paris that reached to Lavoisier in the mid eighteenth century. The introduction of medical chemistry at the University of Copenhagen followed a similar course. Since the early seventeenth century, when Christian IV set up a royal laboratory at Rosenborg under the direction of the Paracelsian chemist Peter Payngk, the kings had supported chemistry in Copenhagen privately. But as was the case at Marburg, but some fifty years later, the ruler's patronage eventually brought chemistry to the university, too.

The first Dane to lecture specifically on chemistry at the University of Copenhagen was Ole Borch, better known by the Latin form of his name, Olaus Borrichius (1626-1690). As a student, Borch had pursued a broad course of study at the University of Copenhagen, laying the foundations for a career as a polymath in the second half of the century. He always considered himself primarily a philologist, but his early contact with medicine strongly stimulated his interest in natural philosophy, which played an important part in his career.[69] In his first treatise touching on medical theory, *De cabala characterali* (1649), Borch denied the medical efficacy of characters, words, seals, or images, and in general refused the Paracelsian claim that the human imagination

---

69 Details of Borch's biography are readily available in H. D. Schepelern's excellent English introduction to the printed edition of Borch's travel diary, *Olai Borrichii Itinerarium 1660-1665: The Journal of the Danish Polyhistor Ole Borch*, ed. H. D. Schepelern (Copenhagen: Reitzel, 1983), pp. vii-xliii. This biographical introduction includes a translation of Borch's autobiography (pp. xv-xxi), which he composed toward the end of his life (1690). E. F. Koch, *Oluf Borck: en litærærhistorisk-biografisk Skildring* (Copenhagen: Jacob Lund, 1866), offers a lengthier biography.

could act directly on the macrocosm. He did not, however, deny the existence of "occult" forces and sympathy between the human body and environmental phenomena. This suggests that Borch's interest in problems of causation, which lie at the base of natural philosophy, began very early in his career.[70]

From 1655-1660 Ole Borch was patronized by Joachim Gersdorff, a powerful Danish noble, who permitted Borch to work in his private laboratory and extensive personal library. Gersdorff and Frederik III had a common interest in metallurgical chemistry, and Borch's expertise in this area probably led to his appointment by the king to an "extraordinary" professorship in 1660.[71] Before settling in as professor at the University of Copenhagen, however, Borch travelled extensively in Europe, receiving his M.D. at Angers in 1664.

Upon returning to Copenhagen in 1666, Ole Borch lectured, conducted organic and inorganic chemical research, and wrote books on chemistry, pharmacology, philology, botany, and on the generation of stones both in man and in the earth.[72] His chemical lectures, for which student notes survive in manuscript, and his active research represent the first attempt to institutionalize chemistry at the University of Copenhagen.[73]

---

70 Borrichius, *Olai Borrichii Itinerarium*, pp. xxiv-xxvi.

71 Ibid., p. xxviii. Borch was appointed ordinary professor of philology and extraordinary professor to teach medical students botany in the summer and chemistry in the winter. See Stig Veibel, *Kemiens Historie i Danmark*, vol. 1 of *Kemien i Danmark* (Copenhagen: Arnold Busck, 1939), p. 58.

72 Tagea Egede Christensen, "Bibliographia Borrichiana," *Mindeskrift for Oluf Borch paa 300-aarsdagen for hans fødsel*, ed. Vilhelm Maar (Copenhagen: Arnold Busck, 1926), pp. 37-64. Koch, *Oluf Borck*, p. 78, notes that Borch was appointed supervisor of the royal laboratory.

73 Copenhagen, Kgl. Bibl., GKS 1721 4° contains "Elementa chemiæ Borrichio attributa," which is supposed to be Borch's lecture notes. NKS 338a, Petrus Jani Lucoppidanus, "Elementa chemiæ in auditorio Academiæ Hafniensis a viro excellentissimo & experientissimo Dn. D. Olao Borrichio ... publice prælecta," corresponds to "Elementa chemiæ Borrichio attributa" very closely. Although there is not a word for word similarity between these two, the order and content is nearly identical, suggesting that they pertain to the same lecture series (ca. 1669-71). Bound with this is Petrus Lucoppidanus' lecture notes for the corresponding botany lectures, suggesting that chemistry and botany were taught seasonally during these three years. Another student manuscript, Copenhagen, Kgl. Bibl., Thott 744 4°, Albertus Achillis Toxotius, "Prælectiones has publicas viri, nobilissimi, ... Dn. D. Olaj Borrichii," is dated 1685. It looks like Toxotius began taking notes mid-course, as it follows the latter half of "Elementa chemiæ Borrichio attributa," and this suggests that Borch repeated the 1669-71 lecture sequence in 1683-85.

What we know about Ole Borch's education and teaching suggests that his interest in chemistry was not so much theoretical as practical and historical. On the other hand, a letter that he wrote to Ambrosius Rhodius 28 February 1660 tells us that Borch was scrutinizing Rhodius' writings, which included a lengthy defense of Severinus' doctrines, when the Swedes attacked Copenhagen and he had to leave his study to man the walls.[74] His winter lectures stressed formulas and techniques useful to the medical student, just as his summer botanizing emphasized identification of medically useful herbs.

Ole Borch's first chemical treatise was published just two years after his return to Copenhagen. Its title, *De ortu et progressu chemiæ dissertatio* (*Dissertation on the origin and progress of chemistry*), aptly describes the fundamentally historical nature of the work. The dedication proclaims Borch's resolve to include nothing in his book that is not based either on experiment or authority, and what actual chemistry is discussed is presented within the treatise's essentially historical structure.[75] Despite his clear disagreement with key Paracelsian ideas, which are expressed in his earlier *De cabala characterali*,[76] the historical treatment of chemistry in *De ortu et progressu chemiæ*, published twenty years later, does not seek to vilify Paracelsian medicine, but strives to recount the contributions of various philosophers and schools from chemistry's ancient beginnings to the present. As a philologist, he drew on traditional myths, etymological arguments, and the contemporary discoveries and publication of hieroglyphs to recreate a history of chemistry that not only tells a story, but conveys something about the essential nature of that art. The importance he attached to this point of view is indicated by his polemic with Hermann Conring, a physician and professor at Helmstedt.

In his 1648 treatise *De hermetica medicina* (*On Hermetic Medicine*), Conring echoed Sennert in recognizing Severinus for making Paracelsus' philosophy somewhat intelligible, and not just compiling the ideas of

---

74 Koch, *Oluf Borck*, p. 28. I have not personally seen this letter, which is supposed to be in Copenhagen, Kgl. Bibl., NKS 590 4°. The treatise he mentioned was probably Rhodius' *Disputationes supra Ideam medicinæ philosophicæ* (1643), which is discussed in chapter nine, below.

75 Koch, *Oluf Borck*, pp. 99-101.

76 Ibid., p. 16.

the master, but using them to create his own doctrine.[77] Specifically, he credited chapter thirteen of the *Idea medicinæ* for developing the concept that diseases have *semina*, an idea that he said is scattered about in the writings of Paracelsus.[78] However, Conring was also sharply critical of Severinus, making fun of him for accepting Paracelsus' ideas too readily. Referring to Paracelsus' statement that "the whole man is the disease," Conring said that anyone who is even slightly more learned than Paracelsus recognizes this to be "shameful ignorance," just as is Severinus' claim that diseases are not in the categories, but the categories in the diseases.[79]

Borch's historical interpretation of chemistry was fundamentally incompatible with the view expressed by Hermann Conring in his *De hermetica medicina*. Conring was strongly anti-Paracelsian and in general doubted both the historical authenticity and doctrinal reliability of "Hermetic" chemistry. *De ortu et progressu chemiæ* was Borch's response to Conring's rejection of the venerable antiquity of chemistry, which Borch traced back to antediluvian sources.[80]

Ole Borch claimed that Petrus Severinus' work had given him the motivation to write *De ortu et progressu chemiæ*, saying that Severinus was his Miltiades (a victorious Greek general), who would not let him sleep until the work was done. Perhaps part of his admiration for Severinus stemmed from the fact that Severinus was a fellow Jutlander. Ole Borch likened his career to that of Severinus: both had come from Ribe Latin school, were appointed professors in the arts faculty at a young age, had traveled abroad, studying natural philosophy and medicine at foreign universities. Both had attained the M.D. and gained international recognition.[81]

---

77 Conring, *De hermetica medicina*, p. 181: "Qui sane inter eos præcipuus est Petrus Severinus Danus, licet videri velit Paracelsicorum hinc inde disjectorum dogmatum compilator, multa tamen Bombastica rejecit, multa ex suo cerebro confinxit, quo informis Paracelsica Ars & Philosophia aliquam doctrinæ effigiem nancisceretur. Iam vero plerique Severinum potius quam Paracelsum sectantur."

78 Ibid., p. 197.

79 Ibid., p. 198. Conring also mentioned Severinus on pp. 184-85, 187, 200, and 212, quoting from both chapters thirteen and fourteen of the *Idea medicinæ*.

80 Koch, *Oluf Borch*, p. 99.

81 Ibid., p. 99; Borrichius, "Dedication to Frederik III," *Dissertatio de ortu et progressu chemiæ*, ff. 3r-4r.

Besides a general disagreement about the historical nature of chemistry, Ole Borch may also have been offended by Conring's outright rejection of Paracelsian doctrine and his scorn for Severinus. We can judge Conring's position from a 1687 tract, *In universam artem medicam*, where he traced all contemporary Paracelsian nonsense back to the pen of Paracelsus:

> It is certain that he [Paracelsus] has perverted all philosophical [illegible] and even to the extent that it is used in medicine. The infinite errors and most false doctrines, even now fostered by a great many people, whether they seem to be Helmontian or otherwise, derive their origin solely from his writings. No one will believe this, unless he reads Paracelsus for himself.[82]

Conring's implication of Severinus in the propagation of these "infinite errors and most false doctrines" is likewise outspoken:

> And indeed no one else from that age is easily found who has openly stuck to the Paracelsian theories, which the Helmontian school has devoured, except that in Denmark, Petrus Severinus has dared to propagate extraordinary, crazy ideas, which a certain William Davidson, a Scot, later undertook to illuminate in his commentaries … But by reading them it is evident that they are pure nonsense, with the result that I am amazed that Borrichius has so prolixly congratulated himself about such predecessors, whose doctrines, though his vestiges remain, he quietly disproves and everywhere condemns as falsehood, by means of his own philosophy, which is sensible and healthier.[83]

---

82 Conring, *In universam artem medicam*, pp. 131-32: "De Paracelso & nos supra pluribus egimus, ad cap II. Certum est omnem philosophicam [Greek word – illegible in the reproduction that I used] atque adeo etiam eam quæ in medicina usum habet eum pervertisse, & infinitos errores & falsissima dogmata, nunc quoque a plurimis foveri, quæ, sive Helmontiana videantur, sive alia, ex ipsius scriptis unice ducunt originem: quod nemo putaverit, nisi qui Paracelsum ipsum evolvat."

83 Ibid., p. 136: "Et ex illis quidem temporibus nemo amplius inventus est facile, qui Paracelsicis dogmatis aperte inhæreret, Helmontiana secta eam absorbente, nisi quod in Dania *Petrus Severinus* mira deliria propagare ausus sit: quæ commentariis illustrare suscepit postea *Wilhelmus* quidam *Davidsonius* Scotus … Sed meras nugas esse facile

→

Conring published this in 1687, after several exchanges between him and Borch had already transpired. He had responded to the criticism in Borch's *De ortu et progressu chemiæ* by bringing out a revised edition of *De hermetica medicina* in 1669, to which was appended an "Apologeticus adversus calumnias et insectationes Olai Borrichii" (An apologetic tract against the calumnies and abuses of Ole Borch).

Ole Borch answered in 1674 with *Hermetis, Ægyptiorum, et chemicorum sapientia ab Hermanni Conringii animadversionibus vindicata per Olaum Borrichium* (*The wisdom of Hermes, the Egyptians, and the chemists, vindicated from the censures of Hermann Conring by Ole Borch*).[84] In this great chemical tract, Ole Borch took Conring to task for neglecting the contributions of the ancients and abusing the memory of the Hermetic philosophers and Paracelsus. Conring may have been genuinely puzzled by Borch's defense of Paracelsian doctrine, since Borch himself eschewed such philosophical systems and preferred time-tested formulas and the experience of the laboratory. However, Borch's *historical attitude* did not permit him to view Paracelsus as the evil creator of an unsound philosophy. Instead he praised Paracelsus for his role in the development of chemical pharmaceuticals.[85] While Conring apparently hated Hermetism and Paracelsianism because they were impious and absurd, Borch's historical perspective allowed him to see the Hermetic philosophers and Paracelsians on an equal footing with the Peripatetics, Galen, and the Arabic physicians.[86] From Borch's point of view, in the second half of the seventeenth century, Paracelsus and Severinus had become historical personages. Borch used them not to polemicize for or against a Paracelsian cosmology, but to defend a view of history and legitimize chemistry.

→ patet legentibus, ut mirer Borrichium de tali antecessore sibi tam prolixe esse gratulatum, cujus tamen dogmata, relictis vestigiis ejus saniore & sobria sua philosophia tacite falsitatis ubique convincit ac damnat." William Davidson's commentaries on Severinus' *Idea medicinæ* are surveyed in chapter ten, below.

84 Debus, "The Significance of Chemical History," p. 2.

85 Koch, *Oluf Borck*, pp. 101-103.

86 Debus, "The Significance of Chemical History," p. 2.

KØNING

In 1663, while Ole Borch was touring Europe, a Norwegian student named Mourits Pederssøn Køning (Mauritius Petri Køning) defended two dissertations in the arts faculty, one on logic and another on natural philosophy. The second of these, *Dissertatio de rerum principiis et mechanica seminum liturgia*, concerns the principles of Paracelsian cosmology and Severinus' disease theory.[87] In the preface Køning tells his readers that the words and doctrines to follow are not his, but those of Paracelsus. He warns us that he has not bothered to alter the vocabulary, which he implies may in fact be appropriate.[88]

The propositions that Køning set out in the eighteen theses of this dissertation are tersely stated, and there are no specific citations or other references that can direct the reader to his sources. However, both the subject matter and the terminology bear a strong resemblance to that of Severinus' *Idea medicinæ*, a third edition of which had been published just three years before. A brief description of Køning's dissertation will serve to illustrate this similarity, which is suggested already by his use of the Severinian phrase *mechanica seminum liturgia* in the title.

87 Køning, *Dissertatio de rerum principiis et mechanica seminum liturgia*. Holger Rørdam, "Bidrag til tre Biskoppers Levned. I. Dr. Mouritz Pedersen Køning, Biskop i Aalborg Stift (d. 1672)," *[Ny] Kirkehistoriske Samlinger*, 4th ser., vol. 1 (1889-91), p. 351, noted a lost manuscript by Køning, "Tractatus de spiritibus mechanicis eorumque foecunda subole, a quibus omnes naturales actiones proficiscuntur, iisque differentibus subtilitate et crassitie secundum actionum analogiam."

88 Køning, *Dissertatio de rerum principiis*, f. 2v: "Mea non sunt, quæ vobis paginæ præsentes exhibent, verba vero et dogmata Theophrasti Paracelsi, qui cum, meo judicio, de naturæ mysteriis multa docte et nervose consignavit, verba ejus, quæ Viri Doctissimi in suis scriptis integra servant, et presse sequuntur, immutanda non putavi. Vocabulorum novitas si quando occurrit, de illa non multum laborabimus, siquidem Philosophis partus suos pro lubitu vestire, et nomina interdum ad rei modum attemperare licet." [The words and doctrines which these present pages exhibit to you are not in fact mine, but those of Theophrastus Paracelsus, who, in my opinion, learnedly and vigorously recorded many things about the mysteries of nature. His words, which very learned men preserve intact in their writings, I have not thought to change. We have not much troubled about the novelty of the vocabulary, whenever it occurs, since philosophers are permitted to dress their offspring at their pleasure, and now and again to fit the names to the nature of the thing.] Severinus also stated the desirability of naming things according to their essences.

The dissertation begins at the beginning, with the planting of seminal reasons in the primeval chaos:

> The Creator placed light and the seminal reasons of all things into four incorporeal, void, empty natures by means of an incomprehensible magic, by virtue of the word and that spirit which was carried above the waters, imparting the principles of bodies, by which the things to be brought forth onto the worldly stage have been clothed.[89]

The placement of this proposition at the beginning of the dissertation probably served aesthetic ends, but it also reinforces the claim that I made in chapter four – that the theological aspects of *semina* theory made it attractive to Christian philosophers.

Køning adopted the Paracelsian-Severinian division of the world into two concentric globes with two of the elements, the "empty natures," dominating in each. These elements he populated with *semina*, which the elements foster, arouse at their predestined times, incite to maturity, and receive when they are spent.[90] The *semina* are by themselves incorporeal, "not at all bound to the restrictions of the dimensions," and are connected to the elements by an "indissoluble link." They come forth from their "abysses" and are "confined to places, and subject to the cycles of the ages, with the result that they fulfill the laws of motions,

---

89 Ibid., f. 3r: "In quatuor naturis, incorporeis, inanibus, vacuis, lucem & seminales rerum omnium rationes incomprehensibili Magia posuit Creator, virtute verbi & Spiritus illius, qui super aquas ferebatur; principia corporum adjungens, quibus induerentur in mundanam scenam proditura." This is quoted verbatim from *Idea medicinæ* pp. 41-42.

90 Køning, *Dissertatio de rerum principiis*, f. 3v: "Quatuor Elementa recte constituit Paracelsus in duos globos distributa." [Paracelsus truly established four elements, distributed in two spheres.] "Sunt enim Elementa loca, matrices & domicilia vitali validaque potestate munita, quæ semina generationi consecrata fovent, digestis temporibus suscitant, ad maturitatem promovent, & emeritis receptacula concedunt." [Moreover, the elements are places, matrices and domiciles fortified with a living and mighty power. They foster *semina* consecrated to generation, arouse them at their appointed times, push them to maturity, and as receptacles they yield to the worn out ones.] The first is a paraphrase of *Idea medicinæ*, p. 41; the second is almost verbatim from pp. 46-47.

generations, and transplantations."⁹¹ As in the *Idea medicinæ*, *semina* are responsible for the sensible properties or signatures of things, and they govern the reception and rejection of outside "impressions" that seek to act on objects, such as, for example, when a celestial star conspires with a terrestrial star to influence the processes of generation (*Liturgiæ generationum*).⁹²

Thesis seventeen of Køning's dissertation provides the best illustration of the similarity between the doctrine he is professing and that of the *Idea medicinæ*, which is undoubtedly his source:

> Briefly, *semina* are the chains of both parts of nature, joining the visibles to the invisibles, in which the laws of motion, predestinations of generations, and processes [*Liturgiæ*] of transplantations and dispensations of the wholly worldly anatomy [*universæ mundanæ Anatomiæ*] are contained, as if in vital powers adorned by an incomprehensible wisdom. In the service [*ministerio*] of these, the impressions of agents are received or refused by patients, the things above are joined to those below, and the sympathy of all nature is watched over. From these proceed the flavors, odors, colors, and vital qualities, forms, and the rest of the signatures, in a mechanical process of generations and transplantations [*in mechanico generationum & transplantationum processu*].⁹³

91 Køning, *Dissertatio de rerum principiis*, f. 4r, thesis 7: "Semina vero ante progressum ex suis Abyssis indissolubili nexu Elementis cohærent, sensuum censuras repudiant, nullis dimensionum vinculis alligata." [In fact, seeds, before going forth from their abysses, adhere to the elements by an indissoluble link, refuse the judgement of the senses, and are not at all bound to the restrictions of the dimensions.] Thesis 8: "Progredientia principiis junguntur, locis includuntur, temporum revolutionibus subjiciuntur, ut absolvant leges motuum, generationum, transplantationum." [Going forth, they are joined to the principles, confined to places, and subject to the cycles of the ages, with the result that they fulfill the laws of motions, generations, and transplantations.] These are loose paraphrases from *Idea medicinæ*, p. 48.
92 In Thesis 11 (Køning, *Dissertatio de rerum principiis*, f. 4v), Køning explicitly stated the Paracelsian-Severinian doctrine that "impressions" from celestial *astra* require the conspiracy of their terrestrial counterparts in order to have any effect on generation. This mechanism provides for the influence of celestial bodies on terrestrial ones, without the consequent astral determinism.
93 Ibid., f. 5r: "Breviter; semina sunt vincula utriusque naturæ, visibilia invisibilibus conjungentia, in quibus motuum leges, prædestinationes generationum, & transplantationum Liturgiæ & universæ mundanæ Anatomiæ dispensationes continentur, tanquam in vitalibus potentiis incomprehensibili sapientia decoratis. Quorum ministerio agentium

→

I have set in brackets particular marked terms that stand out in the *Idea medicinæ* and derivative texts in order to emphasize that Køning used the very words that Severinus had employed in presenting these ideas. And, given that several of the passages that I have quoted here from Køning's dissertation are close paraphrases of corresponding passages from the *Idea medicinæ* – and in some cases almost verbatim quotations – it is evident that Køning must have closely read Severinus' book, even though he does not cite it, or else he lifted the ideas from somebody who had.

The chronology of Køning's education and travels would seem to preclude any long-term contact with Ambrosius Rhodius, who was probably more familiar with Severinus' ideas than anyone else in Norway when Køning was a student. Køning was sent to Latin school in Viborg (Denmark) instead of to Christiania's gymnasium, where Rhodius was a lecturer, and could only have met Rhodius casually, either when visiting Norway or when Rhodius came to Copenhagen in 1658. There is, in any case, no evidence for such contact and no reason to suppose Køning's interest in Paracelsian doctrine came from Rhodius. After several years in Copenhagen, Køning studied in Germany and England for three years, and might well have encountered Severinus' ideas abroad. From England he apparently returned to Norway, where he allegedly had an early version of his dissertation published.[94] By this date, Rhodius was imprisoned at Vardøhus fortress, well above the arctic circle. Whatever interest Mourits Køning may have had in Paracelsian philosophy, it left no mark on his subsequent writings or career. He joined the theological faculty at the University of Copenhagen as an adjunct in 1666, was appointed professor of theology by the king in 1667, and was elevated to Bishop of Aalborg the following year.[95]

→ impressiones a patientibus admittuntur, vel repelluntur, summa infimis conjunguntur, & totius naturæ sympathia custoditur; ex quibus sapores, odores, colores, & qualitates vitales conformationes & signaturæ cæteræ in mechanico generationum & transplantationum processu procedunt." Quoted almost verbatim from *Idea medicinæ*, pp. 58-59.

94 Mauritius Petri Køning, *Nova quædam, sed vera et genuina logices principia* (Christiania: Michael Thomassøn, ca. 1662-63), is now lost. See Holger Rørdam, "Bidrag til tre Biskoppers Levned," p. 350.

95 Bjørn Kornerup, "Køning, Mourits," *DBL*, vol. 8 (1981), p. 412. A couple of days after his appointment as adjunct he was given the rights and responsibilities of a Doctor of Theology by royal order. With absolute monarchy, the kings of Denmark acquired the right to create professorships at will, and Køning was the first such *doctor bullatus*. See Rørdam, "Bidrag til tre Biskoppers Levned," p. 355.

Aside from Ole Borch's references to Severinus and Køning's use of the *Idea medicinæ*, little notice was taken of the *Idea medicinæ* or its chief doctrines in the Danish medical literature after 1650, until the nineteenth century, that is, when Andreas Bremer made extensive use of the *Idea medicinæ* for his treatment of Paracelsian doctrine in his *Dissertationis de vita et opinionibus Theophrasti Paracelsi particula posterior* (1836), for which he was promoted to *Doctor in Medicina*.[96] However, the *Idea medicinæ* was probably still being read in the second half of the seventeenth century, and perhaps an occasional reader took notes on it in private, as did Nicholas Steno. Even so, by then Severinus' influence on medical thought was doubtless waning in Scandinavia just as it was abroad.[97] He was mentioned briefly by Thomas Bartholin in a 1673 tract on the "transplantation" of diseases, but only to acknowledge that transplantation was possible. Bartholin's explanation is in no way Severinian, and Severinus is not referred to at all in subsequent treatises on this subject by Hermann Grube (1674) and Johann Frederik Grynæus.[98] In Denmark, Severinus and his book had, for all practical purposes, passed out of current debate and into medical history.

SWEDEN

Judging by the number of surviving manuscripts and the social prominence of their authors, Paracelsianism was much more acceptable in Sweden than in Denmark in the seventeenth century.[99] One of the earliest proponents of Paracelsianism in Sweden was an eager student

---

96 Andreas Fredericus Bremer, *Dissertationis de vita et opinionibus Theophrasti Paracelsi particula posterior* (Copenhagen: Trier, 1836).

97 Steno mentioned the *Idea medicinæ* in his so-called "Chaos Manuscript," according to Gustav Scherz, *Vom Wege Niels Stensens: Beiträge zu seiner naturwissenschaftlichen Entwicklung*, Acta historica scientiarum naturalium et medicinalium 14 (Copenhagen: Munksgaard, 1956), p. 33. See also Bastholm, *Petrus Severinus*, p. 24.

98 Thomas Bartholin, *De transplantatione morborum dissertatio epistolica* (Copenhagen: Daniel Paulli, 1673), p. 14; Hermann Grube, *De transplantatione morborum. Analysis nova* (Hamburg, 1674); and Johannes Fredericus Grynæus, *Disputatio medica inauguralis de morborum transplantatione et cura sympathetica* (Copenhagen, 1708).

99 Swedish Paracelsianism is the subject of Lindroth, *Paracelsismen i Sverige*.

of occult literature named Johannes Bureus (1568-1652). His scholarly interests can, however, be better described as theosophical than medical, insofar as he mined the works of Paracelsus and his followers primarily for their mystical, cabalistic content, rather than applying himself to chemical philosophy and medicine. If his thought shows any traces of Severinian doctrine, they likely came to him indirectly, through reading texts such as Heinrich Khunrath's *Amphitheatrum*.[100] Sweden and Denmark were fierce economic and political rivals in the early modern period and were several times at war, which discouraged intellectual as well as economic commerce. Not surprisingly, many intellectual stimuli came to Sweden directly across the Baltic, from German and Polish lands. However, some direct influence of Danish Paracelsianism on Swedish Paracelsianism is conceivable insofar as several active scholars were highly mobile and served as philosophical couriers. Such was the case with Joachim Morsius, who visited Bureus on several occasions to discuss heretical religious doctrine.[101]

Joachim Morsius (1593-1642?) was a seventeenth-century pansophist and Rosicrucian, who traveled frequently to Denmark and was very interested in Severinus' unpublished manuscripts.[102] He was born in Hamburg and studied at Rostock and other German universities during the formative years of the Rosicrucian movement (1610-1613) before taking a position as university librarian at Rostock. From 1616 on he seems to have traveled almost incessantly in Germany, Denmark, Belgium, Holland, France, Italy, and England. In 1619 he was at Cambridge, where he allegedly studied chemistry.[103] His frequent visits to Denmark and numerous, well placed contacts there (including Jonas Charisius, Severinus' son-in-law) make it plausible that he helped keep interest in

---

100 Ibid., p. 113.

101 Ibid., pp. 173ff. Bureus was very receptive to the ideology of the Rosicrucian movement and even published tracts in their name. Not surprisingly, then, he was also well read in works by authors of the "outsider Lutheran" tradition, e.g. Valentin Weigel and Johan Arndt and their followers. On the connection between the "outsider Lutheran" or "outsider Protestant" heterodoxy and Paracelsian doctrines, see Shackelford, "A Reappraisal of Anna Rhodius," p. 376.

102 On Morsius see Lindroth, *Paracelsismen i Sverige*, p. 173. See also R.J.W. Evans, *Rudolf II and his World* (Oxford: Clarendon, 1973), p. 284.

103 Ferguson, *Bibliotheca Chemica*, vol. 2, p. 111.

Paracelsianism alive in Severinus' native land during the years after 1616, when such views were increasingly suspect. At any rate, we know that Morsius, who published Paracelsian tracts, knew and praised the *Idea medicinæ*, so perhaps the reputation of Severinus' ideas was first brought to Sweden by him.[104] It is even possible that Severinus' unpublished manuscripts found their way into Swedish hands with the help of Andreas Hoberweschelius, another wandering cosmopolitan Rosicrucian. However, owing to accidents of geography and the chronic hostilities between Stockholm and Copenhagen, scholarly communication flowed into and out of Sweden by way of northern Germany more often than via Denmark.

Paracelsian ideas first generated interest among academics at the University of Uppsala toward the middle of the seventeenth century.[105] Isaac Isthmenius, professor at Uppsala from 1642 on, was among the first Swedish academics to take an interest in Paracelsian chemical doctrines, which he considered in various disputations. In one of these, *Disputatio physica de mistione* (1651), he discussed the Severinian doctrine of *semina*, but evidently relied on Sennert's *De chymicorum ... consensu et dissensu* as his source.[106] In 1627 a Bohemian Paracelsian, Johannes Raicus (d. 1632), joined the medical faculty at Uppsala, where he remained until he went to Dorpat (Tartu, Estonia) to oversee the organization of a *gymnasium* there. According to Sten Lindroth, the influence of the *Idea medicinæ* on Raicus' medical philosophy, most evident in his *Tractatus de podagra medico-kimicus* (1621), likely stemmed from his university days at Wittenberg, where he had been a student of Sennert, who, despite his critical attitude toward Paracelsianism,

104 Bastholm, *Petrus Severinus*, p. 26. According to Ferguson, *Bibliotheca Chemica*, vol. 2, p. 112, Morsius published works by Nollius, Drebbel, and Suchten as well as his own lengthy catalogue of alchemical, medical, philosophical, and theosophical literature. Furthermore, we know from his plea to the Rosicrucian Andreas Hoberweschelius, urging him to have the Paracelsian manuscripts in his possession published, that he was concerned about the fate of Severinus' unpublished manuscripts.

105 Lindroth devoted an entire chapter of *Paracelsismen i Sverige* to Paracelsianism at the University of Uppsala, where there were several professors who were either Paracelsian or sympathetic to Paracelsianism.

106 Isacus Isthmenius, *Disputatio physica de mistione* (Uppsala, 1651), theses 8 and 19, according to Lindroth, *Paracelsismen i Sverige*, pp. 271-2. I have not been able to see Isthmenius' treatise and rely on Lindroth's account.

introduced his students to Severinus' doctrines.[107] Thus, Raicus and Ambrosius Rhodius, perhaps the most enthusiastic supporter of Severinus' ideas in seventeenth-century Scandinavia, were both students of Daniel Sennert and serve as examples of his influence as a writer and teacher.

While at Uppsala, Raicus published a dissertation on a kind of phthisis or consumption that the Paracelsians regarded as caused by "tartarus." Paracelsus had attributed a whole class of diseases to tartar, a mucilaginous impurity similar to the residues in wine casks. But this particular kind of tartar was a vitriolic salt, which Raicus held accountable for the chronic behavior of phthisis. Citing chapter twelve of the *Idea medicinæ* as a source, Raicus wrote that the disease is aggravated by particular foods, especially fish and eel, which contain quantities of dissolved sulphur impurities that are mixed with mercurial and tartarous impurities and are associated with the origin of abscesses. The treatment is to rid the body of the tartarus with diaphoretics, diuretics, and expectorants. For these, Raicus recommended various recipes attributed to Paracelsus, Croll, and other chemists.[108] This reference indicates that Severinus' theory was at least known at Uppsala and applied to specific illnesses, in this case phthisis.

Despite the importance of Paracelsianism in Sweden in the first half of the seventeenth century, Severinus' ideas did not have as broad an influence there as in Denmark. Still, there are indications that his book was available. The inventory of Edmund Gripenhielm's library includes the *Idea medicinæ* along with other influential Paracelsian texts by Croll, Penotus, Khunrath, and others. As in the case of England and elsewhere, Severinus' conception of *semina* as exogenous causes of disease was the most durable of his doctrines. In Sweden this theory lived on into the

107 Lindroth, *Paracelsismen i Sverige*, pp. 328-30, 353, 370, 374, and 384. The biographical information given for Raicus by Gustav Neander, *Ur Lungsotens och Lungsotsbehandlingens äldre Historia i Sverige* (Stockholm: Norstedt, 1924), p. 36, does not wholly agree with that given by Lindroth. Neander reports that Raicus studied medicine at Elbing, came to Sweden in 1625, was appointed at Uppsala in 1627 and at Dorpat in 1630, where he died in 1631.

108 Johannes Raicus, *De Phthisi ex Tartaro* (Uppsala: Eskil Mattson, 1628). I have not been able to see this treatise, but have relied on the Swedish translation given in Neander, *Ur Lungsotens Historia*, pp. 151-197.

second half of the century in the pansophism of George Stiernhielm (1598-1672).[109]

Severinus was also known to the Swedish chemist and metallurgist Urban Hjärne (1641-1724), who ran the *Laboratorium Chymicum* that had been set up for the Swedish Department of Mines (*Bergskollegium*).[110] Hjärne was sympathetic to chemical philosophy and was moved by the wholesale rejection of Paracelsian ideas and by the vilification of Paracelsus by Conring and other antiparacelsians to defend the "Teutonic Philosopher."[111] The main points of Hjärne's defense were aimed to reveal Paracelsus as a pious and able adept, whose theory did not seriously conflict with the teachings of Luther. He mentions Severinus only briefly, as one who, in the company of Michael Toxites, Dorn, Andreas Solea, Quercetanus, Moffet, Van Helmont, Davidson, and George Starkey, understood both chemistry and philosophy better than did Erastus, Libavius, Conring, and the other antiparacelsians.[112] Three years later, Hjärne cited chapter eight of the *Idea medicinæ* along with Davidson's *Philosophia pyrotechnica* to support the thesis that things of this world are produced by the three Paracelsian principles and the four Aristotelian elements, to which they are joined.[113] His quotation makes it clear that Severinus' book was still being read in Stockholm at the end of the seventeenth century.

109 Ibid., pp. 176 (note 8), and 477.

110 On Urban Hjärne, see Sten Lindroth, "Hiärne, Block och Paracelsus. En redogörelse för Paracelsusstriden 1708-09," *Lychnos* (1941): 191-292; "Urban Hiärne och Laboratorium chymicum," *Lychnos* (1946-47): 51-116.

111 Urban Hjärne, *Defensionis Paracelsicæ Prodromus. Eller, Kort Föremäle af then uthförligare Förswars Skrift för den stora Philosophus Theutonicus Theophrastus Paracelsus, som nyligen medelst en hård Beskyltning uthan någon Orsak är worden antastad* (Stockholm: Julius G. Matthiæ, 1709).

112 Ibid., p. 5.

113 Urban Hjärne, *Acta et tentamine chymica in regio laboratorio Stockholmiensi, elaborata et demonstrata, in decades redacta atque divisa una cum præmissa parasceve seu prævia manuductione ad experimenta rite perficienda* (Stockholm: Johan Werner, 1712), p. 97.

I have attempted to document references to Petrus Severinus, to the *Idea medicinæ*, and to the chief doctrines expressed in it as fully as practical within the scope of four chapters in order to establish the importance of his work to the history of ideas. Severinus' teachings were known at least casually to a diverse educated public, impinging on medical theory, poetry, and geology. His reputation as a Paracelsian medical philosopher was truly international, inasmuch as those who owned and cited his work lived in all the major nations in western, central, and northern Europe, and in one case, New England. His doctrine of the seminal origin for things, diseases in particular, was especially influential, although it is true that these references conform to the genres of medical literature that are relatively easy to identify and peruse, and this fact has no doubt made my survey somewhat selective. However, it is not a mistake to look for something first in those places where you expect to find it, and then to widen the search later. Even so, echos of *semina* theory turned up not just in the Paracelsian medical literature, but in more general discussions of natural philosophy by Pierre Gassendi and Kort Aslakssøn, for example, and the logical conclusion is that this was indeed Severinus' most influential doctrine.

Severinus was one of the earliest learned authors to build a philosophical system around Paracelsus' ideas, and for this reason he was enormously important to the dissemination of Paracelsian theory. Most of the authors mentioned in these four chapters were either Paracelsian sympathizers, physicians interested in incorporating chemical philosophy into an eclectic method of healing, or critics hostile to Paracelsus. The critics' perspectives are perhaps most salient to the modern eye, on account of the rhetorical power that is invested in them. The earliest discussion of Severinus' work that I have found was in fact part of Thomas Erastus' 1572 assault on Paracelsian philosophy, which focussed attention on Paracelsian doctrines. Often these critics devoted considerable time and space to commentary on Severinus' ideas, the prime example of which is Andreas Libavius' attack on Severinus' philosophy as expounded by Libavius' rival, Johannes Hartmann. However, by far the lengthiest treatments of Severinus' ideas are to be found in treatises devoted specifically to explaining, defending, and applying Severinus' work. These are the subject of the next two chapters.

PART FOUR

READING THE
IDEA MEDICINÆ PHILOSOPHICÆ

Chapter Nine

"A MAPPE OF MEDECYNE" AND AMBROSIUS RHODIUS' DEFENSE OF THE *IDEA MEDICINÆ PHILOSOPHICÆ*

𝕴T HAS BEEN amply demonstrated in the foregoing chapters that Severinus' *Idea medicinæ philosophicæ* was a widely read and influential book. As one of the earliest scholars to give Paracelsian medical philosophy a learned exposition and metaphysical basis, Severinus was lauded by those who favored chemical philosophy and medicine, men such as Guy de la Brosse and Thomas Moffet, and he was criticized by those who opposed the Paracelsians, especially by Thomas Erastus and Andreas Libavius. But most people who left specific comments concerning Severinus and the *Idea medicinæ* in print or incorporated recognizable bits of Severinus' theory into their own work reacted with greater equanimity than was the case with authors who, like those mentioned above, represented extreme doctrinal positions. This was generally the situation in the seventeenth century, when time put greater distance between Severinus and the intense debate over Paracelsianism that had begun in the last quarter of the sixteenth century.

As previous chapters have shown, most references to Severinus in the literature of the period were rather brief, indicating specific interest in his *semina* theory or merely citing the *Idea medicinæ* as a source of Paracelsian doctrine. These references provide important clues as to how widely Severinus' ideas spread and give us some grasp of the variety of contexts into which they found their way – contexts as diverse as Johannes Hartmann's medical theory and Edward Jorden's balneology. They were incorporated into the "Mosaic physics" of Kort Aslakssøn and received passing mention by John Donne and Edward Herbert, to repeat but a few of the intellectual traces of the *Idea medicinæ* that were identified in previous chapters. Identification of these references and the contexts in which they occur give us a good conception of who was reading the *Idea medicinæ*, or at least knew something of its content, and inform us about the variety of uses to which Severinus' ideas were put. However, to understand better how the book as whole was read we must examine several lengthier treatments of the *Idea medicinæ*, especially the commentaries devoted specifically to it, in this chapter and the next.[1]

There are three printed books that can be classified as dedicated commentaries on Severinus' work. One was composed by a student of Daniel Sennert and Ole Worm named Ambrosius Rhodius, who married Severinus' granddaughter, Anna Frederiksdatter Severinus. The remaining two were written by William Davidson of Aberdeen, whose interest in Severinus' philosophy was mentioned already in chapter five. Davidson's treatises will be characterized in the next chapter on account of their length. But before turning to study these commentaries, it is useful to consider two additional means of assessing how the *Idea medicinæ* was read. The first of these is a text, if one can call it that, consisting of the marginalia in a particular copy of the 1571 edition of the *Idea medicinæ*. A quick survey of these marginal annotations will illuminate what one anonymous reader found interesting about Severinus' medical philosophy. The second "text" is actually a draft of an English translation of the *Idea medicinæ* that was given the title "A Mappe of Medicyne." Although a translation is not formally a commentary, this manuscript offers clues to what the translator found new or perplexing in Severinus' book, and this provides insight into how it was understood.

---

1 It might well be argued that Libavius' criticism of Severinus' theories (which he says were repeated by Johannes Hartmann) constitutes a commentary on the *Idea medicinæ*. However, since this matter has already been discussed in chapter seven, it will be omitted here.

ONE READER'S MARGINALIA

My attention was first directed to the copy of the *Idea medicinæ* that resides in the Beineke Library at Yale University because it was alleged to have once belonged to the great English natural philosopher and occultist, John Dee. This copy later found its way into the hands of one of New England's early adepts and the first governor of Connecticut, John Winthrop, Jr.[2] The many marginalia, said to be in Dee's hand, promised to reveal what the famous Elizabethan magus made of Severinus' medical philosophy. But after close study of these annotations, I am in doubt about the reported history of the book and the identification of the marginalia with John Dee. Nevertheless, this copy of the *Idea medicinæ* is quite heavily annotated and provides an opportunity to see what one late sixteenth or seventeenth-century reader found noteworthy, whoever he or she may have been.[3]

It is evident that the annotator began to read the *Idea medicinæ* systematically, rather than consulting it casually for particular information, because the marginalia begin already on page four and continue rather consistently until p. 124, where they break off abruptly, implying that the annotator quit reading the book closely at that point. Of these first 124

---

2 New Haven, Connecticut, Yale University, Beinecke Yna31 571s. Ronald Wilkinson identified this book as having belonged to John Dee. See Wilkinson, "The Alchemical Library of John Winthrop," p. 182 (cf. ch. 6, n. 85 above).

3 Several of John Dee's books are known to have been in John Winthrop, Jr.'s collection, some of which were annotated and underlined by Dee. Others have been identified as having belonged to Dee, but were annotated by someone else. The catalogue that John Dee made of his books and manuscripts indicates that he did indeed own a copy of the *Idea medicinæ* as well as Severinus' now very rare *Epistola*, both of which he marked to take with him to the continent in 1583. However, the Beinecke copy of the *Idea medicinæ* is one of several Paracelsian and alchemical books given to Yale by F.B. Winthrop and is not marked with any of John Dee's usual marks of ownership. I agree with Julian Roberts and Andrew G. Watson, eds., *John Dee's Library Catalogue* (London: The Bibliographical Society, 1990), p. 89, that the annotations do not seem to be his; Certainly the hand does not clearly resemble any of the samples of Dee's handwriting that they reproduced. Perhaps more telling, the "pointing hands" in the Beinecke copy are of a distinctly different style: the one reproduced on p. 74 of the catalogue has a round cuff and a continuous hand, whereas those in the Beinecke *Idea medicinæ* have a cuff formed by two lines, one of which is part of the thumb line, which is itself sometimes discontinuous from the rest of the hand, unlike the samples from Dee's books.

pages, eighty six, or about seventy percent, contain marginalia. Often the annotations consist of words or phrases extracted from the adjacent text, which is sometimes underlined. This kind of marginal note serves as a topic heading or reference to the content of Severinus' text and usually comprises peculiarly Paracelsian terms (e.g. *Rellolaceæ qualitates, Iliaster, Cagastrum, Cherionia*) or concepts especially characteristic of Severinus' theory, such as *"fructus firmamenti"* (the fruits of the firmament) and *"seminum natura diversa"* (the diverse nature of the *semina*).[4] Some of these headings refer to specific discussions, such as *"officium sulphuris,"* found adjacent to a passage listing some of the functions of sulphur.[5] Several terms are marked on the top outside corner of the page, suggesting that they deserve special attention, either because of their part in Severinus' doctrine or because they are unusual. For example, *"seminis definitio"* (the definition of seed) is penned in at the top left (outside) corner of p. 96 and repeated in the margin adjacent to the passage beginning "therefore the seed is the vital principle," which is underlined.[6] At the upper right (outside) corner of the following page, *Nox Orphei, Orcus Hippoc., Abyssus Mojsis*, and *Iliadum Paracel.* are enumerated, refering to the introduction of these unusual terms in the text.

Longer marginal annotations consisting of several words or a short sentence are more typical and often summarize key points of Severinus' philosophy: "Innate heat is greatest in living things"; "Medicine resides in the balsam of all dead things"; "Bodies come from and are resolved into spirits"; "What is visible in the heavens is also in the other elements"; "Forms are generated from within," not infused by a *dator formarum*, which is underscored in the adjacent text; "Mechanical spirits are the links of the visible and invisible"; "Internal spiritual bodies are vehicles for the seminal reasons"; and so on.[7]

---

4 *Idea medicinæ*, Beinecke Yna 31 571s, pp. 19, 108, 45, and 95.
5 Ibid., p. 119.
6 Ibid., p. 96: "Semen itaque est vitale Principium … rei producendæ."
7 Ibid., p. 22: "Innatum calidum in crescentibus plurimum"; p. 25: "In Balsamo morborum omnium medicina viget"; p. 26: "Ex spiritibus prodeunt corpora et in spiritibus resoluuntur corpora"; p. 53: "Quæ in coelo conspiciuntur in cæteris elementis continentur"; p. 81: "Forma uniuscuiusque rei αὐτοφυὴν"; p. 98: "Spiritus mechanici sunt vincula visibilium et invisibilium"; and p. 113: "Corpora interna spiritualia sunt rationum vehicula."

Often the reader's marginalia illuminate a passage in the text that he or she has underlined, and sometimes these offer a glimpse of the reader's interpretation. For example, next to Severinus' statement on generation, "this multitude will spring up from one seed, with the passage of time," the reader wrote "multitude emanates from unity," which suggests that the he or she placed Severinus' comment in a larger Platonic context.[8] Perhaps the reader also misinterpreted Severinus' words: adjacent to Severinus' observation that the generation of metallic *semina* is comprehended with difficulty by those who have not tasted the cabalistic sources (*fontes*), the reader noted "the mysteries of the metals lie hidden in the source of the cabalistic," which suggests a more literal interpretation than Severinus may have intended.[9]

It is interesting to observe that several of the annotations indicate that the religious implications of Severinus' ideas were important to the reader. On page 34, Severinus' contention that the physician must know the general and particular laws of both terrestrial and celestial nature evoked the handwritten marginal annotation "the whole sphere of nature would be comprehended by the human soul." A pointing hand adds additional emphasis.[10] A comment written at the bottom of page 41, underneath the text, notes that the first incorporeal receptacles of nature took light and seminal reasons from the word of God, revealing the reader's interest in Severinus' Paracelsian interpretation of Genesis.[11] On page 107, Severinus' statement that every herb reflects the presence of God is underlined, and the reader's comment in the margin – "Light of Nature; all things are full of Jove" – indicates that the Paracelsian

---

8 Ibid., p. 107: "Ex unitate Multitudo emanat."
9 Ibid., p. 121: "Mysteria metallorum in Cabalisticæ fonte latent." The annotator's wording suggests that he took Severinus' words literally, rather than referring to the need to study the cabalistic (i.e. alchemical) literature for information on this topic. For the sixteenth-century use of the term cabala to refer to alchemy and other occult sciences, see Harkness, *John Dee's Conversations with Angels*, p. 87, where the author analyzes John Dee's distinction between "vulgar cabala" (a traditional Hebrew scriptural exegesis) and "real cabala," which was the study of God's word as written in the Book of Nature. I believe that her insightful conclusions about Dee on this distinction apply more generally to his contemporaries.
10 *Idea medicinæ*, Beinecke Yna 31 571s, p. 34: "Tota Naturæ sphære ab humana anima comprehendatur."
11 Ibid., p. 41.

concept of the Light of Nature, which reveals the divine plan to man through his study of the natural world, was of interest in the context of divine immanence.[12] The reader's concern for the religious ramifications of Paracelsian doctrine would also explain marginalia referring to passages about the Paracelsian conception of predestination as a kind of law that is built into the very essences of things and his or her interest in the consequence of this for Severinus' *semina* theory, namely that when the predestinations of the seminal reasons are completed, the world will be at an end.[13]

Among the various marginalia there are two explicit references to other authors, and from these we can gain some insight into the reader's assimilation of Severinus' ideas. The first reference is to page 94 of Paracelsus' *Aurora thesaurusque philosophorum* (Basel, 1577), which presumably illuminates Severinus' assertion that there can be no generation unless there is first an agreement or harmony between the principles, so that heat is not overcome by cold, nor wetness by dryness, which the annotator underlined in the adjacent text.[14] If we then turn to page 94 of the *Aurora*, we find the Paracelsian claim that salt is a mediating principle between mercury and sulphur, which unifies those opposites into one common subject.[15] This note reveals to us that the reader was familiar with at least one other Paracelsian work and that the annotations must have been made after 1577, when the *Aurora* was published. It also implies that the reader was placing Severinus' rather general observation that generation requires cooperation and harmony, which is imposed by a spiritual agent, into a very specific Paracelsian context, which assigned this function to salt. The second citation is of a passage attributed to Hermes, which is indicated by a pointing hand: "And just as all things were made by one meditation of the One, so all things were produced from this one thing by adaptation." This serves as a gloss to Severinus'

---

12 Ibid., p. 107: "Lumen Naturæ; Jovis omnia plena."

13 Ibid., pp. 92 and 78.

14 Ibid., p. 43.

15 Paracelsus, *Aurora thesaurusque philosophorum, Theophrasti Paracelsi, Germani philosophi, & medici præ cunctis omnibus accuratissimi. Accessit Monarchia Physica per Gerardum Dorneum, in defensionem Paracelsicorum principiorum, a suo præceptore positorum* (Basel: Palmaguar, 1577). According to the pagination of Yale's copy of this book, the part quoted by the annotator is actually from the treatise by Dorn.

PHILOSOPHICAE.   53

placet, etiam feminarias uirtutes & fœcunditates, ex
cœlo inconfideratè deduxerunt. At certè, quæcunq̃
in cœlo explicata confpiciuntur, in cœteris quoq̃ Elementis, uirtute et uitali poteftate continētur: à quibus
actiones proficifcuntur : in quibus Scientiæ mecha-
niciq̃ rerum proceſſus uigent : in quibus temporum
decreta momenta cuftodiuntur. Corpora ubiq̃ mortua funt. Sic æftatis, hyemis, ueris, autumni fydera, in
Terra continentur, in Aqua & Aere: quæ nifi confpi-
rarent cum aftris Firmamenti, fteriles cœleftium im-
preſſiones utiq̃ accufaremus, fi temporum Tranf-
plantationes, & confluentiarum præuaricationes an-
nonæ calamitates pariunt. Mutua enim feminum
confpiratione, familiaritate, nutricatione, totius Naturæ fœcunditas ftabilitur : impreſsionum reciproca
uiciſsitudine nexus conferuatur. Harum legibus ui-
tiatis fterilitates & defectus fequuntur. Sed quæ-
nam funt illa corpora aftralia inferiorum Elementorum? Sanè duplicata funt. Puriori, quæ cœleftium
perfectionem æmulantur, in confpectum non ueni-
unt, nifi artificū induftria, diuina adaptatione ab ad-
iunctis feparentur. Poteftatem, uitam, actionum ui-
gorem ubiq̃ demonftrant. Quemadmodum uerò
inter fe differunt femina, officijs & proprietatibus: ita
hæc quoque corpora differre aſſerimus: herbarum
corpora ab arborum, animalium, mineralium, metal-

G 3   lorum,

The annotations on this page of a copy of Petrus Severinus' Idea medicinæ philosophicæ *reveals the reader's interest in the religious implications of his theory. This
copy may have come to America in the early seventeenth century. Courtesy of the
Beinecke Rare Book and Manuscript Library, Yale University.*

statement that things in nature are separated by divine adaptation, *divina adaptione* being doubly underscored in the *Idea medicinæ*.[16]

The overall impression that the reader's comments give is that he or she was primarily interested in the metaphysics in Severinus' book and not in how it illuminates medicine per se. The annotations generally refer to the fundamentals of Severinian theory and place them in a larger context of Neoplatonic, probably Hermetic thought, and reinforce the contention that Paracelsian literature was of interest to people who were engaged with the religious aspects of natural philosophy. The consistency in the hand, the abrupt breaking off of the marginal comments, and the uniform color of the ink imply that the reader read systematically and with persistence rather than coming back to the text intermittently over an extended period of time.

"A Mappe of Medicyne"

There is in the Sloane Collection at the British Library a lengthy English manuscript (Sloane MS. 11) bearing the title "A Mappe of Medicyne or Philosophicall Path Conteininge The groundes of all the doctrines of Paracelsus, Hippocrates & Galen Compiled by Peter Severine a Dane." It is a draft of a translation of the entire *Idea medicinæ* made by an unknown scholar at an undetermined time, but most likely in the seventeenth century. The title page carries the name Anthony Bartlet, but signs of erasure next to the name suggest that he may not have been the original owner. The translation is not complete in the sense of being polished, but it does cover the entirety of the Latin original. There are signs of editing – strikeouts and new terms or new text inserted between lines – but overall the manuscript gives the impression of a first draft that

---

16 *Idea medicinæ*, Beinecke copy, p. 53: "Hermes. Et sicut res omnes fuerunt ab uno medi-
tatione unius: sic omnes res natæ fuerunt ab hac una re adaptatione." This comes almost
verbatim from the third statement of the *Emerald Table* of Hermes, the Latin text of
which is printed in Julius F. Ruska, *Tabula Smaragdina: Ein Beitrag zur Geschichte der
Hermetischen Literatur* (Heidelberg: Carl Winter's Universitatsbuchhandlung, 1926),
p. 2. See also Wayne Shumaker, *The Occult Sciences in the Renaissance: A Study in Intellectual Patterns* (Berkeley: University of California Press, 1972), pp. 179-80.

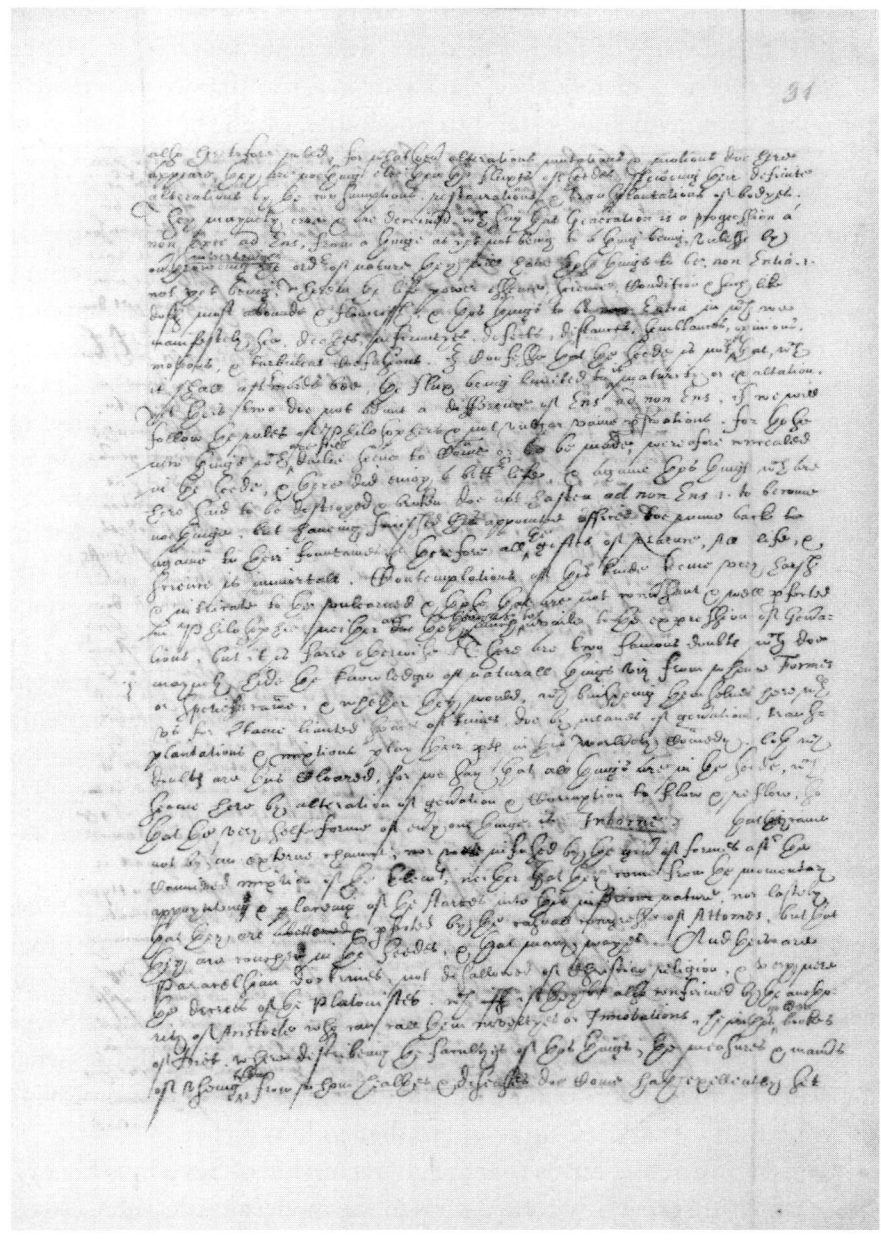

An English translation of Petrus Severinus' Idea medicinæ philosophicæ *under the title "A Mappe of Medicyne or Philosophicall Path" is preserved in the Sloane collection at the British Library. Courtesy of the British Library.*

was somewhat emended in the writing but not yet reworked for publication. In the absence of further evidence we cannot know if "A Mappe of Medicyne" was merely a scholar's personal translation, or intended for publication, which is certainly a possibility, given the popularity of English Paracelsian tracts in the seventeenth century.

Three features of the manuscript argue for its being readied for publication. First, there are sporadic marginal headings, suggesting that repeated use or circulation was expected. Second, whereas Severinus wrote in Latin and included occasional Greek terms and quotations, the translator rendered the Latin into English, but in many instances translated the Greek into Latin! This implies that the reader was expected to be unable to read Greek, and Latin only with difficulty. In this way the exotic and authoritative nature of the quotations could be retained in an otherwise vernacular edition. However, in some instances the Greek phrases were simply omitted, sometimes with space left in the manuscript, as if the translator had passed over the Greek with the intention of coming back to it later. Third, the summaries that Severinus often integrated into the final paragraphs of each chapter, which were set off from the surrounding text by the use of all capitals, were extracted and placed as abstracts before the chapters in the manuscript, implying that the writer of Sloane MS 11 was restructuring Severinus' format for eventual publication. Whatever the purpose behind Sloane MS 11, it is clear that a great deal of time and effort went into this lengthy translation of such a difficult Latin text.

It may seem odd to look at a translation for clues as to how a book was read, since "A Mappe of Medicyne" in fact offers no gloss or other commentary beyond the translated text of the *Idea medicinæ*, yet the information it yields reveals one English reader's interpretation of Severinus' idiom and terminology. Strikeouts and rewordings tell us what concepts the translator found difficult to render and therefore provide us insight into what ideas were unfamiliar to him or her.[17]

Consider the chief terms that are characteristic of Severinus' theory, those which are especially conspicuous to the modern reader, like *scientia*

---

17 It is entirely possible that the translator was a woman, since – at least in Denmark – women were active in vernacularizing texts of particular interest. However, for convenience I shall refer to the translator as he.

mechanica, lithurgia, Orcus, dona, signa, insignia, signatura, domesticus, minera, anatomia, officina, hospes, fomites, and even *idea.* Most of these terms were discussed in previous chapters in the context of Severinus' use of them. A thorough grasp of the translator's understanding of Severinus' philosophy is not possible without a complete comparison of the English text with the Latin, which lies beyond the scope of this study, but we can acquire a sense of the novelty of some of the major concepts presented in the *Idea medicinæ* by sampling how some of these terms were rendered. Page references to the Latin terms, given in parentheses below, refer to the 1571 edition of the *Idea medicinæ.* References to the English translations are given as folium numbers of the corresponding "A Mappe of Medecyne."

Severinus used the term *mechanica* and its variants chiefly as an adjective modifying a noun, but rarely as a substantive.[18] Usually the translator merely Anglicized the word, as in his rendering of *"spiritus mechanici ventriculi"* (p. 260) as "the mechanick spirits of the stomacke" (f. 82v), and *"radicum proprietates ac mechanicas progressiones"* (p. 234) as "the properties and mechanicke processes of Rootes" (f. 75v). There are many such instances, for example "mechanicke spirits" (f. 35v), "mechanicke art" (f. 36r), and "mechanicke methode" (f. 41r), implying that the translator either did not know an alternate meaning, or else assumed the reader would know what "mechanick" meant in these contexts. However, in a couple of passages where *mechanica* modifies *lithurgia* or *processus,* alternative words are presented, suggesting that "mechanicke" did not convey an obvious meaning. For example, *scientiæ mechanicique rerum processus* (p. 53) is rendered "the sciences and usuall [mechanick] processes of things" (f. 22r), where "usuall" was underlined and "mechanick" was added in above the line. A similar case, where *dona sunt plurima, Scientiæ & mechanici processus* (p. 63) is translated as "there be many guifts, sciences, & vitall [ordenary] mechanick processes" (f. 26r), points to the translator's uncertainty about what *mechanici* meant. In this case, both "ordenary" and "mechanick" are above the line, marked for insertion after "vitall," but "ordenary" appears to have been lined out. This implies that the

---

18 For example, *artificiosa mechanica* (Severinus, *Idea medicinæ,* p. 100), where *artificiosa* modifies what must be the substantive, *mechanica.*

translator initially opted for "vitall," but supplemented that with "ordenary" and then "mechanick." Note, too, the literal translation of *dona* and *scientiæ*, a practice that is also characteristic of Sloane MS 11. On one page, *mechanicos* was translated as both "ordenary" and "workeing," in both cases with "mechanicke" put in above the line.[19]

The term *lithurgia* is translated variously. Sometimes it is taken to mean process, but can also mean method, as for example, *"Non enim Generationis Mechanicam lithurgiam … intelligunt"* (p. 162), which became "They understand not that mechanick method of generation" (f. 55v), or *"Lienis mechanicam lithurgiam"* (p. 174), which became "the mechanick methode of the spleene" (f. 60r). In one case *lithurgia* and *methodorum* appear in the same sentence and were both translated "methods."[20] *Lithurgia* might mean progress, as in "the mechanick progresse of generations and transplantations" (f. 73v) or even orders, as in "mechanicke orders of spirits in the progress of generations & transplantations" (f. 78r).[21] These various renderings suggest that the translator had an idea that *mechanica lithurgia* involved ordinary processes or functions, but that he was not too confident about the translation.

Several of the arcane terms that Severinus used were left untranslated in Sloane MS 11, indicating that their uses were peculiar to this kind of theory and did not have a wider meaning – or at least the translator did not bother to assign them a more general meaning. Included in this group are *Orcus* (Anglicized to "Orke") and *minera*, as in "from the myneras of their rootes" (f. 86r).[22] This contrasts with the treatment of another peculiar term, *fomites*. *Fomites* had been used in a medical sense by Fracastoro to denote the microscopic bits of matter that spread contagion. Severinus did not adopt the concept as a fundamental part of his theory of disease, which was not essentially a materialist theory, but he did occasionally use the term, as when he described diseases

19 Severinus, "Mappe," f. 35r: "the ordenary [mechanicke] processes of generations" and "the workeing [mechanicke] spirits & tinctures." This corresponds to Severinus, *Idea medicinæ*, p. 96.

20 "Vide calamitatem sensibilium Methodorum in occulta Naturæ lithurgia" (Severinus, *Idea medicinæ*, p. 207) became "Behold the calamitie of sencible methods in the secret methodes of nature" ("Mappe," f. 69r).

21 These are translations of "Generationum ac Transplantationum mechanica lithurgia" (Severinus, *Idea medicinæ*, p. 227) and "spirituum mechanicas lithurgias in Generationum & Transplantationum progressu" (Ibid., p. 244) respectively.

22 Ibid., p. 272: "a radicum mineris."

"which have their rootes & fomites in the Anatomye of the stomack" (f. 74v).[23] In this case *fomites* was untranslated, but in other instances it was rendered as "nurtures" and "enticements," suggesting that the translator was going to the root (*fovere*, to warm or foment) in search of a more general meaning.[24]

Certain terms the translator must surely have known, yet he refrained from translating them, perhaps because he wished them to signal an unusual connotation in the context of the *Idea medicinæ*. For example, there are instances where the Latin *ens* and *entia* are retained as "Ens" and "Enses."[25] Similarly, the peculiar Paracelsian use of the term *astra* to refer both to the "stars" that are in terrestrial matter and to the more familiar celestial bodies is retained by rendering *astra* as "asters," even though "starres" is also used, and the distinction is not consistent.[26] One explanation is that the translator understood that Severinus used the term in an uncommon way and sought to distinguish this special use from the ordinary use, but had not yet applied this policy throughout the draft. Inconsistencies such as this give the manuscript an uneven quality, which tends to vitiate judgements about the translator and his intended audience. Nevertheless, as mentioned before, certain formalities observed in Sloane MS 11 indicate that the translator was not merely making an English version of the *Idea medicinæ* for his own use, but had an audience in mind, one which was perhaps familiar with medicine but uncomfortable with Latin – say apothecaries or healers without the benefit of a university education, or maybe even the gentleman *curioso*. Although there are many instances where terms were merely Anglicized from their Latin or Latinized Greek forms, such as "cedmatick" (f. 85v), "pontagious" (f. 76v), "Endimyan," "Epidemyall," and "Epidemick" (f. 90v), there are many other instances where an attempt was made to find the native English translation, espe-

23 Ibid., p. 230: "quæ in ventriculi Anatomia radices sive fomites habeant."
24 For example, ibid., p. 200: "fomites & mineras habent" ("have nurtures & mineraes" – "Mappe," f. 66r), and p. 229: "Natura … manus dat & hospitem admittit peregrinum, cujus radices, mineræ vel fomites, in certa quadam Anatomia corporis recepti" (Shee [i.e. Nature] admits this stranger, this guest, & entertanes him with a seemeing frendlynes, whose rootes, minerals, or enticements being found in some certaine Anatomie of the bodie" – "Mappe," f. 74r).
25 For example, "Mappe," ff. 21r, 22r, 59r, and 68r.
26 For example, ibid., f. 21v, where "Asters" are internal phenomena, and "celestiall stars" are also mentioned. Compare with "visible Asters" and "celestial Asters" (f. 22r), and "Starres" (f. 44r).

cially for the established medical terms for diseases and drugs, for example "hawkeweede," "prymerose," "coweslip," and "gowte." Sometimes both classical and vernacular forms were used, such as "tythymalus or milkethistle" (f. 87v) for *tythymallorum* (p. 279) and "wolfe-banely or nappellous" for the adjective *nappellosa* (p. 285).

One could continue an analysis of the peculiarities and inconsistencies of translation in Sloane MS 11 at length and come up with an increasingly more nuanced impression of the translator, but since the manuscript is really a draft, perhaps the results would be no more definite. This brief survey shows that the translator really did understand some of the peculiarities of Paracelsian and Platonist expressions, insofar as he often translated them into English. Yet he balked at others, suggesting that these had not been properly digested by physicians. His handling of decidedly Paracelsian terms like *Rellollaceum*, translating "*Rellollaceis qualitatibus*" (p. 19) as "passive dead quallityes" (f. 10r), shows an easy familiarity with Paracelsian texts and meanings, yet *minera* defied easy translation.

One final point of translation deserves comment here, and that pertains to the interpretation placed on the Greco-Latin word *idea*, a key to understanding the title of Severinus' book and therefore the meaning of its contents. In chapter twelve, the phrase "*unam communemque Ideam*" (p. 249) was translated as "one generall or commune Idea and patterne" (f. 79v), indicating that the translator, a seventeenth-century reader of the *Idea medicinæ*, clearly understood Severinus' book to offer a general theory or pattern for medicine, that is, an idealization. This is best summed up by his translation of another passage from chapter twelve, which may have given the title "A Mappe of Medicyne or Philosophicall Path" to Sloane MS 11: "We doe not here promise an absolute & perfect description of Diseases, but a patterne, or path which in some measure disposeth the Philosophicall truthe" (f. 74v).[27]

---

27 Severinus, *Idea medicinæ*, pp. 230-31: "Non enim perfectam morborum descriptionem hoc loco pollicemur: Sed Ideam & adumbrata vestigia Philosophicæ veritatis." Here "idea" is clearly identified with a form or sketch, much as the outline of a foot is left behind in the footprints, a series of which form a path. One is reminded of the illustration of a man following Nature's footprints with the aid of a lantern, which is the emblem for "the secrets of nature" (emblem XLII) in Michael Maier, *Atalanta fugiens, hoc est, Emblemata nova de secretis naturæ chymica* (Oppenheim: Hieronymus Gallerus, 1618; facsimile reprint, Kassel and Basel: Bärenreiter Verlag, 1964), p. 177.

AMBROSIUS RHODIUS

The first actual commentary on the *Idea medicinæ* is a little known, rather uncommon Latin treatise written in Norway during the Thirty Years' War and published in Copenhagen in 1643. Its title, *Disputationes supra Ideam medicinæ philosophicæ Petri Severini*, or more fully and in translation, *Debates over Petrus Severinus' Idea medicinæ philosophicæ, ... in which obscure and difficult passages of that book are illuminated, opponents are refuted, and many discourses taken from Nature's innermost recesses are brought up for consideration,*[28] reveals the author's knowledge of the controversial reception that Severinus' book had encountered and suggests a defense of his ideas. Indeed, Ambrosius Rhodius, the author of this commentary, systematically presented the major doctrines of the *Idea medicinæ* and provided supporting information and different points of view drawn from a wide variety of sources, to provide a contemporary context for understanding Severinus' ideas. The commentary thus offers us a valuable opportunity to see how the *Idea medicinæ* was read approximately seventy years after it was published.

Ambrosius Rhodius is almost unknown to modern scholarship and warrants an introduction here. He was a Saxon, born 10 November 1605 in Kemberg, near Wittenberg, where his father, Jacob Rhodius, was a parish priest.[29] His uncle, also named Ambrosius Rhodius, was a profes-

28 Ambrosius Rhodius, *Disputationes supra Ideam medicinæ philosophicæ Petri Severini Dani Philosophi & Friderici II Daniæ & Septentrionalis Regis Archiatri olim felicissimi, Quibus loca illius Libri obscura & difficilia illustrantur, adversarij refutantur, & multi discursus ex intimis Naturæ adytis deprompti moventur* (Copenhagen: Salomon Sartorius, 1643).

29 The earliest source of biographical information is Ambrosius Rhodius' autobiography, written in 1654, when the outbreak of plague apparently caused him to reflect on his life. Although this autobiography is not known to exist today, the text was preserved by Rhodius' first biographer, Gottlieb Müller, a priest in Kemberg, in his 1760 work "Lebensgeschichte eines für die Krone Dännemark merkwürdigen Sterndeuters Ambrosius Rhodius." Although this was supposedly published, according to A.G. Kästner, "Ambrosius Rhodius," in *Geschichte der Mathematic* (Gøttingen, 1800), no printed copy has been found. Müller's manuscript exists in Copenhagen, Kgl. Bibl., NKS 2088 4°. The autobiographical text itself has been published in Emmerich Ingerslev, *Ambrosius Rhodius og Hans Hustru* (Copenhagen: Vilhelm Tryde, 1916), pp. 13-19. On the Rhodiuses see Shackelford, "A Reappraisal of Anna Rhodius." Another important source is Johan Scharffenberg, "Bidrag til de norske lægestillingers historie før 1800," *Norsk Magasin for Lægevidenskaben*, 5th series, vol. 2 (1904), pp. 1329-1384. General biographical and bibliographical information can be found in *NBL*, vol. 11 (1952), pp. 409-410; H. Ehrencron-Müller (ed.), *Forfatterlexikon omfattende Danmark, Norge og Island indtil 1814*, vol. 7 (1929), pp. 7-8.

sor of mathematics at Wittenberg. He had been an assistant to Tycho Brahe at Prague in 1600 and later distinguished himself as the author of a lengthy treatise on optics.[30] Young Ambrosius received an excellent education at home, where he was by his own account "diligently instructed in the fear of God and the Latin and Greek languages" before being sent to Grimma Fürstenschule at age fifteen.[31] In 1626 the plague closed the doors of the aristocratic academy, interrupting his studies. The following year Rhodius' parents sent him to the University of Wittenberg, where he studied mathematics under his uncle Ambrosius, medicine under Daniel Sennert, anatomy and botany under Gregory Nymann, and physics under Johan Sperling.[32] He was promoted to *magister philosophiæ* in 1629, after which he pursued the study of medicine and was educated "in botany, anatomy, chemical operations, astrology, and whatever else belongs to the medical curriculum."[33] In 1632 he left Wittenberg and went to the University of Königsberg, where he became an adjunct in the philosophical faculty and lectured on physics and mathematics.[34] By this time Saxony was engulfed in the Thirty Years' War, and Rhodius, wishing to see Denmark, Holland, France, Italy, and other lands, set off for Copenhagen in April of 1635, the beginning and end of his grand tour of the continent. He began to study at the University of Copenhagen with the intention of attaining an M.D. degree, but the ravaging of Saxony had deprived him of family support, and he lacked

30 Ambrosius Rhodius, *Optica* (Wittenberg: Sauberlich, 1611). The elder Ambrosius was apparently very interested in aspects of Kepler's work in optics, insofar as he directed (and after the custom of the time, probably authored) a thesis defended in 1608 by Daniel Conrad, *Exercitationes opticæ* (Wittenberg: Henckel, 1608). This thesis took up key aspects of Kepler's light metaphysics. See Jiri Marek, "The response to Kepler's book *Ad Vitellionem* ... in the thesis of Daniel Conrad in 1608," *Atti Fondazione Giorgio Ronchi* 23 (1968): 352-62.

31 See Rhodius' autobiography, in E. Ingerslev, *Ambrosius Rhodius*, p. 14: "In der Gottesfurcht, lateinischen und griechischen Sprache fleissig unterrichtet."

32 Ibid., p. 15, n. 1. Years later Ambrosius Rhodius, *Disputationes supra Ideam medicinæ philosophicæ*, p. xiii, referred to Sennert as his former teacher ("meum qvondam præceptorem"). Judging from the many references to Sennert and citations of his works, to be found in all Rhodius' treatises, he must have been a great influence on Rhodius.

33 E. Ingerslev, *Ambrosius Rhodius*, p. 15: "in Botanicis, Anatomicis, chymicis operationibus, Astrologicis, und was mehr ad studium Medicum gehören mag."

34 Jens Christian Berg, "Efterretninger om det af Kong Christian den Fjerde stiftede Gymnasium i Christiania, og Sammes Lærere," *Budstikken*, vol. 3 (1822), col. 441. According to his autobiography, Rhodius was offered promotion to doctor, but could not afford the costs of promotion.

the money to pay the costs associated with formal promotion.[35] Unable to afford extended residence where he had been staying, he moved into the house of a physician in Copenhagen named Frederik Severinus, the son of Petrus Severinus.

Rhodius quickly gained acceptance in the elite learned "family" at the University of Copenhagen, many of whom were in fact related by blood or by marriage. In particular he ingratiated himself with one of Denmark's leading theologians, Jesper Brochmand (Dr. Theol., and Bishop of Sjælland after 1638), Dr. Henning Arnisæus (Royal Physician to Christian IV), and Ole Worm. Later that year (1635) Rhodius published and defended a thesis on scurvy under the direction of Ole Worm, dedicating it to Brochmand and Arnisæus.[36] Ambrosius Rhodius defended yet another thesis in December, *Disputatio astrologica de astrorum influxu* (Astrological disputation concerning the influence of the stars), the subject of which is the effect of the stars on the generation of disease in man.[37] Rhodius frequently cited the works of Daniel Sennert, his former teacher, who was no doubt a major source for his views, but clearly he was also familiar with Severinus' *Idea medicinæ*, which he explicitly cited in Thesis 22. Furthermore, the arguments he presents in this thesis reveal that by 1635 he had already read and reflected on the main doctrines of the *Idea medicinæ*: that the generation of new forms, for instance diseases, begins with a progression from *semina*, and that certain constellations can force a new impression on a growing organism, displacing the one provided by the seed, and in this way cause disease.

By his own account, Rhodius became so well known at the university, both for lecturing and disputation (*legendo et disputando*), that he was offered promotion to a doctorate in the medical faculty. Again lacking pecuniary means, he was unable to secure the degree.[38] Perhaps also

---

35 E. Ingerslev, *Ambrosius Rhodius*, p. 16.
36 Ambrosius Rhodius, *Theses medicæ de scorbuto* (Copenhagen: Salomon Sartorius, 1635).
37 Ambrosius Rhodius, *Disputatio astrologica de astrorum influxu, quomodo homines ad certas constellationes morbis fiant obnoxij* (Copenhagen, 1635). This he dedicated to his patron, Dr. Mads Jensen, who was Ole Worm's father-in-law. See also J.C. Berg, "Efterretninger," col. 443.
38 Rhodius' autobiography, in E. Ingerslev, *Ambrosius Rhodius*, p. 16.

because of the cost, Rhodius chose not to continue his planned European tour, although the hospitality of Frederik Severinus' house may also have played a role in his decision to stay: while living there Ambrosius became engaged to Frederik's daughter, Anna Severinus. Meanwhile, Rhodius' benefactors were seeking to place him professionally, and when the position as physician to Christian IV's Children's Hospital (Børnehuset) was vacated, Rhodius was appointed by Chancellor Friis, no doubt through the influence of Ole Worm and Henning Arnisæus.[39] He held this position until 14 May 1637, when he was appointed to teach natural philosophy at Christiania's gymnasium, in the provincial capital of Norway.[40]

The gymnasium's charter called for "a *physicus* and *mathematicus*, who is also a good *medicus*," and to fill this need, Christopher Urne, the *Statholder* or Governor of Norway, selected Ambrosius Rhodius and wrote to the Consistory to verify his qualifications.[41] Even before the Consistory replied favorably, Rhodius' position was secured by a royal letter to Christopher Urne (14 May 1637). The salary for the professorship was 200 rigsdaler annually, with the promise of a canonry when one was vacated. Rhodius received this in 1646.[42] After moving to Christiania to take up his new position in June of 1637, Ambrosius returned to Copenhagen and married Anna 6 May 1638 and thus became a member of Copenhagen's leading medical family, which included the Severinuses, the Worms, the Finckes, the Bartholins, and the Charesiuses.[43]

39 The letter appointing Rhodius physician at the Børnehus and at Bremerholm (18 June 1636) is printed in *Kjøbenhavns Diplomatarium*, ed. O. Nielsen, vol. 3 (Copenhagen: Gad, 1877), p. 164. On the history of the Børnehus, see Olaf Olsen, *Christian IVs tugt- og børnehus*, 2d ed. (Højbjerg: Wormianum, 1978), p. 97; and Otto Sperling, *Selvbiografi 1602–1673*, ed. Sophus Birket Smith (Copenhagen, 1885).

40 Einar Høigård, *Oslo Katedralskoles Historie* (Oslo: Grøndahl, 1942), p. 30. Christiania's gymnasium replaced the cathedral school in Oslo, the medieval town that Christiania supplanted. In 1636 the gymnasium was formally funded with chairs in theology, philosophy (logic and metaphysics), and natural philosophy (physics and mathematics).

41 Quoted by E. Ingerslev, *Ambrosius Rhodius*, p. 24: "en Physicus och Mathematicus, den ochsaa er en goed Medicus." See also ibid., p. 25. The ruling elite of Norway at that time was generally drawn from the Danish nobility, and it is therefore likely that the king or one of Rhodius' patrons recommended him to *Statholder* Urne.

42 Ibid., p. 25. Scharffenberg, "Bidrag til de norske lægestillingers historie," p. 1338, reports that Rhodius obtained the canonry by royal letter of 9 June 1647.

43 See Rhodius' autobiography, E. Ingerslev, *Ambrosius Rhodius*, p. 18.

Few records from which we might learn of Rhodius' life in Christiania during the late 1630s and early 1640s survive. Ole Worm congratulated him on his successful practice in a letter written in the spring of 1640, so he must have become fairly well established in a short time.[44] This was Rhodius' most prolific period as a writer, in which he published two lengthy treatises. In the first of these, *Dialogus de transmigratione animarum Pythagorica* (Dialogue on the Pythagorean transmigration of souls), he gave the *semina* theory a greater exposition than he had in his 1635 *De influxu*.[45] The second treatise, *Disputationes supra Ideam medicinæ philosophicæ*, which is of particular interest here, is a chapter by chapter summary of Severinus' major tenets with a discussion and defense of them. This tract offers us the opportunity to see how Rhodius, a well educated, mid-seventeenth-century iatrochemist, read and interpreted Severinus' work. Full treatment of Rhodius' analysis would require a book by itself, but we can examine his introductory statements for clues to his reasons for studying and defending the *Idea medicinæ* and then sample a couple of chapters to see how he dealt with his subject, and in this way we may gain an impression of the whole commentary.

Disputationes supra Ideam medicinæ philosophicæ

Ambrosius Rhodius was likely attracted to Petrus Severinus' *Idea medicinæ* for several reasons. He had lived in the house of his son, Frederik Severinus, and was now married to his granddaughter, Anna Frederiksdatter Severinus, whose family reputation would stand to gain by renewed praise of her grandfather's *Idea medicinæ*. Furthermore, Severinus had been a client of Christian IV and his father, Frederik II, to whom the *Idea medicinæ* was dedicated. It only made sense, from the standpoint of seeking patronage, to write a commentary on this book and dedicate it to the king. He was acknowledging past and current

---

44 Worm, *Breve*, vol. 2, p. 176.
45 Ambrosius Rhodius, *Dialogus de transmigratione animarum Pythagorica* (Copenhagen: Salomon Sartorius, 1638). Rhodius dedicated this tract to Christopher Urne, Norway's governor.

favors and at the same time fishing for continued support for his career and his scholarship. Rhodius stated this quite plainly in the preface to the *Disputationes*.[46] But aside from these practical considerations, it is clear that the subject matter of the *Idea medicinæ* itself attracted Rhodius, whose interest in Platonism is evident from his previously published tracts.

As a student of medicine under the guidance of Daniel Sennert, whom he identified here as "my former teacher," Rhodius no doubt had encountered the principle themes of the *Idea medicinæ* many times before. The dedication, however, suggests that Rhodius was particularly captivated with the changeableness and imperfection of this world; with political instability, destruction, disease, and death – topics especially well suited to the Thirty Years' War. He opened the dedication to Christian IV with a statement of gratitude for having been spared the fate of his homeland: "While my German fatherland perishes in war, most powerful king, most merciful lord, I live safe in Norway. God has rescued me and delivered me into the protection of your most serene, most merciful royal highness."[47] I think that Rhodius was genuinely grateful to the king for appointing him, an exile, to what were rather lucrative posts at a time when he was especially vulnerable. He had lost his patrimony in the war that was ruining Germany and therefore he lacked the means to finish a doctor's degree, which was a usual prerequisite for a professorship or appointment to court. He again refers to this at the closing of the dedication, where he asks for the king's continued favor and acknowledges his importance in maintaining peace in a time of war, which was completely destroying his native land – a peace that enables scholars to contemplate God's creation and turn their minds to spiritual matters.[48] Remember, by 1643 war had afflicted Europe for a quarter of a century, with no end in sight. It is therefore not surprising that Rhodius' mind would be captivated by the vicissitudes of fate, of change and stability, and of generation and corruption in the world. These concerns are manifest in his preface:

46 Rhodius, *Disputationes*, p. vi.
47 Ibid., p. i: "Dum mea Patria Germania bello perit, Rex Potentissime, Domine Clementissime, in Norvvegia tutus vivo. Eripuit me Deus, & Vestræ Serenissimæ Reg. Majestatis Clementissimæ protectioni tradidit."
48 Ibid., p. vii.

For just as God turns the fortunes of men by a wondrous change, so too do natural things play under the changeable condition of fate on this world stage. One thing disappears, another comes back. … During the time one compound is dissolved, another living one is born. For mixable things begin to exist by themselves. Soon these once more suffer their fate and are mixed with the earth. From the earth they are again attracted by plants and they also undergo remarkable changes. Worms appear from decaying plants, and from these are born chrysalides and butterflies, and other little animals from them. All things undergo this changeable spectacle as if they are acting out a theatrical play.[49]

Rhodius sought to know more about the metaphysics of change and, specifically, the generation, stability, and disappearance of diseases. Quite likely he hoped to discern an underlying order to medicine. "Yet how changeable are transplantations in the generation of diseases?" he wrote.[50] It was evident to him that the distinctions between diseases were often blurred, because the impurities that produce disease mix among themselves and give rise to new transplantations or hybrids: "Thus we often see podagrical catarrhs, leprous paralyses, abscesses, jaundices, and consumptions that are polluted with ulcerous properties, and arthritic, paralytic, and catarrhal fevers that are prone to leprous predestinations."[51]

Severinus' *Idea medicinæ* directly addressed issues such as these and

---

49 Ibid., pp. ii-iii: "Sicuti enim Deus mirabili conversione fortunas hominum versat, ita etiam sub varia sortis conditione in hac mundana scena res naturales ludunt. Hoc abit, illud revertitur. … Dum compositum dissolvitur, aliud vivens nascitur. Nam miscibilia per se incipiunt existere. Mox hæc rursum sua fata patiuntur, terræque miscentur. Ex terra rursum a plantis attrahuntur, adeoque mirabiles subeunt vicissitudines. Ex plantis putrescentibus prodeunt vermes, ex his nascuntur chrysalides ex istis papiliones, & alia animalcula. Omnia tam vario spectaculo peraguntur, ac si lusum scenicum agerent." On the theme of *lusus* in nature, see Paula Findlen, "Jokes of Nature and Jokes of Knowledge: The Playfulness of Scientific Discourse in Early Modern Europe," *Renaissance Quarterly* 43 (1990): 292-331.

50 Rhodius, *Disputationes*, p. iii: "Quam variæ etiam fiunt Transplantationes in morborum generationibus?"

51 Ibid: "Ita sæpe conspiciuntur catarrhi podagrici, paralyses leprosæ, apostemata, icteritiæ, cachexiæ, ulcerosis proprietatibus inquinatæ, febres arthriticæ, paralyticæ, catarrhosæ, ad prædestinationes leprosas inclinatæ."

offered an explanatory theory that Rhodius found satisfactory. Like Severinus and every other university educated physician, Rhodius had cut his teeth on Aristotle and Galen, and like Severinus, Rhodius found the discrepancies between Galenic theory and Mosaic physics to be troubling. If we are to believe Rhodius' dedication, his study of the *Idea medicinæ* provided answers to some of the problems vexing him:

> Here a new kind of philosophizing was presented to me, different in very many ways from Aristotle and Galen, and in agreement in many ways with Paracelsus. At first sight, these things appeared to me to be complete riddles, most especially concerning the doctrine of the elements, which I thought even Oedipus would not have solved. But as I continued, a new day began to shine on me, gradually dispersing the shadows that had covered my mind.[52]

The better he came to understand Severinus' ideas, the more unjust he regarded the judgements of the Dane's critics, and he determined to refute them, or at least correct their errors.

Like Severinus, Rhodius sought to avoid open polemic and chose as a format a dialogue between three friends, in which the principle doctrines of the *Idea medicinæ* could be presented, clarified, and defended without directly confronting any one author or philosophical school. "Friends," he began his preface to the reader, "resort to speaking together openly."[53] He stated his desire for a balanced, amiable consideration of Severinus' ideas more clearly a few pages later:

> In disputing, I provoke no one with insults, although the author [Severinus] was received and treated here and there by envious and malevolent persons, and especially badly by Erastus. For I believe this to be unsuitable for Christians, and all those who strive to raise the value of

---

52 Ibid., pp. iv-v: "Hic novum mihi exhibitum fuit Philosophandi genus, ab Aristotele & Galeno in plurimis diversum, cum Paracelso in multis consentiens. Visa sunt mihi primo intuitu mera ænigmata, & potissimum circa Elementorum doctrinam, quæ ne Oedipo solvenda putavi. Sed pergenti novus illuxit Sol, nebulas animo suffusas paulatim discutiens."

53 Ibid., p. viii: "Amici colloquentes, Lector candide, in medium revertuntur."

their reputation by this manner of proceeding generally suffer a loss of good reputation among good men.[54]

Although Rhodius did not choose to write a defense of Paracelsian ideas *per se* and thereby enter the continued, vicious debate between the Aristotelians and the chemical philosophers, he did believe that there were useful ideas to be found in Severinus' book, which needed to be exposed and vindicated. Rhodius concluded his preface with a plea to the reader to examine what he has written for what is "true and agreeable to nature," but not to confuse obscurity with nonsense: "When the truth is hidden under the covers, do not at once imagine that it is absent. Draw back the covers."[55] It is instructive at this point to draw back the covers of Rhodius' commentary and examine selected pieces of the underlying text, beginning with the beginning and then sampling chapters from each of the three main divisions of the book.

A FRIENDLY DISCUSSION OF THE *IDEA MEDICINÆ*

Rhodius organized his analysis of the *Idea medicinæ* as a three-day discussion between three friends, Theophilus, Philomusus, and Theodosius. Each of the three "days" comprises a short introduction followed by a sequential consideration of several chapters of the *Idea medicinæ*.[56] The introductory comments serve to orient the reader to what follows, but

54 Ibid., p. xiii: "In disputando neminem convitiis lacesso, licet passim a malevolis & invidis, potissimum vero ab Erasto male acceptus, & tractatus sit Author. Nam a Christianis hoc alienum puto: quique hoc procedendi modo famæ suæ dignitatem extollere nituntur, apud bonos bonæ famæ jacturam plerumque faciunt."

55 Ibid., xiv: "Sententias percense, proba, examina, & quæ sunt vera & Naturæ consentanea retine. Unum hoc exopto. At si veritatem quibusdam in locis non statim agnoscis, diligentius inquire. Ubi sub pallio sese occultat, absentem statim putare noli. Detrahe velamen."

56 The "Colloquium of the First Day" examines chapters one through seven; on the second day chapters eight through twelve are covered; on the third day chapters thirteen through fifteen. The dialogue was a prose form that was well suited to presentation of controversial topics and not uncommon among Rhodius' contemporaries. See Principe, *Aspiring Adept*, pp. 68-69 for a brief discussion of the significance of Boyle's choosing the dialogue as a format for writing about transmutational chemistry.

also provide Rhodius a ready forum for drawing attention to particular problems. The preamble of the Colloquium of the First Day, for example, introduces the reader to the roles of the three interlocutors and to basic difficulties presented by Severinus' text. The first speaker is Theophilus, who represents Rhodius.[57] He begins by introducing the *Idea medicinæ* as a book that contains many things at variance with Aristotelian and Galenic doctrine, which aroused very bitter opponents against its author. However, Theophilus claims that Severinus was misunderstood and that his critics have badly corrupted and twisted his words into meanings that he would not have imagined. Accordingly, the purpose of their friendly debate is to bring these misunderstandings to light and to clarify Severinus' ideas. Philomusus, the second speaker, replies that he has read through the *Idea medicinæ* as Theophilus requested, "but did not find anything that could satisfy a mind eager for truth." Its contents seem wholly absurd, or at best riddles that are concealed so well as to defeat the best attempts to discover them.[58] Just consider his theory of the elements, Philomusus says. Severinus claimed that the elements are fortified with vital power, foster the seeds of generation, promote them to maturity, and provide refuge for them when they are worn out. The elements are places, therefore they are empty and incorporeal. "I don't know what he is saying," continues Philomusus, "for I have never heard any Aristotelian philosophize in such a manner." Rhodius thus began his commentary at a fundamental point of disagreement between chemical philosophy and Aristotelian philosophy, a point that Severinus had specifically addressed: the nature of the elements and principles and how *semina* guide the cycles of generation and corruption of all things.[59]

Philomusus admits that he was confused by Severinus' confounding of the Aristotelian elements, when he spoke of terrestrial fire, terrestrial water, celestial earth, fiery air, and so on, thus producing sixteen elements from the original four. Furthermore, Severinus claimed that

---

57 Theophilus begins by introducing the *Idea medicinæ* as a text that he mentioned several times in his previous discourse *On the Pythagorean Transmigration of Souls*. Since Rhodius really published such a tract in 1638 (see n. 45, above), he is clearly identifying himself with the fictional Theophilus.

58 Ibid., p. 1: "Sed quod animum veritatis cupidum possit explere non inveni."

59 Ibid., p. 2: "Ego quid loquatur, nescio. Neque enim ullum unquam Aristotelicum tali modo Philosophantem audivi."

each element was two-fold, namely visible and invisible, increasing their numbers further:

> In another place he says that bodies come to be from non bodies. And there are a great many other things with which that book bulges and overflows. Not without reason did Libavius write about it in his *Examination of Hartmann's Philosophy*: "The good man says many things as if he had recently taken them from the depths and treasuries of nature and has seen them all naked – but he demonstrates nothing."[60]

For Libavius and others, the *Idea medicinæ* and Paracelsian philosophy in general seemed to be empty words, and even the words were strange. As an example of this, Philomusus points to Severinus' multiplex use of the term anatomy,

> which he everywhere treats contrary to the accustomed meaning. In chapter two he writes: the anatomy and power of the whole seed abounds in the radical moisture; In chapter four: much in the world anatomy is doubted and misunderstood; In chapter twelve: those things seem to conduct the anatomy of health. In another place he writes that the seed flows together to the anatomy of the testes.[61]

Philomusus goes on to identify tincture as another problematic word, along with "other monstrous terms" such as *relollaceum, Iliadus,* and *Archeus,* concluding with a quotation from Galen: "He who confuses the uses of terms confuses the ideas of the things themselves."[62] We see

---

60   Ibid.: "Alio loco dicit, ex incorporeis fieri corporea. Et quæ quam plurima sunt alia, quibus scatet & turget iste liber. Non immerito Libavius *in Examine Philos. Hartmann.* de eo scribit: Bonus vir multa dicit, quasi nuper ex thesauris & abyssis Naturæ prodiisset, et omnia nuda vidisset; sed nihil probat."

61   Ibid.: "Quod ubique præter consuetudinem tractat. *Capite 2.* scribit: In radicali humiditate totius seminis Anatomia & potestas viget. *Cap. 4.* Multa in Mundana Anatomia dubia & incomprehensa. *Capite 12.* Quæ sanitatis Anatomiam gerere videntur. Alio loco, semen ad testium Anatomiam confluere scribit."

62   Ibid.: "Conturbatus nominum usus, & rerum ipsarum cognitionem conturbat." The quotation is attributed to Galen, *De simplicium medicamentorum temperamentis ac facultatibus,* book 3, chapter 12. In the modern edition, Claudius Galen, *Medicorum Græcorum Opera quæ extant,* ed. Karl Gottlob Kühn (Leipzig, 1826), vol. 11, p. 569, we find "His ergo occasionibus perturbatus nominum usus rerum quoque una perturbat notitiam."

from this that Rhodius was perplexed by Severinus' use of Paracelsian neologisms, much as was the anonymous reader of the *Idea medicinæ* who was discussed previously.

The third discussant in the dialogue is Theodosius, who initially favors traditional philosophy, but is not hardened into a doctrinal position. He enters the dialogue with a brief summary of the fundamental tenets of Galenic theory, which he says was modeled on geometry. He notes that Galen deduced "with compendious subtlety the causes and ways of the symptoms and cures of all the elemental diseases" from the humors, elements, and the primary and secondary qualities, caustically concluding that Libavius' comment about Severinus, that the good man says much and demonstrates nothing, could not be applied to Galen![63] "Should we now abandon Galen," says Theodosius, "and go over to the camp of Paracelsus, who has called forth I don't know what kind of monsters from his *Iliaster* and *Cagastrum*?" He cites Sennert, who accused Paracelsus of writing without any supporting reasoning, as if he were "a dictator or emperor of literature," so that his treatises "seem more like a jumble of twigs than books."[64] He declares that whoever dares to demonstrate these monstrous "doxomanias" must be considered to be without judgement and blinded by love of Paracelsus and he concludes "I cannot wonder enough that Severinus wanted to extol Paracelsus to such a degree with extraordinary praises and to consider him to be among the foremost physicians and philosophers."[65]

Next Philomusus takes up Theodosius' criticism of Paracelsus by repeating the by then familiar attack on Paracelsus' character, which was based on a letter ostensibly written by Johannes Oporinus to Johann Wier. But Theophilus rebuts Philomusus' account by citing Michael

---

63 Rhodius, *Disputationes*, p. 3: "Quatuor humores Elementorum qualitatibus primis & secundis insignitos adjunxit: ex quibus subtilitate compendiosa morborum omnium Elementalium, Symptomatum, Curationumque causas & modos deduxit." Rhodius' ironic point here is that Galen, by relying on Euclid's demonstrative geometry as a model for medicine, "demonstrates" much, but says little that is true or useful in medicine.

64 Ibid.: "Deficiamus jam a Galeno, & transeamus in castra Paracelsi? qui nescio quæ portenta ex suo Iliastro & Cagastro excitavit. Et hæc nullis rationibus adductis, sed quasi Dictator & Imperator rei literariæ, ut Sennertus scribit, promulgavit, & pleraque ita confuse & inepte scripsit, ut scopæ dissolutæ potius quam libri videantur."

65 Ibid.: "Non satis possum mirari, quod tam egregiis laudibus Paracelsum Severinius velit extollere, & inter Principes Medicos & Philosophos referre."

Toxites' account, which relates that Oporinus later expressed remorse over having written such bad things about his former teacher, whom he only afterwards recognized to have been extraordinarily learned.[66]

It is easy for an antagonist to find fault with Paracelsus, Theophilus continues, but yet conceal what is praiseworthy. In defense of Paracelsus, Theophilus quotes extensively from Severinus' *Epistola*, which he claims to have seen among Severinus' manuscripts.[67] Theophilus' very faithful replication of Severinus' text devolves into a paraphrase toward the very end. Here Severinus is reported to have written that Paracelsus may have erred in some ways, just as he showed human weakness in his personal behavior. However, man should imitate the bees and work collectively, using various interpretations of nature to approach a true understanding, and not rely solely on the strength of one individual philosophy.[68] Severinus himself, says Theophilus, behaved no differently and willingly sought out what was valuable in Paracelsus' writings: "His writings apply better to what Paracelsus wrote than do those of any other man."[69] In due course, his opinion of the elements will be shown not to be absurd. As for his terminology, he follows Paracelsus in coining new words for things. Here we should be "good natured," Theophilus appeals, and accept that different terms, like different kinds of money, have value if only their value can be agreed on.[70] Take the terms anatomy and tincture, for instance: "Sometimes he employs this word [anatomy] for the analysis and resolution of a thing; sometimes for the location of a thing." "He uses the term tincture for the property of a thing, by which its power of acting flows, or for the power of acting itself." Thus, when Severinus says that certain foods "are endowed with powerful tinctures," he means that "they are furnished with powerful faculties." Similarly, *Relollaceum* means powerless, sterile; *Iliad* is the same as Hippocrates' *Orcus*, the abyss of potentiality; and the *Archeus*

---

66 Ibid., p. 4.
67 The fidelity of Rhodius' quotation to the printed text of the *Epistola* suggests that he was working from it or from a manuscript draft that closely resembles it. Discrepancies are easily accounted for by Rhodius' modifications of Severinus' text to fit the dialogue format.
68 Ibid., p. 9.
69 Ibid., p. 10: "Cujus scripta ad Paracelsi lectiones plus, quam ullius alterius conferunt."
70 Ibid.

is a natural spirit that serves a natural faculty. Likewise, context can easily explain other terms, Theophilus continues, so the proper way to proceed is to examine the *Idea medicinæ* in detail, chapter by chapter.[71] And this is what they do.

Each chapter is introduced by a short summary of its content, which is set in large type, followed by a smaller print discussion by the three interlocutors, in which they bring in opinions of other authors to clarify or contest various points. These vary considerably in length. The presentation of chapter three consists of a one-page summary and two and a half pages of dialogue. At the other extreme, chapter two is highlighted in two pages of text, followed by thirty six pages of discussion! The difference in space allotted to consideration of these chapters reflects how the author has chosen to treat the material as well as which particular topics he wished to stress. Chapter Four of the *Idea medicinæ*, which offers a general outline of the whole of Severinus' theory, is summarized in two pages, but receives only brief dismissal from Philomusus: "In this chapter is contained a sketch of those things that are treated in later ones. Therefore, it will be better to look into each one in its own place, and immediately to take up examining the following chapter."[72] On the other hand, chapter fifteen, on the different kinds, properties, compositions, and preparations of remedies, receives a one page summary and elicits no response on the grounds that it is not at all controversial and lies beyond the scope of the present discussion: "I find nothing in this last chapter that offends me," Theodosius says with a play on the dual meaning of the verb *offendere* (to find or come upon and to offend). "We have [already] treated the greater part of the things that are contained here one place or another. But it is better that we should undertake a specific discourse on the composition of medicaments," that is, at another time.[73]

---

71 Ibid.: "Interdum pro rei ἀναλύσει, & resolutione hanc vocem usurpat; Interdum pro rei loco." "Sic vocabulo Tincturæ pro rei proprietate, a qua vis agendi fluit, seu ipsa potestate agendi utitur. Nam quando Cap. 9. dicit: Alimenta validis tincturis esse imbuta, idem est, ut ipse explicat, ac validis facultatibus prædita."

72 Ibid., p. 60: "In hoc capite continetur adumbratio eorum, quæ in sequentibus pertractantur. Satius igitur erit unumquodque suo loco videre, & statim caput sequens assumere excutiendum."

73 Ibid., p. 213: "In hoc ultimo capite nihil offendo, quod me offendat. De plerisque, quæ hic continentur hinc inde egimus. De compositione vero medicamentorum, satius est, ut peculiarem discursum instituamus."

The discussion of chapter twelve offers an example of the kinds of doctrine that Rhodius thought needed extended explanation and merits description in depth, especially since that chapter contains some of the chief novelties to be found in the *Idea medicinæ*. Study of Rhodius' commentary can provide us insight into which of Severinus' ideas he found particularly difficult or supposed that his contemporaries would find especially hard to understand properly. If Rhodius' education can be assumed to be similar to that of his peers, then this sampling from his commentary can plausibly illuminate how other students of medical literature in the mid-seventeenth century read the *Idea medicinæ*.

A FATAL BLOW TO GALENISTS

Rhodius' explication of chapter twelve of the *Idea medicinæ* (On the Generation and Transplantation of Diseases) is longer than that of other chapters, save chapter two (What is Medicine and What Foundations does it have in Nature). This comes as no great surprise, since Severinus' seminal pathology was of primary interest to most readers of the *Idea medicinæ*, as this study has shown. However, Rhodius indicates another reason for giving chapter twelve special attention; it delivers, in the words of the interlocutor Theodosius, a fatal blow to the medical theory of the Galenists.[74]

The principal issues that the three discussants take up in this chapter are the proper definition of disease, that is, its ontology, and the correct understanding of the relationships between diseases, their causes, and their symptoms. The discussion begins with a review of the chief philosophical opinions about disease. The Aristotelians viewed disease as a privation. It does not have positive essence, but is rather the lack of correct functioning. The Platonists were concerned with the good, the ideal, and since disease was regarded as bad, they devoted no special attention to it. The physicians, by which he must mean medical authors between Hippocrates and Galen, eschewed speculation and were content

---

74 Ibid., p. 166: "Hoc caput Galenicis est lapis offensionis, quo frangitur cerebrum."

to arrive at an understanding of causes and effects on the basis of observation. A brief introduction to the fine points of logic follows: obstructions of functions are causes and diseases are effects, at least in the real
world. The remote cause is the disease's genus, the proximate cause its
species, and the effect or apparent manifestation is the individual speci-
men of the disease. But the nominal ordering of things is the opposite:
the disease is the most general category (genus), the obstruction is the
species, and the obstructing impurity is the individual.

Against this background of categories and definitions, Severinus'
theory of disease as *ens morbi* is introduced. Rhodius makes a point of
explaining that pathogenic *semina* are not fixed in particular disease
bodies, but rather adhere to the roots of host entities. He also notes
that they have specific disease characteristics and cannot simply be
classified as excesses, humors, or obstructions. Diseases generate and
decay as do all other seminal orders. Theodosius explains that this is
a main discrepancy between Severinus and the Galenists, and cites
Sennert, who thought Severinus' system was absurd because it failed
to distinguish causes from effects. Rhodius' response to this criticism
is to attempt to interpret Severinus' doctrine in terms that academic
philosophers will understand: Theophilus explains that the Galenists
classify an excess of a humor, say blood, as the cause of a disease. The
humor is not the disease – there is nothing specifically or essentially
pathogenic about blood – but its removal (by bloodletting) eliminates
the disease. Severinus, however, views a disease as caused by the presence of specific impurities, for example in the blood. These impurities,
inasmuch as they carry in them the potential for generating a specific
disease, are disease in potency. If they are removed, then the disease as
an actualization cannot occur. The model Theophilus offers is that a
disease is like a flower: whether blossoming (in act) or still incipient, as
a shoot (in potency), it is nevertheless a flower. Philomusus adds that
Severinus used such terms because he wanted to fit the names of things
to the actual things, rather than forcing the things to fit the convenient
verbal categories of the logicians.[75]

Rhodius develops this line of investigation by setting up a comparison between the causation of fever and the heating of water by fire. Is

75 Ibid., pp. 167-70.

there a transfer of form, that is, does a quality wholly leave one subject and enter another? Or does it remain in its root cause (the shoot) even as it flows forth as a fruit (the blossom)? Theodosius admits that in the case of water being heated, the quality, namely the hotness of the fire, must be transferred to the water with the substance of the fire, its root. Philomusus generalizes the point: "Accidents do not move from subject to subject," and where there are characteristics of a being, the being must also be.[76]

Theophilus extends this model to disease. In the case of fever, the nitrosulphurous impurity is the pathogenic when it is exalted, it produces the symptoms of fever. The nitrosulphurous impurity is therefore the subject of the febrile heat, just as fire is the subject of the heat in water. Just as fire penetrates the water, heating it throughout, so too fevers and poisons produce symptoms that are immediate everywhere in the body. Theodosius denies that the febrile symptoms are actually in the nitrosulphurous impurity, to which Theophilus responds that Severinus did not mean that they were *actually* in the impurities, but rather present in them as virtues. The confusion arose because Severinus referred to all stages of the generation of a disease as the disease. The nitrosulphurous impurity does not become feverish, but rather causes the body it affects to become feverish. When Severinus stated that he had seen a fever thrown up by vomiting, he did not mean that the fever itself was in the vomit, but rather that its roots were there, and that once the febrile roots (the nitrosulphurous impurities) were removed from the body, the fever also disappeared, because the febrile heat, a quality, cannot be separated from its subject. The heat that was in potential in the nitrosulphurous impurity was the same heat that made the fever patient hot; when the impurity was thrown up, the fever abated, much as water begins to cool when the fire is removed. In this sense the impurity is said by Severinus to be the disease.

To this Theodosius objects. Severinus confuses a substance with an accident. The heat is not the fire, but flows from the form of the fire, and therefore is categorically distinct. Theophilus counters this Aristotelian objection with an argument that sounds like something Nicholas of Cusa

---

76 Ibid., p. 171: "Nam accidentia non migrant de subjecto in subjectum. Et ubi sunt propria alicujus rei, ibi adest & ipsa res."

might have uttered: Theodosius' logic does not apply to this situation because the disease potential in the roots is not yet specialized, since it can become different disease manifestations under different circumstances. Therefore, since it is indeterminate, it is not a substance, and it cannot be categorized. The antecedent cause, the disease, and the symptoms are not essentially distinct, but constitute different modes of one subject.[77]

This explanation does not wholly satisfy Theodosius the Galenist; It is still wrong to confuse cause and effect. A bladder stone may cause a failure to urinate, but the stone and the prevented function (a privation) remain categorically distinct. This time Philomusus attempts to clarify Severinus' position. The mucilages existing in the foods we consume constitute the most general genera, because they contain all the information or blueprints (*rationes*) for all their possible disease manifestations. When accumulated in a particular part of the body, their scope is restricted, and they constitute subalternate genera. Once an impurity is exalted, it becomes a species and brings about a specific disease individual.[78]

The modern historian looking back on this philosophical impasse between Severinus' view and the Galenist-Aristotelian ontology will see that the argument goes back at least to the fifteenth century. Severinus' developmental (seminal) model agrees with Cusa's idea of a Neoplatonic continuum of existence from the most general to the most concrete explication. Looking at it from this perspective there is no meaningful ontological distinction between an idea and its specific realization, a point the peripatetics would not concede. For Severinus, the bladder stone is a disease waiting to appear on the world stage. But it would seem from Rhodius' effort to explain the *Idea medicinæ* in terms familiar to any university student that he judged the gap between Galenist and Severinian conceptions of disease to be bridgeable.

At this point in the discussion Philomusus changes the topic. An earlier comment by Theodosius reminded him that Severinus' definition of disease as a substance is regarded by some as unsound doctrine: "Our author is considered to be a heretic and accused of Manichæism

77 Ibid., pp. 174-75.
78 Ibid., p. 176.

in this matter."[79] Theodosius reviews Severinus' doctrine about how pathogenic tinctures, released after the Fall of Adam, supervened on the *semina* that were created in the beginning, making them pathogens. These *semina* now have substantial existence and can cause diseases in man. Such ideas, says Theodosius, are too close to the madness of the Manichæans.[80] Next Philomusus reviews Sennert's position on Severinus' disease ontology, summarizes Augustine's opinion on the matter, and asserts that God in any case rested on the seventh day. Whatever he created was created before that. But Theophilus defends Severinus, pointing out that he did not introduce the idea that God created a substantial evil. It is not the seminal being, but rather the supervening tinctures that were evil. Theodosius objects: new tinctures imply a new creation, hence the creation of evil, and consequently the doctrine is Manichæan.[81]

Indeed, although Severinus surely did not view his theory as implying any heresy, it is easy to see that it was open to this interpretation, as Erastus had made clear. Severinus never answered Erastus in print, so the charge stood. Rhodius must have understood the importance of resolving this issue if he were to make Severinus' ideas more acceptable. To this end he came up with a new tactic: Theophilus gets Theodosius to admit that there are contrary natures in the created world, including man, and that these must have been created in the beginning. However, these opposites did not attack each other at first, because they were part of a harmonious whole. It was only after the contraries became distinct – independent and salient – that contrariness appeared in nature. Theophilus argues that contrary *tinctures*, that is, ones contrary to health, were also created, but lay hidden until they received a higher command. God's curse, visited upon Adam and Eve, thus dissolved the friendly concord between opposites and permitted the contrary tinctures to invade others and supervene, displacing the other tinctures. Thus, every substance is good inasmuch as it is a substance. A substantial change comes about with the supervening evil tinctures. Evil is therefore only accidental

---

79 Ibid., p. 177: "Et memini a Theodosio Authorem hic pro hæretico habitum, & Manichæismi insimulatum."

80 Ibid., p. 177-78.

81 Ibid., p. 179.

to things. To illustrate this point, Theophilus asserts that poisons are essentially good, but poisonous (evil) to man. (This idea, incidentally, fits well with Paracelsus' contention that toxic substances were good sources for powerful medicines, if only the poisonous qualities could be removed.) Since Severinus also believed these evils to be accidents, he cannot be regarded as a Manichæan, Theophilus concludes.

Theodosius is not contented with this explanation and points out that Severinus specifically stated that everything was initially created pure, free from corruption and death, and that he said nothing at all about primaeval, harmonious mixtures of contraries. Theophilus counters by saying that Severinus really meant that there was initial concord, with the pure completely prevailing over and subordinating the admixed impurity. At that point Rhodius left off further discussion of Erastus' charge of heresy. It is, however, worth noting that Rhodius' attention to the fine points of this doctrine suggests that he was concerned for the theological integrity of Severinus' philosophy in the 1640s.[82]

Returning to the main "stone of offense" against Galenism, namely Severinus' view of disease, Theodosius baits discussion by asserting that disease is still best explained in terms of humoral pathology, as Hippocrates, Galen, and Avicenna had done. There is, therefore, no need for Severinus' Paracelsian novelties. But, Theophilus asks, what qualities of the humors can explain the corrosiveness observed in various ejecta from the sick? Theodosius noted that the ancients attributed qualities other than the four primary ones to the humors, citing Hippocrates, who attributed hotness *and* saltiness to the humors, and so on. In this way Rhodius sets up a discussion of Severinus' use of chemical qualities to describe diseases and causes.

In response to Theodosius, Theophilus stated that Severinus *did not* reject the humors, merely argued that it was not the humors or their Galenic qualities that produced disease, but rather it was the pathogenic *semina* within the humors that were responsible. The *semina* produce the manifest qualities. Theophilus cites Hippocrates (as had Severinus) to support Severinus' contention that neither hot nor cold cause disease, but rather the "dynameis" in the body. Furthermore, Severinus did not

---

82 Ibid., pp. 179-81.

discount the role of the humors entirely, since he regarded them as wombs for the *semina*. Turning the argument against Galen, Theophilus points out that Galen did not mean just one thing by the term bile, but used it to refer to various substances with diverse characteristics. One must therefore look below the humor to its specific properties, which are æruginous, mercurial, opiate, etc.[83]

Much of the remainder of the commentary on chapter twelve is devoted to an application of this chemical nomenclature to the specific cases of inflammations and ulcerations, both of which can be internal or external and therefore offer some problems for Severinus' theory. Theodosius summarizes what Severinus has written about the generation of inflammations: the seminal roots of inflammations reach various wombs in the body in both liquid (resolved) and vaporous (spiritual) forms. They are then digested by fermentation and await separation and maturity. At maturity they erupt or "boil over" (ebullition) from incorporeal potencies to become corporeal and endowed with the specific qualities, which are the signatures of the disease. When their time has expired the spirits disappear, and the body's vital balsam cleans up the residual impurities, returning things to normal. Specific kinds of inflammations arise from specific chemical roots. Sulphurous spirits cause prunelles; arsenical spirits result in bubos and pestilential inflammations; and auripigmental ones cause pleurisies, no matter where in the body they might occur. Thus, extravasation of blood may lead to inflammation, insofar as the accumulating blood may contain the seeds of an inflammation, which then give rise to inflammations if they are brought to ebullition. According to this theory, extravasation of the blood merely provides an opportunity for the potential disease to express itself.[84]

Theodosius also cites Sennert's criticism of this theory and his defense of the Galenic humoral account of inflammation. In the first place, falling down (i.e. bruising oneself) causes the generation of inflammations in everybody, as do other external causes. Severinus' theory does not well explain what would seem to be a mechanical causation. Second, the Galenic theory that inflammation is brought about by corrupt, extravasated blood fits well with observation. It is known that nature attempts

83 Ibid., pp. 181-85.
84 Ibid., pp. 185-86.

to rid the body of corrupt humors through the available passageways, but that when this fails, humors are expelled through the bursting of glands and buboes and other extraordinary means.

Philomusus and Theophilus respond by trying to accommodate the old and new theories. Philomusus asks if, when flint is struck to make fire, it is the striking itself or rather some sulphur in the flint that causes the fire. Theodosius responds that no fire is generated without the striking. Philomusus wonders why striking ordinary rocks together does not produce fire. Theodosius answers that not all stones are suited to yielding fire. "Therefore," concludes Philomusus, "sulphur would be the proximate cause, and the striking only the necessary cause, which kindles the sulphur into burning. And the smell well proves the presence of sulphur."[85] Theophilus explains that falling down is an external cause, like the striking of the flint. One must take care to distinguish between the proximate and the necessary causes. As far as the extravasation of blood is concerned, Severinus would not dispute that matter accumulated in "foreign anatomies" is corrupted, resolved, and dispersed. But, if that extravasated blood is pure, the symptoms will be much different from when it is imbued with foreign seeds. Here Rhodius has reduced the apparent disagreement between the Galenist position and Severinus' theory to a matter of misunderstanding: Severinus was speaking at a higher level – "he does not deny what you think he denies," says Theophilus.[86] The problem is that the Galenists do not correctly discern the importance of *semina* in the accumulated humors. Their view, according to Rhodius, is too materialistic.

Turning to consider ulcerations as another example of diseases that can be explained by Severinus' theory, Theodosius lists the necessary conditions for ulcerations and how they develop: If the body's vital balsam is congenitally deficient or weakened for some reason, if the diet has been improper, if there is an imperfect separation of the nutriments, where the resulting residual impurities contain corrosive salts with powerful tinctures of corrosive *semina*, and if the mumia of the blood or some

---

85 Ibid., p. 187: "Erit ergo sulphur causa proxima, & concussio tantum causa sine qua non, quæ sulphur ad inflammationem incitat. Nam & odor præsentiam sulphuris satis probat."

86 Ibid., pp. 187-88: "Non igitur hæc negat, quæ Ipsum putas negare."

other location is transplanted, then the roots of disease are introduced. Once the disease is rooted, it is nourished by corresponding impurities and produces fruit at the appropriate times. As with inflammations, specific roots or corrosive salts give rise to specific diseases – ferruginous salts result in cancers, æruginous salts in herpes and lupus, aluminous salts in hydropsical ulcerations, nitrous salts in the itch, and vitriolic salts in scabies. However, Theodosius has doubts about all this. Why are these diseases not produced when those corrosive salts are applied to the skin? Theophilus replies that although the chemical natures of salts being applied externally are the same as when they are present internally ("they never forget their nature"), there are circumstantial differences that effect how they behave. For example, chemicals applied to the skin differ from chemical *semina* in the blood in terms of the circumstances of their location, not in their substance. Much depends on the wombs that the *semina* take root in, and so on.[87]

This last discussion reveals that Rhodius clearly understood Severinus' chemical nomenclature not merely as an abstract analogy but as specifying an observable, direct relationship between pathogenic impurities and laboratory chemistry. Thus, what might be viewed as a complex Paracelsian system of signatures and correspondences between the macrocosm and microcosm is in this case a more direct association of the observable, corrosive properties of certain salts with the ulcerations and inflammations that they generate.

The third "day" of discussion between Rhodius' three friends is the shortest, comprising only about nine percent of the treatise. The preamble, however, is of particular interest. It opens with Philomusus recalling a passage from the Hermetic corpus about a spiritual force that penetrates all substance, which many believe to refer to a universal spirit that gives each thing its specific form. He now wonders if this is the same thing that the Platonists mean by a World Spirit or World Soul, which the Aristotelians wholly reject as an old wives' tale. He asks Theophilus to elaborate on this idea, since he (i.e. Rhodius) has written on the subject before, in the hope that it will help explain Severinus' theory.

---

87 Ibid., pp. 188-89.

Theophilus obliges and explains that the Platonists conceived of a world spirit that was a kind of matter impregnated with the *rationes* of the World Soul. This "seedlike nature, as if a preserver of seeds, a propagator," as they call it, is the intermediary between the Archetypes and the corporeal world. Philomusus judges that this is what Severinus meant by the term "universal medicine." Theodosius objects that this cannot be, because it was said before, in the discussion of chapter two, that if the inner nature of something were poisonous, it could not be changed and must be rejected as a poison. Theophilus clarifies that there is a universal nature common to things, which becomes specified by supervening forms. In itself this universal nature is good, even divine:

> For, just as God universally flows in the actions of all natural things, and we are, live, and move in God (Acts 17), so too he wished to place an example of his divine majesty in nature, from the contemplation of which we would be able to learn his omnipotent cooperation. Just as the angels, those governing spirits, are in God immediately, so every living and moving corporeal creature moves and lives in God by means of this universal nature.[88]

Through Theophilus, Rhodius has equated Severinus' vital balsam or universal spirit with a divine principle that is immanent in nature. This spirit is subject to supervening forms that give it diverse specific characteristics, such as laxative, sweet, or poisonous. To illustrate, Theophilus brings forth the example of the philosophers' stone. Without a ferment it agrees with all forms indifferently. It is, properly speaking, what the ancients called prime matter: "It is ungenerated, incorruptible, and is the subject of generation and corruption."[89] In the human body it joins

88 Ibid., pp. 191-2: "Nam quemadmodum Deus universaliter influit in omnium rerum naturalium actiones, & in Deo sumus, vivimus & movemur *Actor. 17.*: ita etiam in Natura divinæ suæ Majestatis exemplum ponere voluit, ex cujus contemplatione possemus Omnipotentem Ipsius cooperationem addiscere. Sicuti Angeli, spiritus illi Administratorii immediate sunt in Deo: ita mediante hac Natura universali, creatura omnis corporea vivens & movens, in Deo movetur & vivit." The Scriptural reference is to Acts 17:28 "For in him we live, and move, and have our being" (King James Version).
89 Ibid., pp. 192-93: "Quæ est ingenerabilis, est incorruptibilis, est subjectum generationis, & corruptionis."

with the innate heat and becomes innate heat, just as it becomes gold when joined with a ferment of gold. Theodosius objects that if indeed the universal spirit is the philosophers' stone, then it is present in all things, and therefore chemists are wasting their efforts to find the proper source. Theophilus rebuts this, saying that while it is true that the universal spirit exists in all things, it is not distributed to them in equal measure and is not as readily extracted from some as from others. One can recognize here Severinus' claim that vital balsam is more easily extracted from minerals and vegetables than from animals, which is one justification for the use of mineral-based chemical preparations.

From our twentieth-century perspective, it seems odd that Rhodius should have devoted considerable attention to aspects of Severinus' theory that impinged on theology. In particular, he showed interest in whether Severinus' account of the origin of disease, which is an evil, can be construed as a Manichæan heresy and also in Severinus' interpretation of nature's vitality as an attribute of a world spirit, which is God manifest in things. But such issues were not out of place in the middle of the seventeenth century. Rhodius lived in a doctrinally charged atmosphere, in which religious matters were contested, and even the act of contesting them could be interpreted as heterodox. For teachers of natural philosophy, as Rhodius then was, the religious consequences of philosophical speculation and vice versa must have been compelling.[90] It is my suspicion that Ambrosius Rhodius was not merely defending the *Idea medicinæ* from past and present detractors, when he wrote the *Disputationes*, but also explaining and defending his own ideas about the nature of the world and God's relationship to it. The *Idea medicinæ* does not speak very directly to these religious issues, since it is primarily a philosophical and medical treatise. Even so, Severinus did associate

---

90 See Shackelford, "A Reappraisal of Anna Rhodius," for consideration of the religious and social milieu surrounding Ambrosius Rhodius in Christiania. On early seventeenth-century educators' concerns for a theology and natural philosophy that are compatible, see Ann Blair, "Mosaic Physics and the Search for a Pious Natural Philosophy in the Late Renaissance," *Isis* 91(2000): 32-58.

seminal knowledge with innate spirit. It reflected God's presence in all living things, which he connected with the Paracelsian Light of Nature.[91]

Severinus' followers and near contemporaries, for example Kort Aslakssøn, had placed his theory in the Neoplatonic mainstream, interpreting spirit and vital balsam as a kind of divinity in things. Another contemporary, Giordano Bruno, was similarly anxious to celebrate the world soul as a divine immanence in nature. Their brand of metaphysics was really a kind of natural theology that bordered on pantheism in its exaltation of the holy spirit. Ambrosius Rhodius, writing half a century later, also emphasized the Neoplatonist aspect of the *Idea medicinæ*. Yet one thing is clear: Rhodius recognized the general application of Severinus' metaphysics as a theory of generation and corruption and did not merely appreciate it as a useful theory of pathogenesis. While he did not really add anything significant to the teachings of *Idea medicinæ*, it is evident that he grasped the significance of Severinus' main ideas and sought to explain them to a new generation. To this end he supported them by means of numerous references to medical authorities – well over fifty of them. The authors that Rhodius cited in his commentary reveal the breadth of his reading in medical literature in general, and his familiarity with Paracelsian and Hermetic texts in particular. Given Daniel Sennert's prominent place in Rhodius' medical education, it is not surprising that Rhodius mentioned him often and that he would attach major importance to Severinus as an interpreter of Paracelsian doctrine, especially since Sennert himself had read the *Idea medicinæ* and reacted to it in print and perhaps also in his teaching. Whether Rhodius encountered the Dane's ideas in Sennert's lectures or in his *De chymicorum cum Aristotelicis et Galenicis consensu ac dissensu*, or whether he first took up the *Idea medicinæ* as an expatriate in Severinus' homeland, cannot readily be determined. However, it is likely that his residence in Frederik Severinus' house and his marriage to Anna Frederiksdatter Severinus contributed a personal motivation to his defense of Petrus Severinus' ideas.

---

91 Severinus, *Idea medicinæ*, p. 107.

Chapter Ten

WILLIAM DAVIDSON'S COMMENTARIES ON THE *IDEA MEDICINÆ PHILOSOPHICÆ*

WILLIAM DAVIDSON of Aberdeen is best known to historians for teaching chemistry at the Jardin des Plantes in Paris in the second quarter of the seventeenth century, where we already met him in chapter five, as part of Guy de la Brosse's program to bring Paracelsian chemistry into pedagogy. His early textbook, *Philosophia pyrotechnica*, which was in part based on his teaching and intended for use by his students, is regarded as a link in the evolution of basic chemical curriculum that began with Andreas Libavius, Jean Bodin, and Oswald Croll and lead to the chemistry of the French Enlightenment. The *Philosophia pyrotechnica* went through a couple of editions and likely found a greater readership among students of chemistry than did Davidson's later works, both of which are highly theoretical and arcane, because it treats chemical laboratory methods and procedures as well as presenting Paracelsian theory, and therefore had practical utility as a laboratory manual. However, to the extent that these later works represent the development of Davidson's philosophy at a more mature stage, they are arguably of greater importance to understanding Davidson himself.[1] Furthermore, since the bulk of his later writing was devoted to

---

1 A careful study of all Davidson's writings has yet to be done. For Davidson's biography see John Read, "William Davidson of Aberdeen," *Ambix* 9 (1961): 70-101, and John Small, "Notice of William Davidson, M.D. (Gulielmus Davissonus), First Professor of Chemistry, and Director of the Jardin des Plantes, Paris, afterwards Physician to the King of Poland," *Proceedings of the Society of Antiquaries of Scotland* 10 (1875): 265-280.

commentaries on Severinus' *Idea medicinæ*, further study of his work is warranted here, as it is the single largest source by which we can judge how Severinus was read and used in the seventeenth century. Since these treatises span several hundred pages of relatively compact, Latin text, a full and balanced treatment is not possible nor appropriate within the present scope. However, it is possible to summarize and highlight the contents of several exemplary chapters and scrutinize the introductory matter to the various sections of these treatises in order to learn how Davidson read and used Severinus' ideas.

William Davidson's brand of chemical philosophy was clearly in-fluenced by his reading of Severinus' *Idea medicinæ* already by the early 1630s, when he was writing the *Philosophia pyrotechnica*. However, even a cursory inspection of his books reveals that he incorporated Severinus' Paracelsian thought into a wider, more mystical and Neopythagorean form of cosmology that is more like that of Michael Maier and Robert Fludd, more Rosicrucian one might say, than was the metaphysics of the *Idea medicinæ*. Already in the *Philosophia pyrotechnica* and in the French version, *Les Elements de la Philosophie de l'Art du Feu ou Chemie*, Davidson made use of emblems to capture and convey meanings and argued the essentially mathematical nature of his chemical philosophy, which he claimed was founded on geometrical (Euclidean) principles.[2] However, if Severinus ever endorsed the diagramatic, emblematic, and numerologi-cal approach later associated with the Rosicrucians, it is certainly not evident in the *Idea medicinæ*, which is devoid of explicit and elaborate hierarchies of the categories of being. Indeed, Severinus accused Galen of having sold out ancient medicine by forcing theory to conform to "geometrical" demonstrations! But where Severinus associated geometry with Euclidean proofs and argument from logic, Davidson's view of mathematics was more Pythagorean, associated with cosmic harmony and reminiscent of Robert Fludd's works. Davidson, therefore, used Severinus' ideas in a context that viewed God's planning as essentially numerical and symmetrical, rather than conceiving creation merely to

---

2 John Read, "William Davidson of Aberdeen," p. 83. I rely here on Read's study of William Davidson, *Les Elements de la Philosophie de l'Art du Feu ou Chemie*, trans. Jean Hellot (Paris, 1651 and 1657) for my interpretation.

This diagram from William Davidson's Philosophia pyrotechnica illustrates his commitment to a Neoplatonic or Gnostic foundation for the generation of the natural world from dark (corporeal) and light (incorporeal) sources. Such ideas underlay the Rosicrucian worldview in the seventeenth century and indicate the wider intellectual context into which Severinus' Paracelsian ideas of body and spirit were incorporated. Reproduced by courtesy of the Department of Special Collections, General Library System, University of Wisconsin-Madison.

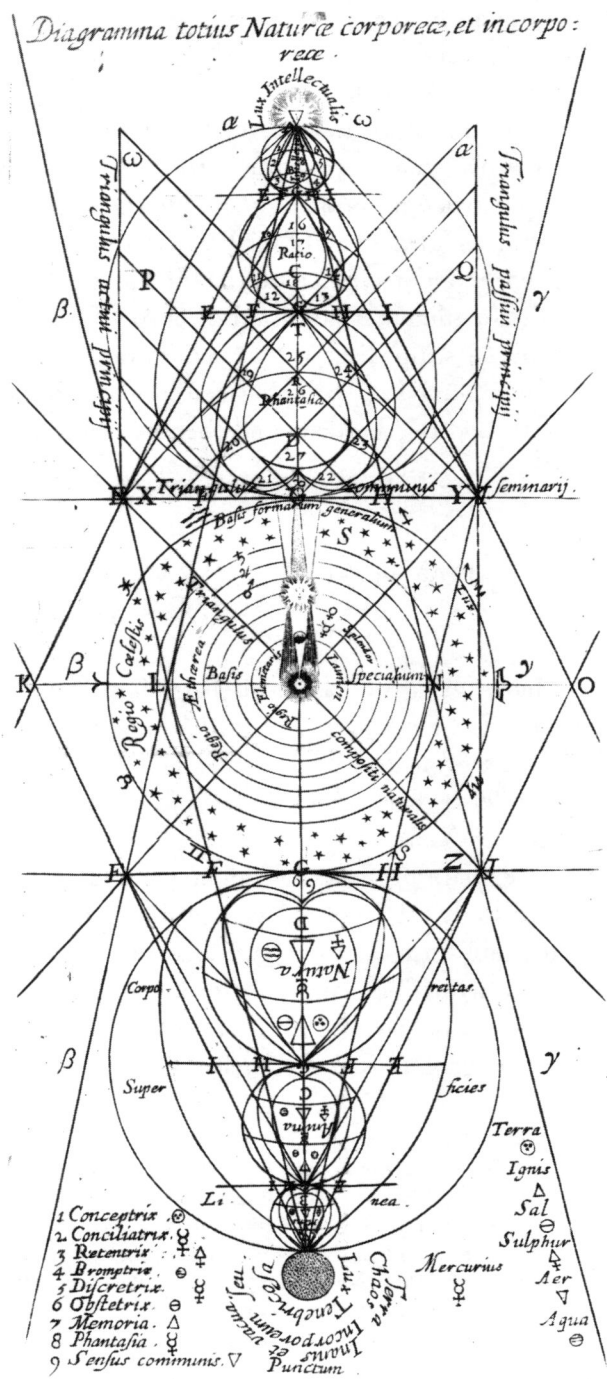

be ordered in the less rigorously mathematical sense of "according to number, weight, and measure."[3]

Davidson's emphasis on the numerical structure of the world and the attempt to capture and convey this structure by emblems and diagrams carried over into his commentaries on the *Idea medicinæ*, which were first published in 1660 and 1663. He apparently continued to work with these ideas for the rest of his life, for in 1668 he had a book printed that allegedly contains indices to the 1660 edition of the *Idea medicinæ* and to his first commentary on it (also 1660).[4] This was a monograph on *plica polonica*, a scalp disease that was associated particularly with Poland, where he served as royal physican from ca. 1659 until 1667 or 1668, when he returned to Aberdeen and then finally to Paris.

DAVIDSON'S FIRST COMMENTARY ON THE *IDEA MEDICINÆ*

William Davidson called his first commentary a *Preliminary Publication for the Commentaries on the Idea Medicinæ Philosophicæ of the Sublime Philosopher and Incomparable Man, Petrus Severinus the Dane*, which I shall refer to here as his *Prodromus*.[5] It opens with an introduction to the reader (*ad lectorem*), which reveals why he has undertaken to publish a text explaining Severinus' doctrine and why the student of medicine should study this book. Davidson shared with Severinus a commitment to reestablishing medicine on ancient Hippocratic and Platonic foundations, which he claimed had long since been abandoned by medical students, who favored both "hypotheses that are unjustly accommodated to geometrical demonstrations and cleverness of speech" over

---

3 While it was commonplace to recall this Scriptural dictum in defense of the order of creation, clearly there were different emphases assigned to the "mathematical" nature of the cosmos by different authors.

4 See Read, "William Davidson of Aberdeen," p. 79, n. 29 on Davidson's *Theophrasti Verdici Scoti Doctoris medici Plicomastix seu Plicæ e numero morborum Apospasma* (Danzig, 1668). I have not seen this book.

5 William Davidson, *Commentariorum in sublimis philosophi & incomparibilis viri Petri Severini Dani Ideam Medicinæ Philosophicæ ... Prodromus.*

COMMENTARIORUM

In ſublimis Philoſophi & incomparabilis Viri

PETRI SEVERINI DANI

IDEAM MEDICINÆ PHILOSOPHICÆ,

Propediem proditurorum

PRODROMUS.

n quo *Platonicæ* doctrinæ explicantur fundamenta, ſuper quæ *Hippocra-*
tes, *Paracelſus* & *Severinus*: nec non ex antitheſi, *Ariſtoteles*
& *Galenus* ſua ſtabilivere Dogmata.

Sub finem Authoris doctrina, febrium exemplo, in
praxim reducitur.

Hiſce ſelectiorum Chemicorum remediorum, *omnibus à Capite ad Calcem*
affectibus appropriatorum, 40 *annorum uſu probatorum*, *ſine*
fuco & jactantia deſcriptorum, *manipulus adjicitur.*

Opera & ſtudio

WILLIELMI DAVISSONI, Nobilis Scoti ;

hriſtianiſſimi Galliarum & Navarræ Regis Conſiliarii & Medici, domus hortique plantarum Medicinalium, qui Pariſiis in ſuburbio S. Victoris eſt, olim Præfecti: nunc
autem S Regiæ Majeſtatis Poloniæ & Sueciæ Senioris Archiatri & Chemici:
S. Reginalis itidem Majeſtatis in vulgari Medicina Perſonæ Medici.

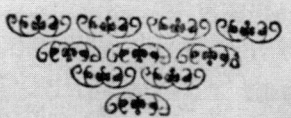

HAGÆ-COMITIS,

Ex Typographia ADRIANI VLACQ.
cIɔ Iɔc LX.

The title page of William Davidson's 1660 commentary on Petrus Severinus' Idea
medicinæ philosophicæ. *Reproduced by courtesy of the Department of Special
Collections, General Library System, University of Wisconsin-Madison.*

the observation and experience of natural things.[6] He does not reject hierarchy in philosophy, which he defines as the ordering of causes and effects, nor demonstrations per se, but believes that a general laziness led physicians to forsake reality for the "remarkable subtlety" of humoral theory, which has failed.

Davidson specifies two developments that indicate the inadequacy of traditional scholastic medicine. First, occult properties were reintroduced to medicine. This is evidence of the insufficiency of a medical philosophy that is restricted to the Galenic qualities and degrees. It has, in effect, pointed medical theory toward the older Hippocratic "powers" once more. Second, it is clear that chemical physicians, even those empirics who merely follow recipes, have succeeded in treating diseases that have eluded the Galenists. Thus, both the Galenic theory and the traditional therapy that it supported were found wanting.

Davidson reveals to the reader that when he was a student he took his professors' complaints about traditional medicine to heart: they felt that Aristotelian theory did not fit medical reality and that therapy that is based on humoral pathology did not succeed in treating the most difficult diseases. While studying in Paris he attended the informal and unauthorized meetings of chemical physicians and began to take a special interest in Platonic philosophy. He observed that the empirical chemists, although they enjoyed a successful practice, did not advance the art of medicine as a coherent method of healing. Therefore, he cast about for a new doctrine that could embrace chemical cures – a task at which the Aristotelians had failed.

The peripatetics and the chemists both handed down an analytic method, he claims, but the method of the former, which is found in the *Meteorology* and other tracts by Aristotle, is flawed. It is speculative and "totally false and diametrically opposed to sensible resolution."[7] Many are the physicians who enlarge their errors under the protection of Aristotle's name. The best physicians, however, are not the chemi-

---

6 Davidson, *Prodromus*, p. i (the first page of the unpaginated *ad lectorem*): "infidas hypotheses Geometricis demonstrationibus, & fucatis linguæ muneribus injuste accommodatas."

7 Ibid., p. v: "qualis est illa Meteororum, quæ tota falsa est, & e Diametro resolutioni sensibili opposita."

cal "empirics" or the Galenist "dogmatics," but those who have been trained in both kinds of medicine, Galenic and chemical. Severinus was one of these eclectics, as were Quercetanus, Phædro, Mayerne, Nolle, Sennert, and Hartmann, to name a few. Despite their differences, all these authors traced chemical physiology and therapy to Hippocrates rather than to Galen.

Davidson tells the reader that he then began to read what chemical philosophers had written, books in which Severinus was praised, but he could make little or no sense out of their "empty chatter about rellolacean qualities, mechanical spirits, the archeus." All these unfamiliar terms struck him as the horrible incantations of magicians.[8] Furthermore, there was disagreement among the various authors, whom he likened to nocturnal animals groping about in the daylight. He found only Severinus to be free of such difficulties. However, to understand the *Idea medicinæ*, one must be well grounded in ancient philosophy, which is why some condemn the book merely by looking at the title. Davidson wishes that those critics had spent as many *months* studying ancient philosophy as they had wasted *years* on learning to recite Aristotle! It is difficult to convince such people of the value of Severinus' theory, since they think they already know everything and therefore resist their own senses in their struggle against the truth. Yet, perhaps they can still benefit from reading this *Prodromus* to Severinus' ideas.

Davidson claims that he is not merely transcribing the *Idea medicinæ*, but rather explaining it on the basis of his own long study and experience. He has read the ancient sources and come to a "genuine sense of this Platonic and chemical author" and he has used Severinus' ideas in teaching his students in Paris.[9] But why is this author so important? Severinus, whom Davidson describes as "one who gave immortality to chemical philosophy," succeeded in framing a metaphysics that made sense out of what the chemical physician understood from experience; the student who learns the "metaphysical composition" of the world from

8 Ibid., p. ii: "Apud tales nihil præterquam vanas de qualitatibus rellolaceis, spiritibus Mechanicis, de Archeo ... quasi horribiles Magicarum incantationum (ut mihi videbantur) voces audiebam."

9 Ibid.: "ut Authoris hujus Platonici & Chemici genuinum sensum & consensum cum Chemica resolutione acciperem."

Davidson's *Prodromus* will know what to expect of its "physical composition," which can only be examined by means of chemical analysis.

Davidson recommends that the student, after learning the material presented in the *Prodromus*, systematically read the works of Proclus, Plato, Iamblichus, Hermes Trismegistus, the fragments of Zoroaster, a compendium of Plato's treatises, and tracts by Alcmaeon, Stobæus, and Lucretius. Among more recent authors, the student is directed to Fortunatus Licentius, Jean Fernel, Leon Hebræus, and Van Helmont.

The ancient writers often wrote in dialogues and fables in order to conceal their meanings, and this is why Severinus did not present his physiology – which he proposed as a plan to advance medicine – in a straightforward style that would be suitable for the beginner. To compensate for this inconvenience, Davidson says that he has written his *Prodromus* so that "every student trained in chemical analysis can scientifically, both metaphysically and chemically, uncover the causes of all natural effects." He wishes for no reward for his effort and expense, other than that the public use the book and benefit from it.[10]

The body of the 1660 *Prodromus* opens with a brief summary of Severinus' doctrine and method, which covers some of the same rhetorical ground as the *ad lectorem* had, only with brevity and greater bombast: Severinus' erudition obviously shines forth in the *Idea medicinæ*, which few today understand, he writes. This is not because of the obscurity of his style and method, but because students of the usual schools have been indoctrinated from their childhood "by the corrupt and evil principles of the Aristotelian school (with considerable damage for all fields of study)" and they are therefore poorly equipped to understand Severinus' words.[11]

Anyone who wishes to be a faithful disciple of Severinus, he continues, must "come forth naked" and suspend his judgement until he has read to the end. He will perceive the author's modesty and deep erudi-

---

10 Ibid., p. v: "qua possit unusquisque in Analysi Chemica versatus causas omnium effectuum naturalium tam Metaphysice quam Chemice, scientifice denodare, si velint."

11 Ibid., p. 1: "Sed iis qui in scholis vulgaribus consenuerunt vix intelligibilem; non propter methodi aut styli verendam obscuritatem, nec tam propter ..., sed propter rudiorum ingeniorum pravum habitum, quem a cunabilis, a corruptis & maleficis Scholæ Aristotelicæ principiis (cum insigni omnium studiorum detrimento) contraxerunt indelibilem."

tion, his elegance of style, the dexterity of his method, and its usefulness. Based on ancient and holy sources, Severinus' theory is diametrically opposed to "ordinary physics." The two, Severinian and Aristotelian, disagree on principles, differ in development, and are in the end discordant. Severinus first lays out the principles, explains the "mechanical" or skillful procedures for acting on them, and then establishes the appointed reasons for the causes of things. These include the "wondrous ordering" between prior and posterior and the relationships by which the lower and weaker orders of things "are preserved, governed, and fostered by the higher and stronger."[12] Everywhere in the *Idea medicinæ* Severinus introduced the judgements of the ancient and more recent philosophers on such matters.

Davidson next gives an exegesis of the title of the book itself, suggesting the thoroughness with which he expects to analyze its contents: The book is called *Idea medicinæ philosophicæ fundamenta continens totius doctrinæ Hippocraticæ, Galenicæ & Paracelsicæ*. The first word, *idea*, is a Platonic term referring to the stable exemplar or model, from which different copies can be made and which forms the basis for an idealization. This is the sense in which medical and philosophical writers have used the term when they refer to idealizations and models (*ideata aut exempla*), whence it follows that the idealization or theory can nowhere be understood unless the underlying idea or exemplar is known.[13] Davidson's implication is that unless we understand the Platonic reality behind medicine, we cannot model it; that the art of medicine must have sound theoretical underpinning.

Continuing this analysis, Davidson says that the book is called an idea "of philosophical medicine" (*medicinæ philosophicæ*) to distinguish it from a treatise on empirical medicine. Philosophical medicine provides principles, the truth of which depends on metaphysics – it provides the certain and inescapable foundations (*fundamenta*) upon which the whole of Hippocratic, Galenic, and Paracelsian medicine is founded. Severinus specified "of Hippocratic doctrine" (*doctrinæ Hippocraticæ*) so that the reader would understand that he meant not

12 Ibid: "Mirandoque ordine, posteriora a prioribus dependere, inferiora a superioribus, debiliora a potentioribus conservari, gubernari & foveri asserit."
13 Ibid., p. 2.

just Hippocrates' treatises, but the whole Hippocratic theory, which embraces the philosophical principles of Democritus, Plato, Empedocles, and Anaxagoras. Finally, although Galen and Paracelsus seem to disagree on many points, it is easy to find agreement and reconciliation between them on many others.[14]

Next Davidson presents what he sees as the principle subject and scope of the *Idea medicinæ*. Severinus wanted nothing less than "to reform and renew ordinary medicine, which long ago fell into base error, on account of the failure of true metaphysics." One ought to proceed to a conclusion on the basis of true, general principles before descending to particulars.[15] In the whole book Severinus imitates Plato, Plotinus, and Iamblichus, but especially Proclus, whose simplicity Severinus concealed in his eloquent and beautiful style. Davidson apparently felt that Proclus' philosophy was crucial to Severinus' work, because he wrote that had he not reread Proclus and his "imitator" Patrizi very often, he would not have devoted so many years of intensive study to the *Idea medicinæ*: "I would have left this author more than shrouded in Cimmerian darkness, to the great loss of philosophers and physicians, but especially of chemists."[16] Indeed, the key to Severinus' philosophy is understanding that it is not new, but renewed – inasmuch as it was cultivated by Proclus and other Platonists.[17]

Under the rubric "the key to the book," Davidson introduces the method that he plans to employ in the *Prodromus*, by way of example. He will use what he calls "Platonic inductions," where a conclusion is inferred from givens, proofs, and specific arguments that are brought to bear on a proposition. For example, if one were to examine the proposition "everything productive of another thing is superior to the nature of the product," first one would identify the possibilities. Either the

---

14 Ibid.

15 Ibid.: "Scopus Severini Dani in hoc libro est reformare & renovare Physicam vulgarem, quæ jam dudum in turpes errores desciverat, propter veræ Methaphysices defectum: … antequam ad particularia descendatur."

16 Ibid., p. 3: "& authorem hunc plusquam Cymeriis tenebris involutum, magno Philosophorum & Medicorum, sed præcipue Chemicorum damno.. reliquissem." Davidson noted Francesco Patrizi's importance as a translator of Proclus' Theology and Physics in the *ad lectorem* (p. iv), but I presume that when he calls him Proclus' imitator he is alluding to Patrizi's *Nova de universis philosophia* (Ferrara, 1591).

17 Davidson, *Prodromus*, p. 3: "utpote a subtili Proclo aliisque Platonicis exculta."

producer is superior, inferior, or equal to the product. There is no fourth alternative. Then, on the basis of axioms that would be introduced in an actual argument, and which are assumed to be true and are conceded by the opponent, it would be demonstrated that the producer is neither inferior nor equal to the product, proving the truth of the proposition by elimination.[18] Once a series of such propositions has been established, the desired conclusions will follow by necessity. Next Davidson will turn this logical structure into a "positive theory" (*doctrina positiva*), which will be used to explain the occult terms that Severinus has woven into his philosophy. Furthermore, this "positive theory" also will be accommodated to Davidson's own metaphysical framework, the sphere of radical beings. It is interesting that Davidson, using this elaborate logical machine, which I suspect Severinus would have rejected as being too "geometrical" and not closely related to experience, hoped to explain Severinus' philosophy by integrating it into his own Neoplatonic scheme. Severinus' doctrine of seminal progression is therefore fitted into a large system of orders and classes of being that are emanating from the One, the uncreated godhead.

Although Davidson's metaphysical system is in principle independent of Severinus' theory, it does provide the background against which Davidson has read the *Idea medicinæ*, or perhaps better stated, it is the general schema into which Davidson has integrated Severinus' ideas. It therefore bears a brief introduction. The system comprises seven orders which each contain seven classes. There is a hierarchical relationship both "horizontally" across the orders and "vertically" within each order. The first order contains the seven classes of radical beings that were conceived at the instant of creation and are therefore the first "unfolding" or emanation of the One, which can be likened to the center of a sphere, unfolding all from within. Each entity within this order is itself unfolded "vertically" from those above it. The first class, Created Being or Prime Metaphysical Mixture, unfolds itself into Life, which unfolds itself into Intellect, Intellect into Soul, Soul into Spirit, Spirit into Form, and Form into Matter.[19] At least this is how it is described

---

18 Ibid., p. 4: "Omne productivum alterius præstantius est natura producti."
19 Ibid., p. 5.

in the "key to the book." In practice Davidson's method is not as orderly
and straightforward as he pretends in the introduction, and when he
sets about treating the order of the seven radical beings or elements
systematically, they are Being, Essence, Life, Intellect, Soul, Spirit (or
nature or form), and Matter.[20]

The second order is the order of seminary reasons, also called *astra*
and spirits. These are the chains between the invisible, incorporeal
world and the visible, corporeal world and they range accordingly from
"space" to "atoms." Davidson assimilated Severinus' *semina* into this
order, which he develops in detail in his commentary on chapter six of
the *Idea medicinæ* (On *Semina*). Similarly, he chose the commentary on
chapter seven (On the Principles of Bodies) to expound on his third
order, the order of hypostatic principles and principles of body, which
appears to be the union of the three Paracelsian principles and the four
Aristotelian elements. However, Davidson divides them differently: the
three hypostatic principles are mercury, fire, and air, and not mercury,
sulphur, and salt, as Quercetanus, Libavius, Sennert, and even Severinus himself had contended. According to Davidson's scheme, salt and
sulphur belong with water and earth as principles or elements of body.
More will be said about this below.[21]

Davidson next shows how his method applies to a specific example,
one actually taken from the commentaries themselves. For illustration,
he chose the eighteenth proposition of his discussion of Life, which
is the third class of the first order: "Every caused thing remains in its
cause, and proceeds from it, and returns to it."[22] In the body of the text
these propositions are stated without any discussion or demonstration.
Therefore, his explication of it here conveys a special status to it. That
he selected this particular proposition, which is basic to Severinus' *semina*
theory, to illustrate the philosophical method he used in the *Prodromus*,
indicates how important the metaphysics of the seminal cycle is for his
theory.

---

20 These are summarized on p. 206 of the *Prodromus*, and are surely the correct ones,
    since they correspond to the diagrams included with the book. Spirit and Form, both
    being incorporeal, are often not distinguished in Davidson's work.

21 Ibid., pp. 5-6.

22 Ibid., p. 6: "Omne causatum manet in sua causa, & progreditur ab illa, & convertitur
    ad ipsam." This is proposition 18 listed on p. 161.

Davidson begins establishing the proposition by introducing three terms for the three stages of causal development: *mansio* (stasis), *progressio* (going forth), and *conversio* (returning). *Mansio* is to be compared to the center of a sphere and characterizes the stability of true beings when they remain in themselves. *Progressio* is the diffusion of being from its center, like the infinite rays emanating from a geometric center, and should be likened to the area of a circle or volume of a sphere. Through *progressio* the radical beings of the first order unfold the reasons of the second. Davidson claims that this first order, collectively, is what Severinus meant when he referred to ideas and exemplars, and they are also known as true beings, radical matter, whole substance, and preserving cause. Their *progressio* is what Hippocrates called *Orcus*, and their *conversio* is what he called *Tenebræ*.

Progressio is especially characteristic of the seven seminal reasons, which are the links between incorporeal beings and the bodies that are continually flowing from them. They are also called *astra* because of their virtue and power (*astrum*) and because, like celestial bodies, they exhibit cycles (full moons and new moons). Severinus also calls them mechanical spirits.

Conversio, the return of a thing to its cause, follows from the sympathy that exists between effect and cause. *Conversio* is understood to apply to incorporeals, because bodies perish as soon as they are abandoned by the mechanical spirits. However, bodies can also be restored by spirits, which convey new powers to them: these incorporeal causes go forth from and return to their divine retreats, where they can rest. The whole process can be likened to systole and diastole. In this way, "bodies emulate eternity through the propagation of individuals and the renewal of bodies."[23]

Having finished discussing proposition eighteen, Davidson next turns to its logical demonstration, which is beyond the scope of the present

---

23 Ibid., p. 8: "per propagationem individuorum, & corporum renovationem, corpora æternitatem æmulantur." This vision of all corporeal reality emanating from incorporeal, spiritual centers is fundamental to Severinus' *semina* theory, but also the metaphysics of Nicholas of Cusa and Plotinus, which explains why Davidson found Proclus useful for understanding Severinus.

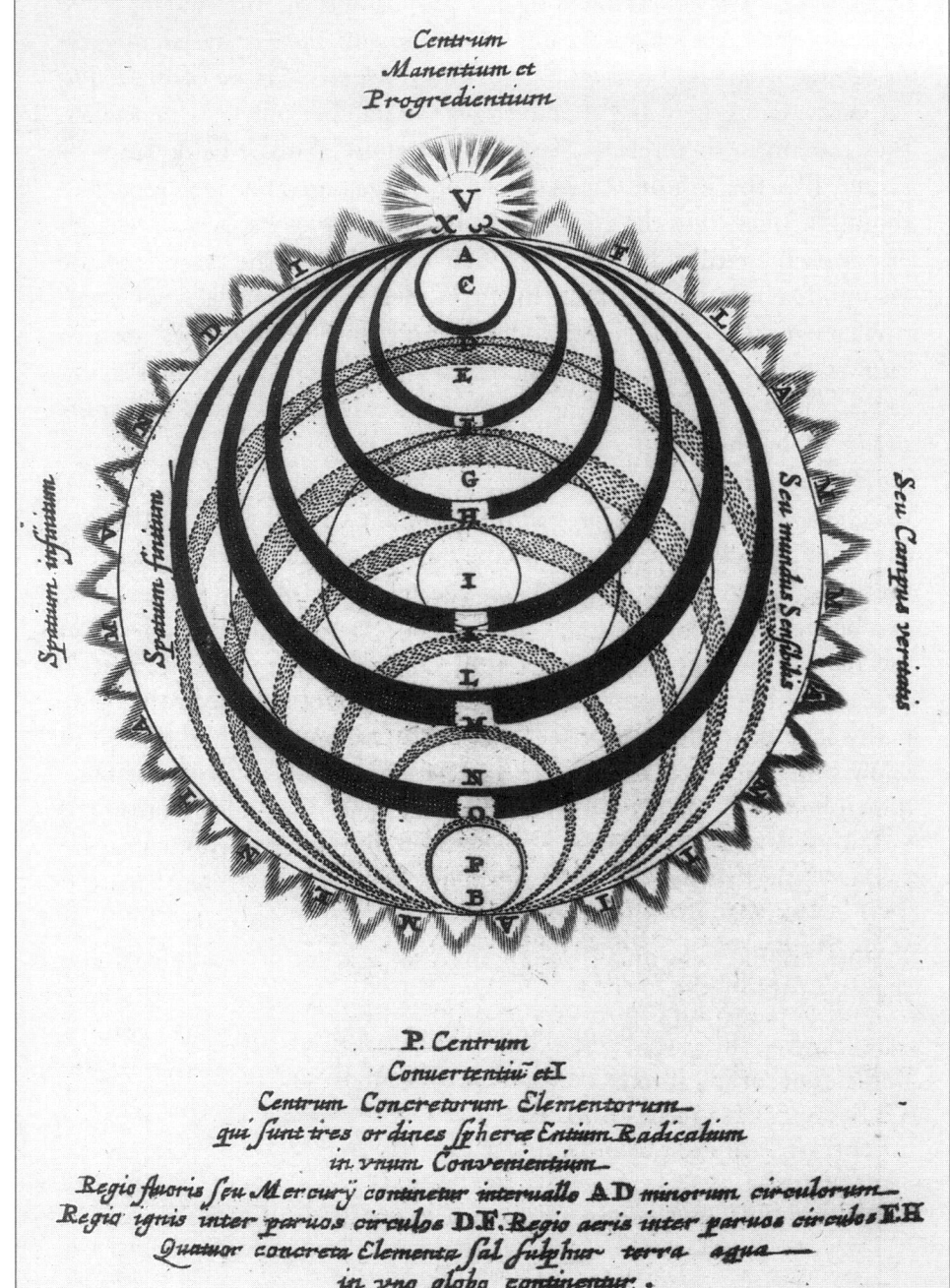

This schema for the generation of the world, from William Davidson's 1660 commentary, suggests a monotheistic light metaphysics of creation, as opposed to the Gnostic, bipolar system portrayed in the illustration from the earlier Philosophia pyrotechnica *(see illustration p. 405). Like the light metaphysics of Robert Grosseteste and Johan Kepler, this system suggests an initial emanation of creation from the divine godhead which creates finite space and, on reflection, creates the sensible world of bodies. However, where the earlier tradition assumed an emanation from the center to the circumference and reflection back to the center, Davidson's model places the divine source at the edge of finite space and envisions the reflection as initiating from a point diametrically opposite. Reproduced by courtesy of the Department of Special Collections, General Library System, University of Wisconsin-Madison.*

analysis. The main point to be gleaned from this survey of his method is that he used the *Idea medicinæ* to provide a structure around which to build his own metaphysics. The choice is a good one, since there are many points of tangency between Severinus' theory and Davidson's, no doubt because they drew on many of the same sources. However, where Severinus developed a system of general metaphysical principles to support generation, transplantation, and corruption and oriented his doctrine to explaining biological function, including pathology, Davidson erected a more elaborate Neoplatonic metaphysics that is replete with analogies drawn from light metaphysics and mathematical theory. Furthermore, he presented it in a much more philosophically rigorous way, with articles and propositions, axioms and demonstrations. In this respect, Davidson has shown himself in this book to be more the philosopher and less the Paracelsian-inspired medical theorist.[24]

24 At least the form of Davidson's presentation gives the appearance of rigorous argument, but I leave it to philosophers to determine if it is in fact any more logically sound than Severinus' text.

The body of the *Prodromus*

The main body of Davidson's *Commentariorum ... prodromus* is divided into two parts, a 470-page commentary on the *Idea medicinæ* itself, and a 52-page application of Severinus' doctrine to the example of fevers, which is built upon the theory of drug action that Severinus had applied to specific types of remedies and diseases in chapter fifteen. The first part comprises analyses of each chapter of Severinus' book. Typically a chapter heading is followed by Severinus' summary of the chapter's content, the *anacephaleosis*, which is reprinted from the italicized summary that Severinus provided at the close of most chapters of the *Idea medicinæ*. Then a long and detailed commentary on some particular part or parts of it ensues. The treatment Davidson gives to each chapter of the *Idea medicinæ* varies greatly in length and approach, as do the original chapters. Chapter four, for instance, receives no commentary at all. The analysis of chapter two includes a one paragraph summary and a seven page commentary. The commentary associated with chapter five, on the other hand, stretches 146 pages and is subdivided into numerous articles, propositions, problems, and other subsections that introduce material not taken from the *Idea medicinæ*, but related to the metaphysical principles found in Severinus' work. For example, Severinus discussed the generation of bodies as a progression or "flowing forth" of being from seminal centers, and once a being's cycle is near the end, it "reflows" back into its seminal domicile. In chapter five Davidson expands this concept to embrace the sequential unfolding of the world in terms of fundamental categories of being. Employing several diagrams that are reminiscent of ones used in Neoplatonic and Rosicrucian literature and quoting the poem "Psyche" from Fracastoro's *De Turris*, Davidson writes of the expansion of the world from a "center of development" (*centrum progredientium*) to fill a finite space, which is a sphere inside an infinite space or "the field of truth."[25] This progression creates a "solid globe of radical beings, of the seminary reasons, and then finally of the concrete elements for delineating the system of the whole world" – in accordance with the teachings of the ancient philosophers.[26]

---

25 Ibid., pp. 105 and 98-99.
26 Ibid., p. 104: "Constructio globi solidi entium radicalium, rationum seminariorum, tum denique elementorum concretorum ad delineandum systema totius mundi, tum ad Hypotheses veterum philosophorum conformandas instituti."

This form of philosophizing is similar in many respects to sixteenth-century Italian natural philosophy, such as it is expressed in the work of Giordano Bruno and Patrizi, a tradition that may have influenced Severinus as well.[27] Whatever the textual origins or philosophical impulses for Davidson's work, it clearly agrees with Severinus' metaphysics on many points, as an inspection of chapter five shows: imperfection receives its cause from perfection; there is nothing in the effect that was not first in the cause; things that are not mixed are prior to things that are; incorruptibles are prior to corruptibles; everything that has dimension is divisible, has parts, and is corporeal as a consequence; every separation of the one is the cause of the many; nothing comes from nothing; and so on. Some of Davidson's statements also clearly express the ideas behind *semina* theory, such as "that which lies hidden in unity is made manifest in multiplication" and "diffusion is separation, separation is the cause of multiplication, multiplication is the cause of progression or progress, and progress is the cause of motion."[28]

Much as Severinus had blurred the boundary between corporeal and incorporeal at the level of seminal generation, Davidson blends the formal and material: "All matter in the incorporeal world is formal, but in the corporeal world, form itself becomes material."[29] However, where Severinus, in the *Idea medicinæ*, restricted his discussion to the metaphysics of life – of generation and corruption – Davidson reaches out to include a more generalized Renaissance philosophy that embraces mathematical axioms, such as "lines drawn from the circumference to the center are indivisible at the center," as well as teleology, e.g. "all things seek the good".[30]

Davidson's commentary on chapter six of the *Idea medicinæ* (On *semina*) illustrates once more how he has interpreted Severinus' ideas

---

27 The content of this part of Davidson's commentary resembles that of Bruno's dialogue *De la causa, principio e uno*, for example, and Davidson himself referred to Patrizi as an influential interpreter of Proclus and also cited Fracastoro.

28 Ibid., p. 134. Article I, axiom #37: "Quod latet in unitate manifestatur in multiplicatione"; Article I, axiom #26: "Diffusio est separatio, & separatio est causa multiplicationis, multiplicatio est causa progressionis, aut progressus, & progressus est causa motus."

29 Ibid., p. 150. Article II, axiom #13: "Omnis materia in mundo incorporeo est formalis, sed in corporeo ipsa forma fit materialis."

30 Ibid., pp. 133 and 134. Article I, axiom #12: "Lineæ a circumferentia ductæ ad centrum, in centro sunt indivisibiles"; Axiom #20: "Omnes res bonum appetunt."

in a large metaphysical structure. Following the established pattern, it opens with a paragraph summary or *anacephalæosis* that is identical (except for punctuation) to the portion of Severinus' text that appears in italics at the end of chapter six, in the third edition (1660).[31] Davidson's analysis of this text (*analysis logica*) begins with a very straightforward, close reading of Severinus: By "*semina*" Severinus does not mean seeds covered by husks, but specific causes – spiritual, incorporeal bodies that are the chains between the incorporeal (the most general kind) and the corporeal (the individual species), as if linking life to death. Comprehended in the *semina* are the dispensations or administrations of the "world anatomy," which Davidson understands as the healing or organic parts of the world. *Semina* develop by a process (*liturgia*) of generation in an orderly and scientific way, governed by the laws of motion and at predestined times. Davidson interprets the term *liturgia* as the continuous and orderly administration of a natural thing.[32] By "vital powers" Severinus meant the essential qualities that existed before bodies, produce bodies, and are wholly incorporeal. A subject cannot exist without them, therefore they are not qualities in the Aristotelian sense, but rather transcendental powers, which is why Severinus called them vital powers. By "adorned with an incomprehensible wisdom" Severinus meant that they are furnished with the divine benevolence that God placed into all things with the Word, willing each to become what he wanted it to be. The mechanical spirits can make use of this wisdom; each thing unfolds itself, yielding its consubstantial and essential characteristics. Once the reader understands these ideas, the rest are easily accessible.[33]

Having provided a gloss on the main ideas of Severinus' chapter summary (*anacephalæosis*), Davidson then gives a more detailed commentary

---

31 The summary that appears in all capitals at the end of the chapter in the 1571 edition of the *Idea medicinæ* appears in italics in the 1660 edition. Davidson's *anacephalæosis* differs from it by one insignificant word inversion and the omission of the clause "quorum ministerio agentium impressiones a patientibus admittuntur vel repelluntur" (Through the service of these, the impressions of agents are admitted or repelled by the things they act upon), for which I have no explanation.

32 Ibid., p. 207: "Per *liturgias* intelligit diuturnas & consuetas administraturas rerum naturalium." Note that this spelling and definition of *liturgia* differ from those given in the 1663 commentary, noted below.

33 Ibid., pp. 207-208.

(*enucleatio*), in which he not only expands his interpretation of specific terms and concepts of the *Idea medicinæ*, but also puts them to his own uses. For example, he begins by explaining why Severinus said that one cannot grasp the nature of the elements without first understanding *semina*, because the latter unfold (*explicant*) the functions of the former. Here, at the outset of this *enucleatio*, Davidson draws attention to a metaphysical structure underlying Severinus' theory, namely the symmetric relationship between two philosophical classes, where the prior and more general explicates or unfolds the posterior and more specific, which in turn implicates or enfolds the prior. This approach to ordering natural philosophy is readily apparent in the philosophy of Nicholas of Cusa and surely informed the thinking of Paracelsus and Severinus, too. But where Severinus was content to use implication and explication in a general way, to sort out the relationships between the ideal causes, seminal reasons, and their corporeal manifestations, Davidson applies it to his entire system of seven metaphysical orders, each with seven parts, which he develops in the course of his commentaries.

Davidson also examines Severinus' use of *semina* as links or intermediaries between the spiritual and the corporeal, between the invisible and visible. He brings in the idea of a non-body (*incorpus*), which he can directly and grammatically oppose to body (*corpus*), and defends this barbarism as necessary if the method of antithesis is to be applied. To *corpora* and *incorpora* he adds *semina*, which link the first two, to form a triad. In terms of Davidson's larger metaphysics, these three correspond to the three primary orders of the seven, namely the radical elemental beings, the concrete elements, and the radical seminary virtues. Where Severinus endowed *semina* with the power and knowledge to unfold being in a general sense, Davidson attributes to them seven specific "seminary reasons" that parallel the seven radical beings or elements from which they unfolded, as he laid out in his commentary on chapter five. These seminary reasons are the stars (*astra*) and chains that bind the radical and concrete elements.[34] They are, in order, Space, Light (*Lux*), Brilliance (*Splendor et Radii*), Illumination (*Lumen*), Innate Heat, Fixed Sulphur, and Atoms or Least Bodies, each of which is described

34 Ibid., p. 213.

in the section on seminary reasons that makes up the balance of the commentary on chapter six of the *Idea medicinæ*.

Thus, the seven seminal or seminary reasons of the second order act as metaphysical chains between the radical elemental beings of the first order and the "hypostatic principles of body" of the third order, which comprises mercury, fire, air, salt, sulphur, earth, and water. Although these "hypostatic principles" seem to be a union of the three Paracelsian principles and the four Aristotelian elements, Davidson has in fact re-ordered and regrouped them, as mentioned above. His division reflects his identification of the first three (mercury, fire, and air) as incorporeal principles and the remaining four (salt, sulphur, earth, and water) as "utterly concrete bodies and evident to the senses."[35]

Just as Severinus at times conflated *semina* and *astra* as links between the corporeal and incorporeal, Davidson also speaks of the *astra* as intermediary chains and notes that Severinus did not understand them as celestial stars but rather as fruits of the radical elements. Again fitting the doctrines of the *Idea medicinæ* to his metaphysics, Davidson explicates the *semina* as inextricably linked to the radical elements, penetrating their depths and administrating the laws of nature. They are endowed with the vital, generative power to make a multitude from unity by means of mixing. The fruits or products of this mixing are the concrete elements and principles of bodies that constitute the third order in his hierarchy.

Davidson notes that Severinus referred to the *semina* as being mechanical, just as he had the *astra* and spirits, and that they contain in them the "dispensations of the general world anatomy."[36] He claims that Severinus took this concept, by analogy, from the anatomists, which is a reasonable interpretation: the good anatomist possesses a knowledge of his subject, which is the lesser world (microcosm). Likewise, the spirit of the greater world assumes the dispensations of the macrocosm for reducing powers, forces, and essences to actions, by virtue of its "anatomical expertise," which can be likened to the "science" or knowledge

---

35 Ibid., p. 209: "Tertius vero ordo erit principiorum hypostaticorum corporis, nempe Mercurij, Ignis & Aeris, Salis, Sulphuris, Terræ, & Aquæ: quorum tria prima sunt incorporea; quatuor vero ultima, prorsus corpora concreta & sensibus obvia."
36 Ibid., p. 211: "universæ mundanæ Anatomiæ dispensationes."

that the Paracelsians considered to be innate in nature.[37] Thus all laws of motion are also in the *semina*, and this point provokes Davidson to make an extended analogy to illustrate how change and stability are reconciled.

There are two kinds of motions, internal and external. Internal motion is active but stable; it is the motion of the spirit. External motion is passive and variable, the motion of the body. Together they can be likened to the movement of a compass or divider: one bow is anchored at a center, and "as from one invisible point" communicates its laws, measures, and ratios – its wisdom – to the other bow, which is extended and mobile. The center is likened to the center of the soul, which while turning about itself remains a dimensionless point, and yet it communicates its inner motion to the body, with the help of the intellect. The extended bow of the divider describes a variable motion that is determined by the center. By analogy, the motion of the seminal reasons is an inner, stable, and active motion that communicates to its fruits the predestinations, including the proper times for germination, growth, and maturity: "For in those *semina* and *astra* the whole force of things to be generated and transplanted is contained and lies hidden, as in vital powers that are equipped with an incomprehensible knowledge." With their help, the impressions that are enfolded in the radical elements of the first order and hidden from the elements of the third order (the principles and concrete elements) are unfolded and either admitted or rejected.[38]

---

37 Ibid. "Per universæ mundanæ Anatomiæ dispensationes; intelligit Entium ministerium, per quæ Mundus hic administratur, vocabulo ab Anatomicis desumpta; nam sicut bonus Anatomicus subjecti humani corporis, ut minoris Mundi, notitiam per se habere debet; sic Natura, forma seu spiritus Mundi universalis, essentiam, partes & dispensationes anatomicas Mundi majoris, hoc est partium essentialium ejus ignorare non debet. Itaque dispensationes mundanæ sumuntur, pro reductione potentiæ, virium & essentiæ, in actum, a Mundi spiritu peritissima Anatomissa." The analogy is plain: both microcosm (man) and macrocosm have souls that guide them, and both have bodies, therefore both have "anatomies." The innate knowledge that governs the generation of the human body, assuring that the organs end up in the proper places, and so on, has a parallel in the "knowledge" innate in the macrocosm.

38 Ibid., p. 212: "In istis enim seminibus & astris, tota rerum generandarum & transplantandarum vis, tanquam in potentiis vitalibus, incomprehensibili scientia decoratis, continetur & delitescit."

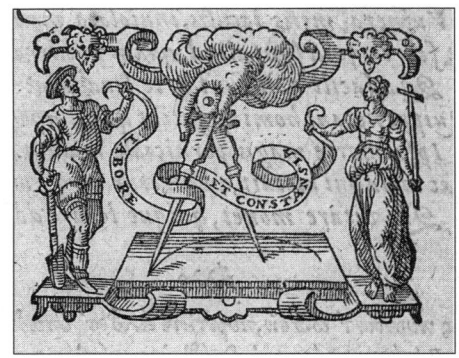

The idea that God is the designer and creator of the natural world was commonplace in early modern Christian natural philosophy. It found expression in the printer's device shown here, from a book published by Christophor Plantin in 1583. The divider and caliper are symbols of the order and measure apparent in nature and therefore are emblematic of the divine presence that is manifest in nature's numeric relationships and harmonies. William Davidson's effort to establish a metaphysics based on the geometric symmetries and harmonies that underlie medical theory and practice is evident in the illustrations that accompany his books. Courtesy of The Danish National Library of Science and Medicine.

THE ACTION OF DRUGS

One of the main purposes of medicine is to treat the ill. The method of treatment, broadly construed, and the theoretical basis that supports it vary considerably between chemical and Galenic practitioners, even if specific therapeutic technologies sometimes do not. Therefore, the actual administration of drugs, together with the theory of disease and cure that guides that administration, form the ultimate proving ground for the legitimacy of a school of medical thought.[39] Consequently, we might expect that the final chapter of the *Idea medicinæ*, in which Seve-

---

39 I do not claim that medical care is the only end or measure of medicine, which may provide a theoretical or explanatory system that satisfies other cultural needs. However, sooner or later most systems of medicine, as systems of medicine, are judged by practitioners on the basis of their ability to relieve the patient efficiently.

rinus applies his theory of generation and transplantation to explain how healing works and how specific drugs act against diseases, would be of great interest to chemical physicians like Davidson. By examining Davidson's reading we can gain insight into how the practicing physician might interpret Severinus' theory and apply it to therapy.

Davidson's commentary on chapter fifteen begins by clarifying that Severinus was addressing his theory to internal diseases rather than to repairing damage caused by wounds, and that the success of medicine in dealing with such diseases depends on the careful correlation of drugs and symptoms. The physician must learn specific drugs and their uses. Consideration of drugs again raises issues of method and epistemology. The learned physician differs from the empiric in that he applies reasoning and a theoretical knowledge of physiology to form a diagnosis and arrive at a therapy (indications and preparations). This method should produce superior results. But the Galenist physician, despite his learning, is less effective than the empiric, because he uses false reasoning, which is based on defective philosophical principles, and also because he ignores the empirical wisdom of collective experience. The difference between Galenic and empirical medicine is most pronounced when it comes to the most serious diseases. For such conditions Davidson would prefer the advice of an experienced peasant to that of the dean of the medical faculty! The better physician draws on both reason and experience, tempering theory with practice and using theory to guide practice. The chemical (Paracelsian) physician might succeed in diagnosing internal, supervening diseases where others fail, because he understands how the observable symptoms relate to the unobservable release of the spirits of the salts and the unseen chemical destruction of the body's natural balsam or radical moisture. Therefore, the knowledge of salts, which is acquired through chemistry, is necessary for understanding the courses of disease and for grasping the nature of the morbific *semina* that lie hidden in the body. If a successful cure depends on resolving these salts, then an indication arrived at by means of qualitative, humoral theory will not avail: here the inexperienced empiric will prevail over the practiced physician.[40]

40 Ibid., pp. 480-482. By supervening diseases I think Davidson means diseases that follow upon other diseases or internal diseases that follow upon external wounds, for example a fever arising from an infected cut.

Davidson's distinction between less serious and more serious diseases is an important one for understanding that Paracelsian medicine did not exclude traditional therapies. "Chemical" medicine, as it was preached by Severinus, was not limited to the use of chemically prepared drugs, but was eclectic and polypharmaceutical, and presumably this flexibility was reflected in his therapy. Indeed, this is affirmed by Johannes Paludan's assessment of Severinus' practice in his letter to Henricus Smetius, which was noted in chapter three above. Davidson explains that Severinus, like Hippocrates, asserted various origins for diseases and different methods for curing them, and that these demanded different remedies. A controlled regimen is sufficient to restore health in some diseases. For these, it is appropriate to apply "natural" remedies, by which he means traditional herbal drugs that have not been artificially prepared or processed. Following Severinus, Davidson labels this class of drugs "alimentary" remedies, because they do not differ in form from ordinary foodstuffs. Thus, diet and regimen were important elements of Hippocratic medicine and remained a part of Paracelsian practice.[41]

"Medicines" or medicaments constitute a second class of drugs. These are based on *materia medica* that induce serious symptoms if taken unmixed and unprepared, that is, they have dangerous side effects. These have powers that exceed those of the "mechanics" of the human body, and for that reason are effective against diseases that have overcome those mechanics and damaged or destroyed the body's vital balsam. Strong diseases require strong remedies, and these must be prepared in such a way as to diminish their side effects while leaving their medical efficacy intact: "The use of these in the most serious diseases is necessary, and medicines of this sort should in no way be applied without chemical preparation, as they do not only require the hand of the expert laborant, but much more the reasoning of the learned chemist."[42]

There are both alimentary drugs and medicating drugs in most classes of *materia medica*; purges, diuretics, diaphoretics, and so on.

---

41 Ibid., p. 482. Severinus classified drugs as alimentary, medicinal, and toxic in chapter fifteen of the *Idea medicinæ*.

42 Ibid.: "Horum usus in morbis gravissimis necessarius est, & talia sine præparatione chemica nullo pacto adhiberi debent, nec enim periti solum artificis manu, sed eruditi chemici ratiocinatione multum indigent."

However, the most powerful of the sleep-inducing drugs (*somnifera*) and anodynes are chemically prepared medicines, chiefly antimonials and mercurials. These are needed in illnesses that are characterized by sleeplessness and pain and against diseases with fixed roots, which do not respond to alimentary drugs. Their use is advocated by necessity and requires chemical compounding and preparation. Specifics of this sort were discovered through experiments or were found to be in use among peasants, who did not have the benefit of instruction in Galenic theory! Indeed, most of the useful drugs mentioned by Galen were taken from the empirics in the first place.[43]

Davidson claims that Galenic humoral medicine merely confused drug theory. For example, medicines that are strengthening (the class *corrobantia*) are sometimes referred to as heating drugs, and they heat and moisten the body by arousing the body's natural balsam. But, it is not the heat and moisture that are the causes and principles of the drugs! The drugs' actions are grounded in the hypostatic principles, for example in their salt and sulphur. Sulphurs come in various kinds with various faculties: attracting, repelling, narcotic, sleep-inducing, anodyne, and so on. Similarly, there are diaphoretic mercury salts that are confortative, mitigating, regenerating, etc. Again, since the actions of these drugs depend on their chemistry, the true physician must have chemical knowledge.

To this end, Davidson exhorts those who have scorned and reviled chemistry to return to the true path. They should embrace the distinctions among natural causes that are advocated by Severinus, apply a pious diligence to chemical preparations, and be grateful that they have such powerful drugs at their disposal. One should study chemical medicine from "select and approved authors," such as Severinus, but not rely on written speculation: The good chemical physician must also learn from his practice. He will use his knowledge of the properties of drugs to prepare remedies that can reach specific illnesses in specific parts of the body; on the basis of his experience, he will assign specific drugs to specific illnesses, from head to toe. One must learn to prepare those drugs oneself and not rely on experts, even if they are friends. The physician must learn to study all things himself, preferably cultivating

---

43 Ibid., pp. 483-84.

this habit from youth, and not put too much faith in books. And when trying out a new medicine, or one that is at any rate new to you, keep the dosage low, below the recommended level, if there is one, until you learn the proper amount for that particular drug and that particular patient. This is the easy way to avoid errors.[44] Thus, Davidson's chemical medicine was in practice much like traditional medicine, insofar as one had to tailor the particular drug to the particular case. But, with chemical drugs, dosage was very important. This was only established by experience and with the help of a fundamental knowledge of the chemical processes that govern change.

GALENISM VS. CHEMICAL MEDICINE
IN THE TREATMENT OF FEVERS

The second part of the body of Davidson's 1660 commentary is devoted to an application of the general doctrine that is presented in the first part to the specific example of fevers. Fevers were of particular importance to early modern medicine because many of the epidemic diseases with high morbidity were classified as fevers and because fevers were not adequately explained by traditional humoral pathology. They often produced violent paroxysms and chills in patients who were manifestly hot. Usually they were characterized by periodic recurrences, which led to their classification as tertian, quartan, quotidian, and so on. Furthermore, the most notorious fevers were obviously epidemic, and this is a property that was not well explained by traditional Greco-Roman medicine, which viewed disease as fundamentally an idiopathic phenomenon that is defined by the individual's temperament, behavior, personal experience, and humoral balance. The search for causes that could explain the cyclical recurrence of infectious fevers led to theories that identified miasmas, contagion, meteorological phenomena, and astrological influences as causes – factors that were common to entire populations that were similarly afflicted within a short period of time.

---

44 Ibid., pp. 485-86.

Still, prior to the development of statistical epidemiology and the germ theory in the nineteenth century, none of these theories was wholly satisfactory. To be a credible alternative to Galenism, chemical medicine needed both to treat fevers more effectively than did traditional therapy and to support this treatment with a coherent chemical pathology, which of course was Severinus' aim. This section of Davidson's *Prodromus* is consequently of great importance to understanding the value he ascribed to chemical medicine and why he believed it to be superior to the Galenic method.

Davidson opens his discussion of fevers by blaming Western medicine for its failure to cope with this "ferocious enemy," which afflicts man more than do other diseases. Myriads of clever books about the essence and treatment of fevers have been written, but with no fruitful result. It is a disgrace to learned medicine that those who escape the hands of physicians, for example the peasants of eastern Europe and some southern peoples, are believed to fare better than do many of the Europeans who are treated by physicians. For these latter, the cure is often worse than the disease.[45]

The reason for the failure of Galenic medicine to treat fevers is clear to Davidson: The whole theory of curative indications is built on false physical foundations, such as matter and form, the primary qualities, and the humors. With all the purgations available to the Galenist, none succeeds in reducing a tertian or quartan fever very much. Indeed, a bad purge does not sufficiently dislodge the morbific matter or *fomes* and has the added liability of further weakening the patient. In over forty years of practice, Davidson has seen physicians who seem very diligent pursue erroneous therapy, and perhaps he has even done so himself. But the fault does not lie with the weaknesses of individual practitioners; where the art is unhealthy and based on the dead letter of written scholarship, there is little hope for a favorable outcome. Moreover, long traditions are not easily changed. Davidson writes that he agrees with Severinus in that the most effective way to reform medicine is to correct errors gradually and to provoke the diligence of physicians rather than attempt to demolish the general laws of healing all at once. By secretly

45 Ibid., p. 486.

(quietly) investigating nature and the properties of those things from which vitality proceeds, the physician will sooner fulfill his duties with greater gratitude.[46]

Next Davidson sets out to define what a fever is. Like Severinus, he would have its name spring from the root idea, from the essence of the thing itself and its internal faculties, rather than "from the common, external, dead, momentary, and relollacean ones."[47] Thus, diseases ought not be defined in terms of hot and cold, but rather in terms of the *causes* of heat and cold, namely impure, foetid, and resolved nitrosulphurous impurities, which are impregnated with a primeval heat or fire. Likewise, "cold" diseases arise from mucilages and the fluid spirits of nitrous salts. The roots of such diseases might be found in the anatomy of the stomach or some other organ, that is, in the dispensation of the functions or duties of that organ, but the fruits of such diseases are the supervening febrile symptoms. When a nitrosulphurous *minera* germinates, it initially sends forth "superficial flowers" and induces coldness, yawning, stretching, shivering, stiffness, and so on. These occur at set times.

Davidson says that Severinus defined fever according to its development from morbific *semina*. It can be said to have a *real* cause, because it arises from a morbific impurity, say a nitrosulphurous mucilage or tartar, which is the "genus" of the disease. The presence of this impurity results from a failed separation and expulsion, which can then be regarded as the disease's "subalternate genus." The morbific matter may block passageways or otherwise damage the body's normal function, which is then the individual "species" of the disease. But a disease can also be defined *nominally*, in which case the damaged or impaired function becomes the genus, the obstruction or blockage the species, and the morbific impurity that is lodged in the organ becomes the individual. Either way, the fever is defined as a nitrosulphurous disease that is aroused by the active faculties of the "seminary reasons" of salt and sulphur, which are exalted, separated, concocted, and inflamed in the heart and then reduced to

---

46 Ibid., p. 487.

47 Ibid., pp. 488-89: "A radicibus ipsis nomina, & definitiones morborum derivari debere ab essentia rei, ab internis facultatibus, non a vulgaribus, externis, mortuis, momentaneis aut relolaceis, ut sunt qualitates primæ & similes signaturæ quæ externas non internas facultates manifestant."

act by a mercurial spirit. This gives rise to dangerous symptoms such as "restlessness, chills, stiffness, and like signatures."[48]

Different sorts of impurities, seated in different parts of the body, produce different effects. Some are inflamed and others are not; some are acute, like the arsenical, plague-causing sort, while others are chronic. Some are sulphurous and therefore inflammable, but others are aluminous or vitriolic, and so on. Therefore, the physician who sees fever as caused by heat, and therefore attempts to counter it with cold, will not succeed. This is because the hotness is only the accident, whereas it is the *subject* of the heat, namely the morbific matter, that must be removed. And indeed, this kind of fever should be called nitrosulphurous, since a thing ought to be named according to the nature of its substance, just as stinging nettle (*urtica*) is so named because it causes a burn (*urit*), even though it is actually a salt in the nettle that causes this effect.[49]

Next Davidson takes up the timing and cyclical nature of fevers, explaining them according to Severinus' theory. Clearly diseases have cycles that include periods of inactivity and crises. Those caused by *semina* in foodstuffs quickly obey regular laws of change, although their "digestion" time, which determines when they appear, will vary according to the kind of disease and where the pathogens are lodged: "For those seeds of diseases that are introduced into the anatomy of the stomach are more quickly fermented and moved forward to effervescence than those that are received in the elements of the liver, kidneys, synovia, blood, and similar parts." Also, a febrile seed will germinate more quickly than colic tinctures in the intestine or stomach, and the roots of a tertian fever will be loosened by digestion more readily than those of a quartan. Ephemeral (acute) fevers rise faster after fermentation than do hectic (fiery) fevers.[50]

---

48 Ibid., p. 491. Severinus also presented the distinction between real and nominal definitions of disease, which was also discussed by Ambrosius Rhodius in his commentary (see chapter nine). Even though Severinus' ontology aimed to render such scholastic distinctions irrelevant, the discussion of the proper genus, species, and individual of a disease implies that the authors sought to explain this theory in terms that would be familiar to the university-educated reader.

49 Ibid., pp. 491-92.

50 Ibid., p. 508: "Citius enim fermentantur & ad effervescentias promoventur, quæ in ventriculi anatomia inseruntur morborum semina, quam quæ in hepatis, renum, synoviæ, sanguinis, & similium partium Elementis recipiuntur."

Although Davidson does not belabor the point here, he notes that the periodicities of fevers are characteristic of the diseases, rather than the disease being characteristic of the patient. This illuminates an important distinction between how the Paracelsians and the Galenists viewed the essence of disease: "The cycles of quartans, tertians, and quotidians remain regular and constant" despite variations in the regions, ages, sexes, foods, and habits of the patients.[51] Therefore, the diseases themselves must have some identity distinguishable from the individual temperament of the patient, an observation that would support an "ontological" concept of disease as an entity. Following Severinus, Davidson identifies the causes of fevers as "febrile seeds and impurities and sulphurous nitrates," which are abundant in wine, bread, beans, meats, fish, oils, fruits – all foods.[52]

Fevers can be said to reside in the body as a whole, and yet there are particular places in which they are generated or lie dormant for long periods. Ephemeral fevers are seated in the body's spirits, putrid fevers in its fluids, and hectic fevers in its disposition (*habitus*). But they can reside elsewhere, and undergo coction in other elements, wombs, and fields, such as in the veins and arteries. Conversely, fevers can arise wherever "coctions" can occur in the body and wherever there are suitable *matrices* (wombs) and elements that are endowed with the properties of febrile *semina*. Of course, the prerequisite seminal reasons for the fever must also be present. All fevers, whether continuous, tertian, quartan, quotidian, spurious, erratic, or hectic, can have seats and *fomites* in the various organs – the stomach, intestines, spleen, liver, kidneys, and mesentery. Therefore, recognizing where the fever is based is important to curing it. A fever rooted in the stomach is rather easily expelled by vomiting, but special arcana are needed to treat fevers seated in the spleen and other organs.[53]

When it comes to chemically treating fevers, Davidson follows Severinus' (and Hippocrates') dictum that nature is the true healer,

---

51 Ibid.: "Quia in febribus tempora digestionum & resolutionum manifestissima sunt, … consideratione dignum est, qua ratione regionum, ætatum, sexuum, alimentorum, consuetudinum, neglecto discrimine, quartani, tertiani & quotidiani circuitus maneant perpetui & constantes."
52 Ibid.: "Semina tandem & impuritates febriles sulphureæque nitrositates."
53 Ibid., p. 509.

and that the physician is merely a minister. Accordingly, the physician should take nature as an example and not seek to destroy diseases by inducing contrary qualities. Rather, he should use medicaments that he himself has prepared by separating them from the admixed impurities and concrete elements. Such medicines do not work by heating, cooling, moistening, and drying, nor by cutting through and removing obstructing matter, but by means of nature's vital principle, which is the balsam that gives life to animals, minerals, and vegetables. The use of this principle to remove the radical diseases that sprout from *semina* in the body constitutes healing.

The common *materia medica* that physicians use are not really medicines any more than are wood or stones. Those kinds of treatments are based on the Galenic perception of diseases as imbalances of the humors, which is faulty, because it ascribes diseases to "external qualities." If these remedies seem at times to work, it is not on account of any such qualities, but because they contain an inner balsam. Aristotle mentioned such an internal balsam, but Galen did not use that idea and instead attributed diseases to "the whole substance," by which he meant a certain mixture of the four qualities.[54]

Davidson explains that the Paracelsian idea of curing with similars rather than with contraries is based on the Hippocratic conception of nature as the true healer. Nature does not desire conflict, which is brought about by contrary qualities, but rather peace, which consists of the proper distribution of nourishment: bony material is properly provided to the bones, membranous matter to the membranes, and so on. Therefore, the first indication for healing is to imitate nature by strengthening similars and expelling contraries. Consequently, the physician has a twofold mission, namely 1) to strengthen the body so that it can free itself of disease and 2) to expel the tartarous impurities that have nitrosulphurous qualities.[55]

Dislodging impurities from the body requires that the physician have an exact knowledge of them. And since we are what we eat, these impurities come into us with our foods. Therefore, the physician should

---

54 Ibid., pp. 523-24. This concept of diseases of the whole substance enjoyed a renaissance in the sixteenth-century work of Jean Fernel. See chapter four, note 115 above.

55 Ibid., p. 527.

have as complete a knowledge of the animal, mineral, and vegetable kingdoms as he can, since there are as many kinds of impurities as there are foods. This knowledge he must acquire from reading and from direct examination of nature. And here Davidson quotes Severinus' advice to abandon personal material wealth and to go forth and seek knowledge in the field and at the furnace, a passage that has been quoted many times since.[56]

Precise knowledge of specific impurities, and therefore diseases, enables the physician to find a remedy that is specific to each disease. However, it may be useful to have a drug that generally purges and eradicates tartarous diseases. Such a medication is good for both acute and chronic disease, and can extinguish a fever within three or four hours. Various antimony derivatives are suitable, for example emetic antimony, which is a nitrosulphurous remedy and contains healing mummy within it. There are also others, such as flowers of antimony and an infusion of glass of antimony. Davidson directs the reader to consult his earlier books and the practice of other chemical physicians for recommendations pertaining to specific drugs.

There are febrifuges other that the antimonials, which cure fevers through vomiting and also through separation (*secessum*). These include mineral-based drugs (e.g. vitriol, salt of vitriol, precipitate of silver) and those prepared from plants (e.g. leaves and roots of hazelwort, decoction of hedge hyssop, *gummi gutta*, and decoction of *verbena*). However, twenty years' experience practicing medicine among the English, French, Germans, and Poles has convinced Davidson that these do not compare with the antimonials for easily and quickly eliminating fevers by benignly provoking two or three vomitings. If they fail to achieve a cure in that way, they also work through separation (*secessum*), sweating, urination, and via insensible transpiration – often accompanied by a sense of euphoria.

In cases where, for some reason or other, these drugs are not desirable, the physician can always return to leaves of sena, rhubarb, and tamarind, or use cassia, manna, or various syrups, all of which have nitrosulphurous indications and can be used effectively against mild

56 Ibid., pp. 527-28. See chapter six, note 51 above.

fevers. "But in desperate and raw fevers, you will sooner move the stones of the sea from their place than remove one atom of morbific cause" by means of these less powerful drugs.[57] For these cases, one will need an antimonial febrifuge, such as one of those described in his *Philosophia pyrotechnica*, which can completely eradicate the fever from the body. Yet there is a second kind of treatment for fevers, which does not actually heal the body by rooting out the febrile agent, but rather strengthens the body to make it stronger against the fever. Medications used for this are called mitigating remedies, and include the anodynes, for example anodyne sulphur of vitriol.[58]

Davidson sees the particular method outlined here, namely using chemical purges, as being especially effective because it imitates and assists nature, which is the true healer. If the body's nature is reacting to a disease by causing a sweat, then the physician uses a diaphoretic to assist sweating. If evacuations are called for, he uses the appropriate kind of medicine for the desired elimination. He uses these drugs to hasten the course of the disease to its natural crisis. They are specifics and directed to specific ends, which prompts Davidson to use a military metaphor: the physician is like a king who directs his troops to attack the enemy by the fastest road. When one foe has been destroyed, they can be again gathered to drive against the next.[59]

The key to curing diseases that arise from morbific impurities is the removal of the matter itself by purging. However, Davidson clearly distinguishes the chemical physician's purging from the traditional approach, both in theory and practice, and returns to this topic again to elaborate. First, purging impurities is manifold and complicated, because each proper place or organ in the body has its own preferred means of separation and expulsion, in most cases unseen transpirations. Since the physician succeeds by imitating nature, he should have a similarly

---

57 Ibid., p. 529: "At in desperatis & crudis febribus, citius saxa maris e loco movebis, quam ut vel atomum unam causæ morbificæ abstuleris." Davidson's use of the term "atom of morbific cause" in what is essentially a Paracelsian, idealist philosophy points to Charles Webster's assertion that the line between mechanical corpuscularian philosophy and a theory based on active principles was sometimes blurred in the seventeenth century. See Webster, *From Paracelsus to Newton*, p. 69.

58 Davidson, *Prodromus*, p. 530.

59 Ibid.

nuanced approach to evacuation, rather than merely purging different humors, which "answers very little to the desired effects." For what does one achieve by purging yellow bile in the case of a tertian fever, black bile in a quartan, and phlegm in a quotidian? The result is that the fever is weakened but a little and the patient more, adding to his burden and increasing his susceptibility.[60]

The physician might justify the removal of an excess humor in cases of fever by observing abnormal coloring in evacuated blood or vomit, which presumably reflects a surfeit of one or another humor. However, Davidson argues, these colors are in truth caused by the medicines that the physician has applied. Purged bile may be classified as yellow, golden, coppery, and greenish-colored, but these colors come from the use of drugs like cassia, tamarind, manna, or rhubarb, which create what they evacuate. Such remedies are not without value, though, since they can effectively purge tartarous fluids that have settled in the intestines.[61]

The Galenic theory behind the therapy of purging defines disease as a qualitative imbalance or intemperance in the patient's body, which results from a correlated surfeit of one or more of the four basic humors (blood, yellow bile, black bile, phlegm), which is associated with an imbalance in the four primary qualities, hot, dry, wet, and cold. Such an imbalance can arise from various causes, e.g. improper diet, and is exacerbated by blockages that obstruct the body's natural efforts to redress the humoral imbalance. The chemical physicians do not disagree with this last point, but classify these obstructions differently, and embed them in a different theory. Rather than being caused by the more fundamental problem, that is, the qualitative imbalance – too much heat, for example – they attribute obstructions to the spirits of the salts that come into the body with various foods. This theoretical difference implies a therapeutic difference. Whereas the Galenist will attempt to counter a disease by applying drugs with qualities that are contrary to the disease, for example by using a cold remedy to cure a hot disease,

60 Ibid., p. 531: "Oportet scire purgationes, quas continuo vulgus celebrat, desideratis effectibus minime respondere, veluti si in tertiana bilem millies purgemus, in quartana melancholiam, in quotidiana pituitam, quid efficimus?"
61 Ibid., pp. 531-32.

the iatrochemist will attempt to dissolve the chemical obstruction by means of a similar chemical spirit or solvent.[62]

The chemical physicians' emphasis on identifying the cause of a disease with the peccant matter and the *semina* contained within it also lies at the root of their disdain for Galenic therapy, which, beyond being ineffective, can cause harm. As noted before, incorrect and immoderate purging of humors can severely weaken the patient without affecting the peccant matter at all, thereby fatiguing his natural healing powers and strengthening the disease. Even when the purging of humors does affect the corrupt, morbific matter, harmless fluids are also bled off, and this results in thirst and weakness. Furthermore, the medications used to promote evacuation of a humor can inhibit natural transpiration and thus induce serious symptoms.

The correct method is to purge the fever wholly from the body, preferably by means of a series of medications, for example in three dosings. However, not every fever can be cured by the same method, and Davidson admonishes the physician to recognize the species of tartar (an example of an impurity) that is responsible and apply the particular remedy that is suited to it. Since the nature of the disease depends not only on the impurity, but also on its location, the physician must account for that, too. Once the cause of the disease and its seat have been determined, the proper purge must be chosen, and here, too, the chemical physician differs from the Galenist.

It is the iatrochemists' use of chemically-prepared, often mineral-based drugs that clearly marked them as distinct from the traditional Galenists, and in many cases debate between these opponents centered on the drugs themselves – whether they were too toxic or even effective at all. Opponents also criticized the chemists for their "empirical" approach, that is, using drugs for which there was no proper theoretical foundation in Aristotelian physics, or else for grounding their use in a fantastic Paracelsian doctrine. However, as is clear from treatises like Davidson's commentaries, chemical physicians believed that the remedies they used were not only safe and more effective against diseases than traditional *materia medica*, but also less unpleasant for the patient.

---

62 Ibid., p. 534.

Here, for example, Davidson warns that "not all vomitives are either agreeable or safe for this task, for the white hellebore of Hippocrates and Galen is terrible, as are also all species of *tithimalus, acipon* or terrible herb, *gummi gutta*, hazelwort, and hedge hyssop, which the judicious physician ought not consider for fevers."[63] These drugs, says Davidson, "excel in wickedness" and disrupt the body's function much more than even the difficult antimonial drugs. In contrast, Davidson has used emetic powder, or the flowers of emetic powder (*flores pulveris emetici*), usually accompanied by twenty grains of sweetened mercury (*mercurius dulcificatus*), "with great success and on the recommendation of my patients." This is because normally it causes little vomiting. However, the physician must expect to put in long hours preparing it.[64]

To purge tartar that is lodged in the intestines, via stools, Davidson says that the proper remedy is diaphoretic antimony that has been chemically prepared with crystals of tartar and *diagredium*, as recommended by Oswald Croll. Tartar in the stomach is treated in another way, using one of several specific mercury compounds. To rid the blood of tartarous impurities, one must resort to phlebotomy, which, on the advice of Severinus, is the only remedy that is suitable for use in all fevers. This is especially true for "symptomatic" fevers, which otherwise should be expelled from the body's disposition (*habitus*) or fleshes by means of a diaphoretic. Diaphoretics may be made from plants, spirit of tartar, flowers of sal ammoniac, spirit of cinnabar or antimony, mineral bezoardicum, and similar substances.

This method, namely the application of specific remedies to expel particular kinds of tartar that are lodged in known places in the body, is the "true and legitimate" one according to Davidson. Yet sometimes the species of tartar is unknown, for they are only recognized through

---

63   Ibid., p. 535: "Tamen omnia vomitiva non sunt ad hoc munus nec accepta nec tuta, terribilis enim est Hippocratis & Galeni Helleborus albus, & omnes species Titimallorum, Acipon, sive herba terribilis, gummi gutta, assarum, gratiola, de quibus in febribus non debet vel cogitare prudens Medicus."

64   Ibid., pp. 535-36: "Semper cum Euphoria usus sum pulvere emetico, floribus pulveris emetici, sed soleo exhibere cum viginti granis Mercurij dulcificati, & semper usus sum cum multa laude, & ægrorum meorum recommendatione." One should recall Severinus' letter to Theodor Zwinger (see chapter three), in which he mentions the length of time needed to prepare a chemical medicine.

long experience. In these cases it would be best to have a general cure, of the sort that he described in his *Philosophia pyrotechnica*, to which the reader can turn.[65]

Adumbratio

As if he thought that 538 pages of commentary on the *Idea medicinæ* had failed to reach the core of Severinus' medicine, Davidson appended a 170-page "sketch of the whole work," in which he claims to expand upon the physiological hypotheses and the meaning of the more profound and unusual passages of the *Idea medicinæ*.[66] Using Severinus' theory, Davidson wished to show how individual afflictions of the human body can be treated by means of medicines drawn from animal, vegetable, and mineral sources. Many of these remedies must be chemically prepared.

Like the body of the 1660 commentary, the appended sketch goes over much of the *Idea medicinæ*, chapter by chapter. Although this time specific diseases and drugs are discussed (for example leprosy, fistula, podagra, butter of antimony, and cinnabar of antimony), and sections are devoted to "coction," therapeutics, and observed practice, Davidson persisted in building theoretical structures that are based on seven-fold divisions and geometrical relationships of the sort one encounters in the works of the Rosicrucian authors. This is readily apparent in his association of the seven concrete elements or bodies with the seven seminary elements or incorporeal bodies that were mentioned earlier.[67] These Neoplatonic hierarchies reveal Davidson's vision of the *Idea medicinæ* as but one expression of a thoroughgoing metaphysical system. The *Prodromus* is, in fact, Davidson's articulation of a Renaissance Platonist cosmology that he believed could accommodate Aristotelian and Para-

---

65 Ibid. The *panacea* was a widely sought drug. Recall Severinus' own efforts to refine such a general drug, mentioned in his letters (see chapter three).

66 "Totius operis Adumbratio," ibid., pp. 539-708.

67 See the diagram on ibid., p. 646.

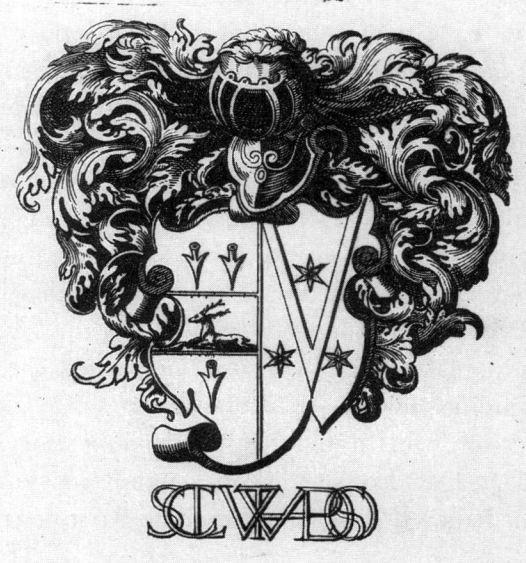

TOTIUS OPERIS
ADUMBRATIO.

In qua Hypotheses Physiologicæ profundiorum & insue-
tarum locutionum sensus, æquivocationum & synoni-
morum denodationes, indicationes diagnosticæ , &
leges curativæ juxta authoris & Hippocratis mentem
expanduntur:

Per quas singuli affectus humani corporis per *Medicamenta è Vegetabilium,*
Animalium, & Mineralium familia desumpta, & pleraque juxta Chemice-
rum modum præparata, legitimum finem sortiuntur.

Operâ & studio illius qui sub sequenti Anagrammate nomen exponit,

sI VIVVs ILLe MVnDo saLVs,

Prævisa valent.

The title page of William Davidson's summary sketch of his 1660 commentary on
Severinus' Idea medicinæ philosophicæ, which comes at the end of the com-
mentary itself. Reproduced by courtesy of the Department of Special Collections,
General Library System, University of Wisconsin-Madison.

celsian philosophy and Galenic and chemical medicine.[68] Perhaps it was this irenic, unifying impulse that first drew him to the *Idea medicinæ*, the title of which promised the foundations of both Galenism and Paracelsianism.

DAVIDSON'S SECOND COMMENTARY

Apparently the *Prodromus* of 1660 did not satisfy Davidson's desire to explicate the doctrine of the *Idea medicinæ*. Despite its length and complexity, the *Prodromus* is still a forerunner or introduction in the sense that it places key Severinian ideas in the context of sixteenth and seventeenth-century philosophy rather than mainly and formally focusing on the elucidation of Severinus' ideas themselves. Davidson's second commentary, the *Commentaria in Idæam medicinæ philosophicæ* (1663), attends to the subject text more closely, unfolding and restating its meanings, and does not as frequently stray into the diagrammatic and emblematic Neoplatonic structures that characterize the 1660 *Prodromus*.[69]

The commentary opens with an admonition to the diligent reader, which explains the purpose of the book and introduces Severinus. Right from the start, Davidson is concerned that readers will be frightened off by the difficulty of reading Severinus' book, because of its length and obscure terminology. But, by reading Davidson's commentary as an introduction, such hindrances can be removed, and the task made sufficiently simpler that the curious reader can learn more in three months than he might otherwise comprehend in ten years' study of many such authors, whose meanings are buried in intricate stories, parables, and analogies.[70] Such texts are worthy of the student's efforts, since by studying them he will "avoid the thousand palliatives, difficulties, and fictions that are found in Aristotle's books on meteorology, the soul, and on generation and corruption." The ideas in those books are entangled in

---

68 Particularly beginning on ibid., p. 674: "De ulteriori Methodo applicandi Doctrinam Severini Dani Aitiologisticam Praxi Galenicæ."

69 Davidson, *Commentaria in Idæam medicinæ philosophicæ Petri Severini Dani, medici incomparabilis & philosophi sublimis.*

70 Ibid., p. 3: "Ad studiosum lectorem Parænesis."

COMMENTARIA

I N

I D Æ A M

MEDICINÆ PHILOSOPHICÆ

PETRI SEVERINI DANI,

Medici incomparabilis &

Philoſophi ſublimis:

Ad faciliorem difficultatum enodationem , quæ in ipſo ,
propter Lectoris in Philoſophia Veterum parum forſan
verſati defectum , apparere videntur , aditum præbentia.

Operâ & ſtudio

WILLIELMI DAVISSONI

Nobilis Scoti; Chriſtianiſſimi Galliarum & Navarræ Regis Conſiliarii & Medici ; domûs hortique
Plantarum Medecinalium, qui Pariſiis in ſuburbio S. Victoris eſt, olim Præfecti : Nunc autem S. Regiæ Majeſtatis Poloniæ & Sueciæ ſenioris Archiatri & Chemici ; S. Reginalis
itidem Majeſtatis Perſonæ Medici.

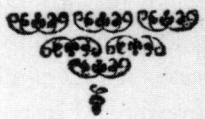

HAGÆ-COMITIS;

Ex Typographia ADRIANI VLACQ.
M. DC. LXIII.

The title page of William Davidson's second commentary on Severinus' Idea medicinæ
philosophicæ, published in 1663. Reproduced by courtesy of the Department of Spe-
cial Collections, General Library System, University of Wisconsin-Madison.

sophistic logic and have blinded the eyes of the peripatetics.[71] Aristotle had great disdain for many of his predecessors and put forth his own doctrines in place of theirs, which he dissuaded his students from reading. But close examination of the writings of the ancients and diligent work with chemical processes have shown how much Aristotle wronged the ancient philosophers. These things cannot be learned at once, or understood from somebody's report of them. But who would deny three months to learn the doctrines of the ancients and the chemists, when it requires two years in the schools of the peripatetics to learn their natural philosophy?[72]

Davidson writes that much of the ancients' knowledge is disguised, woven into their fables and stories, or else it is buried in the lore of the chemists, which may sometimes be corrupted with false observations. But these difficulties ought to be overcome – "only humility and a genuine confession of ignorance will provide easy access for those who would advance in the art."[73]

The method that the ancients used in speaking and teaching, that is, by constructing fables, was both analytical and synthetic. The analytic part reveals divine wisdom, which is knowledge of things that are inaccessible to the senses, through allegories and obscure ways of speaking. This way is very old and works by making analogies and images. It was devised by the ancients – and by the chemists – because men are more easily taught by means of stories. Davidson documents examples of these at length: the fables about Porus and Penia in Plato's *Symposium*, about Prometheus in *Gorgias*, about the Fates in book ten of the *Republic*, and so on. Plato, Proclus, the Pythagoreans, and others cloaked their philosophies in such stories about the gods, their nectar and ambrosia, etc., all of which needs interpretation. Nectar, for example, corresponds to a kind of boundlessness (*infinitas*). It is a moisture, a supplement to the natural boundlessness, fertility, and never failing abundance in things. Ambrosia, on the other hand, is a kind of boundary. It is constant

---

71 Ibid.: "Mille palliationes, difficultates, commenta, quæ in libris Aristotelis *acroaseos*, meteororum, de anima, de generatione & corruptione reperiuntur, Sophisticis Logicæ circuitibus intricata evitabunt."

72 Ibid.

73 Ibid., p. 4: "Sola humilitas, & ingenua ignorantiæ confessio aditum facilem progressuris in arte præbebit."

perfection, solid, a supplement to the steadfast intelligence in things.[74] Fables about such things contain a wisdom that is accessible to those who possess the keys to their meaning, that is, those who "possess some tincture of the holy literature," by which these meanings are altered. These meanings are accessible because all things below contain a spark of divine wisdom, which they have retained.[75]

Davidson further elaborated these ideas in the preface, drawing out his schema of radical elements, seminary elements, and concrete elements from the cast of divine characters and their associated guardians (*tutelares*). He also related the legends of heroes and semi-divines to the development of natural philosophy, implying an overlap between pagan stories and Biblical stories: A large number of gods arose because some men, who were perceived to be wiser and more clever at the arts and sciences, were thought to have descended from heaven, as one reads about St. Paul and Barnabas in the *Acts of the Apostles*, or else they were supposed to have shared a kind of divine spark while they were alive and were then assumed to have become gods after they died. Eventually the idea of men becoming gods or going to the gods was generalized to becoming or going to one God.[76]

Davidson anchored the seven-fold groupings of philosophical elements, which characterize his work, in the early mythological and scriptural sources. Orpheus had put seven souls in control of the seven spheres, and placed Bacchus and a muse in charge of these souls. Each soul was given two powers: a formal and masculine one for understanding, doing, unfolding, and animating, which was represented by Bacchus, and a material, feminine, and passive one, which was represented by a muse. "And what else do these stories seem to insinuate than, as was said, that those divine and manifold powers at first lay hidden in infinite space, in the potency of the first cause, namely Jove, that is, the first uncreated being, and in the exemplars of the thing to be made."[77] Here

---

74 Ibid., pp. 4-5.
75 Ibid., p. 6: "qui sacrarum literarum tincturam aliquam habebant."
76 Ibid., p. 8.
77 Ibid.: "Quæ fabula quid aliud insinuare videtur, quam quasi diceretur istas facultates Divinas & multifarias primo in potentia primæ causæ, nempe Jovis, hoc est primi entis increati, & exemplaribus rerum faciendarum in spatio infinito latuisse."

Davidson expounded a basic Christian Platonist cosmogony – that God created the world from himself by sowing seminal reasons or exemplars into the void.

In addition to the seven spheres mentioned by Orpheus, there are many sevens in the ancient and sacred literature: seven metals, seven atmospheric phenomena (meteors), seven steps to the entrance of God's house (*Ezechiel* 40: 22), seven days of creation, seven flavors, seven precious stones, and so on. The house of wisdom was erected on seven pillars, as mentioned in *Proverbs* 9: 1, so it comes as no surprise that Davidson arranged his seminary, concrete, and radical elements in groups of seven, since "this number seemed to be chosen by the holy spirit" and is also customary among men. Besides the number seven, the number three and of course unity are important.[78]

Much of Davidson's preface is devoted to developing these sevenfold and three-fold correlations, which were commonplace in Hermetic philosophy at that time. For example, he associates three kinds of fire (burning, vivifying, and loving) with the three regions of the world (elemental, celestial, and supercelestial) and assigns each of the seven metals to a planet and a major organ. All of these classes and harmonies come together in man, who is for that reason called the microcosm. Like Robert Fludd and other authors that we might term Hermetic or Rosicrucian, Davidson held that the microcosm participated in the intelligible, supercelestial world by means of the spirits in his brain; The spirits perpetually moving the heart and the blood were linked to the constant virtues of the stars; Man's participation in the world of generation and corruption were at once evident in the parts of his body lying below the diaphragm. His body is elemental, his spirit is celestial, and his intellect is from God.[79]

Davidson claimed to have digressed on the ancients' "synthetic" way of conveying wisdom in stories because he believed that the chemists' methods of teaching were similar to those used in antiquity and also like those used by the Platonists – but opposed to those handed down among the Aristotelians.[80] The chemists also believed that seven metals

78 Ibid., p. 9: "Numerus hic electus a spiritu sancto videbatur."
79 Ibid., pp. 9-10.
80 Ibid., p. 10.

were linked to the seven planetary spheres and had formal and material virtues (nectar and ambrosia), which acted in man. Since man eats animals and vegetables, which are themselves nourished by vegetables and minerals, he has within him metallic and vegetable spirits that ordinary medical physiology (*Physiologia Medicina vulgaris*) does not take into consideration, but instead refers them to "a thousand varieties of bile and phlegm that are impossible to distinguish in man, which our author [Severinus] more aptly, easily, and correctly assigns to varieties of minerals, metals, and vegetables."[81] Therefore the reader ought to study chemistry in order to learn how the human body is formed and how it is destroyed. Furthermore, he should always have at his fingertips the *Idea medicinæ*, which contains "the true theories of Hippocrates and ancient medicine."[82]

The body of Davidson's second commentary is a chapter by chapter explication of short sentences or phrases from the *Idea medicinæ*, each followed by a comment expanding on its significance. Brief descriptions of his treatment of chapters five and eight will amply illustrate his method. The analysis of chapter five begins thus:

> *Elements are places, wombs, & dwellings.* This is the summary [Anacephaleosis] of the fifth chapter, containing his chief conclusions, the first text of which is: *The doctrine of the elements is entangled in confusion, error, and a great diversity of opinions.*[83]

In this instance, Davidson chose not to further comment on the *anacephalæosis*, but proceeded directly to the first phrase to be glossed. This *textus primus* comprises the opening words of chapter five of the *Idea medicinæ* and it occasions a six-page commentary. Next a *textus secundus* is introduced, followed by a commentary on it, and so on. The com-

---

81　Ibid., p. 11: "Sed referuntur ad mille species bilis & pituitæ hominibus distinctu impossibiles, quas Author noster ad mineralium, metallorum, & vegetabilium species aptius, facilius, & verius deducit."

82　Ibid., p. 11: "Oportet ergo de necessitate Chemiam colere, ut ab ea dignoscantur omnes potentiæ ... oportet etiam Authorem hunc in quo vera Hippocratis & antiquæ Medicinæ theoremata continentur, jugiter præ manibus habere."

83　Ibid., p. 53: "Caput V. *Elementa sunt loca, matrices, & domicilia.* Hæc est Anacephalæosis quinti Capitis, præcipuas ejus conclusiones continens, cujus Textus Primus est: *Tanta opinionum varietate, confusionibus, & erroribus implicata est doctrina elementorum.*"

mentary to the third text (*Esseque in natura*) of chapter five is short and exemplifies Davidson's reading:

> Here Sennert accuses Severinus of increasing the number of the elements when he said that in nature there is an earthy fire, earthy air, earthy water, and then again a celestial earth; likewise a fiery earth, aerial water, and finally an aerial fire and an earthly water. Meanwhile, he does not think that Severinus used the great Hippocrates as his source. For he attested in his book on affects that all kinds of faculties lie hidden in earth, that is, bitter, salty, bland, just as they do in bile and phlegm. Therefore, if there are in earth so many different faculties, terrestrial rivals of fire, air, and water, either they do not judge earth to be a true simple element, or they would show me elementary earth without using the art of the chemists. Otherwise, all the most absurd things are imposed on Hippocrates. Consequently, from this argument they should conclude that the number of the elements is multiplied excessively.[84]

In this example Davidson merely incorporated and sustained Sennert's criticism of Severinus without further comment.

Davidson's analysis of chapter eight provides another illustration of his methodical approach to reading the *Idea medicinæ*. Again, the commentary begins with a reprise of the opening line of the *anacephalæosis* of the chapter, in this case presenting the key to Severinus' doctrine, namely that "generation is the development of *semina*."[85] The gloss on this phrase explains briefly what Severinus meant by generation and the role he assigned to the *semina* and their knowledge or skill in the

---

84 Ibid., p. 62: "Accusat hic Severinum Sennertus, quod numerum elementorum augeat, dum ait esse in natura ignem terrestrem, aerem terrestrem, aquam terrestrem, & rursum terram coelestem: similiter terram igneam, aeriam aquam, & postremo ignem aerium, aquam terream: non cogitat interea Severinum habere divinum Hippocratem pro Authore. Is enim in libro de affectibus testatur omnigenas Facultates in terra latere, hoc est, amarum, salsum, & insipidum, sicut in bile & pituita. Si igitur in terra sint tot facultates diversæ, ignis, aeris, & aquæ, terrestris æmulæ, aut terram pro vero elemento simplici non estimant, aut absque Chemicorum arte terram elementarem mihi monstrent, alioquin absurdissima quæque Hippocrati imponentur: Proinde ex hoc argumento elementorum numerum multiplicari pessime concludent."

85 Ibid., p. 150: "Itaque generationem esse progressionem seminum."

mechanical process of bringing forth the rudiments of bodies. Davidson notes that Severinus employed the term "mechanical" to draw an analogy between the seminal inner agent (*archeus*) and the expert craftsman and that he also used the term *"lithurgia"* as "a metaphor taken from the mechanical arts."[86] Davidson's choice to spell this word with an "h" and to explain it as drawn from the crafts tradition contrasts with his earlier interpretation, in the 1660 commentary (see above), of *liturgia* as an administrative process, and this may have led Walter Pagel to trace the term to lith-urgy or stone cutting.[87] However, there is an important distinction between the craftsman and the *archeus*, namely that the latter shapes matter from within according to the seminal archetype, rather than from without. Davidson describes this as an orderly mechanical process, much as Severinus had, but now calls it "scientific," no doubt reflecting Severinus' use of the term *scientia* to refer to the seminal plan that is used by the *archeus* to carry out the seminal predestination.[88]

Davidson places Severinus' use of the *archeus* or inner craftsman to explain seminal development in a Scriptural context by drawing an analogy between the divinely inspired seed and the craftsman Bezeleel, whom God infused with the divine spirit and instructed to construct the tabernacle. Likewise, the "seminary spirits" were instructed by God the Creator after he brought them forth from the boundless abyss of potential by means of the word *fiat*. They received their orders much as had Bezeleel. By means of the *semina*, God bound an incorporeal nature to bodies and insured their continuity and reproduction according to the divine exemplar. Further, Davidson likens the progression of *semina* from potency to developed body and back to potency again to the wanderings of travelers: having completed their assigned functions they begin to wonder at their foreign lodgings and contemplate returning to their origin (cause), "as if to their ancestral fatherland," so that they might learn the reason for their departure and receive new orders for a new mission.[89] Davidson was long resident in France, and at the

---

86 Ibid. "Metaphora ab artificibus Mechanicis desumpta."
87 Severinus spelled it *lithurgia*. See the discussion of this in chapter four.
88 Ibid., p. 151: "Ordinata corporum explicatione Mechanico & scientifico processu."
89 Ibid.: "donec absolutis officiis, & fructibus quasi expositis, mirari incipiant tam peregrina diversoria, … tandem progressum terminant ad causam quasi avitam patriam."

time this commentary was published he was living in Poland. Was he already contemplating a return to his native Scotland?

Following this explication of the *anacephalæosis*, which amounts to a survey of the fundamentals of *semina* theory, Davidson glosses thirty texts from chapter eight of the *Idea medicinæ*, each introduced by the beginning words of a sentence extracted from that chapter.[90] These texts are italicized quotations and serve as rubrics, signaling an important subject. Several of these glosses are quite short, clarifying one concept. For example, the eighth text, *Quod si catenam auream Homeri*, gives Davidson an opportunity to point out the agreement between Severinus' philosophy and ancient wisdom. In this case, Severinus called the connection between the visible, corporeal part of the world and the invisible, incorporeal realm the golden chain of Homer, imparting to it an ancient lineage. The idea of a chain of being underlies all Hermetic and Neoplatonic philosophy, namely what is weaker is supported and nourished by what is stronger, the inferior by the superior, the lower by the higher, and so on. This assertion of the logical priority of the cause to the effect is basic to Severinus' theory, and he affirmed it many times in the *Idea medicinæ*.

Davidson's commentary on the seventh text is longer and touches on the heart of Severinus' theory: *Semen itaque est vitale principium* (Therefore the seed is the vital principle). However, the result is more rhetorical than illuminating. First, Davidson claims that Severinus defined three ways of acquiring knowledge, namely by 1) defining something that is essential, 2) deducing effects from causes, and 3) demonstrating properties that are essential to something. Then Davidson introduces the idea that *semina* have contents, which establish bodies that are suitable to generate and preserve them, and that these *semina* are the roots, matter, and foundations of these bodies. Which of the three kinds of knowledge acquisition this statement represents is not explained – indeed, Davidson praises Severinus for ignoring "the precepts of dialectical definitions" in defining *semina*.[91]

---

90 The thirty extracted sentence fragments represent most of the twenty seven pages occupied by chapter eight in the 1660 edition of the *Idea medicinæ*. With only one exception, they are the first words of a sentence.

91 Ibid., p. 155.

The subject of dialectical reasoning leads Davidson further away from the text at hand, and he finishes with a diatribe against "those who wish to measure physical truth by logical subtleties," namely the Aristotelian philosophers. Many of these seem to prefer to "destroy truth" (ignore physical reality) "rather than put aside the syllogistic and counterfeit praise of the shaded truth."[92] People of this sort create irreconcilable quarrels and controversies in theology as well as in medicine and physics. Such a physician would prefer to cover a wound prematurely rather than suffer his "syllogistic faith" to be humiliated. For this reason, namely that the Aristotelian sophist raises dialectic above what the senses reveal about reality, Davidson considers Aristotle to be "the most dangerous enemy of the Christian faith." There is no easier path to the destruction of religion and learning, he writes, than the careful cultivation of Aristotle's logic by less acute minds.[93]

Davidson's handling of this text shows that he aims not just to explain Severinus' meaning in this commentary, but also to defend chemical medicine and attack its detractors. Although these critics generally remain anonymous in his text, he does make specific references occasionally. In his commentary on text twenty six (*Restant mineralium generationes*), for example, Davidson summarizes Severinus' claim for the seminal origins and life of minerals, as also for animals and vegetables, and then defends the idea against criticism by Daniel Sennert: Minerals, too, are recipients of the eternal cause, which "is the divine force and power that is diffused throughout the lower world – what the ancients called the spirit or soul of the world."[94] The ancient philosophers and the Platonists incorporated the world soul into their cosmologies. Even Aristotle did not deny it. The church fathers confirmed it, and holy scripture demonstrates it to us. The Creator introduced this world soul or spirit into the *semina* by his divine benediction, so that they might

92 Ibid.: "Qui ab argutiis Logicis veritatem Physicam metiri volunt, & ut cum moerore dicam multi malunt ipsam amicam veritatem perdere, quam Syllogisticam & fucatam veritatis umbratilis laudem deponere."

93 Ibid.: "Nulla alia minus salebrosa via relicta fuit Aristoteli fidei Christianæ infensissimo hosti, qua religionem, & rem literariam susque deque destrueret, quam ut Logicam suam ingeniis minus perspicacibus excolendam insinuaret."

94 Ibid., p. 170: "Æterna autem ista causa est vis & potentia Divina diffusa per inferiora, quam veteres spiritum mundi aut animam nominabant."

"imitate eternity" and be aware of the first cause by their development and preservation. Davidson stops short of pantheism in this account by excepting the human rational soul from the initial ensouling of the world. In this matter, he contends, he refuses to hold an opinion that differs from what the Christian church teaches. Thus, Davidson, like Rhodius, shows sensitivity to the vulnerability of Severinus' theory to attacks on its consequences for religion.

In part, Davidson's recapitulation of the compatibility of Severinus' theory with accepted interpretations of *Genesis* is directed at the critics of the *Idea medicinæ*. Here he singles out "the very learned Sennert," who disagreed with Severinus' ascription of the divine spirit to the seminal abysses and faculties. Sennert also criticized Severinus for "multiplying new entities" and, more generally, accused the chemists of novelty. But, Davidson points out, these are ancient doctrines and only appear to be novelties because Severinus used new names to demonstrate ancient concepts that were subsequently blotted out of philosophy by the stupidity of scholars. Just because one cannot see *semina*, does not mean that they do not exist. If anyone were to ask Severinus when he had actually seen *semina* developing from those abysses and blessed retreats, he would have responded by saying that we have corporeal eyes so that we might see corporeal matter, but must see the invisible with the eyes of our mind. As regards the ascription of a soul, and therefore life, to minerals, nobody who had reflected on the composition of the minerals or on the ordered arrangement of their veins would doubt that they have life and partake of its phenomena, including periods of development and maturity. Moreover, if they are living, then they are also liable to diseases and death. Thus, minerals also have *semina* lying hidden in their abysses, which at the appointed times join with spirits and construct mineral bodies.

The final example from Davidson's commentary on chapter eight that will be examined here is the gloss on *Unumquodque Elementum*, which refers to the unity of various regions of the cosmos. This unity is accomplished by the vital principle of generation, which is found in the *semina* and *astra* of all regions and imposes a stability on forms. Although *astra* are only visible in the heavens, they were placed in all the concrete elements by the Creator. Davidson claims that this text and other passages taken from the *Idea medicinæ* formed the basis upon which Michael Sendivogius built his theory in *Novum lumen chymicum*. This is interesting to us because it establishes an intellectual connection between Severinus and Sendivogius, whose book was very influential among late seventeenth-century natural philosophers, including Isaac Newton.[95]

✤

This brief characterization of William Davidson's commentaries on Severinus' *Idea medicinæ* cannot claim to have much more than scratched the surface of what is contained in these lengthy books, a fuller appreciation of which must await a monographic study devoted to Davidson and his work. Nevertheless, the portions that I chose to present here demonstrate his approach, his method of organizing his commentaries, and his close reading of the *Idea medicinæ*. Judging by these texts and also by his earlier *Philosophia pyrotechnica*, I conclude that Davidson grappled with the theory presented in Severinus' book for much of his adult life. Certainly the main ideas presented by Severinus run through Davidson's work. Furthermore, by examining the introductions to these commentaries, it is possible to learn why Davidson spent so many hours of his life on the *Idea medicinæ* and on the medicine to which it pertained.

First, Davidson clearly believed that traditional, Galenic medicine was insufficient for the diseases of the time, which required chemically-prepared drugs. But a wholly empirical drug therapy alone was not satisfactory for a learned physician, a problem that many physicians no doubt encountered when trying to justify the use of empirical remedies. In the *Idea medicinæ* Davidson found a theoretical basis for chemical therapy that also made sense in light of what the ancient philosophers had written. To integrate Severinus' theory more fully into the Platonic schemes of the late sixteenth and seventeenth centuries, Davidson elaborated a logical framework that accommodated Severinus' *semina* and *astra* to a larger Neoplatonic hierarchy. In this sense, Davidson's explanation of Severinus' ideas is even more esoteric than the material

---

95 Ibid., p. 172. Richard S. Westfall, *Never at Rest: A Biography of Isaac Newton* (Cambridge, Cambridge University Press, 1980), p. 291 notes Newton's use of Sendivogius' *Novum lumen chymicum, e natura fonte et manuali experienta depromptum* (Cologne, 1614).

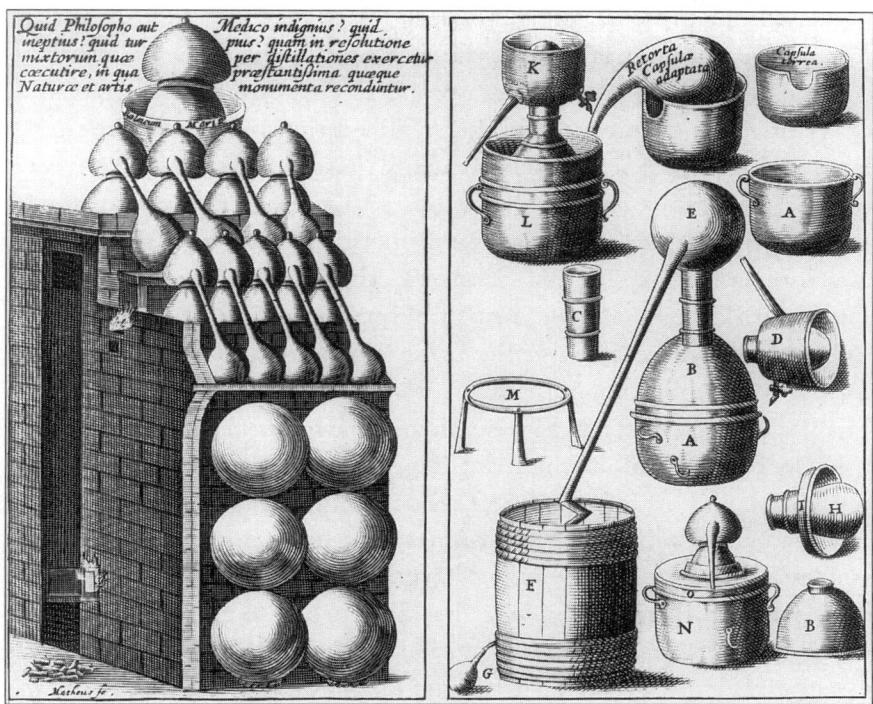

Illustration of apparatus for iatrochemical preparations from William Davidson's Philosophia pyrotechnica. *Reproduced by courtesy of the Department of Special Collections, General Library System, University of Wisconsin-Madison.*

presented in the *Idea medicinæ* itself. However, Davidson also showed how the general principles that Severinus laid out could be applied to particular diseases, namely fevers. He recognized this class of diseases and the ways of curing them as decisive evidence for the superiority of Paracelsian medicine over traditional methods. This is of particular importance, inasmuch as Paracelsian medicine has often in the past been seen as composed of chemical drug therapy and an overlying chemical philosophy, which was easily stripped off by those who sought to use the drugs in an otherwise Galenic practice. Davidson's example proves that early modern physicians believed that the theory itself had value in explaining and directing therapy in ways that traditional methods of curing did not. The use of chemically-prepared drugs was only one aspect of Paracelsian medical practice.

Davidson's presentation and explication of the chief doctrines of the *Idea medicinæ* is quite faithful to the source, although many of Severinus' concepts are restated and further explained. He admired Severinus' style of writing and deep erudition, but realized that this made the theory inaccessible to most students, particularly those indoctrinated in the ways of Aristotle. However, Davidson did not merely paraphrase or repeat Severinus, nor did he always accept uncritically what he had written, as his repetition of some of Sennert's criticisms shows. Furthermore, Davidson's varied understanding of Severinus' use of the term *lithurgia* indicates that his analysis of the Dane's theory had not reached a final form by the publication of the first commentary, but continued to evolve. His frequent use of terms like "seminary" (*seminarius*), which Fracastoro used much more often than did Severinus, who preferred "seminal" (*seminalis*), and his references to Fracastoro and other sixteenth-century physicians and philosophers indicates that he was constantly making connections between the work of Severinus and a larger body of theory. This larger picture, along with his digressions to provide analogies, explains his diagrams and his citation of poetry and reveals what was essentially a more synthetic use of the *Idea medicinæ* than what Ambrosius Rhodius had done in his commentary. Where Rhodius was eager to explain what Severinus had meant and defend it against his critics, Davidson used Severinus' theories to build a grand metaphysical edifice. Neither treatment seems to have elicited much comment from posterity, although Davidson's reputation as a didactic chemical author and royal physician probably ensured that his books would be sought out more readily than the obscure German expatriate, Rhodius, whom history has hitherto remembered mainly for his fateful marriage to Anna Frederiksdatter Severinus.[96]

---

96 Prior to my own work on Rhodius, the longest published study to consider Anna and Ambrosius Rhodius – and the only extensive one – was E. Ingerslev's *Ambrosius Rhodius og Hans Hustru* (Ambrosius Rhodius and His Wife), which focuses primarily on Anna's legal struggles with the Norwegian and Danish authorities and the resulting imprisonment of the couple. Ambrosius Rhodius' interest in Paracelsian theory was incidental to that study.

Conclusion

PETRUS SEVERINUS
AND THE HISTORY OF IDEAS

THE INTELLECTUAL tradition that is connected with the name
Paracelsus has a well established place in the history of medicine,
both as a reaction to medieval scholastic medicine and as an enticing
foreshadowing of the importance that chemistry would come to play in
modern therapeutics. Roughly contemporary with Nicolaus Copernicus
and Andreas Vesalius, who have been credited with initiating an inquiry
that resulted in the permanent abandonment of medieval Aristotelianism, Paracelsus is also held up as an example of a new attitude toward
natural philosophy – one that revolutionized the way science was done
over the next two hundred years. Yet many scholars have pointed to his
barbarisms, the medieval character of his thought, and the decidedly
religious context of his vision of medicine and, indeed, the whole world.
It is this dual nature of Paracelsus and the importance of his work that
stymies his easy placement in a grand narrative of European intellectual
development and both frustrates and intrigues students of the history
of science and medicine.

While it is becoming generally recognized that there was no abrupt
discontinuity in the development of natural philosophy that would
warrant the use of the term "revolution" in the sense that political historians use the term, the idea that there was an important reorientation
of world-view in early modern Europe is still accepted, and it is fair
enough to retain the term "scientific revolution" for this process, if one
bears in mind that there was no sudden, univocal, or necessarily progressive change in the content of knowledge and how that knowledge was
constructed. Revolution in this qualified sense can denote a profound

metamorphosis, even if the rate and direction of this transformation is not clearly defined. Even given this revised framework for understanding the emergence of early modern science, the location of Paracelsian philosophy within the long-term changes in scientific thinking that constitute the scientific revolution continues to defy consensus. In part this has resulted from the traditional emphasis by historians of early modern science on revolutionary developments in the exact sciences, the application of mathematics and quantification to theory, and the containment of speculation by means of a scientific method that stressed experiment and physical demonstration. Paracelsus does not comfortably sit in any of these categories, and neither do many of those who followed him.

The scientific revolution, construed as a fairly clear shift from one set of models and modes of inquiry to another, has had its center on well-studied discoveries and theoretical innovations within astronomy, physiology, and physics. The role assigned to Paracelsus in these grand changes is twofold: he is a troublesome iconoclast, rattling the cages of entrenched university teaching, and a pioneer in chemistry, a field that failed to find closure in the revolutionary process until Antoine Lavoisier set it on the path toward modernity in the late eighteenth century. Thus, Paracelsus is sometimes portrayed as an undisciplined and unsystematic thinker, who blundered upon powerful new chemical substances, for which he gave cloudy theoretical explanations that flew in the face of received and rational opinion. He has been easily marginalized within the scientific revolution as a symbol of a Renaissance spirit that subjected medieval authority to scrutiny, but failed to produce any substantial contribution to science. However, the better acquainted scholars become with the full breadth and variety of theories aired in the sixteenth and seventeenth centuries, the clearer it becomes that important topics for scientific debate lay not only in astronomy, mathematics, and physics, but also in matter theory and medicine, where the presence of Paracelsus cannot easily be ignored.

Even if Paracelsus has not been well assimilated into the history of science, Paracelsian scholars have been alert to his importance as a stimulus to doctrinal change for a long time now and have acknowledged his followers' contributions to the intellectual dialogue from which the "new science" of the seventeenth and eighteenth centuries emerged. Recently it has even been suggested that Paracelsus may be *the* key figure in the early stages of a general revolution in science.[1] Yet Paracelsus has remained in the shadows, a quirky European intellectual on the periphery of the great synthesis. Despite pronouncements that historians must study the past in its own terms and avoid "whiggish" judgement of early modern thinkers on the basis of how modern their science seems, the agenda of who and what to study in the scientific revolution remains anchored in a developmental sequence, in part because it is the movement toward the end that is of interest. There is a vestigial whiggism that relegates people like Paracelsus to the context, while the Galileos and Newtons – now understood in their proper historical frames as courtiers and alchemists – remain the stuff of the text of the revolution itself. And it is no wonder. The more one comes to know Paracelsus and his ideas, the less modern he seems, and the less motivation there is for understanding him as an integral part of scientific change. Recent study of Isaac Newton and the general interest in alchemy among the virtuosi of Restoration England has shown that there is at least a chronological overlap between alchemical and Paracelsian thinking and the mechanistic hypotheses of Descartes and Gassendi, and plausibly there are intellectual connections as well. But if, as Charles Webster has suggested, Isaac Newton has more and more come to resemble Paracelsus in certain respects, then those respects have not been fully digested by historians of science and are still often regarded as vestiges of metaphysical confusion that clouded what is really of value in Newton's thought.

Abused for centuries by his portrayal as an unsavory and uneducated drunkard, who meddled in dark commerce with unclean spirits, Paracelsus remains alien and unlikeable. His treatises are hardly clearer to us than they were to his contemporaries, who found them perplexing and contradictory. Even when sifted and winnowed for intelligible kernels of wisdom, Paracelsus' words have a peculiar ring and do not, by themselves, put forth a lucid view of how the world operates and

---

1   Allen Debus says as much in the closing sentence of the second chapter ("The Chemical Key") of *Man and Nature in the Renaissance* (Cambridge: Cambridge University Press, 1978). William R. Newman's recent opinion on the importance of Paracelsus was noted in the introduction, above.

what our place within it is.[2] I doubt that this impression will change appreciably, since no amount of honest historical work can alter the fact that Paracelsus was not a modern thinker and his ideas were not anchored in anything like a modern intellectual frame. As a historical *persona* he is perhaps best left as an impression, a spectral presence that is unsettling to the world of rational science and medicine, as one finds him in George Ryga's modern play.[3]

To understand how Paracelsus' ideas affected the construction of science, one must look not to Paracelsus, but to the many students, scholars, adepts, and philosophical dilettantes who read Paracelsus and shaped his vision into credible philosophical systems and put this theory to use in chemistry, medicine, and religion. Petrus Severinus was one of the earliest of those who went beyond locating Paracelsus' manuscripts and seeing them printed and actually took Paracelsus' ideas and elaborated them into a coherent and cogent body of doctrine. Consequently, he holds a prominent place among those who, in effect, created Paracelsianism and gave it force of persuasion at a time when European intellectuals were looking for alternatives to Aristotelian natural philosophy and Galenic medical theory. If we are to grasp this process and understand the place of Paracelsian ideas in the genesis of a new natural philosophy, the new science, then we must read the books produced by the Paracelsians and reconstruct the intellectual milieu of their authors; We must assess the influence of Paracelsian ideas and the interplay of these ideas with other philosophies of the early modern republic of letters. This is at times a tedious path to tread: We must follow the terms, phrases, and concepts of Paracelsian doctrines from one text to another, in order to assess how they were transmitted and transformed. And, wherever possible, we should see how these ideas were applied to medical practice, to religion, to pharmacology, and to the art and literature of early modern Europe.

Eventually ideas become so transformed that they are no longer readily identified with a particular source. To some extent this happened

2 Consider, for example, the impression that one gets from sampling Paracelsus' ideas in *Paracelsus: Essential Readings*.

3 George Ryga, *Two Plays: Paracelsus and Prometheus Bound* (Winnepeg, Manitoba: Turnstone Press, 1982).

in the work of J. B. van Helmont, so that those who followed his lead were no longer construed as Paracelsians, but as Helmontians. Some of the Helmontian concepts were in due course again transmuted by Walter Charleton and Robert Boyle and their generation into several of the metaphysical piers upon which corpuscular philosophy was constructed, and this change was so complete that their heritage is only now being reconstructed. Consideration of Paracelsian contributions to corpuscularian philosophy, which on the surface bears little resemblance to anything written by Paracelsus, therefore requires careful study of how Paracelsian ideas were shaped and reshaped by the generations of authors between Paracelsus and Boyle – for example how key concepts were augmented, adapted, and fit into new contexts by these intermediaries, and why they appealed to succeeding generations at all. Van Helmont was one of these intermediaries, and Severinus was another. Andreas Libavius and Daniel Sennert realized this when they referred to some of their contemporary Paracelsians as Severinians, followers of a Severinian school of thought. The *Idea medicinæ* must, consequently, be viewed in the first instance as a Paracelsian tract, as a book that explains selected concepts that Severinus took from Paracelsus and interpreted in a theoretical framework that was created by Severinus from his reading of Hippocrates and Neoplatonic writers, what he learned from his training as an academic physician, from his observations at the bedside and in the laboratory, and also from his assessment of what other sixteenth-century authors thought.

A Paracelsian metaphysics

Ultimately, the significance of Severinus and his work must be judged in the context of those who read the *Idea medicinæ*, commented on Severinus' ideas, and incorporated them into their own work. This is the historiographical assumption that has guided the construction of this study. However, another way to assess Severinus' place within the development of Paracelsian medical theory is to see what he believed he had accomplished with the publication of the *Idea medicinæ*. We can gain some insight into this by examining the final portions of the *Idea medicinæ*, the *peroratio* or conclusion and the *anacephalæosis* or summary, both of which Severinus used to locate his philosophy within the world of medicine.

The *peroratio*, coming as it does at the end of fifteen chapters of theoretical discourse, is particularly important, because it is Severinus' last attempt to reach the reader and shape his or her opinion of the significance of his work. He began by placing the *Idea medicinæ* in relation to the state of sixteenth-century medicine and the authority of the ancients. He said that he had proposed an ideal or brief survey of philosophical medicine, in which he has demonstrated that the methods of his age, i.e. of Galenic medicine, are not at all grounded in the consensus of Hippocrates and the ancient philosophers. He thought that Galen had not exhausted the "light of nature" – using the Paracelsian idea that divine wisdom is vested in the natural world – but that some of nature's secrets still lay hidden, awaiting the proper time and place of discovery. The implication is that Galen did not, could not have known all that there is to know and that it is the duty of each age to correct the errors and improve on the methods of the past. This attitude places Severinus in the spirit of sixteenth-century medical humanism, and in keeping with that tradition, Severinus wanted to assert his right to question and criticize Galen and to find the common truths that underlay the various schools of medical thought.

In his own composition, Galen had relied on the intellectual freedom to dispute the teachings of Archigenes, Asclepiades, Herophilus, Protagoras, Erasistratus, and also his own teacher, Quintius – he had even disputed against Moses, "the prophet of living philosophy," Severinus wrote. Therefore, why should he not be permitted to dispute Galen's teachings? Why, Severinus asked, should Galen's writings "be venerated as if evangelical prophecies"?[4] No physician should have a stranglehold on medical investigation. Severinus therefore made a plea for intellectual freedom and the right to investigate and interpret nature: "Men ought

---

4 Severinus, *Idea medicinæ*, p. 406: "Proinde, si iudicij libertate fretus, contra Archigenem, Asclepiadem, Herophilum, Protagoram, Erasistratum, Quintium Præceptorem suum, etiam contra Mosen, viventis Philosophiæ interpretem, sæpe frivole disputauit: quæ religio est, ipsius scripta, quæ nobis non magis quam ursis & apris destinavit, tanquam Evangelica oracula venerari?"

not take away from [other] men the freedom of human genius, the light of nature, and the power for distinguishing, for judging."[5] This, he felt, is what blind adherence to Galen had done. "The monarchy of the Greeks has ended," he declared, implying a decisive break with medieval scholasticism.[6]

Severinus' words should be read in the light of the heady resurgence of humanism, also medical humanism, which was given an acceptably Christian form and mission by Philipp Melanchthon, whose influence suffused the educational system of Lutheran Germany and Denmark and left its mark on an entire generation of Danish students. Perhaps Severinus had absorbed the spirit of Philippist humanism already as a student at Ribe Latin School, which was in the intellectual watershed of Wittenberg. If not, then he was surely immersed in it at the University of Copenhagen, where Niels Hemmingsen's views set the tone of the continuing Reformation.

For Lutherans, the focus of faith and salvation was on the individual, who was obliged to personally confess an interpretation of the articles of faith. Likewise, for the Paracelsians, the success of the physician depended on his qualities and knowledge as an individual, including his personal piety. Thus, when Severinus demanded the right to interpret medical knowledge, independent of the medical establishment, he was extending to natural science the Protestant demand that the individual be free, in principle, to interpret Scripture independent of the ecclesiastical establishment.

Severinus did not consider himself to be breaking decisively with Galenism in all respects, but rather correcting certain errors and bringing the whole into accord with the "living philosophy" that persuaded the Hermetic doctors of his generation. "I praise Galen's diligence and admire the subtleness and swiftness of his genius," he wrote; "I admit his observations, too ... and I do not despise all the indications for cures or the diagnoses of affected places that he himself proposed."[7] It

---

5 Ibid.: "Libertatem humani ingenij, Naturæ lumen, discernendi, iudicandi facultatem, homines hominibus, eripere non debent."

6 Ibid.: "Desiit Monarchia Græcorum."

7 Ibid: "Laudo industriam Galeni, ingenij subtilitatem, & celeritatem admiror: observationes quoque ... admitto: neque omnes curationum Indicationes vel locorum affectorum dignotiones, quas ipse proposuit, contemno."

was not Severinus' intention abruptly to destroy traditional medicine, which was what the Galenists suspected in the Paracelsian challenge. Instead, he wrote that it was prudent to correct the errors of Galenism gradually and inspire physicians to investigate the properties of things for themselves, to learn the properties of things "and bring them forth in secret, for thus their duty will be accomplished with greater gratitude" – greater, that is, than if they were openly to challenge the Galenic establishment all at once.[8] This would seem to be a clear statement of the old Pythagorean dictum, which medieval alchemists and Paracelsian physicians had adopted, that knowledge is best revealed in its entirety only to those who are adequately prepared for it, namely the adept. This was a sentiment that was repeated with approval ninety years later by William Davidson in his commentary on the *Idea medicinæ*. Yet there is a practical wisdom in this attitude, too. Severinus' generation was witness to the strong reaction that the introduction of chemical drugs and the consequent growing interest in Paracelsus' treatises had aroused among university-educated Galenic physicians, particularly those connected with the medical faculty at Paris. Paracelsian medicine, as medicine, was very controversial in the decade before Severinus' book was printed, and during this time Severinus was studying in Paris, and probably other places in France, as well as in Italy and maybe at German and Swiss universities, too. Had he known that Paracelsian medicine, and even his own version of it, would be attacked on religious grounds, he would have done well to be even more secretive. But those issues reached print only after the *Idea medicinæ* was available at the book fairs, if we are correct in seeing Erastus as the vanguard of that kind of criticism.

Severinus claimed in the *peroratio* that he was content to let the old doctors persist in their Galenic ways, since he knew that they would pay him no heed, anyway. Besides, Severinus claimed that in treating many of the common diseases, they could do but little harm. He was, however, concerned that a new generation of physicians be able to withstand the scorn and opposition of "those who have now grown old in the art,"

---

8 Ibid., pp. 406-407: "Tutius est consilium, paulatim errores corrigere, Medicorum indus-triam strenue excitare, ad Naturæ & Proprietatum inquisitiones, a quibus sanationes, & omnes vitales actiones procedunt, clanculum adducere: ita enim officium, maiori gratitudine absolvetur."

and not be frightened away from pursuing new avenues of inquiry. Apparently Severinus understood that his defense of Paracelsian medicine would be controversial and sought to encourage others to follow his lead. "I know what disturbances I have exposed myself to," he wrote; He had seen the weapons of his adversaries and has "thrown up a shield that will easily dull their edges." He did not believe the Galenists to be invincible. If enough students of medicine could rally against the foes of change and conspire to find new medicines and erect a new method, then they could turn the cowardly herd of traditional physicians before they reached the precipice of disaster, and in so doing they might free the Truth, which has long been imprisoned in the shadows.[9] It is clear from Severinus' rhetoric that he viewed himself as one of the new generation of medical philosophers who would save the world, and they would follow a Paracelsian course to do it. He admonished his readers to

> investigate the mysteries of nature more carefully. Learn the properties of the salts, the sulphurous species, and the mercuries. Abandon those deadly hypotheses of hotnesses and complexions, discovered in the ruins of all of medicine. Arise from your slumber, for life is vigilance.[10]

At first glance this activist program for scientific progress would seem to conflict with the millenarian note on which Severinus ended the *peroratio*. He called on God to bring together those who had strayed from the true path, reconcile their disunity, and dispel the darkness of intellectual disharmony "so that we may embrace that blessed Unity that He displayed in His son, become members and citizens of the heavenly Jerusalem, and rejoice in the eternal knowledge of Truth."[11] It is not a coincidence that Severinus closed his text with an admonition

9 Ibid., p. 407: "Proinde, qui nunc in Arte consenuerunt ... Prudentiores enim sunt, quam ut meis admonitionibus, in hoc negocio egeant. ... Scio & ego, quantis fluctibus me obiecerim. Sed tela adversariorum prævisa sunt: minus ferient. Scutum obieci quod aciem facile retundet."

10 Ibid.: "Diligentius Naturæ mysteria inquirite. Proprietates Salium, Sulphurearum specierum & Mercuriorum addiscite. Relinquite fatales illas Hypotheses Caliditatum & Complexionum, in perniciem totius Medicinæ inventas. Surgite a somno. Vita enim vigilia est."

11 Ibid., p. 408: "ut beata illa Unitate, quam filio suo unigenito proposuit, adepta, Socij & Cives coelestis Hierusalem redditi, æterna Veritatis cognitione gaudere possimus."

to investigate nature tirelessly, followed by an expectation that the new Jerusalem is attainable. Historians have seen this juxtaposition before, in Paracelsus and in Francis Bacon, for instance, and have come to accept that the revolution in scientific thinking was rooted in a larger ideological transformation that found expression in Protestant millenarianism as well as the vision of better living through scientific and technological innovation. We must constantly be reminded that Paracelsian medical philosophy was vested in Paracelsian religious thought, and that both supported a world-view embraced by physicians, poets, and lay religious leaders.

Severinus affixed a summary or *anacephalæosis* to the body of the *Idea medicinæ*, in which he recapitulated the chief points of his philosophy, as he saw it, and they are easily identifiable as Paracelsian. First, he recognized that there are medicines for all diseases to be found in nature. Or, to be more precise, there exists in nature *a medicine* that can be used to cure all diseases, and that is because it contains the vital balsam or radical matter, which is the basis of all activity in the natural world. This vitality ought therefore to be studied by the physician.

Following Paracelsus, and a line of reasoning that is well supported by Aristotelian hylomorphism, Severinus thought of the material world as the *matrix* or womb in which the implanted seminal forms grew into bodies. Specifically, he considered the four Aristotelian elements to be wombs or dwellings that are fortified with the vital balsam or principle of activity that fosters the *semina* or seeds located within them. Since these elements are essentially *places* (*loci*), they are not bodies. However, they are bounded by the limits placed on them by the vital balsam.[12]

Severinus defined *semina* as the necessary links joining the world of ideas to the world of bodies, connecting the invisible to the visible. They contain the laws of motion, the predestined cycles that all things manifest, and the processes or "liturgies" that constitute generation and transplantation – and indeed the dispensations of the general world anatomy. *Semina* govern the reception of impressions and safeguard the harmony of nature. That is, they maintain the integrity of the species, and in instances when this integrity breaks down, and transplantation results, the *semina* determine this process, too. Things in Severinus'

12   Ibid., pp. 409-10.

world do not happen by chance or in a chaotic manner. He envisioned the generation of all bodies as a material realization of knowledge contained within *semina*, which assures that the unfolding of individuals happens in an orderly, harmonious way that protects the continuity of the species. He analogized generation as a liturgy, in which what was incorporeal becomes corporeal, with all the "functions, colors, flavors, odors, hotnesses, coldnesses, wetnesses, drynesses, sizes, locations, forms, harmonies, durations, appointed timings, and all the trappings" that are appropriate to the thing.[13] Such a theory would have been attractive to the early modern speculative natural philosopher, and it is not hard to imagine Severinus' theory appealing to the student of medicine, who might have been pondering the special function and location of organs within the body, or to the taxonomist, who might have been wondering at the seeming fixity and continuity of species and why hybrids and monstrous births occasionally occur. Severinus' answer to these questions was his doctrine of seminal expression, in which beings are constructed from elements and principles that are mixed according to the "mechanical" knowledge inherent in the seed. However, sometimes other, foreign knowledge intervenes, bringing with it another mixture, and this is transplantation.

Transplantation occurs in all orders, Severinus wrote. It might be that an individual's properties are only slightly altered by transplantation, by means of a weak supervening pattern, which Severinus called a tincture, or an individual might be so affected by a strong tincture that it comes to "demonstrate the signs of a new family."[14] Such powerful transplantations accompany the "resolutions" of the *astra* (stars) that are hidden in things. Transplantations account for what appear to be deviations in the normal pattern of development, and this explains the occurance of diseases as well as the occasional birth of monstrosities and the persistence of weeds, no matter how carefully the seed has been selected.

---

13   Ibid., p. 411: "Generatio, progressio est seminum, in qua ... Individuorum renovatione, specierum perpetuitatem custodiunt: fiuntque in hac lithurgia ex invisibilibus visibilia, ex incorporeis corporea, ... Cuius efficientia, Elementa, & corporum Principia officijs consentanea, colores, sapores, odores, caliditates, frigiditates, humiditates, siccitates, magnitudines, situs, conformationes, consensus, durationes, digesta tempora, & omnia corporum ornamenta, admirando ordine producuntur."
14   Ibid., p. 412: "novæ familiæ insignia demonstrent."

Human procreation is just one variation of the general pattern of seminal generation that Severinus developed. In keeping with the "two seed" theory that medieval medical writers had inherited from Hippocrates and Galen – in contrast to Aristotle's theory – Severinus believed that the vital balsam, which is contained in every part of the body, both in males and females, flows to the reproductive organs of both sexes. When the male seed meets the female seed in the womb, by means of a "natural impulse," the vital balsam "effervesces" and generation commences. The mechanical spirits within the seeds then set about constructing a new human body, drawing on the elements and principles in whatever foodstuffs are available, and using them to fashion parts according to the innate knowledge. The result is an ordered embryological development, in which the right organs end up in the right places. Tinctures that supervene during the process of generation alter it and produce sexual distinctions, which occur in a continuous spectrum from wholly masculine to wholly feminine.[15] Implicit within this theory is the common (and Paracelsian) notion that "impressions" received by a pregnant woman may affect the development of her unborn child, which Severinus has generalized.

Seminal progression or development, since it results in the creation of diverse parts, produces diverse functions or concoctions, which are chemical processes in which impurities are separated from some crude material. This is an idea that is characteristic of Paracelsian pathology, which assigns many kinds of disease to the improper digestion and expulsion of impurities, and therefore is fundamentally incompatible with Galenic humoral pathology. "The generation of the four humors – blood, bile, phlegm, and melancholia – in the liver is imaginary," wrote Severinus.[16] He believed that disease is not a result of a humoral imbalance, but rather the product of a morbific development of seeds within the blood and other substances of the body. The *semina morborum*, seeds of disease, are foreign to the body and can cause disease to root and grow in it by forcing a hostile transplantation of the normally harmonious function. In this way, diseases can be said to grow from seeds that adhere

---

15 Ibid., p. 412.
16 Ibid., p. 413: "Generatio quatuor humorum, sanguinis, bilis, pituitæ, melancholiæ, in hepate, phantastica est."

to the roots of other essences. The seeds of diseases were not created that way, namely morbific, from the beginning of time, but resulted from the tainting of originally pure *semina* as a consequence of man's disobedience and the divine curse. These seeds are joined to the things that we eat. Morbific *semina* unfold in the body in various places, and as they do they produce various symptoms with characteristic timings. These can be used to identify the diseases.[17]

Cures are of two kinds, general (perfect) and particular. General cures or panaceas are preferred, but not easily obtained. Often particular remedies will suffice, however. There are three classes of these, distinguished by the intensity of their pharmacological activity: alimentary, medicinal, and poisonous. One cannot judge the action of these remedies on the basis of simple Aristotelian qualities, but one can learn about a drug's properties by analyzing it chemically to determine its principles. The physician may need to use poisonous medicines in extreme cases, and these must be chemically prepared before use. Their crudeness must be matured, impurities separated from the pure substance, the corporeal nature broken up, and the spiritual parts restored. Characteristics that are harmful and unpleasant must be mitigated and removed from such drugs without harming the curative virtues.[18]

In retrospect, Severinus' brief summary of the *Idea medicinæ* fits well with what posterity found most attractive about the book, namely that the theory of seminal causation of diseases – as a theoretical explanation for chemical therapy – was an organizing principle that a reformed medical philosophy needed. Indeed, Severinus' concept of *semina morborum* did attract wide interest for a century after its publication, as has been amply demonstrated in the foregoing chapters. What Severinus apparently did not foresee was that his book would be used by many as their introduction to Paracelsianism, as a "map of medicine," as the anonymous English translator called it, by which the student could be guided into the world of chemical philosophy.

17 Ibid., pp. 413-14.
18 Ibid., pp. 415-16.

PARACELSIANISM IN DENMARK

This study has demonstrated that the *Idea medicinæ* was a key document in the European development and disemination of Paracelsian
doctrine and, as I have argued above, it should be evaluated within
the textual tradition of Paracelsianism. Severinus' book represents one
juncture, albeit an important one, at which the streams of Paracelsus'
ideas were joined by tributaries flowing from other philosophical and
medical traditions to give rise to the powerful current that Paracelsianism became in the early seventeenth century. However, Severinus' ideas and the circumstances of his life also inform us about the
broader social and intellectual setting in which Paracelsian doctrines
were evaluated and accepted, modified, or rejected. Specifically, they
give us insight into what purpose Paracelsian medicine served in the
learned culture of Denmark at the time of Tycho Brahe. Severinus
and his fellow medical student, Johannes Pratensis, most likely first
encountered Paracelsian medicine while studying at the universities
of Germany, France, and Italy. We can suppose that they found Paracelsian doctrines interesting and intellectually persuasive and were
convinced that the application of these ideas would benefit their
practice of medicine. But it is also likely that their choice to become
proponents of Paracelsian medicine was based on its attractiveness to
patrons at home, for indeed they were patronized by the royal court
of Denmark and by the Danish nobility. Severinus became the king's
personal physician and Pratensis was appointed to a chair in medicine
at the university; Paracelsian medicine was a valued discipline in late
sixteenth-century Denmark, and the advantage of being on the cutting edge of intellectual change probably occured to them while they
were students.

During the very years that Severinus and Pratensis were traveling and
studying, first at the University of Copenhagen and then abroad, Tycho
Brahe was also a student. Although Tycho's social rank precluded him
from an academic career, his world was shaped by an education similar
to theirs, inasmuch as he also became acquainted with the fundamentals
of medicine, chemistry, and a humanist curriculum. All three shared
a commitment to a Hermetic-Platonist world view, which stressed the
personal experience of nature and the power of poetry and demanded

that natural philosophy and Holy Scripture, when properly interpreted, put forth a coherent account of man, nature, and God.

We catch a glimpse of such an integrated scientific and religious philosophy in the work of Tycho's student research assistant, Kort Aslakssøn. In creating a "Mosaic physics" that was compatible with chemical philosophy, Aslakssøn was following a Protestant tradition of finding explanations for Christ's being, his incarnation and resurrection, the presence of divinity in nature and man, and other doctrinal issues, which could be rationalized in terms of natural philosophy. Such solutions remained hot spots of confessional strife even when the more obvious fires of internecine conflict appeared to be dowsed. This, too, was in the Paracelsian tradition, inasmuch as Paracelsus believed that true medicine must be grounded in personal piety and a Christian vision and not taken unquestioned from pagan and Islamic sources. Severinus felt the same way, when he criticized his contemporaries for placing Galen above Hippocrates and other ancient sages, whose philosophy was more genuinely Christian. In fact, we have seen that Severinus built his ideal of philosophical medicine around a metaphysical framework that was amenable both to Christian Platonism and to a chemical interpretation of *Genesis*. His theory that *semina* house the *rationes seminales* that God sowed into prime matter in the beginning was an incorporation of Augustine's creation-metaphysics into medical theory. It is hard to imagine that this was an unconscious accommodation of philosophical medicine and Christian theology. Certainly Severinus' most vehement critics and also his apologists interpreted his theory in the light of its consequences for religion. And if Severinus was taken aback by the severity of Erastus' criticism, it cannot be that he did not foresee that his theory had religious implications. For, Severinus and Tycho Brahe lived in an intellectual world that valued agreement between theology and natural philosophy.

Like Severinus and Pratensis, Tycho was also enmeshed in a network of patronage and exchange that embraced Paracelsian ideas. His fame today rests on his achievements as an astronomer, yet by his own account, he valued "terrestrial astronomy" – the study of the stars within the mundane world – as much as the celestial kind, and both were at the forefront of discussion in early modern natural philosophy. Tycho was a member of the nobility and must be viewed as both client and patron, and consequently his pursuit of the two astronomies should be understood in terms of their value to the small segment of society that funded and conducted the business of reforming science. His research and production of chemical medicines falls within a late Renaissance milieu of noblesse oblige – the aristocrat's obligation to succor his dependents – and the exchange of the products, arts, and knowledge that then fascinated the great noble houses. When we examine Tycho's relationship to the royal court, we must bear in mind that chemistry was one of the currencies of the aristocratic economy. Tycho worked at alchemy at his uncle's manor before building his own laboratory on Hven. He said he was returning from the laboratory when he first observed the "new star" that would bring him fame as an astronomer. And, while it is true that he was patronized by King Frederik II as an astronomer, and was awarded fiefdoms to entice him to remain in Denmark, it is also the case that the crown supplied him with the means to build and fuel a first rate chemical laboratory, which was also a desireable addition to the realm. Not much more than a decade after Tycho dismantled the laboratory at Uraniborg, King Christian IV established a royal laboratory at Rosenborg Castle and hired a Paracelsian physician, Peter Payngk, to run it. Therefore, for Tycho Brahe, as for Severinus and Pratensis, Paracelsian medicine and philosophy must be evaluated in relation to the king's desire to further these subjects and maintain a "staff" of expert consultants available to serve the needs of the government and university.

Tycho Brahe made few references to Paracelsian medicine, and Johannes Pratensis left little written record of any kind. But the surviving evidence supports the view that Tycho held Paracelsian opinions and was perhaps even interested in Paracelsus' religious views. What little we know about Pratensis, a close personal friend of Tycho Brahe, indicates that he taught a medicine at the University of Copenhagen that included Paracelsian ideas. The historical circumstances that Tycho, Severinus, and Pratensis shared, the personal contact, common educational background, and mutual dependence on the network based around the court of Frederik II, all argue for a common intellectual vision. This vision likely guided life at Uraniborg, where symbolic diagrams and profound epigraphs adorned the walls and provided a philosophical framework to edify a generation of Danish students of astronomy and medicine, who worked and studied there in the early stages of their scholarly careers. Kort Aslakssøn was one of these, but Paracelsian ideas also left their mark on Peder Jacobsen Flemløse and Christian Sørensen Longomontanus. To the extent that this intellectual milieu shaped the *Idea medicinæ*, study of the natural philosophy expressed in it can inform us about Tycho Brahe's intellectual world. Likewise, Severinus was a part of the social and political sphere in which Tycho's fortunes were maintained and ultimately permitted to decline. Only four years after Tycho's alienation from the government of King Christian IV had led to his abandonment of Uraniborg and eventually Denmark, Severinus also contemplated leaving royal service, to return to the university. But whereas Tycho Brahe was moved to leave his homeland and offer his services to the Holy Roman Emperor – services that apparently required a chemical laboratory as well as an observatory – Severinus remained in Denmark. He was a survivor, but not for long. By the time of his death in 1602, Tycho Brahe was also dead in Prague, and their dear friend Pratensis had been dead for a quarter of a century. But the world-view that these men discussed and debated in their youth – a philosophy which was informed by the ideas of Paracelsus and destined to shake up academic discourse – did not die with them. It lived on in the work of their students and colleagues and helped shape the natural knowledge and disciplinary developments of seventeenth-century Denmark. As is evident from the many scholars, chemists, physicians, and poets who read the *Idea medicinæ*, Severinus' ideas reached abroad as well and fed the intellectual melting pot that produced a new approach to natural philosophy.

Table of Abbreviations and Standard Works

DBL – *Dansk Biografisk Leksikon*. Ed. Carl Frederik Bricka. 19 vols. Copenhagen: Gyldendal, 1887-1905; 2d ed. 27 vols. Copenhagen: J. H. Schultz, 1933-; 3d ed. Ed. Svend Cedergreen Bech. 16 vols. Copenhagen: Gyldendal, 1979-84.

DDLH – Oluf Friis. *Den Danske Litteraturs Historie*.

DDKH – Bjørn Kornerup and Hal Koch. *Den Danske Kirkes Historie*.

DNB – *Dictionary of National Biography*. 22 vols. 1885-1901; London: Oxford University Press, 1967-68.

DRA – Det Danske Rigsarkiv, Copenhagen.

DSB – *Dictionary of Scientific Biography*. Ed. Charles Coulston Gillispie. 18 vols. New York: Scribner, 1970-90.

GKS – Gammel Kongelig Samling, Kgl. Bibl. Copenhagen.

KUH – *Københavns Universitets Historie*.

NBL – *Norsk Biografisk Leksikon*. Ed. Edvard Bull, Anders Krogvig, and Gerhard Gran. 19 vols. Kristiania (Oslo): H. Aschehoug, 1923-83.

NKS – Ny Kongelig Samling (Kgl. Bibl. Copenhagen).

NRA – Norges Riksarkiv, Oslo.

SAO – Statsarkiv, Oslo.

TBDOO – *Tychonis Brahe Dani opera omnia*.

Bibliography of printed works and manuscripts cited and selected background studies

For alphabetization, leading articles and the Latin prepositions "de" and "ad" have been ignored. "ø" has been treated as "oe."

PRINTED PRIMARY SOURCES

Altes und Neues von Gelehrten Sachen aus Dännemark. Vol. 2. Copenhagen and Leipzig, 1768.

Amwaldus (Georg am Wald). *Bericht und Erklerung … wie und was Gestalt das new von jhm erfunden Terra Sigillata und universal Artzney, wider die Pestilenz und dero Zufellen … zugebrauchen*. St. Gallen: L. Straub, 1582.

Andernachus, Johannes Guintherius. *De medicina veteri et nova tum cognoscenda, tum faciunda commentarii duo*. Basel: Henricpetri, 1571.

Apothecken Taxt: Hvorledis Medicamenta, simplicia oc composita, som hoss begge Privilegerede Apotheckere her i Kiøbenhaffn tilkiøbs findis / effter denne tids oc steds lejlighed selges. Copenhagen: Salomon Sartorius, 1619.

Apothecken Taxt: Hvorledis Medicamenta, simplicia oc composita, som hoss tre Privilegerede Apotheckere her i Kiøbenhaffn / saa vel som hoss andre Apotheckere herudi Kongerig tilkiøbs findis / effter denne tids oc steds lejlighed selges. Copenhagen: Georg Lamprecht, 1645.

Apoteker Taxt, 1672. See *Catalogus medicamentorum officinalium*.

Ashmole, Elias. *Theatrum Chemicum Brittanicum*. 1652; reprint, New York: Johnson Reprint, 1967.

Aslakssøn, Kort (Cunradus Aslacus Bergensis). *De natura caeli triplicis libelli tres*. Siegen, 1597.

—. *Physica et ethica Mosaica, ut antiquissima, ita vere christiania, duobus libris comprehensa*. Copenhagen, 1613.

Aubertus, Iacobus. *De metallorum ortu et causis contra chemistas breuis et dilucida explicatio*. Lyons: I. Berion, 1575.

Aubrey, John. *Brief Lives*. 3rd ed. Ed. O.L. Dick. London: Secker & Warburg, 1958.

B., R. (Robert Bostocke). *The Difference between the Auncient Physicke … and the latter Physicke*. London, 1585.

Bacon, Francis. *The Works of Francis Bacon.* Ed. James Spedding, Robert Ellis, and Douglas Heath. 8 vols. London, 1857-74; reprint, New York: Garret Press, 1968.

—. *The Masculine Birth of Time.* See Farrington.

Baker, George. *The Composition or making of the moste excellent and pretious oil called Oleum Magistrale.* London, 1574.

Barchusen, Johann Conrad. *Historia medicinæ.* Amsterdam: Jansonius-Wæsbergii, 1710.

—. *De medicinæ origine et progressu dissertationes.* Trajecti ad Rhenum: Paddenburg and Croon, 1723.

Bartholin, Caspar. *Oratio de ortu, progressu, et incrementis Regiæ Academiæ Hafniensis.* Wittenberg: Michael Wendt, 1645.

—. *De studio medico inchoando, continuando, et absolvendo.* Copenhagen, 1628. See Conring, Hermann. *In universam artem medicam.*

Bartholin, Thomas. *Cista medica Hafniensis.* Copenhagen: Haubold, 1662.

—. *De transplantatione morborum dissertatio epistolica.* Copenhagen: Daniel Paulli, 1673.

Bartholin, Thomas, ed. *Dispensatorium Hafniense.* Copenhagen: Georg Lamprecht, 1658.

Behrend, C. "En Dagbog fra en Rejse i Danmark 1588." *Danske Magazin* 6th ser., 1 (1913): 334-44.

—. "En Dagbog fra en Rejse i Danmark i Aaret 1588." In *Fra Archiv og Museum,* pp. 294-310. Copenhagen, 1913.

Borrichius, Olaus (Ole Borch). *Dissertatio de docimastice metallica.* Copenhagen: Godicchenius, 1677.

—. *Dissertatio de ortu et progressu chemiae.* Copenhagen, 1660.

—. *Hermetis, Ægyptiorum et chemicorum sapientia ab Hermanni Conringii animadversionibus vindicata per Olaum Borrichium.* Copenhagen, 1674.

—. *Lingua pharmacopoeorum.* Copenhagen: Haubold, 1670.

—. *Olai Borrichii Itinerarium 1660-1665: The Journal of the Danish Polyhistor Ole Borch.* Ed. H. D. Schepelern. Copenhagen: C.A. Reitzel, 1983.

Boyle, Robert. *The Works of the Honourable Robert Boyle, in Six Volumes.* Ed. Thomas Birch. Vol. 4. London, 1772.

Brahe, Tycho. *De nova stella.* 1573; facsimile edition, Brussels: Culture et Civilization, 1969.

—. *Instruments of the Renewed Astronomy.* Ed. Alena Hadravova, Petr Hadrava, and Jole R. Shackelford. Clavis Monumentorum Litterarum (Regnum Bohemiae) 2, Facsimilia – Translationes 1. Prague: Koniasch Latin Press, 1996.

—. *Tycho Brahe's Description of his Instruments and Scientific Work as given in Astronomiæ Instauratæ Mechanica.* Ed. Hans Ræder, Elis Strømgren, and Bengt Strømgren. Copenhagen: Det kongelige danske videndkabernes selskab, 1946.

—. *Tychonis Brahe Dani opera omnia.* Ed. J. L. E. Dreyer. 15 vols. Copenhagen: Det Danske Sprog- og Litteratur-Selskab, 1913-29.

Bremer, Andreas Fredericus. *Dissertationis de vita et opinionibus Theophrasti Paracelsi particula posterior.* Copenhagen: Trier, 1836.

Bruno, Giordano. *Cause, Principle and Unity.* Trans. Jack Lindsay. New York: International, 1964.

—. *The Expulsion of the Triumphant Beast.* Trans. Arthur D. Imerti. New Brunswick, NJ: Rutgers University Press, 1964.

—. *De rerum principiis et elementis et causis.* In *Jordani Bruni Nolani opera Latine conscripta*, ed. F. Tocco and H. Vitelli. Vol. 3. Florence, 1891.

Catalogus medicamentorum officinalium cum Taxa pharmaceuticæ hafniense 1672. Copenhagen: Georgius Gødianus, 1672. The title on the title page differs somewhat from that on the cover: *Catalogus & valor medicamentorum simplicium & compositorum in officinis hafniensibus prostantium*, and in Danish: *Apoteker Taxt paa alt hvis i Kiøbenhaffn hos de fire Privilegerede Apotekere til Kiøbs findis.*

Charleton, Walter. *Physiologia Epicurio-Gassendo-Charletoniana.* London: Thomas Newcomb, 1654.

—. *Spiritus Gorgonicus.* Leiden: Elsevier, 1650.

Christian IV. *Kong Christian den Fjerdes Egenhaendige Breve*, ed. C. F. Bricka, and J. A. Frederica. Vol. 4. 1882; reprint, Copenhagen: Selskabet for udgivelsen af kilder til dansk historie, 1969.

Chronich, Niels Svendsøn. *Tre Aandelige Sange.* Ed. J.C. Tellefsen. Christiania (Oslo): Thronsen, 1882.

de Clave, Etienne. *Paradoxes, ou Traittez Philosophiques des Pierres et Pierreries, contre l'opinion vulgaire.* Paris: Pierre Chevalier, 1635.

Collett, Alf. "Gaarde Mandtal udi Christiania taxerit og forfattedt den 14. 15. oc 16. August Anno 1661." *Personalhistorisk Tidsskrift* 2d. ser., 4 (1889): 177-211.

Conrad, Daniel. *Exercitationes opticæ.* Wittenberg: Henckel, 1608.

Conring, Hermann. *De hermetica Ægyptiorum vetere et Paracelsicorum nova medicina liber unus.* Helmstädt: Henningius Mullerius, 1648.

—. *In universam artem medicam singulasque ejus partes introductio.* Helmstadt: Hammius, 1687. Includes Caspar Bartholin's *De studio medico inchoando, continuando, et absolvendo.*

Crato von Crafftheim, Johann. *Consiliorum et epistolarum medicinalium Io. Cratonis a Kraftheim; nunc primum a Laurentio Scholzio … in lucem editis.* Vol. 3. Frankfurt, 1671.

Croll, Oswald. *Admonitory Preface.* In *Philosophy Reformed and Improved in Four Profound Tracts.* Trans. H. Pinnell. London, 1657.

—. *Basilica chymica.* Frankfurt: Godofridi, 1609.

—. *Royal Chymistry.* In Oswald Croll and Johann Hartmann, *Bazilica Chymica, & Praxis chymiatricæ, or Royal and Practical Chymistry in Three Treatises.* London, 1670.

Davidson, William. *Commentaria in Idæam Medicinæ Philosophicæ Petri Dani, Medici incomparabilis & Philosophi sublimis.* Den Haag: Vlacq, 1663.

—. *Commentariorum in sublimis philosophi & incomparibilis viri Petri Severini Dani Ideam Medicinæ Philosophicæ … Prodromus.* Den Haag: Vlacq, 1660.

—. *Les Elements de la Philosophie de l'Art du Feu ou Chemie.* Trans. Jean Hellot. Paris, 1651 and 1657.

—. *Philosophia pyrotechnica seu curriculus chymiatricus.* Paris: Bessin, 1633-35.

—. *Theophrasti Verdici Scoti Doctoris medici Plicomastix seu Plicæ e numero morborum Apospasma.* Danzig, 1668.

Dessenius Cronenburgius, Bernard. *Medicinæ veteris et rationalis, adversus … Georgii Fedronis, ac universæ sectæ Paracelsicæ imposturas, defensio.* Cologne, 1573.

Donne, John. *Ignatius his Conclave.* London, 1611.

Drechssler, Johann Gabriel. *Disputatio I, De metallorum transmutatione.* Leipzig: Wittigau, 1673.

Duchesne, Joseph. See Quercetanus.

Erastus, Thomas. *Disputationum de medicina nova Philippi Paracelsi pars prima.* Basel: Perna, 1572.

—. *Disputationum de medicina nova Philippi Paracelsi pars altera.* Basel: Perna, 1572.

—. *De occultis pharmacorum potestatibus.* Basel: Perna, 1574.

Fernel, Jean. *De abditis rerum causis libri duo.* Frankfurt: Andreas Wechel, 1574.

Fichard, J. E. von, and Baur von Eyseneck. *Frankfurtisches Archiv für ältere deutsche Litteratur und Geschichte.* Vol. 2. Frankfurt am Main: Gebhard, 1813.

Ficino, Marsilio. *Opera omnia.* Torino: Bottega d' Erasmo, 1959.

Fjelstrup, August. "Peter Payngk: 'Rapsodia Vitæ Theophrasti Paracelsi'." *Janus* 13 (1908): 545-63.

Fludd, Robert. "Declaratio Brevis." Trans. Robert A Seelinger, Jr. In William H. Huffman and Robert A Seelinger, Jr. "Robert Fludd's 'Declaratio Brevis' to James I." *Ambix*, 25 (1978): 69-92.

Franckenberg, Abraham von. *Gemma magica oder magisches Edelgestein.* Amsterdam, 1688.

Friis, Frederik R. *Tyge Brahes Meteorologiske Dagbog, Holdt Paa Uraniborg for Aarene 1582-1597.* Copenhagen: H.H. Thiele, 1876.

Galen, Claudius. *Medicorum Græcorum opera quæ extant.* Ed. Karl Gottlob Kühn. Vol. 11. Leipzig, 1826.

Garboe, Axel. *Ole Worms Stambog.* Copenhagen, 1920.

Gassendi, Pierre. *Opera omnia.* Lyons, 1658; Facsimile reprint, Stuttgart-Bad Cannstatt: Friedrich Frommann, 1964.

—. *Tychonis Brahei vita.* Paris, 1654.

Gouron, Marcel. *Matricule de L'Université de Médecine de Montpellier (1503-1599).* Geneva: Droz, 1957.

Gohory, Jacques (Leo Svavius). *Theophrastus Paracelsi philosophiæ et medicinæ … compendium.* Basel: Perna, 1568.

Grube, Hermann. *De transplantatione morborum. Analysis nova.* Hamburg, 1674.

Grundtvig, Johan. "Et lidet Bidrag til D. Niels Hemmingsens Historie." *[Ny] Kirkehistoriske Samlinger* 2d ser., 4 (1867-68): 742-53.

Grynæus, Johannes Fredericus. *Disputatio medica inauguralis de morborum transplantatione et cura sympathetica.* Copenhagen, 1708.

Guintherius Andernachus, Johannes (Winter von Andernach). *De medicina veteri et nova tum cognoscenda, tum faciunda commentarii duo.* Basel: Henricpetri, 1571.

Hartmann, Johann. *Opera omnia medico-chymica.* Ed. Conrad Johrenius. 7 vols. Frankfurt am Main: Balthas. Christophori Wursti, 1684.

—. *Practical Chymistry.* In Oswald Croll and Johann Hartmann, *Bazilica Chymica, & Praxis chymiatricæ, or Royal and Practical Chymistry in Three Treatises.* London, 1670.

Helmont, Jean Baptiste van. *Opvscvla medica inaudita.* Amsterdam: Elsevier, 1648; reprint, Brussels: Culture et Civilisation, 1966.

—. *Oriatrike; or, Physick Refined.* Trans. J.C. London: Loyd, 1662.

—. *Ortus medicinæ. Id est, initia physicæ inaudita. Progressus medicinæ novus, in morborum ultionem, ad vitam longam.* Amsterdam: Elsevier, 1648.

—. *Ternary of Paradoxes, Of the Magnetick Cure of Wounds, Nativity of Tartar in Wine, Image of God in Man.* London: James Flesher, 1650.

Herbert of Cherbury, Edward. *The Life of Edward, First Lord Herbert of Cherbury, Written by Himself.* Ed. J. M. Shuttleworth. London: Oxford University Press, 1976.

Hester, John, ed. and trans. *A hundred and fourteen experiments and cures of the famous Phisition Philippus Aureolus Theophrastus Paracelsus.* [London, 1584?]. (Contains translations of works by Quercetanus and Penotus).

Hippocrates. *On Ancient Medicine.* In *Hippocrates I.* Trans. W. H. S. Jones. The Loeb Classical Library, vol. 147. 1932; reprint, Cambridge, MA: Harvard University Press, 1984.

Hjärne, Urban. *Acta et tentamina chymica in regio laboratorio Stockholmiensi, elaborata et demonstrata, in decades redacta atque divisa una cum præmissa parasceve seu prævia manuductione ad experimenta rite perficienda.* Stockholm: Johan Werner, 1712.

—. *Defensionis Paracelsicæ Prodromus. Eller, Kort Föremäle af then uthförligare Förswars Skrift för den stora Philosophus Theutonicus Theophrastus Paracelsus, som nyligen medelst en hård Beskyltning uthan någon Orsak är worden antastad.* Stockholm: Julius G. Matthiæ, 1709.

Hofmeister, Adolph, ed. *Die Matrikel Der Universität Rostock.* Rostock, 1889.

Horst, Gregor. *De morborum differentiis et causis, exercitatio I.* Geissen: Caspar Chemlinus, 1612.

—. *De natura humana libri duo … Cum præfatione de Anatomia vitali & mortua pro conciliatione Spagyricorum & Galenicorum plurimum inseruiente.* Frankfurt am Main: Erasmus Kempfer, 1612.

Horst, Gregor, Jr. *Operum medicorum tomus primus.* Nuremberg, 1660.

Isthmenius, Isacus. *Disputatio physica de mistione.* Uppsala, 1651.

Jones, John. *The Arte and Science of Preseruing Bodie and Soule in Healthe, Wisdome, and Catholike Religion.* London, 1579.

—. *The Benefit of the auncient bathes of Buckstones.* London, 1572.

Jorden, Edward. *Discovrse of Natvrall Bathes, and Minerall Waters.* London: Thomas Harper, 1631; reprint, Amsterdam: Theatrum Orbis Terrarum, 1971.

—. *A Discourse of Naturall Bathes, and Minerall Waters.* London: Thomas Harper, 1632.

Kaae, Bue, ed. *Peder Hegelunds Almanakoptegnelser 1565-1613.* 2 vols. Ribe: Historisk Samfund for Ribe Amt, 1976.

Kancelliets Brevbøger. Ed. C. F. Bricka. 24 vols. Copenhagen: C. A Reitzel, 1885-1968.

Kepler, Johannes. *Ad Vitellionem paralipomena.* In *Johannes Kepler Gesammelte Werke*, ed. Walther von Dyck and Max Caspar. Vol. 2, ed. Franz Hammer. Munich: C. H. Beck, 1939.

Kirkeordinansen av 1607 og Forordning om Ekteskapssaker gitt 1582. Facsimile reproduction of the 1607 original. Oslo: Norsk Historisk Kjeldeskrift-Institutt, 1985.

Køning, Mauritus Petri. *Dissertatio de rerum principiis et mechanica seminum liturgia.* Copenhagen: Godicchenius, 1663.

Kolding, Jonas. *Daniæ descriptio nova.* Frankfurt am Main: Feyarbendt, 1594.

Kozak, Johann Sophron. *Anatomia vitalis microcosmi in qua naturæ humanæ proprietates ... explicantur.* Bremen: Berthold Villerian, 1636.

Krag, Anders. *Laurea Apollinarea Monspeliensis.* Basel: Henric Petri, 1586.

Kroman, Erik, ed. *Ribe Rådstuedombøger 1527-1576 og 1580-1599.* Copenhagen: Selskabet for udgivelse af kilder til dansk historie, 1974.

de La Brosse, Guy. *De la nature, vertu, et utilité des plantes.* Paris, 1628.

Libavius, Andreas. *Alchymia.* Frankfurt, 1606.

—. *Analysis Confessionis Fraternitatis de Rosea Cruce.* Frankfurt am Main, 1615.

—. *Appendix necessaria Syntagmatis arcanorum chymicorum.* Frankfurt, 1615.

—. *Gegenbericht von der Panacea Amwaldina.* Frankfurt: Kopff, 1595.

—. *Lapis philosophicus dogmaticorum.* Paris: Doulceur, 1608.

—. *Neoparacelsica.* Frankfurt: Kopff, 1594.

—. *Panacea Ambaldina victa et prostrata.* Frankfurt: Kopff, 1596.

—. *Rervm chymicarum epistolica forma ad philosophos et medicos qvosdam in Germaria.* Vol. 3. Frankfurt: Petrus Kopffius, 1599.

—. *Syntagmatis selectorum undiquaque et perspicue traditorum alchymiæ arcanorum tomus primus.* Frankfurt, 1615.

—. *Wolmeinendes Bedencken von der Fama und Confession der Bruderschafft dess Rosen Creutzes.* Frankfurt, 1616.

Lipenius, M. Martinus. *Bibliotheca Realis Medica.* Frankfurt am Main, 1679.

Longomontanus, Christianus Severinus (Christian Sørensen). *Disputatio prima astronomica.* Copenhagen, 1611.

Maar, Vilhelm, ed. *Holger Jacobæus Rejsebog 1671-1692.* Copenhagen: Gyldendal, 1910.

Maier, Michael. *Atalanta fugiens, hoc est, Emblemata nova de secretis naturæ chymica.* Oppenheim: Hieronymus Gallerus, 1618; facsimile reprint, Kassel and Basel: Bärenreiter Verlag, 1964.

Mangeti, Joannis Jacobi. *Bibliotheca scriptorum medicorum veterum ac recentiorum.* Vol. 2. Geneva, 1731.

Martin Zeillers Neue Beschreibung der Königreiche Dennemarck und Norwegen. Ulm, 1648.

Mercklini, Georg Abraham. *Lindenius Renovatus sive Johannes van der Linden de Scriptis Medicis.* Nuremburg, 1686.

Mersenne, Marin. *Correspondance du P. Marin Mersenne Religieux Minime.* Ed. Tannery, Paul. Vol. 3. Paris: Presses Universitaires de France, 1946.

Moffet, Thomas. *De iure et præstantia chemicorum medicamentorum dialogus apologeticus.* Frankfurt: Wechel, 1584.

—. *Nosomantica Hippocratea.* Frankfurt, 1584.

Moller, O.H. *Cimbria literata sive scriptorum ducatus utriusque Slesvicensis et Holsatici historia literata tripartita.* 3 Vols. Copenhagen: G. F. Kisel, 1744.

Morin, Jean Baptiste. *Astrologia Gallica principiis & rationibus propriis stabilita atque in xxvi libros distributa.* Hague: Vlacq, 1661.

Morsius, Joachim (Anastasius Philaretus Cosmopolita). *Magische Propheceyung Aureoli Philippi Theophrasti Paracelsi.* Philadelphia, 1625.

Nielsen, Ingrid, ed. *Ribe Bys Jordebog: Grundlagt i 1450erne og videreført til omkring 1600.* Esbjerg: Sydjysk Universitetsforlag, 1979.

Nielsen, O., ed. *Kjøbenhavns Diplomatarium.* Vol. 3. Copenhagen: Gad, 1877.

Norlind, Wilhelm. *Ur Tycho Brahes Brevväxling.* Lund: Gleerup, 1926.

Nye Danske Magazine. 2d ser., 3 (1810), p. 71. Letter from Rhodius to [Peter Charisius?] 23 February 1661.

Paracelsus. *Aurora thesaurusque philosophorum, Theophrasti Paracelsi, Germani philosophi, & medici præ cunctis omnibus accuratissimi. Accessit Monarchia Physica per Gerardum Dorneum, in defensionem Paracelsicorum principiorum, a suo præceptore positorum.* Basel: Palmaguar, 1577.

—. *Dritter Theil der Bucher ... Paracelsi genannt.* Basel: Conrad Waldkirch, 1589.

—. *The Hermetic and Alchemical Writings of ... Paracelsus.* Trans. A. E. Waite. Vol. 2 London: James Elliott, 1894.

—. *Les XIV Livres des Paragraphes de Ph. Theoph. Paracelse Bombast, Allemand ... Prince des Medecins Hermetiques & Spagyriques.* Ed. C. de Sarcilly. Paris: Jean Guillemot, 1631.

—. *Medici Libelli ... Theophrasti Paracelsi.* Cologne: Arnold Birckman, 1567.

—. *Opera omnia medico-chemico-chirurgica*, ed. Bitiskius. 3 vols. Geneva: de Tournes, 1658.

—. *Paracelsus: Essential Readings.* Ed. and trans. Nicholas Goodrick-Clarke. Wellingborough, Northamptonshire, England: Aquarian Press, 1990.

—. *Sämtliche Werke.* See Sudhoff, Karl (below).

Patrizi, Francesco. *Nova de universis philosophia.* Ferrara, 1591.

Paulsen, Henning, ed. *Sophie Brahes Regnskabsbog 1627-40.* Århus: Jysk selskab for historie, sprog, og litteratur, 1955.

Penotus (B. G. a Portu Aquitano). See Hester, John. *A hundred and fourtene experiments.*

Petræus, Heinrich. *Nosologia harmonica.* Marburg, 1614-16.

Philiatros, or The Copie of an Epistle, wherein sundry fitting considerations are propounded by a young Student of Physicke. London, 1615.

Primerose, James. *Popular Errours or the Errours of the People in Physick.* Trans. Robert Wittie. London: Wilson, 1651.

Quercetanus, (Joseph Duchesne). *A Breefe Aunswere of Iosephus Quercetanus to the Exposition of Iacobus Aubertus Vindonis concerning the Original and Causes of Metalles.* Trans. John Hester. London, 1591.

—. *Centum quindecim curationes experimentaque.* See Hester, John. *A hundred and fourtene experiments.*

—. *Ad Iacobi Auberti ... responsio.* Lyons, 1575.

—. *Liber de priscorum philosophorum veræ medicinæ materia.* Geneva: Vignon, 1603.

—. *Spagericke Antidotarie for Gunshot.* See Hester, John. *A hundred and fourtene experiments.*

Raicus, Johannes. *De Phthisi ex Tartaro.* Uppsala: Eskil Mattson, 1628.

Resen, Peder Hansen. *Inscriptiones Hafniensis Latinæ.* Copenhagen: Godicchenius, 1668.

—. *Kong Frederichs den Andens Krønicke.* Copenhagen, 1680.

Reusnerus, Hieronymus. *Diexodicarum exercitationum liber de scorbuto.* Frankfurt: Patheniana, 1600.

Rhodius, Ambrosius (the elder). *Optica.* Wittenberg: Sauberlich, 1611.

Rhodius, Ambrosius. *Dialogus de transmigratione animarum Pythagorica.* Copenhagen: Sartorius, 1638.

—. *Disputatio astrologica de astrorum influxu, quomodo homines ad certas constellationes morbis fiant obnoxij.* Copenhagen, 1635.

—. *Disputationes supra Ideam medicinæ philosphicæ Petri Severini Dani Philosophi & Friderici II Daniæ & Septentrionalis Regis Archiatri olim felicissimi, Quibus loca illius Libri obscura & difficilia illustrantur, adversarij refutantur, & multi discursus ex intimis Naturæ adytis deprompti moventur.* Copenhagen: Sartorius, 1643.

—. *Supra visiones anno 1657.* Christiania (Oslo), 1660. Reprinted in E. Ingerslev, *Ambrosius Rhodius.*

—. *Theses medicæ de scorbuto.* Copenhagen: Salomon Sartorius, 1635.

Roberts, Julian, and Andrew G. Watson, eds. *John Dee's Library Catalogue.* London: The Bibliographical Society, 1990.

Rørdam, Holger F., ed. "Bidrag til de filippistiske Bevægelsens og til D. Niels Hemmingsens Historie." *[Ny] Kirkehistoriske Samlinger* 2d ser., 4 (1867-68): 252-326.

—. "Efterretninger om Frederik den Andens Bibel." *[Ny] Kirkehistoriske Samlinger* 2d ser., 1 (1857-59): 203-221.

—. "M. Morten Pedersens historiske Kalenderantegnelser." *[Ny] Kirkehistoriske Samlinger* 2d ser., 3 (1864-66): 483-505.

—. "Uddrag av Acta Consistorii 1573-80, især angaaende D. Niels Hemmingsen." In "Bidrag til de filippistiske Bevægelsens og til D. Niels Hemmingsens Historie." *[Ny] Kirkehistoriske Samlinger* 2d ser., 4 (1867-68): 252-326.

—. "Uddrag af Konsistoriets Forhandlinger 1543-1599." *[Ny] Kirkehistoriske Samlinger* 2d ser., 1 (1857-59): 3-67.

—. "Uddrag af Konsistoriets Forhandlinger 1590-1599." *[Ny] Kirkehistoriske Samlinger* 2d ser., 5 (1869-71): 63-118.

—. "Uddrag af Præsten Christiern Nielsen Juels Aarbog." *[Ny] Kirkehistoriske Samlinger* 2d ser., 5 (1869-71): 342-377.

Ryga, George. *Two Plays: Paracelsus and Prometheus Bound.* Winnepeg, Manitoba: Turnstone Press, 1982.

Seip, Jens Arup, ed. *Dombok for 1661*. Vol. 2 of *Norske Herredags-Dombøger.* 4th series (1652-1664). Oslo: Norsk Historisk Kjeldeskrift-Institutt, 1945. Contains the high court case records against Anna and Ambrosius Rhodius.

Sendivogius, Michael. *Novum lumen chymicum, e natura fonte et manuali experienta depromptum.* Cologne, 1614.

Sennert, Daniel. *De chymicorum cum Aristotelicis et Galenicis consensu ac dissensu liber.* Wittenberg, 1619.

Severinus, Petrus (Peder Sørensen). *Epistola scripta Theophrasto Paracelso, in qua ratio ordinis et nominum, adeoque totius Philosophiæ Adeptæ methodus compendiose et erudite ostenditur a Petro Severino Dano Philosophiæ et Medicinæ Doctore.* Basel: Henric Petri, [1570?]. Reprinted in Paracelsus, *Opera omnia* (1658).

—. *Idea medicinæ philosophicæ fundamenta continens totius doctrinæ Paracelsicæ, Hippocraticæ et Galenicæ.* Basel: Henric Petri, 1571; 2nd ed., Erfurt; 3rd ed., The Hague: Vlacq, 1660.

Simpson, William. *Hydrologia Chymica.* London, 1669.

—. *Philosophical Dialogues.* London: T. Hodgkin, 1677.

—. *Zymologia Physica.* London, 1675.

Sperling, Otto. "Ottho Sperlings Levnet." *Nye Samlinger til den danske Historie* 3 (1792-95): 197-226.

—. *Selvbiografi 1602-1673.* Ed. Sophus Birket Smith. Copenhagen, 1885.

Statholderskabets Extraktprotokol af Supplicationer og Resolutioner 1642-1650. Vol. 1 (1642-1646). Christiania (Oslo): Det Norske Rigsarkiv, 1906.

Statholderskabets Extraktprotokol af Supplicationer og Resolutioner 1662-1669. Vol. 1 (1662-1664). Christiania (Oslo): Det Norske Rigsarkiv, 1910.

Stockfleth, Henning. *De Sande Leffuendes Liv oc Løn (Likpreken over Greggers Krabbe 1656).* Søro: Georg Hantssch, 1656.

Sudhoff, Karl. *Theophrast von Hohenheim genannt Paracelsus Sämliche Werke.* Vol. 10. Munich: Oldenbourg, 1928.

Sydenham, Thomas. *The Works of Thomas Sydenham, M.D.*, trans. R. G. Latham. Vol. 1. London: The Sydenham Society, 1848.

"Tychonis Brahe, Ioh. Pratensis, … Epistolæ ad Petrum Severinum." In *Altes und Neues von Gelehrten Sachen aus Dännemark.* Vol. 2. Copenhagen and Leiden, 1768.

Toepke, Gustav, ed. *Die Matrikel der Universität Heidelberg von 1386- bis 1662.* Vol. 2. Heidelberg, 1886.

W., I. *The copie of a letter sent by a learned Physician to his friend, wherein are detected the manifold errors used hitherto of the Apothecaries.* London, 1586.

Wackernagel, H.G., ed. *Die Matrikel Der Universität Basel.* Vol. 2 (1532/3-1600/1). Basel: Universitätsbibliothek, 1956.

Wad, Gustav Ludvig, ed. *Breve til og fra Herluf Trolle og Birgitte Gjøe.* 2 vols. Copenhagen: Thaning & Appel, 1893.

Webster, John. *The Displaying of Supposed Witchcraft.* London: J.M., 1677.

—. *Metallographia: Or, An History of Metals.* London: A.C., 1671.

Wessel, A. B. *Gamle Breve som Aktstikker til Finmarkens Historie.* Tromsø: Nordlys, 1617.

Wier, Johannes (Weyer). *De præstigiis dæmonum et incantantibus, ac veneficiis.* Basel: Oporinus, 1563.

——. *Witches, Devils, and Doctors in the Renaissance: Johann Weyer, De præstigiis dæmonum.* Trans. John Shea. Binghamton, NY: Medieval & Renaissance Texts & Studies, 1991.

Wimpinæus, Johannes Albertus. *De concordia Hippocraticorum et Paracelsistarum libri magni excursiones defensivæ.* Munich: Adam Berg, 1569; Strasbourg, 1615.

Worm, Ole. *Breve fra og til Ole Worm.* Ed. H. D. Schepelern. 3 vols. Copenhagen: Det danske sprog- og litteraturselskab, 1965-68.

——. *Laurea philosophica summa.* Copenhagen: Henrik Waldkirch, 1619.

——. *Olai Wormii et ad eum Doctorum Virorum Epistolæ.* Ed. Hans Gram. Copenhagen, 1751.

——. *Questiones miscellarum decas.* Copenhagen, 1622.

Zetzner, Lazarus, ed. *Theatrum Chemicum.* Vol 2. Argentorati, 1659.

Zwinger, Jacob. *Principiorum chymicorum examen ad generalem Hippocratis, Galeni cæterorumque Græcorum et Arabum consensum institutum.* Basel, 1606.

Secondary Sources

Aggebo, Anker. "Hans Philipsen Pratensis 1543-76." *Arosia* 17, no. 1. Århus, 1938.

Andersen, Birte. *Adelig Opfostring: Adelsbørns opdragelse i Danmark 1536-1660.* Copenhagen: Gad, 1971.

Applebaum, Wilbur, ed. *Encyclopedia of the Scientific Revolution From Copernicus to Newton.* New York: Garland, 2000.

Armstrong, A.H. *The Architecture of the Intelligible Universe in the Philosophy of Plotinus.* Cambridge: Cambridge University Press, 1940.

Arnold, Gottfried. *Unpartheyische Kirchen- und Ketzer-Historie.* Vol. 4. Frankfurt: Frisch, 1729.

Bastholm, Eyvind, and Hans Skov. *Petrus Severinus og hans Idea medicinae philosophicae.* Acta historica scientiarum naturalium et medicinalium, vol. 32. Odense: Odense Universitetsforlag, 1979.

Berg, Jens Christian. "Efterretninger om det af Kong Christian den Fjerde stiftede Gymnasium i Christiania, og sammes Lærere." In *Budstikken, et Maanedsskrift* (Christiania) 2d ser., 3. Oslo: Grøndahl, 1822.

Berggrav, Jan. *Oslo Katedralskole: Schola Osloensis gjennom 800 Aar.* Oslo: Gyldendal, 1953.

Bianchi, Massimo L. "The Visible and the Invisible from Alchemy to Paracelsus." In *Alchemy and Chemistry in the 16th and 17th Centuries*, ed. Piyo Rattansi and Antonio Clericuzio, pp. 17-50. International Archives of the History of Ideas, vol. 140. Dordrecht: Kluwer, 1994.

Biographie Universelle, Ancienne et Moderne. Vol. 20. Paris: Michaud, 1817.

Birkeland, Michael. "Ambrosius Rhodius." In *M. Birckeland Historiske Skrifter,* ed. Fr. Ording. Vol. 3, pp. 220-247. Oslo: Den norske historiske Forening, 1925.

Blair, Ann. "Mosaic Physics and the Search for a Pious Natural Philosophy in the Late Renaissance." *Isis* 91(2000): 32-58.

Bloch, Olivier Rene. *La Philosophie de Gassendi: Nominalisme, Materialisme et Metaphysique.* International Archives of the History of Ideas, vol. 38. Den Haag: Martinus Nijhoff, 1971.

Brady, Jules M. "St. Augustine's Theory of Seminal Reasons." *New Scholasticism* 38 (1964): 141-58.

Breger, Herbert. "Elias Artista: A Precursor of the Messiah in Natural Science." In *Nineteen Eighty-Four; Science between Utopia and Dystopia.* Sociology of Science, vol. 8. Dordrecht: Reidel, 1984.

Bricka, C.F. "Fortegnelse over Danske og Norske, som ere Immatrikulerede ved Leydens Universitet i det første Aarhundrede af dets Bestaaen (1575-1674)." *Personalhistorisk Tidsskrift* 1st ser., 2 (1881): 104-135.

Brickman, Benjamin. "An Introduction to Francesco Patrizi's *Nova de universis philosophia.*" Ph.D. Diss., Columbia University, 1941.

Broeckx, C. "Le Premier Ouvrage de J.-B. van Helmont, Seigneur de Mérode, Royenborch, Oirschot, Pellines, etc., Publié pour La Première Fois." *Annales de L'Académie D'Archéologie de Belgique* 10 (1853): 327-392; 11 (1854): 119-191.

Bull, Edvard. "En Læge i det ældste Kristiania: Mag. Ambrosius Rhodius' bo." *St. Halvard, Tidsskrift for Oslos By og Kristianias Historie* 4 (1920): 261-75.

—. *Kristianias Historie.* Vol. 2 (1624-1740). Oslo: Cappelen, 1927.

Bull, Francis. *Norges Litteratur Historie.* Vol. 2. Oslo: Aschehoug, 1928.

Burckhardt, Albrecht. *Geschichte der Medizinischen Fakultät zu Basel 1460-1900.* Basel: Universitatsdruckerei, 1917.

Cadden, Joan. *Meanings of Sex Difference in the Middle Ages: Medicine, Science, and Culture.* Cambridge: Cambridge University Press, 1993.

Cedergreen Bech, Svend, ed. *Københavns Historie.* Vol. 2. Copenhagen: Gyldendal, 1980.

Christensen, Tagea Egede. "Bibliographia Borrichiana." In *Mindeskrift for Oluf Borch paa 300 aarsdagen for hans fødsel,* ed. Vilhelm Maar, pp. 37-64. Copenhagen: Arnold Busck, 1926.

Christiansen, Carl S. "Udsigt over en Del af Brevstoffet i Jens Bircherods Dagbøger." *Personalhistoriske Tidsskrift* 3d ser., 3 (1894): 131-140, 194-214.

Christianson, John R. "Cloister and Observatory: Herrevad Abbey and Tycho Brahe's Uranienborg." Ph.D. Diss., University of Minnesota, 1964.

—. *On Tycho's Island: Tycho Brahe and His Assistants, 1570-1601.* Cambridge: Cambridge University Press, 2000.

—. "Tycho Brahe at the University of Copenhagen, 1559-1562." *Isis* 58 (1967): 198-203.

—. "Tycho Brahe: Past and Future Research." *History of Science* 11 (1973): 270-282.

—. "Tycho Brahe's German Treatise on the Comet of 1577: A Study in Science and Politics." *Isis* 70 (1979): 110-40.

Clemedson, Carl-Johan. "Något om Tycho Brahe och hans medicinska verksamhet." In *Sydsvenska medicinhistoriska sällskapets årsskrift 1972*, pp. 38-59. Lund: Sydsvenska medicinhistoriska sällskapet, 1972.

Clericuzio, Antonio. "A Redefinition of Boyle's Chemistry and Corpuscular Philosophy." *Annals of Science* 47 (1990): 561-589.

—. "From Van Helmont to Boyle: A Study in the Transmission of Helmontian Chemical and Medical Theories in Seventeenth-Century England." *British Journal for the History of Science* 26 (1993): 303-334.

—. "Robert Boyle and the English Helmontians." In *Alchemy Revisited*, ed. Z. R. W. M. van Martels, pp. 192-99. Proceedings of the international conference on the history of alchemy at the University of Groningen 17-19 April 1989. Leiden: Brill, 1990.

Clulee, Nicholas. *John Dee's Natural Philosophy: Between Science and Religion*. London: Routledge, 1988.

Cohen, I. Bernard. *Revolution in Science*. Cambridge, Massachussets: Harvard University Press, 1985.

Cold, Daniel Henrik Otto. *Lægevæsenet og Lægerne under Christian IV's Regiering (1588-1648)*. Copenhagen: C.G. Iversen, 1858.

Collett, Alf. *Gamle Christiania-Billeder*. Christiania (Oslo): Cappelen, 1893.

Cook, Harold J. *The Decline of the Old Medical Regime in Stuart London*. Ithaca, New York: Cornell University Press, 1986.

Copleston, Fredrick. *A History of Philosophy*. Vol. 2, pt. 1. 1950; reprint, Garden City, New York: Doubleday, Image Books, 1962.

Coucheron, P. "Om Mag. Niels Svendsen Krønikes Stridigheder med Præsteskabet i Christiania i Aarene 1642-1652." *Theologisk Tidsskrift for Den Evangelisk-Lutherske Kirke i Norge* 1 (1858): 234-98; and 2 (1859): 46-67. Christiania: P. T. Malling, 1858-59.

Daae, Ludvig. *Det Gamle Christiania 1624-1814*. Christiania (Oslo): Cappelen, 1891.

Debus, Allen G. "The Chemical Debates of the Seventeenth Century: The Reaction to Robert Fludd and Jean Baptiste van Helmont." In *Reason, Experiment, and Mysticism in the Scientific Revolution*, ed. M. L. Righini Bonelli and William R. Shea, pp. 18-47. New York, 1975.

—. "The Chemical Philosophers: Chemical Medicine from Paracelsus to Van Helmont." *History of Science* 12 (1974): 235-259.

—. *The Chemical Philosophy: Paracelsian Science and Medicine in the Sixteenth and Seventeenth Centuries*. 2 Vols. New York: Science History Publications, 1977.

—. "Edward Jorden and the Fermentation of Metals: An Iatrochemical Study of Terrestrial Phenomena." In *Toward a History of Geology*, ed. Cecil J. Schneer, pp. 100-121. Proceedings of the New Hampshire Inter-Disciplinary Conference on the History of Geology, September 7-12, 1967. Cambridge, MA: MIT Press, 1968.

—. *The English Paracelsians*. London: Oldbourne, 1965.

—. *The French Paracelsians: The Chemical Challenge to Medical and Scientific Tradition in Early Modern France*. Cambridge: Cambridge University Press, 1991.

—. *Man and Nature in the Renaissance.* 1978; reprint, Cambridge: Cambridge University Press, 1986.

—. "Mathematics and Nature in the Chemical Texts of the Renaissance." *Ambix* 15 (1968): 1-28.

—. "The Paracelsian Compromise in Elizabethan England." *Ambix* 10 (1962): 108-18.

—. *Science and Education in the Seventeenth Century. The Webster Ward Debate.* London: Macdonald; New York: American Elsevier, 1970.

—. "The Significance of Chemical History." *Ambix* 32 (1985): 1-14.

Debus, Allen G., ed. *Science, Medicine, and Society in the Renaissance; Essays to Honor Walter Pagel.* New York: Science History Publications, 1972.

Debus, Allen G. and Michael T. Walton, eds. *Reading the Book of Nature: The Other Side of the Scientific Revolution.* Sixteenth Century Essays and Studies, vol. 41. Kirksville, Missouri: Sixteenth Century Journal Publishers, Inc., 1998.

Degn, Ole. *Rig og fattig i Ribe: Økonomiske og sociale forhold i Ribe-samfundet 1560-1660.* Aarhus: Universitetsforlaget, 1981.

—. *Ribe 1500-1950.* Trans. Shiela and Jørgen Peder Clausager. Scandinavian Atlas of Historic Towns, vol. 3. Odense: Odense University Press, 1983.

Deurs, C. van. "Dr. med. Cold's Afhandling for Doctorgraden: 'Lægevæsenet og Lægerne under Christian den 4des Regjering'." *Bibliothek for Læger* 4th ser., 14 (January-April, 1859): 168-213.

Dreyer, John Louis Emil. *Tycho Brahe: A Picture of Scientific Life and Work in the Sixteenth Century.* Edinburgh: Adam and Charles Black, 1890.

Eamon, William. "Arcana Disclosed: The Advent of Printing, the Books of Secrets Tradition and the Development of Experimental Science in the Sixteenth Century." *History of Science* 22 (1984): 11-150.

—. "From the Secrets of Nature to Public Knowledge." In *Reappraisals of the Scientific Revolution,* ed. David C. Lindberg and Robert S. Westman, pp. 333-365. Cambridge: Cambridge University Press, 1990.

—. *Science and the Secrets of Nature: Books of Secrets in Medieval and Early Modern Culture.* Princeton: Princeton University Press, 1994.

Ehrencron-Müller, H., ed. *Forfatter-lexikon omfattende Danmark, Norge og Island indtill 1814.* 13 vols. Copenhagen: Aschehoug, 1924-39.

Elmer, Peter. "The Library of Dr. John Webster: The Making of a Seventeenth-Century Radical." *Medical History* Supp. 6. London: Wellcome Institute for the History of Medicine, 1986.

Emerton, Norma. "Creation in the Thought of J.B. van Helmont and Robert Fludd." In *Alchemy and Chemistry in the 16th and 17th Centuries,* ed. Piyo Rattansi and Antonio Clericuzio, pp. 85-101. International Archives of the History of Ideas, vol. 140. Dordrecht: Kluwer, 1994.

"En Statsfange på Akershus." *St. Halvard* 28, no. 5 (1950): 2-18.

Evans, R.J.W. *Rudolf II and His World.* Oxford: Clarendon, 1973.

Farrington, Benjamin. *The Philosophy of Francis Bacon.* Liverpool: Liverpool University Press, 1964.

Faxe, W. Ekdahl. *Forlemningar af Tycho Brahes Stjerneborg och Uranienborg på Ön Hven, aftäckte åren 1823 och 1824.* Stockholm: Johan Hørberg, 1824.

Ferguson, John. *Bibliotheca Chemica: A Catalogue of the Alchemical, Chemical and Pharmaceutical Books in the Collection of the Late James Young.* 2 vols. Glasgow: Maclehose, 1906.

Ferrari, Marco. "Alcune vie di diffusione in Italia di idee e di testi di Paracelso." In *Scienze, Credenze Occulte, Livelli di Cultura. Convegno Internazionali di Studi (Firenze, 25-30 Giugno 1980),* pp. 21-29. Florence: Olschki, 1982.

Feustking, Johann Heinrich. *Gynaeceum Haeretico Fanaticum.* Frankfurt and Leipzig: Christian Gerdes, 1704.

Figala, Karin. "Tycho Brahes Elixir." *Annals of Science* 28 (1972): 139-176.

Findlen, Paula. "The Economy of Scientific Exchange in Early Modern Italy." In *Patronage and Institutions: Science, Technology, and Medicine at the European Court 1500-1750,* ed. Bruce T. Moran, pp. 5-24. Woodbridge, Suffolk: Boydell, 1991.

—. "Jokes of Nature and Jokes of Knowledge: The Playfulness of Scientific Discourse in Early Modern Europe." *Renaissance Quarterly* 43 (1990): 292-331.

Fjelstrup, August. *Dr. Peter Payngk: Kong Kristian IV's Hofkemiker.* Copenhagen: A. Giese, 1911.

—. *Guldmagere i Danmark i det XVII Aarhundrede.* Copenhagen: Branner, 1906.

Flood, Bruce P. "The Medieval Herbal Tradition of Macer Floridus." *Pharmacy in History* 18 (1976): 62-66.

Flood, Ingeborg and Leif Brendel, eds. *Norges Apotek og Deres Innehavere.* Vol. 3. Oslo: A. W. Brøgger, 1954.

Flood, Jørgen. *Norges Apothekere i 300 Aar (1588-1889).* Christiania (Oslo): Brøgger, 1889.

Fordyce, C. J., and T. M. Knox. "The Library of Jesus College, Oxford; With an Appendix on the Books Bequeathed Thereto by Lord Herbert of Cherbury." In *Oxford Bibliographical Society; Proceedings and Papers.* Vol. 5, pt. 2. Oxford: Oxford University Press, 1937.

Frank, Robert G. *Harvey and the Oxford Physiologists: Scientific Ideas and Social Interactions.* Berkeley: University of California Press, 1980.

Fredericia, J.A. *Adelsvældens Sidste Dage: Danmarks Historie fra Christian IV's Død til Enevældens Indførelse (1648-1660).* 1894; reprint, Copenhagen: Selskabet for udgivelse af kilder til dansk historie, 1969.

French, Peter J. *John Dee: The World of an Elizabethan Magus.* London: Routledge and Kegan Paul, 1972.

Friedensburg, Walter. *Geschichte der Universität Wittenberg.* Halle: Max Niemeyer, 1917.

Friis, Frederik R. "Et par optegnelser om Uraniborg 1894, Kjøbenhavn." In Kgl. Bibl. Copenhagen, "Afhandlinger om Tycho Brahe, Samlet af J. Dreyer".

—. *Peder Jakobsen Flemløs, Tyge Brahes første Medhjælper, og hans Observationer i Norge.* Copenhagen: Gad, 1904.

—. *Sophie Brahe Ottesdatter.* Copenhagen: Gad, 1905.

—. *Tyge Brahe: En Historisk Fremstilling.* Copenhagen: Gyldendal, 1871.

Friis, Oluf. *Den Danske Litteraturs Historie.* Vol. 1. Copenhagen: Hirschsprung, 1945.

Galluzzi, Paolo. "Motivi Paracelsiani nella Toscana di Cosimo II e di Don Antonio Dei Medici: alchimia, medicina 'chimica' e riforma del sapere." In *Scienze, Credenze Occulte, Livelli di Cultura*, pp. 31-62. Florence: Olschki, 1982.

Garstein, Oskar. *Cort Aslakssøn: studier over dansk-norsk universitets- og lærdomshistorie omkring år 1600*. Oslo: Lutherstiftelse, 1953.

Gascoigne, John. "A Reappraisal of the Role of the Universities in the Scientific Revolution." In *Reappraisals of the Scientific Revolution*, ed. David C. Lindberg and Robert S. Westman, pp. 207-260. Cambridge: Cambridge University Press, 1990.

Gaunø-Jensen, V. "Wilhelm Reymann: Undersøgelser over Peder Sørensens Liv og Lære." *Bibliotek for Laeger* 166 (1974): 105-131.

Gelbart, Nina Rattner. "The Intellectual Development of Walter Charleton." *Ambix* 18 (1971): 149-68.

Gilly, Carlos, "'Theophrastia Sancta' – Paracelsianism as a Religion, in Conflict with the Established Churches." In *Paracelsus. The Man and His Reputation, His Ideas and Their Transformation*, ed. Ole Peter Grell, pp. 151-185. Leiden: Brill, 1998.

Greengrass, Mark, Michael Leslie, and Timothy Raylor, eds. *Samuel Hartlib and Universal Reformation: Studies in Intellectual Communication*. Cambridge: Cambridge University Press, 1994.

Grell, Ole Peter, ed. *Paracelsus. The Man and His Reputation, His Ideas and Their Transformation*. Leiden: Brill, 1998.

Grimm, Harold J. *The Reformation Era 1500-1650*. New York: Macmillan, 1954.

Guerlac, Henry. "Guy de La Brosse and the French Paracelsians." In *Science, Medicine and Society in the Renaissance*, ed. Allen G. Debus, pp. 177-199. New York: Science History Publications, 1972.

Gunnoe, Charles, Jr. "Erastus and Paracelsianism: Theological Motifs in Thomas Erastus' Rejection of Paracelsian Natural Philosophy." In *Reading the Book of Nature: The Other Side of the Scientific Revolution*, ed. Allen G. Debus and Michael T. Walton, pp. 45-65. Sixteenth Century Essays and Studies, vol. 41. Kirksville, Missouri: Sixteenth Century Journal Publishers, Inc., 1998.

—. "Thomas Erastus and his Circle of Anti-Paracelsians." In *Analecta Paracelsica: Studien zum Nachleben Theophrast von Hohenheims im deutschen Kulturgebiet der frühen Neuzeit*, ed. Joachim Telle, pp. 127-48. Heidelberger Studien zur Naturkunde der frühen Neuzeit 4. Stuttgart: Franz Steiner, 1994.

Haeser, Heinrich. *Lehrbuch der Geschichte der Medicin und der epidemischen Krankheiten*. Jena: Gustav Fischer, 1881.

Hankins, James. *Plato in the Italian Renaissance*. 2 vols. Leiden: Brill, 1990.

Hannaway, Owen. *The Chemists and the Word: The Didactic Origins of Chemistry*. Baltimore: Johns Hopkins, 1975.

—. "Laboratory Design and the Aim of Science." *Isis* 77 (1986): 585-610.

Harkness, Deborah E. *John Dee's Conversations with Angels: Cabala, Alchemy, and the End of Nature*. Cambridge: Cambridge University Press, 1999.

Harrison, John. *The Library of Isaac Newton*. Cambridge: Cambridge University Press, 1978.

Hauberg, Poul. "Tycho Brahes Opskrifter paa Lægemidler." *Dansk Tidsskrift for Farmaci* 1, no. 6 (December 1926): 205-212.

Heiberg, Johan Ludvig. *Johan Ludvig Heibergs Prosaiske Skrifter.* Vol. 9. Copenhagen: Reitzel, 1861.

Heidorn, Günter, Gerhard Heitz, Johannes Kalisch, et al., eds. *Geschichte der Universität Rostock 1419-1969.* Berlin: Deutscher Verlag der Wissenschaften, 1969.

Henry, John. "Occult Qualities and the Experimental Philosophy: Active Principles in Pre-Newtonian Matter Theory." *History of Science* 24 (1986): 335-381.

Herholdt, Johan Daniel. "Om Professores medicinæ ved Kjøbenhavns Universitet fra dets Stiftelse af i Aaret 1478 indtil 1588." *Archiv for Lægevidenskabens Historie i Danmark.* Vol. 1. Copenhagen, 1823.

Herholdt, Johan Daniel, and Frederik V. Mansa, eds. *Samlinger til den danske Medicinal-Historie.* Vol. 1. Copenhagen: Gyldendal, 1835.

Høigård, Einar. *Oslo Katedralskoles Historie.* Oslo: Grøndahl, 1942.

Hofmeister, Adolph, ed. *Die Matrikel der Universität Rostock.* Rostock, 1889.

Howard, Rio. *Guy de la Brosse: The Founder of the Jardin des Plantes in Paris.* Ann Arbor, Michigan: University Microfilms International, 1981.

Hovesen, Ejnar. *Lægen Ole Worm 1588-1654: En medicinhistorisk undersøgelse og vurdering.* Aarhus: Aarhus Universitetsforlag, 1987.

Hvolbek, Russell H. "Seventeenth Century Dialogues: Jacob Boehme and the New Sciences." Ph. D. Diss., University of Chicago, 1984.

Ingerslev, Emmerich. "Ambrosius Rhodius og Hans Hustru." *Medicinsk-Historiske Smaaskrifter,* ed. Ed. Vilhelm Maar. Vol. 14. Copenhagen: Vilhelm Tryde, 1916.

Ingerslev, Vilhelm. *Danmarks Læger og Lægevæsen fra de ældste Tider indtil Aar 1800.* Vol. 1. Copenhagen: E. Jespersen, 1873.

Jensen, Christian Axel. *Riberhus Slotsbanke.* Copenhagen: Gyldendal, 1942.

Jones, Rufus M. *Spiritual Reformers in the 16th and 17th Centuries.* London: Macmillan & Co., 1914.

Kästner, A.G. "Ambrosius Rhodius." *Geschichte der Mathematic.* Gøttingen, 1800.

Kaplan, Barbara Beigun. *"Divulging of Useful Truths in Physick." The Medical Agenda of Robert Boyle.* Baltimore: Johns Hopkins, 1993.

Koch, E. F. *Oluf Borck, en literærhistorisk-biografisk Skildring.* Copenhagen: Jacob Lund, 1866.

Kocher, Paul H. "John Hester, Paracelsian (fl. 1576-93)." In *Joseph Quincy Adams Memorial Studies,* ed. James G. McManaway, Giles E. Dawson, and Edwin E. Willoughby, pp. 621-38. Washington: The Folger Shakespeare Library, 1948.

—. "Paracelsian Medicine in England: The First Thirty Years (ca. 1570-1600)." *Journal of the History of Medicine* 2 (1947): 451-480.

Kornerup, Bjørn. *Biskop Hans Poulsen Resen: Studier over Kirke- og Skolehistorie i det 16. og 17. Aarhundrede.* Vol. 1. Copenhagen: Gad, 1928.

—. "Cort Aslaksen. I Anledning af Oskar Garsteins Disputats," *Kirkehistoriske Samlinger,* 7th ser., 2 (1954-56): 346-84.

—. *Ribe Katedralskoles Historie: Studier over 800 Aars dansk Skolehistorie.* 2 vols. Copenhagen: Gyldendal, 1947 & 1952.

Kornerup, Bjørn, and Hal Koch, eds. *Den Danske Kirkes Historie.* Vol. 4. Copenhagen: Gyldendal, 1959.

Krabbe, Otto. *Die Universität Rostock in fünfzehnten und sechzehnten Jahrhundert.* Rostock: Stiller, 1854.

Krause. "Levinus Battus." *Allgemeine Deutsche Biographie.* Vol. 2, p. 135. 2d ed. Berlin: Duncker & Humbolt, 1967.

Kristeller, Paul Oskar. *Eight Philosophers of the Italian Renaissance.* Stanford, CA: Stanford University Press, 1964.

Lessing, Michael Benedict. *Handbuch der Geschichte der Medizin.* Vol. 1. Berlin: August Hirschwald, 1839.

Lind, H.D. *Kong Kristian Den Fjerde og Hans Mænd paa Bremerholm.* 1889; reprint, Copenhagen, 1974.

Lindberg, David C. "The Genesis of Kepler's Theory of Light: Light Metaphysics from Plotinus to Kepler." *Osiris* 2d ser., 2 (1986): 5-42.

Lindberg, David C. and Robert Westman, eds. *Reappraisals of the Scientific Revolution.* Cambridge: Cambridge University Press, 1990.

Lindroth, Sten. "Hiärne, Block och Paracelsus. En redogörelse för Paracelsusstriden 1708-09." *Lychnos*, 1941, 191-292.

—. *Paracelsismen i Sverige till 1600-tallets mitt.* Lychnos Bibliotek 7. Uppsala: Almqvist & Wiksell, 1943.

—. "Urban Hiärne och Laboratorium chymicum." *Lychnos*, 1946-47, 51-116.

Lonie, I. M. "The 'Paris Hippocratics': teaching and research in Paris in the sixteenth century." In *The Medical Renaissance of the Sixteenth Century*, ed. A. Wear, R.K. French, and I. M. Lonie, pp. 155-174. Cambridge: Cambridge University Press, 1985.

Louthan, Howard. *The Quest for Compromise: Peacemakers in Counter-Reformation Vienna.* Cambridge: Cambridge University Press, 1997.

Marek, Jiri. "The response to Kepler's book *Ad Vitellionem* … in the thesis of Daniel Conrad in 1608." *Atti Fondazione Giorgio Ronchi* 23 (1968): 352-362.

Matthiessen, Hugo. *Gamle Huse i Ribe.* Copenhagen: Reitzel, 1937.

McKeough, Michael J. "The Meaning of Rationes Seminales in St. Augustine." Ph.D. Diss., Catholic University of America, 1926.

Meinel, Christoph. "Early Seventeenth-Century Atomism: Theory, Epistemology, and the Insufficiency of Experiment." *Isis* 79 (1988): 68-103.

Mejborg, Reinhold. *Borgerlige Huse, særlig Kjøbenhavns Professor-Residentser 1540-1630.* Copenhagen: Gad, 1881.

Michel, P.H. *The Cosmology of Giordano Bruno.* Trans. R.E.W. Maddison. Paris: Hermann, 1973.

Møller-Christensen, Vilhelm. "Steno's Copenhagen." *Analecta Medico-Historica* 3 (1968): 97-108.

Møller-Christensen, Vilhelm, and Albert Gjedde. "Det medicinske Fakultet 1479-1842." In *Københavns Universitet 1479-1979*, ed. J. Melchior, et al. Vol. 7. *Det Lægevidenskabelige Fakultet*. Copenhagen: Gad, 1979.

Moesgaard, Kristian. "Cosmology in the Wake of Tycho Brahe's Astronomy." In *Cosmology, History, and Theology*, ed. Wolfgang Yourgrau and Allen D. Breck, pp. 293-305. New York: Plenum, 1977.

Moran, Bruce T. *The Alchemical World of the German Court: Occult Philosophy and Chemical Medicine in the Circle of Moritz of Hessen (1572-1632)*. Stuttgart: Franz Steiner, 1991.

—. "Der alchemistisch-paracelsische Kreis um den Landgrafen Moritz von Hessen-Kassel (1572-1632)." *Salzburger Beiträge zur Paracelsusforschung* 25 (1987): 119-45.

—. *Chemical Pharmacy Enters the University: Johannes Hartmann and the Didactic Care of Chymiatria in the Early Seventeenth Century*. Madison, WI: The American Institute of the History of Pharmacy, 1991.

—. "Court Authority and Chemical Medicine: Moritz of Hessen, Johannes Hartmann, and the Origin of Academic Chemiatria." *Bulletin of the History of Medicine* 63 (1989): 225-46.

—. "Libavius the Paracelsian? Monstrous Novelties, Institutions, and the Norms of Social Value." In *Reading the Book of Nature: The Other Side of the Scientific Revolution*, ed. Allen G. Debus and Michael T. Walton, pp. 67-79. Sixteenth Century Essays and Studies, vol. 41. Kirksville, Missouri: Sixteenth Century Journal Publishers, Inc., 1998.

—. "Privilege, Communication, and Chemistry: The Hermetic-Alchemical Circle of Moritz of Hessen-Kassel." *Ambix* 32 (1985): 110-26.

—. "Wilhelm IV of Hessen-Kassel: Informal Communication and the Aristocratic Context of Discovery." In *Scientific Discovery: Case Studies*, ed. Thomas Nickles, pp. 67-96. Dordrecht: Reidel, 1980.

Moran, Bruce T., ed. *Patronage and Institutions: Science, Technology, and Medicine at the European Court 1500-1750*. Woodbridge, Suffolk: Boydell, 1991.

Multhauf, Robert. "Medical Chemistry and 'The Paracelsians'." *Bulletin of the History of Medicine* 28 (1954): 101-26.

Næss, Hans Eyvind. *Trolldomsprosessene i Norge pa 1500-1600 tallet: en retts- og sosialhistorisk undersøgelse*. Oslo: Universitetsforlaget, 1982.

Neander, Gustav. *Ur Lungsotens och Lungsotsbehandlingens äldre Historia i Sverige*. Stockholm: Norstedt, 1924.

Newman, William R. "The Alchemical Sources of Robert Boyle's Corpuscular Philosophy." *Annals of Science* 53 (1996): 567-585.

—. "Alchemical Symbolism and Concealment: The Chemical House of Libavius." In *The Architecture of Science*, ed. Peter Galison and Emily Thompson, pp. 59-77. Cambridge, MA: MIT Press, 1999.

—. "Boyle's Debt to Corpuscular Alchemy." In *Robert Boyle Reconsidered*, ed. Michael Hunter, pp. 107-117. Cambridge: Cambridge University Press, 1994.

—. "The Corpuscular Theory of J. B. Van Helmont and its Medieval Sources." *Vivarium* 31 (1993): 161-191.

—. *Gehennical Fire: The Lives of George Starkey, an American Alchemist in the Scientific Revolution*. Cambridge, Massachusetts: Harvard University Press, 1994.

Nicholl, Charles. *The Chemical Theatre*. London: Routledge and Kegan Paul, 1980.

Niebyl, Peter. "Sennert, Van Helmont, and Medical Ontology." *Bulletin of the History of Medicine* 45 (1971): 115-37.

Nielsen, Lauritz. *Danmarks Middelalderlige Haandskrifter*. Copenhagen: Gyldendal, 1937.

—. *Tycho Brahes Bogtrykkeri*. Copenhagen: Valdemar Pedersen, 1946.

Nissen, R. Tonder. *De nordiske kirkers historie*. Christiania (Oslo): Steen, 1884.

Nordström, Johan. "Lejonet från Norden." *Samlaran* 15 (1934): 1-66.

Norlind, Wilhelm. *Tycho Brahe: en levnadsteckning*. Lund: Gleerup, 1970.

—. *Tycho Brahe: Mannen och Verket*. Lund: Gleerup, 1951.

Norrie, Gordon. *Kirurger og Doctores; et Kritisk Bidrag til Lægeuddannelsens Historie i Danmark før 1800*. Copenhagen: Levin & Munksgaard, 1929.

Norvin, William. *Københavns Universitet i Reformations og Orthodoxiens Tidsalder*. Vol. 2. Copenhagen: Gyldendal, 1940.

Nutton, Vivian. "The Seeds of Disease: An Explanation of Contagion and Infection from the Greeks to the Renaissance." *Medical History* 27 (1983): 1-34.

—. "The Reception of Fracastoro's Theory of Contagion: The Seed that Fell among Thorns?" *Osiris* 2d ser., 6 (1990): 196-234.

Olsen, Olaf. *Christian IVs tugt og børnehus*. 2d ed. Højbjerg: Wormianum, 1978.

O'Malley, Charles Donald. *Andreas Vesalius of Brussels 1514-1564*. Berkeley: University of California Press, 1964.

O'Toole, Christopher J. "The Philosophy of Creation in the Writings of St. Augustine." Ph.D. Diss., Catholic University of America, 1944.

Osler, Margaret. "The Intellectual Sources of Robert Boyle's Philosophy of Nature: Gassendi's Voluntarism, and Boyle's Physico-Theological Project." In *Philosophy, Science, and Religion in England 1640-1700*, ed. Richard Kroll, Richard Ashcraft, and Perez Zagorin, pp. 178-98. Cambridge: Cambridge University Press, 1992.

—. "Providence and Divine Will in Gassendi's Views on Scientific Knowledge." *Journal of the History of Ideas* 44(1983): 549-560.

Ozment, Steven. *Mysticism and Dissent: Religious Ideology and Social Protest in the Sixteenth Century*. New Haven: Yale University Press, 1973.

Pagel, Walter. *Joan Baptista Van Helmont: Reformer of Science and Medicine*. Cambridge: Cambridge University Press, 1982.

—. *Paracelsus: An Introduction to Philosophical Medicine in the Era of the Renaissance*. 2d ed. Basel: Karger, 1982.

—. "Paracelsus and the Neoplatonic and Gnostic Tradition." *Ambix* 8 (1960): 125-166.

—. "The Prime Matter of Paracelsus." *Ambix* 9 (1961): 117-135.

—. "Recent Paracelsian Studies." *History of Science* 12 (1974): 200-211.

—. "Religious Motives in the Medical Biology of the XVIIth Century." *Bulletin of the Institute of the History of Medicine* 3 (1935): 97-312.

—. "The Religious and Philosophical Aspects of van Helmont's Science and Medicine." *Bulletin of the History of Medicine.* Supp. 2. Baltimore: Johns Hopkins Press, 1944.

—. *The Smiling Spleen: Paracelsianism in Storm and Stress.* Basel: Karger, 1984.

—. *William Harvey's Biological Ideas.* New York: Hafner, 1967.

Palmer, Richard. "Pharmacy in the Republic of Venice in the Sixteenth Century." In *The Medical Renaissance of the Sixteenth Century.* Ed. Andrew Wear, et al., pp. 100-117, 303-312. Cambridge: Cambridge University Press, 1985.

Panckouche, ed. *Dictionaire des Sciences Medicinales. Biographe Medicale.* Vol. 7. Paris, 1825.

Panum, P.L. "Vort medicinske Fakultets Oprindelse og Barndom: et Bidrag til Kundskab om Lægevidenskabens og Naturvidenskabernes Udvikling i Danmark." In *Festskrifter udgivne af Det Lægevidenskabelige Fakultet ved Kjøbenhavns Universitet i Anledning af Universitetets Firehunderedaarsfest Juni 1879.* Copenhagen: Gyldendal, 1879.

Pérez-Ramos, Antonio. *Francis Bacon's Idea of Science and the Maker's Knowledge Tradition.* Oxford: Clarendon, 1988.

Petersen, Carl S. *Det Kongelige Biblioteks Haandskriftsamling.* Offprint from *Bogens Verden.* Copenhagen: Nielsen & Lydiche, 1942.

Peuckert, Will Erich. *Die Rosenkreutzer.* Jena: Eugen Diderich, 1928.

Prandtl, Wilhelm. *Die Bibliothek des Tycho Brahe.* Vienna: Herbert Reichner, 1933.

Principe, Lawrence M. *The Aspiring Adept: Robert Boyle and His Alchemical Quest.* Princeton, N J: Princeton University Press, 1998.

Pumfrey, Stephen. "The Spagyric Art; Or, the Impossible Work of Separating Pure from Impure Paracelsianism: A Historiographical Analysis." In *Paracelsus: The Man and His Reputation, His Ideas and Their Transformation.* Ed. Ole Peter Grell, pp. 21-51. Leiden: Brill, 1998.

Rattansi, P.M. "The Helmontian-Galenist Controversy in Restoration England." *Ambix* 12 (1964): 1-23.

Read, Conyers. *Mr. Secretary Walsingham and the Policy of Queen Elizabeth.* 3 vols. Oxford: Clarendon Press, 1925.

Read, John. *Through Alchemy to Chemistry: A Procession of Ideas and Personalities.* London: G. Bell and Sons, 1957.

—. "William Davidson of Aberdeen." *Ambix* 9 (1961): 70-101.

Rees, Graham. *Francis Bacon's Natural Philosophy: A New Source.* Chalfont St. Giles: British Society for the History of Science, 1975.

—. "Francis Bacon's Semi-Paracelsian Cosmology." *Ambix* 22 (1975): 81-101.

Richardson, Linda Deer. "The Generation of Disease: Occult Causes and Diseases of the Total Substance." In *The Medical Renaissance of the Sixteenth Century,* ed. Andrew Wear, et al., pp. 175-94. Cambridge: Cambridge University Press, 1985.

Rørdam, Holger F. "Bidrag til tre Biskoppers Levned. I. Dr. Mouritz Pedersen Køning, Biskop i Aalborg Stift (d. 1672)." *[Ny] Kirkehistoriske Samlinger* 4th ser., 1 (1889-91): 346-379.

—. "Charles de Danzay, fransk Resident ved det danske Hof." In *Historiske Samlinger og Studier vedrørende danske Forhold og Personligheder, især i det 17. Aarhundrede*, ed. Holger Rørdam, pp. 252-333. Vol. 3. Copenhagen: Gad, 1898.

—. "Efterretninger om M. Tyge Asmundsen, Biskop i Lund." *[Ny] Kirkehistoriske Samlinger* 2d ser., 4 (1867-68): 326-358.

—. *Kjøbenhavns Universitets Historie fra 1537 til 1621.* 4 vols. Copenhagen: B. Luno, 1868-77.

—. "Magistre creerede ved Kjøbenhavns Universitet fra Reformationen indtil 1660." *Personalhistorisk Tidsskrift* 1st ser., 3 (1882): 117-143.

Rosenberg, Carl. *Nordboernes Aandsliv: Fra Oldtiden til vore Dage.* Vol. 3. Copenhagen: Samfundet til den danske literaturs fremme, 1885.

Rossi, Paolo. *Francis Bacon: From Magic to Science.* Trans. Sacha Rabinovitch. London: Routledge and Kegan Paul, 1968.

Ruska, Julius F. *Tabula Smaragdina: Ein Beitrag zur Geschichte der Hermetischen Literatur.* Heidelberg: Carl Winter's Universitatsbuchhandlung, 1926.

Sargent, Rose-Mary. *The Diffident Naturalist: Robert Boyle and the Philosophy of Experiment.* Chicago: University of Chicago Press, 1995.

Schaeffer, Aage. "Studier til dansk Apothekervæsens Historie: Hofapotekere og Hofke-mikere i Danmark ca. 1540-1660." *Theriaca: Samlinger til Farmaciens og Medicinens Historie.* Vol. 8. Copenhagen: Danske Farmacihistorisk Selskab, 1963.

Scharffenberg, Johan. "Bidrag til de norske lægestillingers historie før 1800." *Norsk Magasin for Lægevidenskaben* 5th ser., 2 (1904): 1329-1384.

—. "Det militære sanitetsvæsen i Norge i midten af det 17de aarhundrede, navnlig under Hannibals-feiden 1643-45." *Norsk Magasin for Lægevidenskaben* 4th ser., 15 (1900): 533-627.

Scharling, Edvard A. *Bidrag til at oplyse de Forhold, under hvilke Chemien har været dyrket i Danmark.* Copenhagen: J.H. Schultz, 1857.

Schepelern, H. D. *Museum Wormianum, dets forudsætninger og tilblivelse.* Aarhus: Worm-ianum, 1971.

Scherz, Gustav. *Vom Wege Niels Stensens: Beiträge zu seiner naturwissenschaftlichen Entwick-lung.* Acta historica scientiarum naturalium et medicinalium, vol. 14. Copenhagen: Munksgaard, 1956.

Schønau, Frederik Christian. *Samlinger af danske lærde fruentimer.* Copenhagen: N.H.M., 1753.

Sessions, William A. "Recent Studies in Francis Bacon." *English Literary Renaissance* 17 (1987): 351-371.

Shackelford, Jole. "The Chemical Hippocrates: Paracelsian and Hippocratic Theory in Petrus Severinus' Medical Philosophy." In *Reinventing Hippocrates*, ed. David Cantor, pp. 59-88. Aldershot, Hampshire: Ashgate, 2002.

—. "Documenting the Factual and the Artifactual: Ole Worm and Public Knowledge." *Endeavour* 23 (1999): 65-71.

—. "Early Reception of Paracelsian Theory: Severinus and Erastus." *Sixteenth Century Journal* 26 (1995): 123-35.

—. "Hans Jochum Scharff: A Paracelsian Apothecary in 17th-Century Norway." *Norges Apotekerforenings Tidsskrift* 95, no. 9 (May 1987): 212-217.

—. "Paracelsianism and The Orthodox Lutheran Rejection of Vital Philosophy in Early Seventeenth-Century Denmark." *Early Science and Medicine* 8 (2003): 210-52.

—. "Paracelsianism and Patronage in Early Modern Denmark." In *Patronage and Institutions: Science, Technology, and Medicine at the European Court 1500-1750*, ed. Bruce T. Moran, pp. 85-109. Woodbridge, Suffolk: Boydell, 1991.

—. *Paracelsianism in Denmark and Norway in the 16th and 17th Centuries.* Ann Arbor, Michigan: University Microfilms International, 1989.

—. "A Reappraisal of Anna Rhodius: Religious Enthusiasm and Social Unrest in Seventeenth-Century Christiania, Norway." *Scandinavian Studies* 65 (1993): 349-89.

—. "Rosicrucianism, Lutheran Orthodoxy, and the Rejection of Paracelsianism in Early Seventeenth-Century Denmark." *Bulletin of the History of Medicine* 70 (1996): 181-204.

—. "Seeds with a Mechanical Purpose: Severinus' *Semina* and Seventeenth-Century Matter Theory." In *Reading the Book of Nature: The Other Side of the Scientific Revolution*, ed. Allen G. Debus and Michael T. Walton, pp. 15-44. Sixteenth Century Essays and Studies, vol. 41. Kirksville, Missouri: Sixteenth Century Journal Publishers, Inc., 1998.

—. "To Be or Not to Be a Paracelsian: Something Spagyric in the State of Denmark." In *The Paracelsian Moment: Science, Medicine, and Astrology in Early Modern Europe.* ed. Gerhild Williams and Charles Gunnoe, Jr., pp. 35-69. Sixteenth Century Essays and Studies 64. Kirksville, MO: Truman State University Press, 2002.

—. "Tycho Brahe, Laboratory Design, and the Aim of Science: Reading Plans in Context." *Isis* 84 (1993): 211-230.

—. "Unification and the Chemistry of the Reformation." In *Infinite Boundaries: Order, Disorder, and Reorder in Early Modern German Culture*, ed. Max Reinhart, pp. 291-312. Sixteenth Century Essays and Studies, vol. 40. Kirksville, Missouri: Sixteenth Century Journal Publishers, Inc., 1998.

Sherlock, T.P. "The Chemical Work of Paracelsus." *Ambix* 3 (1948): 33-63.

Shumaker, Wayne. *The Occult Sciences in the Renaissance: A Study in Intellectual Patterns.* Berkeley: University of California Press, 1972.

Siraisi, Nancy. *Avicenna in Renaissance Italy: The* Canon *and Medical Teaching in Italian Universities after 1500.* Princeton: Princeton University Press, 1987.

—. "Giovanni Argenterio and Sixteenth-Century Medical Innovation: Between Princely Patronage and Academic Controversy." *Osiris* 2d ser., 6 (1990): 161-180.

Small, John. "Notice of William Davidson, M.D. (Gulielmus Davissonus), First Professor of Chemistry, and Director of the Jardin des Plantes, Paris, afterwards Physician to the King of Poland." *Proceedings of the Society of Antiquaries of Scotland* 10 (1875): 265-280.

Smith, Wesley. *The Hippocratic Tradition.* Ithaca: Cornell University Press, 1979.

Snorrason, Egill. "The History of Medicine in and about Denmark: Sources and Bibliography." *Nordisk Medicinhistorisk Årsbok*, 1968, 218-228.

Sprengel, Kurt. *Versuch einer pragmatischen Geschichte der Arzneikunde.* Vol. 3. 2nd ed. Halle, 1801; 3rd ed. Halle, 1827.

Steneck, Nicholas H. *Science and Creation in the Middle Ages.* Notre Dame: University of Notre Dame Press, 1976.

Stevenson, Lloyd G. "'New Diseases' in the Seventeenth Century." *Bulletin of the History of Medicine* 39 (1965): 1-21.

Sudhoff, Karl. *Bibliographia Paracelsica, Besprechung der unter Hohenheims Namen 1527-1893 erschienen Druckschriften.* Graz: Akademische Druck- und Verlagsanstalt, 1958.

Sverre, Nicolai Aagaard. *Et studium av farmasiens historie.* 2d ed. Oslo: Norges Apoteker-forening, 1982.

Temkin, Owsei. *Hippocrates in a World of Pagans and Christians.* Baltimore: Johns Hopkins University Press, 1991.

Thoren, Victor. *The Lord of Uraniborg: A Biography of Tycho Brahe.* Cambridge: Cambridge University Press, 1990.

—. "Tycho Brahe as the Dean of a Renaissance Research Institute." In *Religion, Science, and Worldview,* ed. M.J. Osler and P.L. Farber, pp. 275-95. Cambridge: Cambridge University Press, 1985.

—. "Tycho Brahe: Past and Future Research." *History of Science* 11 (1973): 270-92.

Thorndike, Lynn. *A History of Magic and Experimental Science.* 2d. ed. 8 vols. New York: Macmillan, 1923-58.

Trevor-Roper, Hugh. "The Court Physician and Paracelsianism." In *Medicine at the Courts of Europe, 1500-1837.* Ed. Vivian Nutton, pp. 79-94. London: Routledge, 1990.

—. "The Paracelsian Movement." In Hugh Trevor-Roper, *Renaissance Essays*, pp. 149-199. London: Secker and Warburg, 1985.

Veibel, Stig. *Kemiens Historie i Danmark.* Vol. 1 of *Kemien i Danmark.* Copenhagen: Arnold Busck, 1939.

Vickers, Brian. "Analogy Versus Identity: The Rejection of Occult Symbolism, 1580-1680." In *Occult and Scientific Mentalities in the Renaissance*, ed. Brian Vickers, pp. 95-163. Cambridge: Cambridge University Press, 1984.

Waite, A.E. *The Brotherhood of the Rosy Cross.* New York: University Books, 1961.

Walker, D.P. *The Ancient Theology; Studies in Christian Platonism from the Fifteenth to the Eighteenth Century.* Ithaca, NY: Cornell Univ. Press, 1972.

—. "Francis Bacon and *Spiritus.*" In *Science, Medicine, and Society in the Renaissance; Essays to Honor Walter Pagel*, ed. Allen G. Debus, pp. 121-130. New York: Science History Publications, 1972.

—. *Spiritual and Demonic Magic from Ficino to Campanella.* London: Warburg Institute, 1958.

Waller, Gary F. *Mary Sidney, Countess of Pembroke: A Critical Study of Her Writings and Literary Milieu.* Salzburg: University of Salzburg, 1979.

Wear, Andrew, Roger K. French, and Iain M. Lonie, eds. *The Medical Renaissance of the Sixteenth Century.* Cambridge: Cambridge University Press, 1985.

Webster, Charles. "Alchemical and Paracelsian Medicine." In *Health, Medicine and Mortality in the Sixteenth Century*, ed. Charles Webster, pp. 302-334. Cambridge: Cambridge University Press, 1979.

—. "Essay Review." *Isis* 70 (1979): 588-592.

—. *From Paracelsus to Newton: Magic and the Making of Modern Science.* Cambridge: Cambridge University Press, 1982.

—. *The Great Instauration: Science, Medicine and Reform 1626-1660.* London: Duckworth, 1975.

—. "Paracelsus and Demons: Science as a Synthesis of Popular Belief." In *Scienze, Credenze Occulte, Livelli di Cultura*, pp. 3-20. Florence: Leo Olschki, 1982.

Weeks, Andrew. *Paracelsus: Speculative Theory and the Crisis of the Early Reformation.* Albany, NY: SUNY Press, 1997.

Werlauff, E.C. *Historiske Antegnelser til L. Holbergs Lystspil.* Vol. 1. Copenhagen: Schultz, 1838.

Wessel, A. B. *Ambrosius Rhodius: en til Finmarken forvist læge i det 17. aarhundrede.* Vardø: Finmarkens boktrykkeri, 1917.

Westfall, Richard S. *Never at Rest: A Biography of Isaac Newton.* Cambridge: Cambridge University Press, 1980.

Wilkinson, Ronald Stearne. "The Alchemical Library of John Winthrop, Jr. (1606-1676) and His Descendants in Colonial America." *Ambix* 11 (1963): 33-51; and 13 (1965): 139-186.

Wilson, William Jerome. "Robert Child's Chemical Book List of 1641." *Journal of Chemical Education* 20 (1943): 123-29.

Wittendorff, Alex. *Tyge Brahe.* Copenhagen: Gad, 1994.

Wollgast, Siegfried. "Zur Wirkungsgeschichte des Paracelsus im 16. und 17. Jahrhundert." In *Resultate und Desiderate der Paracelsus-Forschung*, ed. Peter Dilg and Hartmut Rudolph, pp. 113-144. *Sudhoffs Archiv*, Beihefte 31. Stuttgart: Franz Steiner Verlag, 1993.

Wulff, Frederik. *Det Kjøbenhavnske Barberlavs Historie.* Copenhagen: Martius Trulsen, 1906.

Yates, Frances. *Giordano Bruno and the Hermetic Tradition.* Chicago: University of Chicago Press, 1964.

—. *The Rosicrucian Enlightenment.* London: Routledge and Kegan Paul, 1972.

Young, John T. *Faith, Medical Alchemy and Natural Philosophy: Johann Moriaen, Reformed Intelligencer, and the Hartlib Circle.* Aldershot: Ashgate, 1998.

Zeeberg, Peter. "Kemi og kærlighed: Naturvidenskab i Tycho Brahes latindigtning." In *Litteratur og Lærdom: Dansk-svenske nylatindage april 1985*, ed. Marianne Alenius and Peter Zeeberg, pp. 149-61. Renaissancestudier, vol. 1. Copenhagen: Museum Tusculanums Forlag, 1987.

—. *Den praktiske muse: Tycho Brahes brug af latindigtningen.* Studier fra Sprog- og Oldtidsforskning, vol. 321. Copenhagen: Museum Tusculanums Forlag, 1993.

—. "Science versus Secular Life: A Central Theme in the Latin Poems of Tycho Brahe." In *Acta Conventus Neo-Latini Torontonensis: Proceedings of the Seventh International Congress on Neo-Latin Studies, Toronto 8 August to 13 August 1988*, ed. Alexander Dalzell, Charles Fantazzi, and Richard J. Schoek, pp. 831-838. Binghamton, NY: Medieval and Renaissance Texts and Studies, 1991.

—. *Tycho Brahes Urania Titani: En Digt om Sophie Brahe.* Renaissance Studier 7. Copenhagen: Museum Tusculanums Forlag, 1994.

Selected Manuscript Sources

BASEL, UNIVERSITÄTSBIBLIOTHEK

Fr. Gr. II 28a, Nos. 338-41. Letters from Petrus Severinus to Theodor Zwinger.

COPENHAGEN, DET KONGELIGE BIBLIOTHEK

"Afhandlinger om Tycho Brahe, Samlet af J. Dreyer." Includes F.R. Friis's pamphlet, "Et par optegnelser om Uraniborg 1894, Kjøbenhavn."

Böllings Brevsamling D 4° 1085. Draft of a letter from Severinus to "doctor Erasmus" [1573?]

Böllings Brevsamling D 4° 1280. Incomplete letter to Severinus from an unknown author, May 1584.

GKS 271 2°. and 272 fol. Peter Payngk's Formulary, two exemplars.

GKS 323 2°. Letters from Ambrosius Rhodius to Laurentius Georgius. 27 February 1658, 20 April 1658.

GKS 1076 2° I. Gramske Samling. Includes "Vale Pratensis ad Danzeum."

GKS 1076 2° II. Gramske Samling. Includes "Registering Wdi M. Ambrosij Rhodij Boe 1662."

GKS 1478 4°. "E. Fleischers Confessio."

GKS 1721 4°. "Elementa chemiæ Borrichio attributa."

GKS 1833 4°. Ambrosius Rhodius, "Typis Eclipsis Solaris iuxta Hypotheses Astronomiæ Danicæ 1654 d. 22. Aug ad Elev. Christian. 59' 4"."

GKS 3410 8°. Niels Svendsen Chronich, "Apologia." Copenhagen 28 June 1658.

NKS 338a 4°. "Elementa chemiæ in auditorio Academiæ Hafniensis a viro excellentissimo & experientissimo Dn. D. Olao Borrichio in publice prælecta."

NKS 1305 2°. Contains a letter from Moffet to Severinus (#2, 5 May 1584), a letter from Hans Svanning to Severinus (#28, 22 September 1598), and a poem from Frederik Severinus to Petrus Severinus (#71).

NKS 1986e 4°. "Jens Birkerøds Dagbøger for 1693."

NKS 1997 4°. "Acta Consistorialia over Mag. Niels Svendsen Chronichius 1655."

NKS 1998 4°. The case against Niels Svendsen.

NKS 2073 4°. "Anlangende M. Trugels Nielson, Sogneprest og Kanike i Opslo som var beskyldt for at have fordansket og publiceret den vederstygelige Knipperdollings og Johan von Leydens Historie 1651."

Rostgaard 33 8°. Ole Worm's iatrochemical notes and copies of treatises.

Rostgaard 33 8° Tillæg. Includes a copy of a recipe attributed to Petrus Severinus, and a letter from Hartmann to Worm.

Thott 744 4°. "Prælectiones has publicas viri nobilissimi ... Dn. D. Olaj Borrichii."

Copenhagen, Universitet

Arnamagnæanske Samling A.M. 191a 8°. "Ex Paracelso Plinio et alijs de magnete."

Copenhagen, Rigsarkiv (DRA)

Danske Kancelli B 159a. Extract- og Resolutionsprotokollet for Danske og Norske Sager 1657-60.

Danske Kancelli C. 20. Norske Tegnelser 1660-1670. Indlæg til Sjælandsk Missive.

"Hoffapotekers Regnskaber & cet."108b 24 a-h.

London, British Library

Sloane MS 11. "A Mappe of Medicyne or Philosophicall Path containinge the groundes of all the doctrines of Paracelsus, Hippocrates & Galen compiled by Peter Severine a Dane, philosopher & physician to Fredericke the II King of Denmarke & the Northerne partes."

Sloane MS 3005, ff. 1r-37v. "Exercitationum liber in qua quæstiones philosophicæ, astronomicæ, medicæ, cabalisticæ explicantur." Dated Paris, July 1657.

Sloane MS 3005, ff. 48r-54v. "De febribus." Extracts.

Index

(æ, see ae; ø, see oe; å, see aa)